PEDIATRIC EMERGENCY MEDICINE

SECRETS

PEDIATRIC EMERGENCY MEDICINE

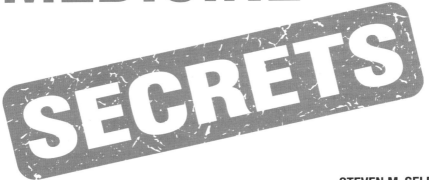

SECRETS

STEVEN M. SELBST, MD
Professor of Pediatrics
Director, Graduate Medical Education
Department of Pediatrics
Sidney Kimmel Medical College at Thomas Jefferson University
Philadelphia, Pennsylvania
Attending Physician
Division of Emergency Medicine
Nemours Children's Hospital, Delaware
Wilmington, Delaware

JILLIAN STEVENS SAVAGE, DO
Clinical Assistant Professor of Pediatrics
Associate Program Director
Pediatric Residency Program
Department of Pediatrics
Sidney Kimmel Medical College at Thomas Jefferson University
Philadelphia, Pennsylvania
Attending Physician
Division of Emergency Medicine
Nemours Children's Hospital, Delaware
Wilmington, Delaware

ELSEVIER

Elsevier
1600 John F. Kennedy Blvd.
Ste 1800
Philadelphia, PA 19103-2899

PEDIATRIC EMERGENCY MEDICINE SECRETS, FOURTH EDITION

978-0-323-93033-8

Notice

Practitioners and researchers must always rely on their own experience and knowledge in evaluating and using any information, methods, compounds, or experiments described herein. Because of rapid advances in the medical sciences, in particular, independent verification of diagnoses and drug dosages should be made. To the fullest extent of the law, no responsibility is assumed by Elsevier, authors, editors, or contributors for any injury and/or damage to persons or property as a matter of product liability, negligence or otherwise, or from any use or operation of any methods, products, instructions, or ideas contained in the material herein.

Previous edition copyrighted 2015, 2008, 2001.

Content Strategist: Marybeth Thiel
Content Development Specialist: Ambika Kapoor
Publishing Services Manager: Shereen Jameel
Project Manager: Beula Christopher
Design Direction: Renee Duenow

Printed in India

Last digit is the print number: 9 8 7 6 5 4 3 2 1

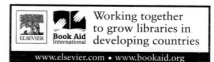

Working together
to grow libraries in
developing countries

www.elsevier.com • www.bookaid.org

To my wife, Andrea.

To my children, Eric, Lonn, and Aarti.

To my grandson, Miles, who brings us immeasurable joy and love every day.

*He reminds us how precious children are, and how rewarding it is
to keep them healthy, happy, and safe.*

Steven M. Selbst

*To my darling children, Emery, Brady, and Drew
who were my greatest advocates throughout this project.
As each of you embark on your wildest dreams, may you always support
and encourage one another, just as you did for me.*

*Jared, thank you for being my constant champion.
I love and appreciate you beyond words.*

*Steve, I cannot thank you enough for always believing in me.
I am forever grateful for your mentorship and friendship.*

Jillian Stevens Savage

CONTRIBUTORS

Beverly Anderson, MD
Fellow, Pediatric Emergency Medicine
Division of Emergency Medicine
Nemours Children's Health, Delaware
Wilmington, Delaware

Linda D. Arnold, MD
Associate Professor
Department of Pediatrics and Emergency Medicine
Yale School of Medicine
Attending Physician
Section of Emergency Medicine
Yale New Haven Children's Hospital
New Haven, Connecticut

Magdy W. Attia, MD
Professor
Department of Pediatrics
Sidney Kimmel Medical College at
    Thomas Jefferson University
Philadelphia, Pennsylvania
Chief, Urgent Care
Nemours Children's Hospital, Delaware
Wilmington, Delaware

Jeffrey R. Avner, MD, FAAP
Chair
Department of Pediatrics
Maimonides Children's Hospital
Brooklyn, New York

Lalit Bajaj, MD, MPH
Professor
Department of Pediatrics
University of Colorado School of Medicine
Denver, Colorado
Chief Quality, Equity, and Outcomes Officer
Children's Hospital Colorado
Aurora, Colorado

M. Douglas Baker, MD
Professor, Executive Vice Chair, Vice Chair for Education
Department of Pediatrics
Robert Wood Johnson Medical School
New Brunswick, New Jersey

Carl R. Baum, MD, FAAP, FACMT
Professor
Department of Pediatrics and Emergency Medicine
Yale School of Medicine
New Haven, Connecticut

Brenda J. Bender, MD
Clinical Assistant Professor
Department of Pediatrics
Sidney Kimmel Medical College at
    Thomas Jefferson University
Attending Physician
Division of Emergency Medicine
Nemours Children's Hospital, Delaware
Wilmington, Delaware

David Bergamo, MD
Pediatric Emergency Medicine Physician
Department of Emergency Medicine
Hackensack Meridian Children's Health at
    K. Hovnanian Children's Hospital
Neptune, New Jersey

Timothy Brenkert, MD, RDMS
Associate Professor
Department of Pediatrics
University of Cincinnati College of Medicine;
Division of Emergency Medicine
Cincinnati Children's Hospital Medical Center
Cincinnati, Ohio

James M. Callahan, MD
Professor of Clinical Pediatrics
Department of Pediatrics
Perelman School of Medicine at the
    University of Pennsylvania
Medical Director
Global Pediatric Education
Children's Hospital of Philadelphia
Philadelphia, Pennsylvania

Kerry S. Caperell, MD, MS, MBA
Associate Professor of Pediatrics
Department of Pediatrics
University of Louisville School of Medicine
Attending Physician
Norton Children's Hospital
Louisville, Kentucky

Hannah Carron, MD
Fellow, Pediatric Emergency Medicine
Division of Emergency Medicine
Cincinnati Children's Hospital Medical Center
Cincinnati, Ohio

Sarita Chung, MD
Associate Professor of Pediatrics and Associate
Professor of Emergency Medicine
Harvard Medical School
Boston, Massachusetts

Kate M. Cronan, MD
Emeritus Clinical Professor
Department of Pediatrics
Sidney Kimmel Medical College at
    Thomas Jefferson University
Philadelphia, Pennsylvania

Jeannine Del Pizzo, MD
Associate Professor of Clinical Pediatrics
Department of Pediatrics
Perelman School of Medicine at the
    University of Pennsylvania
Attending Physician
Division of Emergency Medicine
Sedation Unit
Children's Hospital of Philadelphia
Philadelphia, Pennsylvania

Andrew D. DePiero, MD
Assistant Professor
Department of Pediatrics
Sidney Kimmel Medical College at
    Thomas Jefferson University
Philadelphia, Pennsylvania
Attending Physician
Division of Emergency Medicine
Nemours Children's Hospital, Delaware
Wilmington, Delaware

Monique Devens, MD
Assistant Professor
Department of Pediatrics
Sidney Kimmel Medical College at
    Thomas Jefferson University
Philadelphia, Pennsylvania
Attending Physician
Division of Emergency Medicine
Nemours Children's Hospital, Delaware
Wilmington, Delaware

Maria Carmen G. Diaz, MD, FAAP, FACEP
Clinical Professor of Pediatrics and Emergency
    Medicine
Sidney Kimmel Medical College at
    Thomas Jefferson University
Philadelphia, Pennsylvania
Medical Director of Simulation
Nemours Institute for Clinical Excellence
Nemours Children's Health, Delaware
Wilmington, Delaware

Sara DiGirolamo, MSN, CRNP, CPNP-AC, SANE-P
Sexual Assault Response Team Coordinator
Emergency Department
Children's Hospital of Philadelphia
Philadelphia, Pennsylvania

Kaynan Doctor, MD, MBBS, BSc
Assistant Professor
Department of Pediatrics
Sidney Kimmel Medical College at
    Thomas Jefferson University
Philadelphia, Pennsylvania
Attending Physician
Division of Emergency Medicine
Nemours Children's Hospital, Delaware
Wilmington, Delaware

Nanette C. Dudley, MD
Professor
Department of Pediatrics
University of Utah School of Medicine;
Division of Pediatric Emergency Medicine
Primary Children's Hospital
Salt Lake City, Utah

Susan J. Duffy, MD, MPH
Professor
Department of Emergency Medicine and Pediatrics
Vice Chair Academic Affairs
Department of Emergency Medicine
Warren Alpert Medical School of Brown University
Attending Physician
Division of Pediatric Emergency Medicine
Hasbro Children's Hospital
Providence, Rhode Island

Yamini Durani, MD
Assistant Professor of Pediatrics
Sidney Kimmel Medical College at
    Thomas Jefferson University
Philadelphia, Pennsylvania
Affiliate Physician
Nemours Children's Health, Delaware
Wilmington, Delaware

Todd A. Florin, MD, MSCE
Associate Professor of Pediatrics
Department of Pediatrics
Northwestern University Feinberg School of Medicine
Director of Research
Division of Pediatric Emergency Medicine
Ann and Robert H. Lurie Children's Hospital of Chicago
Chicago, Illinois

Eron Y. Friedlaender, MD, MPH
Professor of Clinical Pediatrics
Perelman School of Medicine at the
    University of Pennsylvania
Attending Physician
Department of Pediatrics
Division of Emergency Medicine
Children's Hospital of Philadelphia
Philadelphia, Pennsylvania

Marla Friedman, DO
Associate Clinical Professor of Pediatrics
Herbert Wertheim College of Medicine
Florida International University
Associate Medical Director, Attending Physician
Division of Emergency Medicine
Nicklaus (Miami) Children's Hospital
Miami, Florida

Susan Fuchs, MD
Professor
Department of Pediatrics
Northwestern University
Feinberg School of Medicine
EMS Medical Director
Division of Emergency Medicine
Ann and Robert H. Lurie Children's Hospital of Chicago
Chicago, Illinois

Payal K. Gala, MD
Associate Professor
Department of Pediatrics
The Perelman School of Medicine at the
	University of Pennsylvania
Attending Physician
Division of Emergency Medicine
The Children's Hospital of Philadelphia
Philadelphia, Pennsylvania

Katie Giordano, DO
Clinical Assistant Professor
Department of Pediatrics
Sidney Kimmel Medical College at
	Thomas Jefferson University
Philadelphia, Pennsylvania
Attending Physician
Division of Emergency Medicine
Nemours Children's Hospital, Delaware
Wilmington, Delaware

Joan Elizabeth Giovanni, MD
Departments of Pediatrics and Emergency Medicine
Children's Mercy Hospital
Kansas City, Missouri

Eric W. Glissmeyer, MD, MBA
Associate Professor
Department of Pediatrics
University of Utah School of Medicine
Director of Pediatric Emergency Expansion
Division of Pediatric Emergency Medicine
Primary Children's Hospital
Salt Lake City, Utah

Deborah L. Hammett, DO
Attending Physician
Division of Emergency Medicine
Nemours Children's Hospital, Delaware
Wilmington, Delaware

Arun Handa, MD
Assistant Professor of Clinical Psychiatry
Department of Psychiatry
Perelman School of Medicine at the
	University of Pennsylvania
Attending Physician
Department of Child and Adolescent Psychiatry and
	Behavioral Sciences
Attending Physician
Division of Pulmonary and Sleep Medicine
Children's Hospital of Philadelphia
Philadelphia, Pennsylvania

Rebecca J. Hart, MD, MSc
Associate Professor
Department of Pediatrics
University of Louisville School of Medicine;
Division of Pediatric Emergency Medicine
Norton Children's and University of Louisville Pediatrics
Louisville, Kentucky

Dee Hodge, MD
Professor of Pediatrics
Department of Emergency Medicine
Washington University School of Medicine
St. Louis, Missouri

Allen L. Hsiao, MD, FAAP, FAMIA
Professor, Interim Chief
Department of Pediatrics and Emergency Medicine
Yale University School of Medicine
Chief Health Information Officer
Yale New Haven Health and Yale School of Medicine
New Haven, Connecticut

Paul Ishimine, MD
Professor
Departments of Emergency Medicine and Pediatrics
University of California, San Diego School of Medicine
San Diego, California

Laurie H. Johnson, MD, MS, FAAP
Associate Professor
Department of Pediatrics
University of Cincinnati College of Medicine
Cincinnati Children's Hospital Medical Center
Cincinnati, Ohio

Priyanka Joshi, MD
Fellow, Pediatric Emergency Medicine
Division of Emergency Medicine
Children's Hospital of Philadelphia
Philadelphia, Pennsylvania

Howard Kadish, MD, MBA
Professor, Vice Chair
Department of Pediatrics
University of Utah School of Medicine
Division Chief, Pediatric Emergency Medicine
Primary Children's Hospital
Salt Lake City, Utah

Caroline G. Kahane, MD
Clinical Fellow
Department of Emergency Medicine
Boston Children's Hospital
Boston, Massachusetts

Susan M. Kelly, MD, MPH, FAAP
Clinical Assistant Professor
Department of Pediatrics
Sidney Kimmel Medical College at
	Thomas Jefferson University
Philadelphia, Pennsylvania
Attending Physician
Division of Emergency Medicine
Nemours Children's Hospital, Delaware
Wilmington, Delaware

Thomas M. Kennedy, MD
Assistant Professor
Department of Emergency Medicine
Columbia University Vagelos College of Physicians and
	Surgeons
New York, New York

Jody C. Kieffer, MD
Assistant Professor
Department of Pediatrics
Sidney Kimmel Medical College at
    Thomas Jefferson University
Philadelphia, Pennsylvania
Attending Physician
Division of Emergency Medicinew
Nemours Children's Hospital, Delaware
Wilmington, Delaware

Jenny Kim, MD
Clinical Professor
Department of Pediatrics
University of California-San Diego School of Medicine;
Division of Hematology/Oncology
Rady Children's Hospital
San Diego, California

Matthew P. Kusulas, MD, MSEd
Assistant Professor
Departments of Pediatrics and Emergency Medicine
Donald and Barbara Zucker School of Medicine at
    Hofstra/Northwell
Emergency Ultrasound Fellowship Director;
    PEM Fellowship Associate Program Director
Department of Pediatrics, Division of Emergency
    Medicine
Cohen Children's Medical Center/Northwell Health
New Hyde Park, New York
Hempstead, New York

Megan Lavoie, MD
Professor
Department of Pediatrics
Perelman School of Medicine at the
    University of Pennsylvania
Attending Physician
Division of Emergency Medicine
Children's Hospital of Philadelphia
Philadelphia, Pennsylvania

John M. Loiselle, MD
Associate Professor
Department of Pediatrics
Sidney Kimmel Medical College at
    Thomas Jefferson University
Philadelphia, Pennsylvania
Chief, Division of Emergency Medicine
Nemours Children's Hospital, Delaware
Wilmington, Delaware

Margarita S. Lorch, MD
Clinical Assistant Professor
Department of Pediatrics
Sidney Kimmel Medical College at
    Thomas Jefferson University
Philadelphia, Pennsylvania
Attending Physician
Division of Emergency Medicine
Nemours Children's Hospital, Delaware
Wilmington, Delaware

Stephen Ludwig, MD
Professor of Pediatrics
Perelman School of Medicine at the
    University of Pennsylvania
Senior Advisor for Medical Education and Global Health
Children's Hospital of Philadelphia
John H. and Hortense Jensen Endowed Chair
Philadelphia, Pennsylvania

Louise Malburg, MD
Assistant Professor of Pediatrics
Washington University School of Medicine
Attending Physician
Division of Emergency Medicine
St. Louis Children's Hospital
St. Louis, Missouri

Ronald F. Marchese, MD
Associate Professor
Department of Pediatrics
Perelman School of Medicine at the
    University of Pennsylvania;
Division of Emergency Medicine
The Children's Hospital of Philadelphia
Philadelphia, Pennsylvania

Danielle N. Mascarenas, MD
Department of Emergency Medicine
University of New Mexico School of Medicine
Pediatric Emergency Medicine Physician
Albuquerque, New Mexico

Constance M. McAneney, MD, MS
Professor of Clinical Pediatrics
Department of Pediatrics
University of Cincinnati College of Medicine;
Division of Emergency Medicine
Cincinnati Children's Hospital Medical Center
Cincinnati, Ohio

Lauren McNickle, MD
Fellow, Pediatric Emergency Medicine
Department of Pediatric Emergency Medicine
Baystate Medical Center
Springfield, Massachusetts

Meghan Meghpara, DO
Attending Physician
Division of Emergency Medicine
Children's Hospital of Philadelphia
Philadelphia, Pennsylvania

Laura Mercurio, MD
Assistant Professor
Department of Emergency Medicine and Pediatrics
Alpert Medical School of Brown University
Providence, Rhode Island

Frances M. Nadel, MD, MSCE, MFA
Clinical Professor
Department of Pediatrics
Perelman School of Medicine at the
    University of Pennsylvania
Attending Physician
Division of Emergency Medicine
Children's Hospital of Philadelphia
Philadelphia, Pennsylvania

Courtney E. Nelson, MD
Clinical Assistant Professor
Department of Pediatrics
Sidney Kimmel Medical College at
    Thomas Jefferson University
Philadelphia, Pennsylvania
Attending Physician
Division of Emergency Medicine
Nemours Children's Health, Delaware
Wilmington, Delaware

Robert P. Olympia, MD
Professor
Department of Emergency Medicine and Pediatrics
Penn State College of Medicine/Penn State Hershey
    Medical Center
Hershey, Pennsylvania

Kevin C. Osterhoudt, MD, MS
Professor
Department of Pediatrics
Perelman School of Medicine at the
    University of Pennsylvania
Medical Director
The Poison Control Center
Children's Hospital of Philadelphia
Philadelphia, Pennsylvania

Brian L. Park, MD
Assistant Professor
Department of Pediatrics
University of California-San Diego School of Medicine;
Division of Emergency Medicine
Rady Children's Hospital
San Diego, California

Elysha Pifko, MD
Assistant Professor
Department of Pediatrics
Sidney Kimmel Medical College at
    Thomas Jefferson University
Philadelphia, Pennsylvania
Attending Physician
Division of Emergency Medicine
Nemours Children's Health, Delaware
Wilmington, Delaware

Erica Y. Popovsky, MD
Assistant Professor of Pediatrics
Northwestern University Feinberg School of Medicine
Attending Physician
Division of Emergency Medicine
Ann and Robert H. Lurie Children's Hospital of Chicago
Chicago, Illinois

Jill C. Posner, MD, MSCE, MSEd
Professor of Clinical Pediatrics
Department of Pediatrics
Perelman School of Medicine at the
    University of Pennsylvania
Attending Physician
Division of Emergency Medicine
Children's Hospital of Philadelphia
Philadelphia, Pennsylvania

Samuel J. Prater, MD, FAAP, FACEP
Adjunct Associate Professor
Department of Emergency Medicine
McGovern Medical School at UT Health Houston
Associate Vice President, Medical Operations
Patient Flow Center
Memorial Hermann Health System
Houston, Texas

William B. Prince, MD
Clinical Assistant Professor
Department of Pediatrics
University of Washington School of Medicine;
Division of Pediatric Emergency Medicine
Seattle Children's Hospital
Seattle, Washington

Joshua Rice, MD
Fellow, Pediatric Emergency Medicine
Division of Emergency Medicine
Nemours Children's Health, Delaware
Wilmington, Delaware

Marisa Riverso, MD
Clinical Assistant Professor of Pediatrics
Sidney Kimmel Medical College at
    Thomas Jefferson University
Philadelphia, Pennsylvania
Attending Physician
Division of Emergency Medicine
Nemours Children's Hospital, Delaware
Wilmington, Delaware

Elisabeth Rogers, MD
Associate Professor of Emergency Medicine
University of Virginia School of Medicine
Chief
Division of Pediatric Emergency Medicine
UVA Health
Charlottesville, Virginia

Nevena Rose, DO
Pediatric Emergency Physician
Christiana Care Pediatric Care Center
Newark, Delaware

Anne Runkle, MD
Assistant Professor of Pediatrics and Emergency
    Medicine
The Ohio State University College of Medicine
Director, Nationwide Children's Hospital ED Outreach
    Program
Associate Director, Ohio EMS for Children State
    Partnership Program
Division of Emergency Medicine
Nationwide Children's Hospital
Columbus, Ohio

Brittney Russell, DO
Fellow, Pediatric Emergency Medicine
Division of Emergency Medicine
Nemours Children's Health, Delaware
Wilmington, Delaware

Christopher J. Russo, MD
Clinical Assistant Professor
Department of Pediatrics
Sidney Kimmel Medical College at
    Thomas Jefferson University
Philadelphia, Pennsylvania
Attending Physician
Division of Emergency Medicine
Nemours Children's Hospital, Delaware
Wilmington, Delaware

Sydney Ryan, MD
Assistant Professor
Department of Pediatrics
University of Utah School of Medicine;
Division of Pediatric Emergency Medicine
Primary Children's Hospital
Salt Lake City, Utah

Stephen Sandelich, MD
Attending Physician
Department of Emergency Medicine
Milton S. Hershey Penn State Medical Center
Hershey, Pennsylvania

Laura Santry, MD
Fellow, Pediatric Emergency Medicine
Division of Emergency Medicine
Nemours Children's Hospital, Delaware
Wilmington, Delaware

Robert E. Sapien, MD
Distinguished Professor
Department of Emergency Medicine
University of New Mexico Health Sciences Center
Albuquerque, New Mexico

Jillian Stevens Savage, DO
Clinical Assistant Professor of Pediatrics
Associate Program Director
Pediatric Residency Program
Department of Pediatrics
Sidney Kimmel Medical College at
    Thomas Jefferson University
Philadelphia, Pennsylvania
Attending Physician
Division of Emergency Medicine
Nemours Children's Hospital, Delaware
Wilmington, Delaware

Richard J. Scarfone, MD
Associate Professor
Department of Pediatrics
Perelman School of Medicine at the
    University of Pennsylvania
Attending Physician
Medical Director, Emergency Preparedness
Division of Emergency Medicine
Children's Hospital of Philadelphia
Philadelphia, Pennsylvania

Robert D. Schremmer, MD
Professor
Department of Pediatrics
University of Missouri-Kansas City
Attending Physician
Department of Emergency and Urgent Care
Medical Director
Center for Pediatric Simulation and Resuscitation
Children's Mercy Hospital
Kansas City, Missouri

Sara A. Schutzman, MD
Assistant Professor
Department of Pediatrics
Harvard Medical School
Senior Physician in Medicine
Department of Medicine
Boston Children's Hospital
Boston, Massachusetts

Sandra H. Schwab, MD, MSCE
Assistant Professor
Department of Emergency Medicine and Pediatrics
Indiana University School of Medicine
Indianapolis, Indiana

Steven M. Selbst, MD
Professor of Pediatrics
Director, Graduate Medical Education
Department of Pediatrics
Sidney Kimmel Medical College at
    Thomas Jefferson University
Philadelphia, Pennsylvania
Attending Physician
Division of Emergency Medicine
Nemours Children's Hospital, Delaware
Wilmington, Delaware

Laura L. Sells, MD
Associate Professor of Pediatrics
Department of Pediatric Emergency Medicine
University of Utah School of Medicine
Salt Lake City, Utah

Suzanne Seo, MD
Assistant Professor
McGovern Medical School at UT Health
Department of Pediatric Emergency Medicine
The University of Texas Health Science Center at Houston
Houston, Texas

Joan E. Shook, MD, MBA
Professor
Department of Pediatrics
Baylor College of Medicine
Chief Safety Officer
Chief Clinical Information Officer
Texas Children's Hospital
Houston, Texas

Sabina B. Singh, MD, FAAP
Assistant Professor of Pediatrics and Emergency
  Medicine
Drexel University College of Medicine;
Division of Emergency Medicine
St. Christopher's Hospital for Children
Philadelphia, Pennsylvania

Nadine Smith, DO
Attending Physician
Division of Emergency Medicine
Nemours Children's Hospital, Delaware
Wilmington, Delaware

Martha W. (Molly) Stevens, MD, MSCE
Associate Professor
Department of Emergency Medicine
Larner College of Medicine, University of Vermont
Attending Physician
Division of Pediatric Emergency Medicine
Burlington, Vermont

Ellen G. Szydlowski, MD
Associate Professor
Department of Pediatrics
Perelman School of Medicine at the
  University of Pennsylvania;
Division of Emergency Medicine
Children's Hospital of Philadelphia
Philadelphia, Pennsylvania

Alexandra A. Taylor, MD, FAAP
Clinical Assistant Professor
Department of Pediatrics
Sidney Kimmel Medical College at
  Thomas Jefferson University
Philadelphia, Pennsylvania
Attending Physician
Division of Emergency Medicine
Nemours Children's Health, Delaware
Wilmington, Delaware

Amy D. Thompson, MD, MSCR
Clinical Associate Professor
Department of Pediatrics
Sidney Kimmel Medical College at
  Thomas Jefferson University
Philadelphia, Pennsylvania
Associate Fellowship Director, Pediatric
  Emergency Medicine
Division of Pediatric Emergency Medicine
Nemours Children's Hospital, Delaware
Wilmington, Delaware

Nicholas Tsarouhas, MD
Professor
Department of Pediatrics
Perelman School of Medicine at the
  University of Pennsylvania
Senior Medical Director
CHOP Transport Team
Attending Physician
Division of Emergency Medicine
Children's Hospital of Philadelphia
Philadelphia, Pennsylvania

Emine M. Tunc, MD
Assistant Professor
Department of Pediatrics
Division of Pediatric Emergency Medicine
UT Southwestern Medical Center
Dallas, Texas

Sarah N. Weihmiller, MD, FAAP
Attending Physician
Department of Pediatric Urgent Care Medicine
Levine Children's Urgent Care
Atrium Health
Charlotte, North Carolina

George A. (Tony) Woodward, MD, MBA
Professor
Department of Pediatrics
University of Washington School of Medicine
Medical Director
Department of Emergency Department and Transport
  Medicine
Chief
Division of Emergency Medicine
Seattle Children's Hospital
Seattle, Washington

Shabana Yusuf, MD, MEd
Associate Professor
Department of Pediatrics
Baylor College of Medicine
Texas Children's Hospital
Houston, Texas

Arezoo Zomorrodi, MD
Associate Professor
Department of Pediatrics
Sidney Kimmel Medical College at
  Thomas Jefferson University
Philadelphia, Pennsylvania
Attending Physician
Division of Emergency Medicine
Nemours Children's Hospital, Delaware
Wilmington, Delaware

PREFACE

Steven M. Selbst and Jillian Stevens Savage

The world is very different since the last edition of *Pediatric Emergency Medicine Secrets*. The COVID-19 pandemic changed us forever. Our priorities were rearranged, and we, perhaps, have a greater appreciation for health care providers on the front lines. However, what never changed is our desire to provide the highest quality emergency care to children across the country. Perhaps even more than ever, clinicians in emergency medicine need rapid access to reliable sources of information to assist in the care of children in the emergency department (ED). *Pediatric Emergency Medicine Secrets* is a unique textbook because of its question-and-answer format. Some questions focus on "fun trivia." Most questions are clinically relevant and provide valuable information about common and unusual pediatric conditions seen in the ED.

Those who care for children in the ED know they will be challenged on every shift. Clinical questions arise with each patient and inquisitive trainees often bring interesting, stimulating queries to bedside discussions of pediatric patients. Physicians rarely have time to sort through lengthy texts or volumes of information to get their answers. This book highlights the difficult questions that arise daily in the ED. It offers succinct, up-to-date answers.

The fourth edition of *Pediatric Emergency Medicine Secrets* is divided into seven sections. The first section addresses life-threatening conditions and immediate stabilization of children. The second section features common chief complaints that are often managed in the ED. Later sections focus on important medical emergencies, surgical emergencies, major and minor trauma, and environmental emergencies. Finally, questions relating to special topics in pediatric emergency medicine (procedural sedation, bio-terrorism, ultrasound, risk management, and the transport of children to specialized centers) are included.

This fourth edition features several new chapters such as Sexual Assault, High-Altitude Illness, Disaster Preparedness, Point-of-Care Ultrasound, and Patient Safety and Quality Improvement. All other chapters have been revised and revamped with new questions and current references. Many chapters have classic photographs and radiographs to enhance learning. Each chapter features Key Points that highlight essential tips and pearls. The Top 100 Secrets have been collated and updated for rapid review and summary.

We recognize how demanding and rewarding it is to care for ill and injured children. We sincerely hope *Pediatric Emergency Medicine Secrets* fourth edition will be very useful to meet the challenges we all face on every shift. We believe the questions and answers in this book will inform and motivate the reader, as do our patients and our trainees.

ACKNOWLEDGMENTS

Steven M. Selbst and Jillian Stevens Savage

We have so many people to thank for their help with the fourth edition of *Pediatric Emergency Medicine Secrets*. Of course, we thank our spouses (Andrea and Jared) our children (Erin, Lonn, Aarti, Emery, Brady, Drew) and grandson, Miles for their encouragement, patience, and understanding as we gave up time with them to work on this textbook. We very much appreciate the help of Marybeth Thiel and Ambika Kapoor at Elsevier Publishing Company. Marybeth was very supportive and helped us to move forward with this latest edition. We especially thank Malvika Shah, Ambika Kapoor, Thilgavathy Mounisamy at Elsevier for their incredible dedication and organizational skills. Malvika, Thilgavathy and Ambika were always so helpful, immediately responsive and understanding while keeping us on course with the production. In addition, we would like to thank Padmavathy Kannabiran from MPS Limited for her expertise and efficiency while pushing this text to publication. We also offer sincere thanks to our many talented colleagues and friends who authored excellent chapters and contributed very important questions for *Pediatric Emergency Medicine Secrets* while caring for children in busy emergency departments across the country. We know that many of the senior authors were devoted mentors to junior faculty who contributed to our book. Thank you to Dr. Kate Cronan, a cherished colleague and friend who was instrumental in the development of *Pediatric Emergency Medicine Secrets* and served as co-editor for the first two editions.

We are especially thankful for John Loiselle, MD who is an outstanding division chief. John has always been very positive and supportive of our efforts while directing a top-quality emergency department. We also acknowledge the very dedicated members of our Division of Emergency Medicine at Nemours Children's Hospital, DE (Magdy Attia, MD, Brenda Bender, MD, Jonathan Bennett, MD, Andrew DePiero, MD, Monique Devens, MD, Maricar Diaz, MD, Kaynan Doctor, MD, Yamini Durani, MD, Katie Giordano, DO, Nicole Green, MD, Susan Kelly, MD, Jody Kieffer, MD, Margarita Lorch, MD, Courtney Nelson, MD, Elysha Pifko, MD, Marisa Riverso, MD, Christopher Russo, MD, John Schneider, MD, Nadine Smith, DO, Alexandra Taylor, MD, Amy Thompson, MD, and Arezoo Zomorrodi, MD). We know we are fortunate to have such wonderful colleagues who are so dedicated to the care of children. We are thankful for our excellent fellows in pediatric emergency medicine (Beverly Anderson, Theresa Barrett, David Bergamo, Melisa Blumberg, Megan Feick, Debbie Hammett, Meghan Meghpara, Joshua Rice, Nevena Rose, Brittney Russell, and Laura Santry) and a very talented core of Physicians Assistants (Jennifer Benko, Victoria Coppola, Megan Donovan, Nicole Pacyna, Kaitlin Pancio, Kara Shewbrooks, Esther Thompson, Allison Tully, and Katie White). We also acknowledge our exceptional office associates, Debbie Campbell, Joan Culver, and Jacklynn Brullo for their invaluable assistance throughout the years. In addition, we recognize the enthusiastic support of Meg Frizzola DO, Interim Chair of the Department of Pediatrics, and David Brousseau, MD, our newly arrived Chair of the Department of Pediatrics at Sidney Kimmel Medical College, Thomas Jefferson University.

Furthermore, we are grateful to the dedicated nurses and clerical staff of our Emergency Department. Finally, we sincerely thank our pediatric residents and the emergency and family medicine residents who come to Nemours to learn about pediatric emergency medicine. They inspire us and motivate us with their passion for education and their commitment to the practice of evidence-based medicine.

CONTENTS

III MEDICAL EMERGENCIES

IV   SURGICAL EMERGENCIES

V   TRAUMA

VI ENVIRONMENTAL EMERGENCIES

VII SPECIAL TOPICS

TOP 100 SECRETS

These secrets are 100 of the key teaching points of *Pediatric Emergency Medicine Secrets, Fourth Edition*. They summarize the basic concepts and principles and most salient details of pediatric emergency medicine.

1. Children commonly develop respiratory failure prior to cardiac arrest. Early intervention, before cardiac arrest, offers the best chance for a successful outcome.
2. The two-thumb method of chest compressions is preferred for newborns, with the depth of compression being one-third of the anteroposterior diameter of the chest—deep enough to generate a pulse. Begin compressions only after optimizing ventilation support. (Heart rate <60 beats per minute despite assisted ventilation for 30 seconds.)
3. Newborn infants do not tolerate cold, and hypothermia can prolong acidosis. Prevent heat loss as much as possible.
4. Respiratory failure may be present without respiratory distress. The work of breathing may appear normal in children with a reduced level of consciousness (ingestion, metabolic derangements, head trauma), neuromuscular dysfunction (muscle disease), or fatigue, despite the presence of significant hypoventilation.
5. If a patient deteriorates after endotracheal intubation, remember DOPE: Displacement of the tube, Obstruction of the tube, Pneumothorax, Equipment failure.
6. Early recognition of shock is essential. The shock state often exists in the presence of "normal" blood pressure. Tachycardia is usually the first compensatory mechanism. Tachycardia out of proportion to the child's clinical picture (i.e., fever, distress) is a red flag.
7. Hypovolemia is the most common cause of shock in children, and this is managed with aggressive volume resuscitation. Avoid vasoactive substances for the treatment of hypovolemic shock.
8. Multisystem Inflammatory Syndrome in Children is a rare complication of SARS-CoV-2 (severe acute respiratory syndrome coronavirus 2) infection in children, presenting weeks after the acute infection. It manifests as fever, diarrhea, rash, and multiorgan dysfunction with hypotension and shock. In addition to fluids, intravenous immunoglobulin and intravenous (IV) steroids are helpful.
9. Magnetic resonance imaging (MRI) is a highly sensitive alternative to a computed tomography (CT) scan in children with suspected appendicitis. The noncontrast study can be completed quickly, often without sedation, avoiding radiation. Do not withhold analgesia from a child with abdominal pain of unknown cause for fear of delaying diagnosis of appendicitis or causing misdiagnosis.
10. In children with altered mental status, do not minimize the extent of the child's illness by assuming the patient missed his nap that day or is difficult to wake up because it is late at night. Do not send children home without seeing them awake and alert.
11. Suspect head trauma or toxicological ingestion in children with altered mental status even when there is no history of either. With the abrupt development of a coma, think trauma (nonaccidental trauma), seizure, or intracranial hemorrhage.
12. Placing babies in the supine sleeping position has decreased the incidence of sudden infant death syndrome. Advise a firm mattress and keep soft bedding (pillows, blankets, bumper pads) and toys out of the infant's sleep area.
13. Respiratory syncytial virus infection can lead to apnea, especially in infants born prematurely, in infants less than 2 months of age, and in those who were ill for less than 5 days.
14. Chest pain in children is rarely related to previously undiagnosed cardiac disease, but children with this symptom deserve careful evaluation. Pediatric chest pain is concerning when it is induced by exercise, associated with fever, syncope, or accompanied by an abnormal finding on physical examination.
15. Crying and irritability in an infant may indicate life-threatening conditions, such as meningitis or abusive head trauma, or benign conditions, such as colic. A careful history and physical examination are essential to detect treatable causes of crying in infancy.
16. Oral rehydration therapy (ORT), when properly administered, is as effective as IV rehydration in the majority of children with mild-to-moderate dehydration due to gastroenteritis. ORT takes less staff time and shortens the length of stay in the emergency department (ED). Offer oral electrolyte solution, 1 mL/kg for mild dehydration and 2 mL/kg for moderate dehydration, every 5 minutes.
17. Button batteries in the ear canal, nose, or esophagus can cause extensive caustic damage in a short period of time and must be removed promptly.
18. A live insect in the ear canal is very painful and distressing. It is best to "paralyze" the insect with a thick viscous solution like mineral oil or lidocaine before removal.

19. Clinical signs such as the age of the child, appearance, and peripheral perfusion are better predictors of serious illness than the height of the fever.
20. Urinary tract infection (UTI) is the most common bacterial infection in febrile infants less than 2 months old.
21. Ingestion of multiple magnets can result in serious complications, including bowel perforation, volvulus, and death. Consider the emergency removal of magnets in the gastrointestinal (GI) tract.
22. Foreign bodies in the nose can often be removed with the "kiss" technique or using a balloon tip catheter (extractor).
23. Consider neuroimaging in children with headaches if there is a history of seizures, an abnormal neurological examination, a recent change in the type of headache, or neurological dysfunction.
24. Brain tumor headaches are worse in the early morning, wake the child from sleep, progressive, and worse with straining or bending forward. Associated findings are vomiting and an abnormal neurological examination.
25. Post–streptococcal glomerulonephritis presents weeks after a streptococcal infection (throat or skin) and presents with "cola"-colored urine, edema, and hypertension.
26. Most neonates with unconjugated hyperbilirubinemia have physiological or breast-feeding jaundice. For infants referred to the ED with unconjugated hyperbilirubinemia, begin phototherapy promptly to prevent encephalopathy and kernicterus. Conjugated hyperbilirubinemia is pathological at any age and requires further diagnostic studies and hospital admission. Jaundice in children older than 3 months is pathological.
27. Slipped capital femoral epiphysis is an orthopedic emergency, and the patient (usually a young teenager with obesity) may present with hip pain or pain referred to the knee or thigh.
28. Neoplastic neck masses are generally painless, firm, and fixed cervical masses. Neck masses that are tender, warm, and erythematous are more likely to have an infectious cause (e.g., cervical adenitis).
29. The rash of Henoch-Schönlein purpura is usually limited to the lower extremities and buttocks, and patients appear well, except for arthralgia and abdominal pain. They may have hematuria and hypertension. Platelet counts are normal, as the condition is related to vasculitis, not thrombocytopenia.
30. A CT scan may help distinguish orbital cellulitis from preseptal cellulitis when the child has severe periorbital edema and eye examination is difficult. Orbital cellulitis is often associated with a sinus infection.
31. Patients with testicular torsion can present with abdominal pain. Always perform a genitourinary examination on a boy with abdominal pain. A history of trauma often confuses the picture.
32. A high "TWIST" score (Testicular Workup for Ischemia and Suspected Torsion) should prompt immediate evaluation by a urologist without waiting for imaging.
33. Children with group A β-hemolytic streptococcus pharyngitis usually do not have a cough or coryza, but submandibular lymphadenopathy is frequently present.
34. Peritonsillar abscess may present in older children and adolescents with a severe sore throat, fever, dysphagia, muffled voice, and a unilaterally enlarged tonsil. There may be a midline shift of the uvula to the contralateral side.
35. Perform a lumbar puncture to rule out meningitis for any child with a stiff neck, fever, and ill appearance. Young infants with meningitis may not have a stiff neck until the infection progresses.
36. Consider retropharyngeal abscess in infants with a stiff neck, fever, and ill appearance. Usually patients with this condition have fullness on one side of the neck and refuse lateral neck movement or have difficulty with neck extension rather than flexion. A lateral neck radiograph is very helpful.
37. Laryngotracheobronchitis (croup) accounts for 90% of ED visits for stridor. Oral dexamethasone is the mainstay of treatment, and nebulized epinephrine is used to reduce airway edema quickly for those in distress.
38. Syncope in children is usually benign and neurocardiogenic in origin. Serious causes must be eliminated with a thorough history, physical examination, and review of an electrocardiogram (ECG). A cardiac abnormality is likely if syncope is recurrent; occurs during infancy, when the patient is in a supine position, or with exertion; or is associated with chest pain or an injury related to the patient's fall. These findings, or a family history of certain cardiac conditions, require further testing, referral to a cardiologist, and possible admission to the hospital.
39. Pelvic inflammatory disease (PID) is often treated as an outpatient with intramuscular or IV ceftriaxone, and 14 days of doxycycline and 14 days of metronidazole. Consider hospitalization of a patient with PID in the following instances: pregnancy, unclear diagnosis, vomiting, peritoneal signs, a young teenager (age <15 years), tubo-ovarian abscess present or suspected, failed outpatient treatment, or the patient's inability to follow the outpatient regimen.
40. Vomiting without a fever or diarrhea may not be due to gastroenteritis. Consider causes outside the GI tract, such as brain tumor, abusive head trauma, and diabetic ketoacidosis.
41. Presume a bowel obstruction for all infants with bilious emesis until proven otherwise. Vomiting due to pyloric stenosis is never bilious.
42. Failure to administer epinephrine (or delayed administration) during anaphylaxis is common and is associated with severe and fatal allergic reactions.

43. If a cyanotic neonate (first 1-2 weeks of life) presents to the ED in distress, begin a prostaglandin drip immediately, given concern for a possible ductal-dependent cardiac lesion.

44. Treat supraventricular tachycardia with vagal maneuvers (ice to the face for infants, Valsalva maneuver for older children), administer adenosine by rapid IV push and saline flush, or consider synchronized cardioversion.

45. There is no need for brain imaging studies or electroencephalography after a simple febrile seizure. Laboratory studies or radiography may be helpful to determine the cause of the fever. Consider a lumbar puncture if the infant has meningeal signs, bulging fontanel, excessive irritability, or lack of immunizations.

46. The development of cerebral edema in patients with diabetic ketoacidosis is associated with severe acidosis, high initial blood urea nitrogen, low arterial carbon dioxide, inadequate increase in serum sodium concentration, age less than 3 years, and bicarbonate administration.

47. Young infants are susceptible to hypoglycemia when ill due to small glycogen stores and high glucose utilization. Rapid identification and treatment (2.5-5 mL/kg of 10% dextrose in water) is crucial. Check a rapid bedside glucose level for any young child with altered mental status if the cause is not immediately obvious.

48. Children with severe dehydration (>10% total body weight loss) typically present in a shock-like state with an "ill" appearance, mottled skin, tachycardia, hypotension, and cool extremities. In children, hypotension is a very late sign of dehydration.

49. Consider cannabinoid hyperemesis syndrome in an adolescent with frequent episodes of nausea and vomiting, often relieved by hot showers. The patient may not admit to regular use of cannabis for an extended period; a drug screen is helpful in diagnosis.

50. Ovarian torsion is more common in postmenarchal females when an ovarian cyst is present, but it can occur in young girls with normal ovaries. A history of recent vigorous activity may provide a clue to the diagnosis of ovarian torsion in a female with a sudden onset of stabbing abdominal pain.

51. Patients with sickle cell disease (SCD) are immunocompromised, and those with fever are at a high risk for bacterial infection. Consider treatment with broad-spectrum antibiotics even if no source of fever is identified.

52. Acute chest syndrome is a serious complication of SCD and can be life-threatening. This syndrome is defined as a new pulmonary infiltrate and chest pain, hypoxia, fever, tachypnea, wheezing, or cough, and often cannot be distinguished from pneumonia. The cause is uncertain but is likely multifactorial.

53. Anticipate tumor lysis syndrome in patients with newly diagnosed leukemia or lymphoma. Aggressive hydration with IV fluids is the mainstay of treatment, with the goal of protecting the kidneys.

54. Admit pediatric patients to the hospital for the treatment of a UTI if: age is less than 2 months, older child with an ill appearance, dehydration, associated chronic disease such as diabetes mellitus or SCD, or a child who is vomiting and cannot tolerate oral medications.

55. Admit pediatric patients to the hospital for the treatment of preseptal cellulitis if: age <1 year, moderate-to-severe illness, inability to rule out extension of infection (orbital cellulitis), toxic appearance and/or signs of meningitis/sepsis, anorexia and/or inability to tolerate oral antibiotics, failure of outpatient management, concerning social situation, or incomplete vaccination (in this case, against *Haemophilus influenzae*).

56. Bats are the leading cause of rabies deaths in the United States. If the bat cannot be caught and tested for rabies, give rabies postexposure prophylaxis when there is a known bite or scratch from a bat or the patient was asleep and a bat was found in the room (may not know if bitten).

57. Emergently treat neonatal conjunctivitis caused by *Neisseria gonorrhoeae* with parenteral and topical antibiotics owing to the risk of corneal perforation.

58. Synthetic opioids, such as fentanyl, are not routinely tested on standard urinary drug screens. Treat fentanyl overdose as you would for other opioid poisonings. For respiratory depression, repeat naloxone as needed every few minutes until there is a clinical improvement. A larger dose of naloxone may be needed with fentanyl overdoses, as it has a higher receptor affinity than morphine (fentanyl is about 100 times more potent than morphine!).

59. Tetrahydrocannabinol (THC) edibles appear similar to common children's snacks and desserts, resulting in increased accidental ingestions. For young children (<6 years old) who ingest edibles with THC, provide supportive care and oxygen therapy. Intubation and critical care monitoring may be necessary, depending on the level of central nervous system depression. For adolescents, primary management includes supportive care, decreasing environmental stimuli, and sometimes the treatment of agitation with benzodiazepines.

60. The most significant risk factors for adolescent suicide include male sex, age older than 16 years, previous suicide attempts, homosexual orientation, mood disorder, substance abuse, poor social support, and access to firearms or other lethal means.

61. The management of bronchiolitis is mainly supportive. Most children do not respond to inhaled β-receptor agonists, and there is no evidence to support the use of corticosteroids or other treatments. Symptoms usually progress over 3 to 5 days and resolve in 2 to 3 weeks.

62. Most pediatric cases of coronavirus disease 2019 (COVID-19) are mild and present with upper respiratory infection symptoms and should be treated with supportive measures. In contrast to adult patients, pediatric patients often have normal chest radiographs, or you may see signs of a viral pneumonia. The American Academy of Pediatrics currently recommends targeted therapy against COVID-19 for specific high-risk patients at risk for severe disease progression (obesity, immunosuppression, neurodevelopmental disorders, medical-technology dependence, SCD, heart disease, chronic kidney disease, chronic liver disease, and diabetes).

63. Consider e-cigarette or vaping product use associated lung injury (EVALI) when an adolescent presents with shortness of breath, chest pain, cough, and possibly fever and chills. Many also have nausea, vomiting, or diarrhea. History reveals recent use of an e-cigarette or vaping product. A chest x-ray shows diffuse hazy opacities; CT scan shows the classic bilateral opacities, typically ground-glass in density.

64. If a child with a tracheostomy tube is in respiratory distress, assume the tube is obstructed or malpositioned. Immediately assess the patient's airway and breathing and be prepared to change the tracheostomy tube.

65. Dental abscesses are a common cause of facial swelling in young children and can be usually managed on an outpatient basis with oral antibiotics and follow-up with a dentist. Consider hospitalization if there is an associated high fever, facial cellulitis, or poor oral intake.

66. Infants and toddlers with intussusception present with episodic bouts of severe abdominal pain (drawing knees to the chest is classic), vomiting that may become bilious, and sometimes profound lethargy. A "currant jelly" stool is a late finding. Ultrasound is the diagnostic test of choice.

67. Strokes are uncommon in the pediatric population, but a high index of suspicion is needed to avoid delay in diagnosis and treatment. MRI with diffusion-weighted studies is most sensitive to make a diagnosis; however, noncontrast head CT is a reasonable first study as it is timelier and usually eliminates the need for sedation. CT will not detect an ischemic event in early stages.

68. Cushing triad (bradycardia, hypertension, irregular respiration) indicates increased intracranial pressure (ICP)—manage this with attention to the child's airway, breathing, and circulation. Rapid sequence induction (RSI) and endotracheal intubation allow for airway protection, and RSI limits further ICP elevation during intubation. Consult neurosurgery immediately and begin treatment with pharmacological agents such as mannitol or hypertonic saline. Reserve hyperventilation for cases of impending herniation.

69. MRI is the imaging test of choice for the diagnosis of osteomyelitis. Plain radiographs are usually normal in patients with this infection.

70. To manage bleeding after a tonsillectomy, attend to the child's airway, breathing, and circulation. Restore intravascular volume. If there is a clot in the posterior pharynx, leave it alone. Removal of this clot could lead to brisk bleeding and even death from aspiration. For severe active bleeding, tamponade the site with gauze and digital pressure until the otolaryngologist arrives.

71. Admit children with urolithiasis if they have evidence of obstruction, including fever, which may indicate infection or possible sepsis. Also, admit those with severe pain, vomiting, or underlying abnormalities of the kidney or genitourinary tract (i.e., renal insufficiency, solitary kidney).

72. Children with facial edema may have nephrotic syndrome rather than an allergy. Check the child's urine for proteinuria and, if present, evaluate renal function, assess for infection, and measure the child's blood pressure.

73. Because of their high velocity and penetrating ability, more than 90% of gunshot wounds to the abdomen will result in organ injury requiring laparotomy. Stab wounds are typically of lower velocity, with less penetrating ability, and can be managed more selectively.

74. Consider tracheal intubation for victims of a fire if there is early-onset stridor, severe burns of the face or mouth, progressive respiratory insufficiency, an inability to protect the airway.

75. Rib fractures, metaphyseal chip fractures, spine and scapula fractures, and complex skull fractures have a high probability of being caused by child abuse.

76. Forensic evidence collection is not recommended for sexual assault of prepubertal children if the assault took place more than 24 hours before presenting to the ED (>72 hours for pubertal children). If forensic evidence is to be collected, instruct patients to leave clothes on, avoid defecating or urinating if possible, and not eat or drink until supplies and personnel are available. Have all necessary team members take a history together to limit the need for the victim to repeat the story.

77. Immediately reimplant an avulsed permanent tooth to preserve tooth viability. If this is not possible, temporarily store the tooth in cool milk, saliva, or balanced salt solutions until an emergent dental consultation can be obtained. Increased extraoral dry time has a poor long-term prognosis.

78. The most common mechanism of pediatric elbow injury is a fall onto an outstretched hand. If there is swelling of the elbow on examination or if elbow radiographs show a posterior fat pad or a displaced anterior fat pad, consider a supracondylar fracture, even if the fracture is not obvious.

79. Chemical burns and suspicion of globe perforation are true ophthalmological emergencies that require immediate recognition and initiation of treatment. Both warrant emergent (same-day) ophthalmological consultation or referral.

80. Pediatric patients with an eye injury may have a globe perforation, but the physical examination can be deceiving. Be suspicious if the mechanism suggests a penetrating foreign body (e.g., hammering or grinding metal) or if the pupil is shaped irregularly (e.g., teardrop pupil).

81. Children older than 2 years with a nonsevere mechanism of injury; normal mental status; no signs of basilar skull fracture; and no history of loss of consciousness, vomiting, or severe headache have a low likelihood of a clinically important intracranial injury. Head imaging can be avoided for those patients.

82. Topical anesthetics such as LET (lidocaine 4%, epinephrine 1:1000, tetracaine 0.5%) are very helpful in reducing pain associated with laceration repair and often preclude the need for injection with lidocaine.

83. Injured children are different from adults. They are more likely than adults to become hypothermic at the scene and during ED resuscitation. Owing to a flexible and less muscular chest wall, rib fractures and flail chest are less common in children, but forces are more easily transmitted to internal organs. Solid organs in the abdomen of children are disproportionately larger and more exposed than in adults. Children have larger heads relative to their bodies and are more likely to land on their heads when they fall; this situation also contributes to cervical spine injuries at a higher level (C2-C3) in children than adults.

84. Steroids are not recommended for most spinal cord injuries in children. Consult a neurosurgeon before administering steroids.

85. Hematuria, a hallmark of genitourinary trauma, is absent, along with some pedicle and penetrating injuries. Contrast-enhanced CT scan is the diagnostic test of choice for stable patients with suspected renal injury (gross hematuria, >50 red blood cells per high power field [RBC/hpf] in blunt trauma, >5 RBC/hpf in penetrating trauma or shock).

86. Tension pneumothorax is diagnosed clinically, without taking time for radiographs, in a child with respiratory distress or cardiovascular compromise. Initial treatment consists of needle decompression performed while the team is preparing for pigtail catheter or tube thoracostomy placement. The placement site is the fifth intercostal space in the anterior or midaxillary line; the traditional second or third intercostal space in the midclavicular line is also appropriate. An immediate release of air should be noted.

87. A child struck in the chest by a pitched baseball may develop commotio cordis and sudden cardiac arrest.

88. Mammalian bites at high risk for infection include puncture wounds, minor wounds of hands and feet, those with care delayed for more than 12 hours, cat and human bites and wounds in immunocompromised children.

89. Observe children in the ED after a submersion injury for at least 4 to 6 hours. Initially asymptomatic, alert patients may develop respiratory distress within a few hours of the submersion. Steroids and prophylactic antibiotics are not indicated.

90. Most children with household electrical injuries are exposed to low voltage and can be discharged from the ED after a brief observation and a normal ECG. Admit patients to the hospital for cardiac monitoring if there is an abnormal EKG, previous cardiac history, loss of consciousness, significant burns, or injury involving high voltage or lightning.

91. The two priorities of treating heat stroke are eliminating hyperpyrexia and supporting the cardiovascular system. Bring the patient to a cool location and remove all clothing. Actively cool the patient by spraying with lukewarm water, positioning fans to blow air across the body, and applying ice packs to the neck, groin, and axilla. IV hydration and diuresis are essential to treat myoglobinuria.

92. Manage frostbite with rapid rewarming of affected body parts in a bath of water (40°C-42°C), splint extremities, separate digits, and give narcotic analgesics while consulting surgical colleagues.

93. Acute mountain sickness (AMS) is very common and can usually be safely managed with analgesics and antiemetics. Acetazolamide may be beneficial but is more helpful in prevention. The preferred treatment for children with moderate-to-severe AMS is descent.

94. Suspect a biologic attack when there is an epidemic presentation in a relatively compressed time frame, especially when the disease is rare or not endemic to the area and when there are particularly high morbidity or mortality rates and more respiratory forms of disease than usual.

95. In the setting of a disaster, children are at increased risk of toxic exposure secondary to multiple factors. Increased minute ventilation causes increased inhalational exposure. An increased heart rate leads to a more rapid systemic spread. An increased skin-to-body mass ratio leads to increased transdermal toxic exposure.

96. Under the Emergency Medical Treatment and Active Labor Act, the referring hospital and clinicians are responsible for ensuring that the quality of care during transport does not diminish and that an unstable patient is not placed in a less-sophisticated environment.

97. Essential information for a handoff in the ED includes relevant medical and surgical history, patient course and current condition, studies obtained and pending, suspected diagnosis, and anticipated disposition.

98. Parents do not have the right to refuse treatment for their child in the ED if a life-threatening situation exists and the emergency physician believes that it is unsafe for a patient to leave the ED to seek care elsewhere, if the patient or parent is under the influence of drugs or alcohol and cannot understand the risks and benefits of receiving or refusing care, or when child abuse is suspected.

99. Ideal staffing for procedural sedation and analgesia in the ED includes a physician experienced in pediatric advanced life support who will administer medications and closely observe the child's response. A second physician should perform the procedure while a nurse documents the patient's response to medications and is available to assist in suctioning and administering oxygen or reversal agents.

100. Point-of-care ultrasound has extensive potential, but most practitioners agree that the best applications in pediatrics include bladder volume evaluation, lung ultrasound to identify pneumothorax or consolidation, focused cardiac ultrasound, and FAST (focused assessment with sonography in trauma) examination to identify free fluid in trauma cases.

Section I ADVANCED LIFE SUPPORT

CHILDHOOD RESUSCITATION

Allen L. Hsiao and M. Douglas Baker

1. **What is the incidence of pediatric cardiopulmonary arrests?**
   Thankfully, cardiopulmonary arrests in children are much less common than in adults but remain an important reason for emergency department (ED) encounters. A prospective study by Ong and associates found an overall annual incidence of cardiopulmonary arrests of 59.7 per million children, with the highest incidence, 175 per million children, noted in the youngest age group (under 4 years). For patients admitted to the hospital, arrests occur in about 0.7% to 3% of pediatric admissions and 1.8% to 5.5% of pediatric intensive care admissions, with a stable estimated 15,200 in-hospital unique patient arrests per year (7100 pulseless, 8100 nonpulseless) based on modeling of American Hospital Association data. The American Heart Association (AHA) estimates there are >5000 out-of-hospital cardiac events per year.

2. **Is the pathophysiology of cardiopulmonary arrest in children similar to that in adults?**
   No. Cardiopulmonary arrests in children most commonly involve primary respiratory failure with subsequent cardiac arrest. Furthermore, cardiopulmonary arrests in children generally follow progressive deterioration and usually do not occur as sudden events. Exceptions to this statement include cases of sudden infant death syndrome (SIDS), major trauma, and certain primary cardiac events.

3. **How does the initial management in children differ from adult cardiopulmonary resuscitation (CPR)?**
   Historically, the initial approach to adult resuscitation was similar to that for children: A (airway), B (breathing), C (circulation/compression), D (drugs), and E (exposure). Attention to proper positioning, oxygenation, and ventilation comes first, and drug therapy comes last. However, in recent years, there has been a strong interest in initiating chest compressions earlier, as each minute of delay may result in a 10% decreased chance of survival. The C, A, and B sequence is now recommended for adult CPR. Because the majority of pediatric arrests are primarily respiratory in nature, adoption of CAB(DE) over ABC(DE) for pediatric patients is not widespread.

4. **What are the common causes of cardiopulmonary arrest in children?**
   Causes of cardiopulmonary arrest in children are numerous, but most fit into the classifications of respiratory, infectious, cardiovascular, traumatic, and central nervous system (CNS) diseases (Table 1.1). Respiratory diseases and SIDS together consistently account for one-third to two-thirds of all pediatric cardiopulmonary arrests.

5. **What is the typical age distribution of pediatric cardiopulmonary arrests?**
   Almost regardless of the underlying disease, the age distribution of cardiopulmonary arrest in children is skewed toward infancy. In a published series on childhood cardiopulmonary arrests, 56% (range, 43%-70%) of patients are younger than 1 year, 26% (range, 21%-30%) are between 1 and 4 years, and 18% (range, 6%-28%) are older than 4 years. For general emergency medicine practice settings, this finding is particularly important. Equipment and skills preparedness for this young age range are crucial to achieving best outcomes.

6. **What are the outcomes of pediatric cardiopulmonary arrests?**
   Survival rates for children who experienced isolated respiratory arrest range from 73% to 97%, and survival rates for children who experienced full cardiopulmonary arrest range from 4% to 28%. One recent comprehensive review of 41 articles on pediatric arrest found that of 5363 out-of-hospital pediatric arrests, only 12.1% of patients survived until discharge and only 4% were neurologically intact. Another study on out-of-hospital pediatric cardiac arrests prospectively followed 474 patients and found that only 1.9% survived until discharge. A multicenter registry of 3419 in-hospital arrests found somewhat better outcomes: 27.9% survived until discharge, but only 19% had favorable neurologic outcomes. The AHA reports a 6.4% to 10.2% survival rate of out-of-hospital cardiac arrests but with favorable neurologic outcomes in as many as 77% of survivors.

7. **What are some prognostic factors for pediatric cardiopulmonary arrests?**
   Some factors that appear to be prognosticators of outcome for arrests include location (in or out of hospital), resuscitation at the scene, presenting rhythm, length of resuscitation, and whether drowning or trauma was involved.

Table 1.1 Common Causes of Cardiopulmonary Arrest in Children	
RESPIRATORY	**CENTRAL NERVOUS SYSTEM**
Pneumonia	Seizures or complications thereof
Near drowning	Hydrocephalus or shunt malfunction
Smoke inhalation	Tumor
Aspiration and obstruction	Meningitis
Apnea	
Hemorrhage	
Suffocation	**Other**
Bronchiolitis	Trauma
Cardiovascular	Sudden infant death syndrome
Congenital heart disease	Anaphylaxis
Congestive heart failure	Gastrointestinal hemorrhage
Pericarditis	Poisoning
Myocarditis	
Arrhythmia	
Septic shock	

For out-of-hospital arrests, bystander or paramedic initiation of resuscitation of witnessed arrest has repeatedly been found to improve survival as much as fourfold compared with initial resuscitation by physicians after patient arrival at the hospital.

Survival of patients presenting with ventricular fibrillation (VF) is much higher than that of patients presenting with asystole, severe bradycardia, or pulseless electrical activity (PEA). Prolonged resuscitation over 20 minutes is often thought to be the strongest indicator of fatality, with chance of survival decreasing by 2.1% per minute in one large study of 3419 pediatric arrests. Overall, trauma- and submersion injury–associated arrests are associated with better survival rates compared with isolated cardiac-origin arrests (21.9% and 22.7% versus 1.1%, respectively). However, those with blunt trauma are about three times less likely to survive compared with those with penetrating trauma.

8. **In general, how can an ED best prepare for the arrival of pediatric patients suffering from cardiopulmonary arrest?**
As previously mentioned, it is relatively rare to have pediatric patients suffering from arrest and requiring CPR. As such, it is of utmost importance to have all the necessary staff, supplies, and medications prepared for this emergency in order to improve survival. Because of the complexities surrounding the care of pediatric patients, the National Pediatric Readiness Project established "Guidelines for Care of Children in the Emergency Department" in 2009. The NPRP group aimed to help EDs improve resuscitation readiness. Recommendations included but were not limited to designation of pediatric physician and nursing coordinators, emergency medical services (EMS) outreach, ongoing quality improvement, documentation of weight in kilograms, weight-based medication dosing, age-specific vital sign notations, adequate transfer policies, and so on. Studies examining guideline adherence noted decreased mortality rates, improved pain control, and decreased radiation for fractures in compliant departments. Adherence to these guidelines requires dedication and ongoing advocacy of ED staff but can absolutely be achieved to provide the best possible care to pediatric patients.

9. **What is the most important task to complete after receiving a call from EMS about a pediatric patient arriving with CPR in progress?**
The team leader should immediately gather the resuscitation team and identify each member's role. An effective resuscitation team should include but is not limited to a physician leader, airway manager, bedside registered nurse (RN), bedside technician, compressor, medication RN, and a timer/recorder. If there is additional preparation time, the team should place a firm surface on the resuscitation bed, ensure means of weight estimation, prepare for intravenous/intraosseous (IV/IO) insertion, calculate resuscitation medications, and prepare airway equipment.

10. **After establishing a clear chain of command and assigning specific duties to all members of the resuscitation team, what is the order of priorities?**
    The order of priorities is as follows:
    1. Maintain chest compressions throughout hand-off from EMS.
    2. Listen to EMS report and record pertinent completed interventions.
    3. Identify the patient's level of responsiveness.
    4. Properly position the patient on a firm surface, considering the potential for head or cervical spine injury.
    5. Establish a patent airway.
    6. Ensure proper oxygenation and ventilation.
    7. Attend to circulation.
    8. Consider drug therapy.

11. **What is the recommended way to establish a patent airway?**
    * The first attempt to establish airway patency should be through *proper airway positioning*. Often, this step alone will be effective. Because most airway obstruction is due to the effect of gravity on the mandibular block of soft tissues, it can be relieved by either a head-tilt chin-lift or jaw-thrust maneuver.
    * Vomitus or other foreign material can also obstruct airways. Inspect the airway for these materials, and *suction early and frequently*.
    * In selected patients with altered levels of consciousness, *nasopharyngeal or oropharyngeal airway stents* are useful. Semiconscious children generally tolerate nasopharyngeal airways better than oropharyngeal airways. Children, such as those in postictal states, who have sustained spontaneous respiratory effort but have upper airway obstruction due to poor muscle tone often benefit from the use of these devices.
    * Although jumping straight to intubation is often tempting, proper positioning with *appropriately sized mask and bag-valve device* is often the most efficacious way to quickly intervene and immediately manage an airway during resuscitations. This may be particularly true for clinicians who infrequently manage pediatric airways and are unaccustomed to intubating smaller and anteriorly positioned tracheas.
    * The *laryngeal mask airway* (LMA) is an often underappreciated and underused supraglottic advanced airway device that may be a very useful tool in managing pediatric airways, providing the competent user a more secure airway without the complexities of endotracheal intubation. Just as with endotracheal tubes (ETTs) and bag-valve masks, appropriate sizing of the LMA for each child is necessary but may be easier to achieve as there are fewer choices based on size.

12. **What is the recommended way to deliver supplemental oxygen to a child?**
    Supplemental oxygen can be delivered to a child by a variety of different means. For the sickest patients, oxygen should be delivered in the highest concentration and by the most direct method possible. Children who demonstrate spontaneous breathing might require less invasive means of administration of supplemental oxygen. Table 1.2 lists some different methods of oxygen delivery with their associated delivery capabilities.
    Children without adequate spontaneous breathing effort require mechanical support. Different bag-valve mask devices have different oxygen delivery capabilities. Self-inflating bag-valve devices are capable of delivering 60% to 90% oxygen, but non–self-inflating devices (anesthesia ventilation systems) deliver 100% oxygen to the patient. Endotracheal intubation offers the most secure and direct means of delivery of 100% oxygen to the patient.

Table 1.2 Methods of Oxygen Delivery and Their Delivery Capabilities
Nasal cannula: 30%-40% oxygen
Simple masks: 30%-60% oxygen
Partial rebreather masks: 50%-60% oxygen
Oxygen tents: 30%-50% oxygen
Oxygen hoods: 80%-90% oxygen
Nonrebreather masks: ~100% oxygen

13. **Which children require intubation?**
    Although the most obvious indication for endotracheal intubation is sustained apnea, a number of other indications exist:
    * Inadequate CNS control of ventilation
    * Functional or anatomic airway obstruction

- Strong potential for developing airway obstruction (e.g., inhalation airway burns and expanding airway hematoma)
- Loss of protective airway reflexes
- Excessive work of breathing, which might lead to fatigue and respiratory insufficiency
- Need for high airway pressures to maintain effective alveolar gas exchange
- Need for mechanical ventilatory support
- Potential occurrence of any of the preceding during patient transport
- Need to place patient in medically induced coma (e.g., intractable status epilepticus and neuroprotective hypothermia protocol)

In many instances, bag-mask ventilation and bag-ETT ventilation are equally effective for the patient. In such circumstances, it is logical to employ the method that the rescuer is best able to deliver. One prospective study randomized the use of bag-mask ventilation and endotracheal intubation by paramedics in 830 out-of-hospital pediatric arrests. There was no significant difference in survival (30% versus 26%, respectively) or good neurologic outcome (23% versus 20%) between the two groups of children. Subsequent studies confirmed that bag-mask ventilation is preferred in the field given the high incidence of intubation-related complications in patients managed by prehospital providers in the United States.

14. **When selecting an ETT, what sizing guidelines are suggested?**
There are a number of ways to ensure selection of properly sized ETTs for children. The most often cited is the following age-based formula:

$$\text{ETT internal diameter (mm)} = \frac{(16 + \text{years of age})}{4}$$

Another "rule of thumb" is really a "rule of finger." Research has demonstrated that the width of the child's fifth fingernail is approximately equal to the outer width of the appropriately sized ETT. Cuffed tubes are generally preferred.

15. **How can I determine if the ETT is appropriately placed?**
Proper depth for ETT insertion from the point of the patient's central incisors can be estimated to be three times the internal diameter of the ETT. Measurement of end-tidal carbon dioxide using a colorimetric detector, observation for symmetric chest expansion, and auscultation for symmetric breath sounds can help ensure proper placement. Confirmation of placement is probably best determined with a chest radiograph. Prior to a chest radiograph, the colorimetric detector offers a rapid bedside determination to detect CO_2 to confirm ETT placement (Fig. 1.1). Alternatively, when available, an end-tidal CO_2 monitor can be connected for expeditious confirmation.

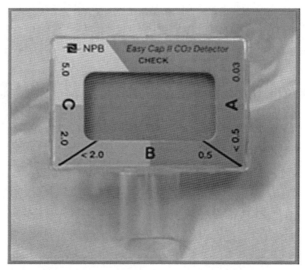

Fig. 1.1 Colorimetric device. Although the image is only reproduced in black and white, in infants and children with a perfusing rhythm, a purple color on the device indicates a problem, whereas a yellow color (detection of exhaled CO_2) implies that the tube is in the trachea.

KEY POINTS: HOW TO DETERMINE THE PROPER PLACEMENT OF THE ENDOTRACHEAL TUBE?

1. Check to see that the tube is inserted at a depth that is three times the internal diameter of the ETT (from the point of the patient's central incisors).
2. Observe for symmetric chest expansion.
3. Auscultate for symmetric breath sounds.
4. Look for distention of the abdomen, indicating misplacement of the tube.
5. Measure end-tidal carbon dioxide using a colorimetric detector. In infants and children with a perfusing rhythm, a purple color on the device indicates a problem, whereas a yellow color implies that the tube is in the trachea.
6. Confirm tube placement with a chest radiograph.

16. **What are the best methods to assess a child's circulatory status?**
    Assessment of a child's circulatory status should always include appraisal of the following:
    - Skin and mucous membrane color
    - Presence and quality of pulses
    - Capillary refill
    - Heart rate and blood pressure
        Always keep in mind that in the instance of acute blood loss, the protective mechanisms of increased heart rate and increased vascular resistance maintain a child's blood pressure within a normal range in spite of losses as high as 25% of total body blood volume.

17. **What is the pediatric assessment triangle (PAT)?**
    The PAT is a visual and auditory assessment tool developed for rapid standardized assessment of pediatric patients. The PAT emphasizes a quick evaluation of a patient in three main areas: (1) appearance, (2) work of breathing, and (3) circulation to skin, to form a general impression of the child's condition (Fig. 1.2). Based on an assessment of normal or abnormal, patients can be categorized in different physiologic categories ranging from "stable" to "respiratory distress" to "decompensated shock" and full "cardiopulmonary failure" (Table 1.3). The PAT is now widely accepted and taught to prehospital specialists in pediatric advanced life support (PALS) as a quick assessment tool.

18. **To whom and how should external cardiac compression be delivered?**
    Apply external cardiac compression to any child with ineffective pulses. The optimal compression-ventilation ratio for two-rescuer CPR is 15 to 2; for single rescuers, it is 30 to 2. It takes a number of compressions to

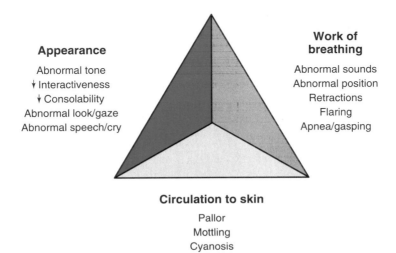

Appearance

Abnormal tone
↓ Interactiveness
↓ Consolability
Abnormal look/gaze
Abnormal speech/cry

Work of breathing

Abnormal sounds
Abnormal position
Retractions
Flaring
Apnea/gasping

Circulation to skin

Pallor
Mottling
Cyanosis

Fig. 1.2 The pediatric assessment triangle.

Table 1.3 Pediatric Assessment Triangle and Patient General Impression

	STABLE	RESPIRATORY DISTRESS	RESPIRATORY FAILURE	SHOCK	CENTRAL NERVOUS SYSTEM/METABOLISM DISTURBANCE	CARDIOPULMONARY FAILURE
Appearance of patient	Normal	Normal/abnormal	Abnormal	Normal/ abnormal	Abnormal	Abnormal
Work of breathing	Normal	Abnormal	Abnormal	Normal	Normal	Abnormal
Circulation to skin	Normal	Normal	Normal/abnormal	Abnormal	Normal	Abnormal

raise coronary perfusion pressure, which drops with each pulse. Interruptions in chest compressions are associated with a decreased rate of return of spontaneous circulation. It is currently recommended that in infants, compressions be applied evenly over the lower half of the sternum with two fingers or two thumbs. The two thumb–encircling hands technique may be preferred for two-rescuer CPR with infants because it produces higher coronary perfusion pressure and more consistently results in appropriate depth of compression. For children and adolescents, compress the lower half of the sternum with the heel of one hand or with two hands, but do not press over the xiphoid process or ribs. Regardless of age, the universal rate of compressions is 100 to 120/minute.

19. **What are the golden rules of vascular access?**
    During resuscitation, procedures should be done by those most talented. Although it is better to have large-gauge vascular access for resuscitation, small-gauge vascular access is adequate to deliver medications and slower infusions of fluids.

20. **What are the options for vascular access in children?**
    There are many options for vascular access in children. Some might not be as available or achievable as others. *Peripheral venous access* is generally preferred over other means. Antecubital, hand, wrist, foot, and ankle veins are the most popular access sites. Saphenous veins in the ankle are deep but often accessible. External jugular veins are also reliably accessible but require difficult positioning of the child to be successful. Scalp veins are potential sites of access in infants but might be difficult to access while managing the patient's airway.

    Central access sites include bone marrow, femoral veins, and subclavian veins. Femoral and subclavian access should be attempted only by those skilled in the procedure. Consider IO access early when venous access cannot be quickly established, especially in the case of apnea and pulselessness in an infant.

21. **Why does IO infusion work?**
    The bone marrow serves as a "stiff" vascular bed. It is composed of interconnected sinusoids that are fed and drained by veins that traverse the cortex of the bone and connect with the central circulation. Fluids infused anywhere into the marrow cavity enter these vascular channels and find their way to the central venous system. Numerous medications and fluids have been shown to be effective when administered via this route.

22. **What are the do's and don'ts surrounding IO infusion?**
    Although there is no age limit for use of IO infusion, it may be easier to accomplish in younger patients, whose bones are less calcified. Remember that IO infusion was developed in the 1930s as a technique of vascular access in adults. Numerous studies using adult patients have demonstrated a cumulative 98% success rate. The preferred site of IO needle placement in children is the proximal tibia, 1 to 3 cm below the tibial tuberosity. Alternate sites include the distal femur, the proximal medial malleolus, and the anterior iliac spine. Any IV fluid or medication can be safely and effectively administered via the IO route. Rates of infusion are limited by needle gauge and length. When infusion is delivered with pressure, flow rates of saline through 20-G needles have been measured as high as 25 mL/minute. Contraindications of IO insertion include fracture, prior puncture of same bone, and overlying infection.

23. **What role does drug therapy play in pediatric resuscitation?**
    Drug therapy during resuscitation is reserved for patients who do not respond adequately to the ABCs. Useful chemical agents include:
    - Epinephrine (to increase heart rate, myocardial contractility, and systemic vascular resistance)
    - Dextrose (to increase glucose)
    - Amiodarone or procainamide (to reverse ventricular arrhythmias)
    - Naloxone (to reverse the effects of narcotics)
    - Adenosine (to abort supraventricular tachycardia)
    - Dopamine (to increase vasoconstriction and blood pressure)
    - Dobutamine (to increase myocardial contractility)
    - Benzodiazepines (to achieve sedation and control seizures)

    Keep in mind that administration of any of these drugs should never be considered as a first line of management. *Oxygenation and ventilation are always the first priorities for any seriously ill child.* Other appropriate supportive measures (e.g., chest compressions for pulselessness or fluid infusion for shock) should precede administration of drugs during resuscitation.

24. **What are the PALS recommendations for pulseless arrest (PEA, asystole)?**
    - Start compressions.
    - Give epinephrine for PEA or asystole intravascularly (IV or IO route) as soon as possible at a standard dose of 0.01 mg/kg (0.1 mL/kg of 0.1-mg/mL concentration) with max of 1 mg. Continue every 3 to 5 minutes throughout resuscitation.

- If unable to obtain IV/IO access, epinephrine may be administered via the ETT at a higher dose of 0.1 mg/kg (0.1-mL/kg or 1-mg/mL concentration).

25. **What are the PALS recommendations for bradycardia?**
    - CPR should be initiated if heart rate is <60/minute despite oxygenation and ventilation.
    - Any intravascularly (IV or IO route) administered epinephrine dose should be given as a standard dose of 0.01 mg/kg (0.1 mL/kg of a 0.1-mg/mL concentration). Repeat every 3 to 5 minutes.
    - In case of inability to establish IV/IO access, one may administer epinephrine via the ETT at a higher dose of 0.1 mg/kg (0.1 mL/kg of the 1-mg/mL solution).
    - Consider atropine if there is evidence of primary atrioventricular (AV) block or increased vagal tone.
    - Consider transthoracic/transvenous pacing.
    - Identify and treat potential underlying causes such as hypothermia, hypoxia, and medications.

26. **Which resuscitation drugs are effective when given via an ETT?**
    The preferred routes of drug delivery for infants and children in cardiac arrest are IV and IO. However, there are four "traditional" resuscitation drugs that are effective when administered through the ETT. Those four are *l*idocaine, *a*tropine, *n*aloxone, and *e*pinephrine. The acronym LANE is an easy way to remember them. *V*ersed (midazolam) is also useful and is effective when administered via the ETT. Adding this drug to the list yields a different acronym: NAVEL. With the exception of epinephrine, endotracheal doses are the same as intravascular doses. All doses of epinephrine given through the ETT should be a higher dose (0.1 mg/kg).

KEY POINTS: DRUGS THAT CAN BE GIVEN VIA THE ENDOTRACHEAL ROUTE

1. Lidocaine
2. Atropine
3. Naloxone
4. Epinephrine
5. Versed (midazolam)—NAVEL

---

27. **Are there minimum dosing requirements for any resuscitation drugs?**
    - **Atropine** (usual dose, 0.02 mg/kg) has a minimum dosing requirement for effective reversal of bradycardia. It appears that at doses lower than 0.1 mg, atropine exerts an effect that might actually worsen bradycardia. Thus, if its use is considered for reversal of bradycardia in a child who weighs less than 5 kg, a minimum of 0.1 mg should be administered.
    - **Dopamine** also has different effects when administered at different doses. At lower doses (1 to 5 μg/kg/minute), dopaminergic effects are seen. When administered at these lower doses, dopamine tends to augment renal blood flow and enhance urinary output. During resuscitation, dopamine typically is used to bolster blood pressure through increased vasoconstriction. For that α-adrenergic effect, higher doses (10 to 20 μg/kg/minute) are required.

28. **What are the recommendations for use of adenosine?**
    Adenosine is the drug of choice in the acute management of supraventricular tachycardia in infants and children with a pulse that does not respond to vagal maneuvers. It is a short-acting agent (half-life of approximately 10 seconds) that slows AV node conduction. To achieve maximum effectiveness, the initial dose is 0.1 mg/kg, given as a rapid intravascular push with an immediate saline flush. For this reason, the team should attempt to place the IV as close to the AV node as possible. If the first dose is properly administered but ineffective, give a larger second dose of 0.2 mg/kg. Usual adult doses are 6 mg (first dose), followed by 12 mg (second and maximum dose). Expect that the first dose might be completely ineffective or only transiently effective. Administration of subsequent higher doses generally yields success.

29. **Does calcium have any usefulness in pediatric resuscitations?**
    The AHA does not recommend the routine use of calcium in pediatric cardiac arrest. Studies have shown worse survival with calcium administration during cardiac arrest resuscitation. However, there remain specific instances when it has significant value. Use calcium to remedy the following situations:
    - Documented hypocalcemia
    - Documented hyperkalemia
    - Documented hypermagnesemia
    - Calcium channel blocker excess

When administered, calcium should be infused slowly. Rapid infusion results in severe bradycardia. Take care to avoid back-to-back infusion of calcium and sodium bicarbonate–containing solutions. If mixed, these agents form calcium carbonate (chalk) in the IV tubing.

30. Does sodium bicarbonate have a role in pediatric resuscitations?

Sodium bicarbonate is not recommended for routine use in pediatric resuscitations. Although it is a useful agent for the reversal of documented metabolic acidosis, it is effective only in the presence of adequate ventilation. When bicarbonate combines with hydrogen, it forms a complex molecule that splits into carbon dioxide and water. The carbon dioxide has only one route of exit, the respiratory tract. Without effective ventilation, this by-product is not removed and the buffering capacity of the bicarbonate is eliminated. A randomized, controlled trial found no benefit from sodium bicarbonate use in neonatal resuscitation, while retrospective data in another study showed survivors were less likely to have received sodium bicarbonate than those who had had longer CPR duration and more pharmacologic interventions; this may reflect heroic attempts to try all available medical interventions. After provision of effective ventilation and chest compressions and administration of epinephrine, one could consider sodium bicarbonate for suspected or confirmed hyperkalemia and sodium channel blocker toxicity (e.g., tricyclics).

31. Is there an easy method to calculate mixtures of constant infusions of drugs?

Several methods are used. Here is one easy method:
- For constant infusion of drugs (epinephrine and isoproterenol) beginning at *0.1 μg/kg/minute*: 0.6 times the weight (in kg) equals the number of milligrams of drug to add to enough water to make a total of 100 mL of solution. The resultant solution is then infused at a rate of 1 mL/hour, delivering 0.1 μg/kg/minute.
- For constant infusion of drugs (dopamine, dobutamine) beginning at *1 μg/kg/minute*: 6 times the weight (in kg) equals the number of milligrams of drug to add to enough water to make a total of 100 mL of solution. The resultant solution is then infused at a rate of 1 mL/hour, delivering 1 μg/kg/minute.

32. What role does defibrillation play in pediatric resuscitation?

Historically, pediatric resuscitation has focused on pulmonary causes; defibrillation is a relatively uncommon intervention in pediatric resuscitation. Although asystole remains the most commonly observed arrhythmia during pediatric cardiac arrests, recent research indicates that VF may occur much more frequently than originally thought. The National Registry of Cardiopulmonary Resuscitation, the largest inpatient pediatric cohort reported to date, found VF occurred in 14% of pediatric arrests. In that study, pediatric patients with VF had a higher survival rate (29%) than those with asystole (24%) or PEA (11%). A study of out-of-hospital pediatric arrests found VF as the presenting rhythm in 17.6% of cases, with children older than 7 years having the highest incidence (38/141, 27.0%). Survival of patients with VF was threefold greater (31.3% versus 10.7%) than in those without a shockable rhythm. These data have prompted advocacy for increased availability of pediatric automated external defibrillators (AEDs).

33. How is defibrillation best accomplished?

In any resuscitation, carefully check the rhythm after airway and breathing are established. Carefully identify a shockable rhythm before defibrillation is attempted.

Defibrillation works by producing a mass polarization of myocardial cells with the intent of stimulating the return of a spontaneous sinus rhythm. Once a shockable rhythm (ventricular tachycardia/VF) is diagnosed in a pulseless patient, prepare the patient for defibrillation and correct acidosis and hypoxemia. High-amplitude (coarse) fibrillation is more easily reversed than low-amplitude (fine) fibrillation. Administration of epinephrine can help coarsen fibrillation.

Defibrillation is most effective with use of the largest paddle that makes complete contact with the chest wall. Using the larger (8-cm diameter) paddle lowers the intrathoracic impedance and increases the effectiveness of the defibrillation current.

Take care to use an appropriate interface between the paddles and the chest wall. Electrode cream, paste, or gel pads are preferred when using paddles. Do not use saline-soaked gauze pads, ultrasound gel, alcohol pads, or bare paddles. Whenever available and if time allows, place and use self-adhesive defibrillation pads instead of paddles, as they allow for safer and more efficient shock delivery and then can be used for cardiac pacing when appropriate.

Whether gel, paste, or pads are used, placement must be meticulous because electrical bridging across the surface of the chest results in ineffective defibrillation and possibly skin burns. When attempting defibrillation, immediate CPR should follow the delivery of one shock, rather than delivery of up to three shocks before CPR. This recommendation is based on the fact that the first shock eliminates VF 85% of the time, and studies have shown long delays typically occur between shocks when AEDs are used. Biphasic defibrillators are preferred as less energy is required and better tolerated. For defibrillation of the pediatric patient, use an initial dose of 2 to 4 J/kg.

34. **Are AEDS useful for children with sudden collapse?**
AEDs have been shown to reliably recognize shockable rhythms in children. PALS guidelines recommend use of AEDs for children 1 year and older. An AED can also be used in infants younger than 1 year if an attenuator is available or when there are no alternatives (i.e., no manual defibrillator is available).

35. **Is induced hypothermia useful in treating children with cardiac arrest?**
Therapeutic hypothermia is recommended for adults following resuscitation from sudden witnessed out-of-hospital VF cardiac arrest but had not been well studied in children. Recently, a pair (in-hospital and out-of-hospital arrests) of randomized, controlled therapeutic hypothermia trials at over 35 children's hospitals showed evidence of increased early postresuscitation hypotension and no improvement in outcomes. However, AHA notes therapeutic hypothermia (32°C-34°C) may be considered for infants and children who remain comatose following resuscitation from cardiac arrest as part of a targeted temperature management plan.

36. **Should families be cleared from the resuscitation room when treating children with cardiac arrest?**
In general, family members should be offered the opportunity to be present during the resuscitation of their infant or child. Multiple studies indicate that parents prefer to be given the option to remain in the room. Many relatives believe their presence is helpful to the patient, and some studies show that being present during the resuscitation helped their adjustment to the family member's death.

37. **Is there a role for telemedicine in pediatric emergencies and resuscitations?**
Pediatric resuscitation is frequently initiated by first responders in the field. Also, resuscitation of children often takes place in general EDs or other settings that are not staffed by pediatric personnel. A recent review of the literature suggests that telemedicine could augment real-time decision-making toward improved quality of pediatric emergency care by facilitating communication between care providers. One fortunate result of the COVID-19 pandemic is the catalyzed adoption of telemedicine and access to cutting-edge software and hardware. While telemedicine cannot replace in-person care and a comprehensive physical exam, it can bridge physical distance and lack of access to pediatric specialists, even just by using mobile telephones. Improved outcomes (significantly shorter time to airway establishment, ventilation, and chest compressions) were demonstrated by Deakin et al. even when CPR advice could only be provided over the telephone, predating the availability of live video-based telemedicine.

BIBLIOGRAPHY

1. Berrens ZJ, Gosdin CH, Brady PW, Tegtmeyer K. Efficacy and safety of pediatric critical care physician telemedicine involvement in rapid response team and code response in a satellite facility. *Pediatr Crit Care Med.* 2019;20(2):172–177. PMID: 30395026.
2. Chen K-Y, Ko Y-C, Hsieh M-J, et al. Interventions to improve the quality of bystander cardiopulmonary resuscitation: a systematic review. *PLoS One.* 2019;14(2):e0211792.
3. Deakin CD, Evans S, King P. Evaluation of telephone-cardiopulmonary resuscitation advice for paediatric cardiac arrest. *Resuscitation.* 2010;81(7):853–856. PMID: 20409630.
4. De Maio VJ, Osmond MH, Stiell IG, et al. Epidemiology of out-of hospital pediatric cardiac arrest due to trauma. *Prehosp Emerg Care.* 2012;16(2):230–236.
5. Dieckmann RA, Brownstein D, Gausche-Hill M. The pediatric assessment triangle: a novel approach for the rapid evaluation of children. *Pediatr Emerg Care.* 2010;26(4):312–315.
6. Fang JL. Use of telemedicine to support neonatal resuscitation. *Semin Perinatol.* 2021;45(5):151423. PMID: 33958229.
7. Fuchs SR, Kannankeril PJ. Out-of-hospital cardiac arrest due to ventricular fibrillation in children-a call to action. *Heart Rhythm.* 2018;15(1):122–123. PMID: 28917566.
8. Gattu R, Teshome G, Lichenstein R. Telemedicine applications for pediatric emergency medicine, a review of the current literature. *Pediatr Emerg Care.* 2016;32(2):123–130.
9. Gausche M, Lewis RJ, Stratton SJ, et al. Effect of out-of-hospital pediatric endotracheal intubation on survival and neurological outcome: a controlled clinical trial. *JAMA.* 2000;283:783–790.
10. Gerritse BM, Draaisma JM, Schalkwjk A, et al. Should EMS paramedics perform paediatric tracheal intubation in the field? *Resuscitation.* 2008;79:225–229.
11. Holmberg MJ, Ross CE, Fitzmaurice GM, Chan PS, et al. American Heart Association's Get With the Guidelines–Resuscitation Investigators Annual incidence of adult and pediatric in-hospital cardiac arrest in the United States. *Circ Cardiovasc Qual Outcomes.* 2019;12(7):e005580 PMID: 31545574.
12. Horeczko T, Enriquez B, McGrath NE, et al. The pediatric assessment triangle: accuracy of its application by nurses in the triage of children. *J Emerg Nurs.* 2013;39(2):182–189. Epub 2012 Jul 24.
13. Lapcharoensap W, Lund K, Huynh T. Telemedicine in neonatal medicine and resuscitation. *Curr Opin Pediatr.* 2021;33(2):203–208. PMID: 33492007.
14. Lubrano R, Cecchetti C, Bellelli E, et al. Comparison of times of intervention during pediatric CPR maneuvers using ABC and CAB sequences: a randomized trial. *Resuscitation.* 2012;83(12):1473–1477. Epub 2012 May 8.
15. Matos RI, Watson RS, Nadkarni VM, et al. Duration of cardiopulmonary resuscitation and illness category impact survival and neurologic outcomes for in-hospital pediatric cardiac arrests. *Circulation.* 2013;127(4):442–451.
16. Meert KL, Donaldson A, Nadkarni V, et al. Pediatric Emergency Care Applied Research Network. *Pediatr Crit Care Med.* 2009;10(5):544–553.

17. Moler FW, Silverstein FS, Holubkov R, et al.THAPCA Trial Investigators Therapeutic hypothermia after in-hospital cardiac arrest in children. *N Engl J Med.* 2017;26;376(4):318–329. PMID: 28118559.
18. Moore B, Shah M, Owusu-Ansah S, et al. Pediatric readiness in emergency medical services systems. *Ann Emerg Med.* 2020;75(1):e1–e6.
19. Ong MEH, Stiell I, Osmond MH, et al. Etiology of pediatric out-of-hospital cardiac arrest by coroner's diagnosis. *Resuscitation.* 2006;68(3):335–342.
20. Pejovic NJ, Trevisanuto D, Lubulwa C, et al. Neonatal resuscitation using a laryngeal mask airway: a randomised trial in Uganda. *Arch Dis Child.* 2018;103(3):255–260.
21. Raymond TT, Stromberg D, Stigall W, et al. American Heart Association's Get With the Guidelines-Resuscitation Investigators Sodium bicarbonate use during in-hospital pediatric pulseless cardiac arrest – a report from the American Heart Association Get With The Guidelines®-Resuscitation. *Resuscitation.* 2015;89:106–113.
22. Scribano PV, Baker MD, Ludwig S. Factors influencing termination of resuscitative efforts in children: a comparison of pediatric emergency medicine and adult emergency medicine physicians. *Pediatr Emerg Care.* 1997;13:320–324.
23. Scrivens A, Reynolds PR, Emery FE, et al. Use of intraosseous needles in neonates: a systematic review. *Neonatology.* 2019;116(4):305–314.
24. Silka MJ, Kobayashi RL, Hill AC, Bar-Cohen Y. Pediatric survivors of out-of-hospital ventricular fibrillation: etiologies and outcomes. *Heart Rhythm.* 2018;15(1):116–121. PMID: 28823600.
25. Stub D, Bernard S, Pellegrino V, et al. Refractory cardiac arrest treated with mechanical CPR, hypothermia, ECMO and early reperfusion (the CHEER trial). *Resuscitation.* 2015 Jan;86:88–94. PMID: 25281189.
26. Topjian AA, Nadkarni VM. Advances in recognition, resuscitation, and stabilization of the critically ill child. *Pediatr Clin North Am.* 2013;60(3):605–620.
27. Topjian AA, de Caen A, Wainwright MS, et al. Pediatric post-cardiac arrest care: a scientific statement from the American Heart Association. *Circulation.* 2019;140(6):e194–e233. PMID: 31242751.
28. Topjian AA, Telford R, Holubkov R, et al. Therapeutic Hypothermia After Pediatric Cardiac Arrest (THAPCA) Trial Investigators Association of early postresuscitation hypotension with survival to discharge after targeted temperature management for pediatric out-of-hospital cardiac arrest: secondary analysis of a randomized clinical trial. *JAMA Pediatr.* 2018;172(2):143–153. PMID: 29228147.
29. Topjian AA, Raymond TT, Atkins D, et al. Pediatric Basic and Advanced Life Support Collaborators Part 4: pediatric basic and advanced life support: 2020 American Heart Association guidelines for cardiopulmonary resuscitation and emergency cardiovascular care. *Circulation.* 2020;142(16_suppl_2):S469–S523. PMID: 33081526.

CHAPTER 2

NEONATAL RESUSCITATION

Constance M. McAneney

1. **What physiological changes take place during the transition from intrauterine to extrauterine life?**

   The cardiopulmonary systems undergo a rapid change from fetal to extrauterine life. With the newborn's first breaths (increasing the neonate's PaO_2 [partial pressure of oxygen] and pH), pulmonary vascular resistance decreases, thereby causing an increase in pulmonary blood flow, which is required for gas exchange. The increase in pulmonary blood flood with lung aeration replaces the dependency on umbilical venous return, which was the source of preload in utero. After the first breaths are taken, the umbilical cord is clamped and systemic vascular resistance rises. Cardiac output increases because of an increase in heart rate. Blood flow through the foramen ovale and the ductus arteriosus reverses direction, and then these structures eventually close. The ductus arteriosus is usually closed functionally by 15 hours of age.

   If the pulmonary vascular resistance does not fall adequately, a persistent right-to-left shunt will occur (persistent pulmonary hypertension). The inability to expand alveolar spaces can cause intrapulmonary shunting of blood (hypoxia).

2. **What preparation is necessary to have for the unexpected emergency department (ED) delivery?**

   Preparation is key, as most ED deliveries are "unexpected." A prearranged plan (which should be simulated periodically to ensure a smooth process and delivery of standard of care) should be set in motion as soon as birth is imminent. That plan should include the assembly of personnel who are best able to take care of the newly born infant. Obtain a brief history, if possible, because it may affect the resuscitation. Equipment and medications specifically for neonatal resuscitation should be kept in a designated tray so they are rapidly available to the resuscitation team (see Table 2.1). Periodic inspection of this equipment for proper functioning and expiration dates of medication should become part of the routine upkeep of the neonatal resuscitation tray.

3. **What are the critical facts in the history that should be elicited, if possible, prior to delivery?**

   The standard maternal history is important but may need to wait until after delivery due to the imminent birth of the infant. Critical information may need to be narrowed to facts that may affect the immediate preparation (equipment and personnel) for the delivery.

   It is important to know if the laboring mother is expecting multiples as there should be a resuscitation area, equipment, and team dedicated to each infant.

   The expected due date is also crucial to determine if the newly born infant will be premature and, if so, approximately how premature. Infants born at less than 36 weeks' gestation are more likely to be born "unexpectedly" and will have an increased risk of needing resuscitation. Depending on the infant's gestational age, smaller caliber equipment may be needed in the case of prematurity.

   If membranes have already ruptured, it will be important to note the color of the amniotic fluid. If the fluid is meconium stained (greenish), anticipate a distressed newly born infant with or without airway obstruction from the meconium. The infant may require intubation with suctioning, though this is no longer routinely recommended for all deliveries with meconium-stained fluid. Equipment should be available and personnel should be prepared to manage this clinical situation.

   Conditions that have significant risk for the need for resuscitation at birth include gestation less than 34 weeks, weight <2 kg, known fetal anomalies or conditions that interfere with respiratory transition, fetal bradycardia, or complications of delivery (i.e., emergency C-section, prolapsed cord, intrapartum hemorrhage, meconium-stained amniotic fluid). If neonatology services are available, early consultation may aid in resuscitation, especially in the setting of a complicated case.

4. **What three basic questions are asked immediately upon the birth of an infant?**
   - Is the newly born infant term gestation?
   - Is the newly born infant crying or breathing?
   - Does the newly born infant have good muscle tone?

5. **If the answers to the three key basic questions are all "yes," how should the infant be managed?**

   The term infant with good tone and normal breathing appears to be transitioning well and can remain with the mother. Secondary to the risk of bradycardia, suctioning of the mouth and nose is avoided in these

Table 2.1 Equipment and Drugs for the Neonatal Resuscitation

Equipment

Gowns, gloves, and masks

Warm towels and blankets

Hat

Plastic bag or plastic wrap ($\leq$32 weeks' gestation)

Radiant warmer

Cardiorespiratory monitor with ECG leads

Pulse oximeter with neonatal probes

Stethoscope

Suction equipment

Bulb syringe

Meconium aspirator

Suction catheters (sizes 5-10 FR)

End-tidal CO_2 detector

Face masks (sizes: premature, newborn, and infant)

Oral airways (sizes: 000, 00, 0)

Oxygen source (tank, wall)

Oxygen blender (set at 21%-30% for neonates <35 weeks, 21% for >35 weeks)

T-piece resuscitator or anesthesia bag with manometer (preferably 500 mL, no larger than 750 mL)

Self-inflating bag (as backup)

Laryngoscope with straight blades (sizes: 0 and 1)

Spare bulbs and batteries

Endotracheal tubes (sizes: 2.5, 3.0, 3.5, and 4.0) and stylet

Laryngeal mask airway

Tape

Umbilical catheters (3.5 and 5 FR)

Umbilical catheter tray

Three-way stopcocks

Nasogastric feeding tubes (8 and 10 FR)

Needles and syringes

Chest tubes (8 and 10 FR)

Magill forceps

Drugs

Epinephrine (0.1 mg/mL)

Naloxone

Normal saline

Dextrose in water 10%

Resuscitation drug chart

ECG, electrocardiogram.

well-appearing infants. Dry the baby, cover in dry linens, and place the infant on the mother, skin-to-skin. Continue to observe breathing, color, and activity. Delay cord clamping for at least 1 minute for newborns not requiring resuscitation.

6. If the answers to any of the three basic questions are "no," how should the team proceed in resuscitation?
Initially, the provider should dry and stimulate the baby, clear the airway, and provide warmth. Place the infant in slight Trendelenburg position, on his or her back with the neck slightly extended. Usually by drying the infant, he/she is adequately stimulated to begin spontaneous and effective respirations. Gentle tactile stimulation includes drying the neonate and rubbing soles of the feet and the back. Clear the airway, *only if necessary*, with a bulb syringe or suction catheter. Duration of the suctioning should not exceed 5 seconds, as vigorous and/or prolonged suctioning will cause bradycardia. Thus if the newly born shows no signs of obstruction or need for positive pressure ventilation, then suctioning, even with a bulb syringe, is not indicated. Warmth can be provided with radiant warmer, plastic wraps, hats, blankets, and warm humidified inspired gases individually or in combination to reduce the risk of hypothermia. Since newly born infants do not tolerate the cold, and hypothermia can prolong acidosis, clinicians must prevent heat loss as much as possible.

7. What is the Apgar score, and how is it utilized in resuscitation?
Assess the newly born infant and assign an Apgar score at 1 minute and at 5 minutes of life (Table 2.2). The Apgar score assesses heart rate, respirations, muscle tone, reflex irritability, and color. It indicates how the infant is doing and/or how the infant is responding to the resuscitation. Apgar scoring should not dictate resuscitative efforts. If the Apgar score is less than 7 at 5 minutes, then the scoring continues every 5 minutes for 20 minutes. *Do not delay resuscitative efforts to obtain an Apgar score.*

8. When should the umbilical cord be clamped?
Cord management has changed over the last decade. For years, the cord was clamped immediately at birth. Studies have found that later cord clamping assists in the extrauterine cardiovascular transition, increases hemoglobin and hematocrit, and improves iron status in early infancy. Of note, delayed cord clamping has also been associated with increased use of phototherapy and polycythemia but not increased rates of exchange transfusions. The current recommendation for term and late preterm ($\geq$34 weeks' gestation) who are vigorous and do not require resuscitation is to delay cord clamping for $\geq$60 seconds. For neonates less than 34 weeks' gestation who do not require resuscitation, it is recommended to delay cord clamping for at least 30 seconds. For term and preterm infants requiring resuscitation at birth, there is insufficient evidence for immediate versus delayed cord clamping. There is insufficient evidence for milking the cord of any newly born infant.

9. How can a very low birthweight premature newborn infant (<1500 g) be kept warm in the ED?
Drying and swaddling, warming pads, increased environmental temperature, hats, and covering with a blanket have been used to keep newborns warm. These techniques have not been evaluated in controlled trials and may not be enough to warm very small newborns. For infants <32 weeks' gestation, a combination of interventions is recommended. These include placing the infant under a radiant warmer, increasing environmental temperature to 74°F to 77°F, warm blankets, heat-resistant plastic wrapping without drying infant, hat, and/or thermal mattress to prevent hypothermia (<36°C). Avoid hyperthermia (temperature > 38°C).

Table 2.2 Apgar Score			
	Score		
SIGN	**0**	**1**	**2**
Heart rate	Absent	Slow (<100/min)	>100/min
Respirations	Absent	Slow, irregular	Good, crying
Muscle tone	Limp	Some flexion	Active motion
Reflex irritability (catheter in nares)	No response	Grimace	Cough, sneezes
Color	Blue or pale	Pink body with blue extremities	Extremely pink

10. **When does the newly born infant need assistance with ventilation?**
Approximately 85% of full-term neonates will breathe within 30 seconds of birth. Another 10% will breathe after drying and stimulation. The remaining 5% of full-term infants require positive pressure ventilation and 2% go on to require intubation. After initial attempts at stabilization by warming, drying, stimulation, and clearing the airway, quickly assess the infant for apnea, gasping respirations, or a heart rate <100/minute. If any of these signs of distress are present, initiate positive pressure ventilation with room air. Place the infant on cardiorespiratory (CR) and oxygen saturation monitoring. Within the first 60 seconds, or the "Golden Minute," the initial steps should be completed and ventilations (if warranted) begun.

11. **What is the best way to determine heart rate in the newly born infant?**
The best way to determine the heart rate of the newly born on physical examination is by auscultation of the precordium. CR and pulse oximetry monitoring are important adjuncts. During resuscitation, CR monitoring is the most accurate measurement of heart rate. Although pulse oximetry is important, changes can be detected more slowly and less accurately during the extrauterine transition. Palpation of pulses can be inaccurate and unreliable.

12. **When is supplemental oxygen indicated?**
The recommendation for the use of oxygen in resuscitation has not changed over the last several years. Not enough oxygen and too much oxygen, even brief exposure to excessive levels during resuscitation, are harmful to the newly born infant. Oxygen saturation level does not reach extrauterine values until several minutes after birth (see Table 2.3), which may result in the appearance of cyanosis. It has been shown that absence of cyanosis is also a poor indicator of oxygenation after birth. Place a pulse oximeter, with a neonatal probe, on the newly born in a preductal location (right wrist or right medial surface of the palm) if resuscitation is anticipated, when positive pressure ventilation is initiated, when cyanosis persists, or when supplemental oxygen is administered.

For the newly born infant ≥35 weeks' gestation that requires positive pressure ventilation, initiate ventilations with room air; do not use oxygen. For the newly born infant <35 weeks' gestation requiring ventilatory support, initiate ventilations with 21% to 30% oxygen. Oxygen concentration can then be titrated based on the goals in the table below. Although it has not been studied, 100% oxygen is utilized when cardiopulmonary resuscitation (CPR) is initiated.

13. **What is the proper technique in assisting ventilations in the newly born infant?**
The mask should fit around the nose and mouth but not cover the eyes or go below the chin. Assisted ventilations should be at a rate of 40 to 60 breaths per minute. An inflation pressure of 20 to 25 cm H_2O may be sufficient but can be increased to >30 to 40 cm H_2O in term infants if needed. In preterm neonates, positive end-expiratory pressure (PEEP) may be helpful, although evidence is limited. All human studies used a PEEP of 5 cm H_2O. Regardless, the effectiveness of the assisted ventilation is judged by the movement of the chest, adequacy of breath sounds, and the heart rate. Poor face mask technique, airway obstruction, movement of the infant, interventions such as removing wet blankets, and distraction of the resuscitator contribute to ineffective mask ventilation. Mask leak and airway obstruction, being the most common reasons, may go undetected unless CO_2 detectors on residual function monitors are used. If the condition of the neonate does not improve, reposition the head, check for patency of the airway, improve the seal of the mask on the face, and increase the inflating pressure of the bag. Use of the T-piece resuscitator over the self-inflating bag is recommended when infants are receiving positive pressure ventilations.

14. **What are the indications for intubation of the newly born infant?**
Indications for intubation vary but are based on the degree of respiratory depression, the success of ventilation efforts, the presence of meconium, the degree of prematurity, and the skill of the health care provider. It is recommended for spontaneously breathing preterm newly born infants with respiratory distress to initiate continuous positive airway pressure (CPAP). CPAP is preferred over intermittent positive pressure ventilation or intubation.

Table 2.3 Target Preductal Oxygen Saturation After Birth	
1 min	60%-65%
2 min	65%-70%
3 min	70%-75%
4 min	75%-80%
5 min	80%-85%
10 min	85%-95%

Endotracheal intubation is indicated if a neonate:
- Has not responded to assisted ventilations with bag-mask ventilation
- Is extremely low birthweight
- Requires chest compressions
- Needs tracheal administration of medications (including surfactant)
- Has signs of respiratory depression and airway obstruction with meconium
- Has special circumstances (diaphragmatic hernia)

Ideally, because ventilator efforts should be maximized prior to chest compressions, endotracheal intubation should occur prior to chest compressions if possible.

15. **How should endotracheal intubation of the newborn be performed?**
Perform the tracheal intubation by the oral route, using an uncuffed endotracheal tube and a laryngoscope with a straight blade (size 0 for premature, size 1 for term). After the endotracheal tube is passed through the vocal cords, check the position by observing symmetrical chest wall movement and listen for breath sounds at the axilla and the absence of breath sounds over the stomach. Confirm tube placement with a CO_2 monitor. Exhaled CO_2 detection is effective for confirmation of endotracheal placement in infants, including very low birthweight infants. Confirm the absence of gastric inflation; watch for condensation in the endotracheal tube during exhalation; and note the improvement in heart rate, color, and activity of the newborn. *A prompt increase in heart rate is the best indicator that the tube is in the tracheobronchial tree and providing effective ventilation.* Confirmation of tube placement by radiograph is also recommended.

The guide for the proper size of the endotracheal tube size is:

$$\text{Endotracheal tube size} = \frac{\text{Gestational age in weeks}}{10}$$

The proper depth of insertion can be estimated by:

$$\text{Insertion depth at lip in cm} = \text{Weight in kilograms} + 6\text{ cm}$$

16. **Are airway adjuncts useful or indicated in the management of the newly born?**
CPAP is widely used in infants who are breathing but exhibiting increased respiratory effort. It has been studied in preterm infants and shown to decrease intubation rates, mechanical ventilation duration, and use of surfactant, but increase rates of pneumothorax. Local expertise and comfort should guide the use of CPAP.

Laryngeal mask airways (LMAs) are adjuncts to airway management and are generally used when tracheal intubation is unable to be attained or face mask ventilation is inadequate. The newly born weighing over 1500 g or $\geq$34 weeks' gestation can be ventilated effectively with LMAs. They have not been studied in infants with meconium-stained fluid, during chest compressions, or for the administration of tracheal medications.

17. **How does the resuscitation of the newly born infant differ if meconium is present in the amniotic fluid?**
It does not differ. Current recommendations no longer advise routine intrapartum oropharyngeal and nasopharyngeal suctioning for meconium-stained infants. Routine endotracheal intubation and direct tracheal suctioning of meconium-stained infants were also shown to be of no value in a randomized control trial. Nonvigorous or "depressed" infants (decreased tone, absent or depressed respirations, poor oxygenation, or a heart rate less than 100 beats per minute) with meconium-stained amniotic fluid require standard resuscitation. If the heart rate falls below 60 beats per minute, perform intubation and initiate positive pressure ventilation. Suction for signs of airway obstruction.

18. **When are chest compressions indicated in the resuscitation of the newly born infant?**
Effective ventilation usually restores vital signs to normal in a newborn, and chest compressions are generally not needed. Because chest compressions make effective ventilations more difficult and heart rate usually responds to assisted ventilation, chest compressions are not initiated until assisted ventilation has been started. The indication for the initiation of chest compressions during the resuscitation of the newly born infant is the absence of heart rate or heart rate less than 60 beats per minute despite adequate assisted ventilation with oxygen for 30 seconds.

19. **What is the proper technique for chest compressions in the newborn?**
Data suggest that the two-thumb encircling hand method may have the advantage of generating peak systolic and coronary perfusion, improved blood pressure, and less provider fatigue. Placement on the chest is at the lower third of the sternum. The rate should be approximately 90 times per minute at a 3:1 ratio with assisted ventilations. Take care not to simultaneously provide a breath while compressing the chest. Compress the chest to one-third of the anteroposterior diameter of the chest. Allow recoil so that the heart can refill. Compressions must be adequate to generate a pulse. Reassess the heart rate every 30 seconds during this time and continue compressions until the heart rate is maintained >60 beats per minute.

KEY POINTS: NEONATAL RESUSCITATION

1. Prevent hypothermia.
2. Intrapartum routine suctioning of the newborn's nose and mouth is not recommended for meconium-stained infants.
3. Delay cord clamping for 60 seconds for term and late preterm (>34 weeks' gestation) infants who are vigorous and do not require resuscitation.
4. If the heart rate falls below 60 beats per minute, perform endotracheal intubation and give positive pressure ventilation.
5. A prompt increase in heart rate is the best indicator that the endotracheal tube is in the tracheobronchial tree and is providing effective ventilation.
6. Begin chest compressions if the heart rate is less than 60 beats per minute despite assisted ventilation for 30 seconds.
7. The two-thumb method of chest compressions is the preferred method, with the depth of compression being one-third of the anteroposterior diameter of the chest.
8. An intraosseous needle can be used for access if the umbilical vein is not readily available.
9. Administer epinephrine if the heart rate remains at or under 60 beats per minute despite 30 seconds of adequate ventilation with 100% oxygen and chest compressions.

20. **What are the most common drugs considered for use in a neonatal resuscitation and when are they indicated?**

Drugs are rarely used in neonatal resuscitation. Bradycardia in the newborn is usually due to inadequate lung inflation and hypoxemia, and thus adequate ventilation is typically a sufficient intervention.

Epinephrine is recommended when the heart rate remains below 60 beats per minute despite adequate ventilation with 100% oxygen AND chest compressions for 30 seconds. Evidence from neonatal models show increased diastolic and mean arterial pressures in response to epinephrine. The current recommended dose for intravenous epinephrine during the neonatal resuscitation is 0.01 to 0.03 mg/kg of a 0.1-mg/mL concentration. High-dose epinephrine is not recommended for neonates because of the rare incidence of ventricular fibrillation and the theoretical risk of a hypertensive response, which could result in intraventricular hemorrhage. The intravenous route is preferred. If vascular access is not available, epinephrine can be given 0.05 to 0.1 mg/kg via the endotracheal tube. Repeated doses should continue every 3 to 5 minutes throughout resuscitative efforts.

Atropine is a parasympathetic drug that decreases vagal tone and is not recommended in neonatal resuscitation. Bradycardia in the neonate is usually caused by hypoxia and therefore atropine is unlikely to be beneficial.

Naloxone is a narcotic antagonist and is not indicated in the *initial* resuscitation of the newly born infant.

Sodium bicarbonate is not recommended for short resuscitations requiring CPR but may be helpful in prolonged resuscitations with adequate ventilator support.

Volume expanders such as crystalloids (normal saline) and blood are indicated for signs of hypovolemia. Signs of hypovolemia in the neonate include pallor, weak pulses, or poor response to resuscitative efforts. The dose for volume expanders is 10 mL/kg, with reassessment after each dose. Isotonic crystalloids are the first choice in volume expanders. Red blood cells (O negative) are indicated in situations of large blood loss.

21. **Where is the best place to obtain intravenous access?**

The easiest and most direct access is the umbilical cord. Any medication, as well as volume expanders, can be given through the umbilical vein. Note that it is not recommended to administer resuscitative drugs via the umbilical artery. Peripheral veins in the extremities and the scalp can also be used, but generally require more skill. Intraosseous lines can be used when no other access can be obtained.

22. **Are there circumstances when resuscitation of the newly born infant may not be the appropriate action?**

Since all ED deliveries are considered "unexpected" and there is no previous relationship with the delivering mother, conversations about withholding resuscitation are difficult at best. Antenatal information can be incomplete or inaccurate. In the ED, it may not be possible to gather this information quickly with precision and reliability. Guidelines should be developed after discussion with local resources, review of the most recent literature, and discussion with parents. Review the guidelines regularly and modify them on the basis of changes in resuscitation and neonatal intensive care practices. If gestational age, birthweight, or congenital anomalies are associated with almost certain death or high morbidity, resuscitation is not indicated. Examples include extreme prematurity (<23 weeks' gestation or birthweight <400 g), anencephaly, and major chromosomal abnormalities incompatible with life.

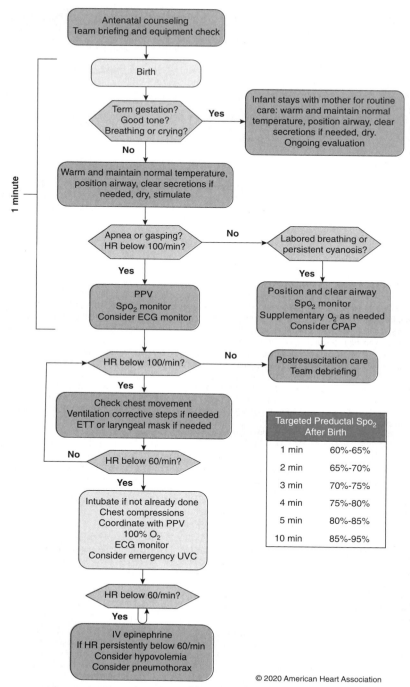

Fig. 2.1 Newborn resuscitation algorithm. *CPAP,* Continuous positive airway pressure; *ECG,* electrocardiogram; *ETT,* endotracheal tube; *HR,* heart rate; *IV,* intravenous; *PPV,* positive pressure ventilation airway pressure; *SpO₂,* oxygen saturation; *UVC,* umbilical vein catheter.

23. **When is it appropriate to discontinue the resuscitation of the newly born?**
Stopping resuscitation of the newly born is obviously a very difficult decision. If no heart rate is detectable after 20 minutes of resuscitation, one may consider stopping the resuscitation. Etiology of the arrest, gestation of the infant, presence of complications, and parents' expressed acceptability of morbidity risk will also play a part in the decision.

24. **How do I put all of this together?**
Refer to the newborn resuscitation algorithm (Fig. 2.1).

25. **What are the top guidelines made by the 2020 American Heart Association Guidelines for Cardiopulmonary Resuscitation and Emergency Cardiovascular Care?**
    1. Newborn resuscitations require preparation and practice, both individually and as a team.
    2. Most newly born infants can be monitored during skin-to-skin contact with mothers and do not require immediate cord clamping or resuscitation.
    3. Ventilation is a priority in newly born infants that require support.
    4. Increase in heart rate is the most important indicator of adequate ventilations and successful resuscitation efforts.
    5. Pulse oximetry should guide oxygen therapy.
    6. Chest compressions are provided only after optimizing ventilation support.
    7. During a resuscitation, monitor the heart rate with electrocardiogram.
    8. Epinephrine is used if the response to chest compression is poor.
    9. Volume is indicated if there is a poor response to epinephrine with history and physical examination consistent with blood loss.
    10. If all resuscitation efforts have failed after 20 minutes, discuss termination of resuscitation with family and the team.

26. **How does one remain competent at neonatal resuscitation?**
Neonatal resuscitation requires knowledge, skill, and behavior acquisition. It is essential to remain competent, and this requires knowledge maintenance and practice, both individually and as a team. Certification requires repeat training every 2 years. Studies show that decay of knowledge and skills can occur within 3 to 12 months of training. Additionally, new standards of care emerge and need to be incorporated into practice. It has been shown that brief and frequent practice improves neonatal resuscitation outcomes. There is no prescriptive interval for intermittent training, but it is recommended that knowledge and skills of the neonatal resuscitation team members be periodically assessed and "boosted" between certifications to sustain competency and achieve the best neonatal resuscitation outcomes.

BIBLIOGRAPHY

Aziz K, Lee HC, Escobedo M, et al. Part 5: Neonatal Resuscitation 2020 American Heart Association Guidelines for Cardiopulmonary Resuscitation and Emergency Cardiovascular Care. *Pediatrics.* 2021;147(suppl 1):10.1542/peds.2020-038505E. e2020038505E. Epub 2020 Oct 21.

Hooper SB, Te Pas AB, Lang J, et al. Cardiovascular transition at birth: a physiological sequence. *Pediatr Res.* 2015;77(5):608–614. 10.1038/pr.2015.21. Epub 2015 Feb 4. PMID: 25671807.

Myers S, Aronson Schniasi D, Nadel F, Gaines S. Cardiopulmonary resuscitation. In: Bachur RG, Shaw KN, Chamberlain J, eds. *Fleisher & Ludwig's Textbook of Pediatric Emergency Medicine.* 8th ed. LWW; 2020:62–73.

Wyckoff MH, Wyllie J, Aziz K, et al. Neonatal Life Support 2020 International Consensus on Cardiopulmonary Resuscitation and Emergency Cardiovascular Care Science With Treatment Recommendations. *Resuscitation.* 2020;156:A156–A187.10.1016/j.resuscitation.2020.09.015. Epub 2020 Oct 21. PMID: 33098917.

Perlman JM, Wyllie J, Kattwinkel J, et al. Part 7: Neonatal Resuscitation: 2015 International Consensus on Cardiopulmonary Resuscitation and Emergency Cardiovascular Care Science With Treatment Recommendations. *Circulation.* 2015;132:S204.

Qureshi MJ, Kumar M. Laryngeal mask airway verses bag mask ventilation or endotracheal intubation for neonatal resuscitation. *Cochrane Database Syst Rev.* 2018;3:CD003314.

Sawyer T, Lee HC, Aziz K. Anticipation and preparation for every delivery room resuscitation. *Semin Fetal Neonatal Med.* 2018;23(5):312–320.10.1016/j.siny.2018.06.004. Epub 2018 Jul 6. PMID: 30369405

Wyckoff MH, Singletary EM, Soar J, et al. 2021 International Consensus on Cardiopulmonary Resuscitation and Emergency Cardiovascular Care Science With Treatment Recommendations: Summary From the Basic Life Support; Advanced Life Support; Neonatal Life Support; Education, Implementation, and Teams; First Aid Task Forces; and the COVID-19 Working Group. *Resuscitation.* 2021;169:229–311.10.1016/j.resuscitation.2021.10.040. Epub 2021 Nov 11.PMID: 34933747.

CHAPTER 3

RESPIRATORY FAILURE

Jody C. Kieffer and Joshua Rice

1. **How is respiratory failure defined?**

   Respiratory failure is defined as an inadequate respiratory response to meet the metabolic demand for oxygen. This can be due to failure of oxygenation or ventilation (excretion of CO_2). More specifically, respiratory failure may be defined as the partial pressure of oxygen (Po_2) less than 60 mm Hg or O_2 saturation less than 93% while receiving greater than 60% of supplemental oxygen. Additionally, Pco_2 greater than 60 mm Hg and/or clinical apnea both indicate respiratory failure.

2. **How commonly do pediatric patients present to the emergency department (ED) with respiratory emergencies?**

   Respiratory symptoms are among the most common reasons that families seek emergency care, accounting for approximately one-third of all visits in the United States. Though most children are well enough to be discharged from the ED, as many as 20% require admission for inpatient care and approximately 3% to 5% end in deaths.

   Respiratory diseases are also the most frequent cause of cardiopulmonary arrest, with especially poor outcomes for patients who develop cardiopulmonary arrest secondary to respiratory failure. The potential for progression of respiratory distress to respiratory failure necessitates prompt and careful evaluation of children with respiratory symptoms. A thorough evaluation with prompt recognition of respiratory distress followed by appropriate interventions improves morbidity and mortality.

3. **When should one anticipate progression from respiratory distress to respiratory failure?**
   - An increased respiratory rate, particularly with signs of distress (e.g., retractions, nasal flaring, seesaw breathing, or grunting).
   - An inadequate respiratory rate, effort, or chest excursion (e.g., diminished breath sounds or gasping).
   - Signs of altered mental status: agitation and restlessness are often early signs of hypoxia, while depressed mental status and lethargy are indicative of hypercarbia and/or severe hypoxia.
   - Cyanosis with abnormal breathing despite supplemental oxygen.

4. **Are there different types of respiratory failure?**

   Respiratory failure can be divided into two categories: hypoxemic and hypercarbic. The hypoxemic type, defined as a Po_2 below 60 mm Hg, is generally caused by mismatch of ventilation and perfusion (V/Q mismatch) in the lung. Hypoxemic respiratory failure from V/Q mismatch is often associated with normal or low Pco_2 as children have compensatory tachypnea and blow off excessive CO_2. In contrast, patients with hypercarbic respiratory failure have an overall decrease in alveolar ventilation that is usually the result of upper airway obstruction, neuromuscular disease, thoracic trauma, or muscle fatigue. These patients have increases in Pco_2 and relatively proportional decreases in Po_2. The physiology in most children with respiratory failure is a combination of these two types, because one type often leads to the other. For instance, an infant with bronchiolitis initially may have hypoxemia from atelectasis and ventilation-perfusion mismatch but may progress to inadequate alveolar ventilation with the onset of respiratory muscle fatigue and increased airway resistance.

5. **Can respiratory failure be present without respiratory distress?**

   Yes. Many etiologies may present without distress and ultimately lead to hypoventilation and failure. For example, toxic ingestions, metabolic derangements, and head trauma may lead to reduced levels of consciousness and cause hypoventilation in the abscess of respiratory distress. Underlying neuromuscular dysfunction (e.g., a child with muscular dystrophy) can also present similarly. Depending upon the duration of symptoms prior to the time of presentation, a child's work of breathing may appear normal in the presence of significant hypoventilation secondary to respiratory muscle fatigue. A high index of suspicion is needed in these cases and a blood gas should be obtained to aid in diagnosis. Elevation of the Pco_2 from hypoventilation may signal worsening fatigue and impending respiratory arrest.

6. **Why are children at greater risk for respiratory failure?**

   Both metabolic and anatomic differences put children at higher risk for respiratory failure than adults. From a *metabolic* standpoint, children—particularly infants—require more oxygen per kilogram of body weight than adults, which accounts for their increased respiratory frequency. *Anatomic factors* also put infants at particularly high risk for respiratory failure. Infants breathe almost exclusively through their noses, so nasal obstruction can

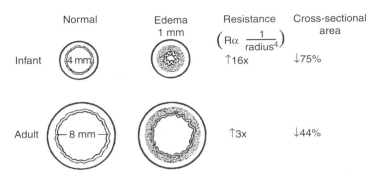

Fig. 3.1 Comparison of the effects of 1 mm of mucosal edema on airway resistance in an infant versus an adult. Resistance is inversely proportional to the fourth power of the radius of the airway for laminar flow and the fifth power for turbulent flow. Airway resistance increases 16-fold in the infant for laminar flow. In a crying infant with turbulent airflow, resistance increases 32-fold. (Reproduced with permission from Cote CJ, Todres ID. The pediatric airway. In: Cote CJ, Ryan JF, Todres ID, Groudsouzian NG, eds. A Practice of Anesthesia for Infants and Children. 2nd ed. W.B. Saunders; 1993.)

quickly cause signs and symptoms of respiratory distress. The caliber of infant airways is small, so respiratory resistance is much higher. Remember that resistance to flow is inversely related to the radius of the airway to the fourth power. Thus even small changes to the airway radius (such as inflammation of the respiratory tree) can lead to large increases in resistance and substantially decreased airflow (Fig. 3.1). Alveoli have less collateral ventilation in infants. Therefore obstruction of small peripheral airways is more likely to lead to atelectasis and hypoxemia. A compliant chest (necessary to facilitate passage through the birth canal) is deleterious to normal breathing, as it provides little opposition to the lung's natural tendency to recoil/deflate and forces children to perform more work than adults to generate the same tidal volume. The diaphragm of infants is also more easily fatigued compared with the diaphragm of older children and adults due to fewer type 1 muscle fibers.

7. **How do I know which of the numerous children with respiratory symptoms will progress to respiratory failure?**
   A detailed history can give information about the vulnerability of the child for respiratory decompensation. Children who are very young, were born prematurely, have chronic pulmonary or cardiac diseases, or have immunodeficiencies are at particular risk.
   Predicting the clinical course is difficult, but most diseases have a typical natural history. If a child is evaluated early in the course of a respiratory infection, that child is very likely to worsen before improvement is noted. Children with significant respiratory effort who appear happy and playful and are maintaining their oxygen saturation and ventilation may worsen suddenly as they become fatigued or as their disease process progresses.
   Young children are more difficult to assess for respiratory problems. Histories are obtained secondhand, as the caregiver interprets behaviors and relays observations that have been made. A careful clinical assessment of risk factors, illness time course, and the current degree of respiratory distress is necessary to identify those patients most likely to develop respiratory failure.

8. **How do I assess respiration in a patient who screams every time I approach?**
   "Stranger anxiety" normally develops around 8 to 9 months of age. The child's alertness to your presence is actually a reassuring sign. Observing the child from across the room provides valuable information. For optimization of the "across the room" evaluation, ensure that a caregiver removes/lifts the gown to expose the chest and neck. General appearance, respiratory rate, nasal flaring, retractions, paradoxical respirations, and grunting can all be appreciated without close proximity to the child. In many cases, the child is more cooperative if your approach is delayed, slow, and accompanied by soothing speech. Attempt to positively interact with the child to maximize the chance of a thorough lung exam.

9. **What are retractions and why do they occur?**
   Normally, inspiration is almost effortless. When airway resistance is high, a child must generate greater negative intrathoracic pressure to draw air into the lungs requiring greater work of breathing, which can be seen as retractions of the neck, chest, and abdominal musculature. When intrathoracic pressure is negative, parts of the chest retract inward. These retractions may be seen just below the costal margin (subcostal), just above the sternum (suprasternal), or between the ribs (intercostal). Retractions are a very important clinical finding even in the absence of wheezing or rales because a child with impending or existing respiratory failure may have

retractions without enough airflow to generate audible abnormal breath sounds. Flaring of the nostrils may also be noted when respiratory distress is severe.

10. **What are paradoxical respirations? Why do they occur?**
The term "paradoxical respiration" is used to describe the aberrant collapse of an infant's compliant chest wall inward (as opposed to typical expansion) as the abdomen moves outward during a breath. Infants who have increased airway resistance generate significantly negative intrathoracic pressures in order to inflate their lungs. As the diaphragm moves downward and the intrathoracic pressure becomes negative, the soft, cartilaginous bones and weak intercostal musculature cannot maintain the thoracic circumference, which leads to the inward collapse seen in paradoxical respiration. Other terms used to describe this phenomenon include *thoracoabdominal asynchrony* or *seesaw breathing*. This can be a sign of impending respiratory failure.

11. **How can one tell if the respiratory failure is caused by an upper airway disease or by a lower airway disease?**
Distinguishing upper from lower respiratory disease can be a difficult part of the clinical evaluation. Many children have disease processes that involve both the upper and lower respiratory tracts simultaneously, for example, bronchiolitis caused by respiratory syncytial virus. In general, respiratory sounds reflecting upper airway inflammation (such as stridor or stertor) are most prominent during inspiration, when negative intraluminal pressure causes fast and turbulent airflow through a smaller diameter airway. Conversely, sounds reflecting lower airway inflammation (such as wheezing or rhonchi) are more prominent during expiration, when positive/inward pressure caused by collapsing of the chest wall compresses intrathoracic airways and again causes turbulent flow through smaller diameter channels.

12. **Is wheezing always present with severe lower airway disease such as asthma?**
No. Audible wheezing requires significant airflow through narrowed small airways. Children with severe obstruction of small airways may have so little airflow that audible wheezing is not present. These children usually have decreased inspiratory breath sounds and increased work of breathing. Administration of bronchodilators to these patients will often increase audible wheezing because there is an overall increase in turbulent airflow as the smooth muscle of the airways relax.

13. **Does the pulse oximeter provide added value to my clinical exam?**
Yes. Hypoxemia is not always obvious from the physical examination. Most children who are hypoxemic from a respiratory illness have signs of respiratory distress, but in some cases, mild-to-moderate hypoxemia is not clinically evident. Hypoxemia is a less potent stimulator of respiratory drive than is hypercarbia. Thus the increase in minute ventilation that occurs with mild hypoxemia is very modest and may be difficult to detect by physical examination. In patients with acute exacerbations of asthma, very poor correlations between asthma score (a measure of respiratory distress) and oxygen saturation have been reported.

Furthermore, visible cyanosis requires 3 to 5 g of unsaturated hemoglobin per deciliter to be visible. If a child has a total hemoglobin of 12 g/dL, cyanosis is not apparent until the oxygen saturation drops below 75%. Pulse oximetry therefore allows clinicians to be aware of hypoxemia before it is severe enough to cause visible cyanosis, which can be helpful in the treatment of acute respiratory distress (Fig. 3.2).

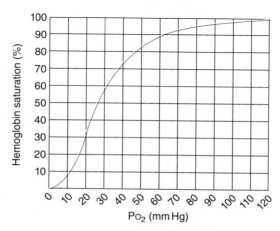

Fig. 3.2 As Po_2 drops below 70 mm Hg, oxygen saturation declines more precipitously.

14. **What causes pulse oximeter readings to be inaccurate?**
    The most common problem is the oximeter probe not consistently registering the pulsatile arterial flow through the skin. This is often caused by movement, poor perfusion of the skin, or bright ambient light. Careful attention to the graphical display of pulsatile flow on the pulse oximeter can almost always distinguish a falsely low saturation due to poor signal capture from true hypoxia. Less commonly, abnormal hemoglobin can cause inaccurate measurements. Carboxyhemoglobinemia will cause a falsely elevated measurement of oxygen saturation by pulse oximetry, while methemoglobinemia can cause a modest lowering.

15. **What is the lowest acceptable oxygen saturation for a child to be discharged?**
    There is often no simple answer to what appears to be a simple question. In healthy awake children, normal oxygen saturation is 97% to 99%. Oxygen saturation below 95% is greater than two standard deviations below the mean (-2 SD). For healthy young infants, -2 SD below the mean is 93%. At altitudes higher than 3000 m (10,000 ft), -2 SD is below 85%. For children with lower airway disease, the American Academy of Pediatrics (AAP) and the World Health Organization (WHO) recommend a target oxygen saturation of 90%, while many clinicians use a threshold of 92% to 94% as a criterion for discharge. These values are largely arbitrary, and there is very little high-quality evidence supporting a specific cutoff, though a recent randomized control study of infants hospitalized with bronchiolitis found that an oxygen saturation target of 90% was as safe and clinically effective as one of 94%.

16. **How do I interpret brief desaturations with feeding or sleeping?**
    Oxygen saturation during feeding or sleeping often dips below the baseline. Feeding and sleeping may be stress tests for desaturation. Normal children monitored during sleep have occasional oxygen saturation nadirs below 93%, and even dipping below 90% is not uncommon. In infants with respiratory illnesses who are asleep, there is no consensus, nor are there data, on whether an oxygen saturation of 90% to 92% for a brief period portends future deterioration or respiratory failure.

17. **What is the significance if the oxygen saturation is 2% to 3% below normal?**
    The relationship between Po_2 and saturation is not linear but sigmoidal, meaning that with each additional percentage decrease from 100% on pulse oximetry, there is a much greater impact on Po_2. That is to say that although there is little difference in Po_2 between saturations of 99% and 96%, there is a substantially greater difference in Po_2 between saturations of 93% and 90%. Oxygen saturation and respiratory rate are objective measures of pulmonary function available to clinicians in most settings. Saturations below 93% in children with respiratory diseases may identify patients with pulmonary/airway inflammation that puts them at risk for developing respiratory failure. Consider oxygen therapy and closer monitoring if the desaturation is persistent (see Fig. 3.2).

18. **Why do some patients with wheezing have a reduction in their oxygen saturation after bronchodilator treatment when they otherwise appear to be improving?**
    Albuterol and other bronchodilators are β-adrenergic agents that are somewhat β₂ selective. β₂-Receptor stimulation and resultant smooth muscle relaxation cause *vaso*dilation along with intentioned *broncho*dilation. One explanation for decreases in oxygen saturation after treatment with bronchodilators is that pulmonary vasodilation results in transiently increased perfusion of poorly ventilated areas of the lung and worsening of ventilation-perfusion matching. This phenomenon is seen in a minority of patients and is not a contraindication to continued, aggressive bronchodilator therapy in children with severe lower airway disease.

19. **What is the value of a chest radiograph in evaluation of a child with suspected respiratory failure?**
    Children with minor respiratory illnesses generally do not require chest radiographs, even if they seek care in an ED. If there is concern about impending or existing respiratory failure, a chest radiograph can be very useful in expanding or narrowing a differential diagnosis. For example, young children with fever and tachypnea may benefit from a chest radiograph, because bacterial pneumonia can be difficult to diagnose by history and physical examination. Foreign-body aspiration, pneumothorax, pneumomediastinum, and cardiac disease are a few of the diagnoses that can also be further evaluated with a chest radiograph.

20. **What is pediatric acute respiratory distress syndrome (ARDS)?**
    ARDS is a common cause of respiratory failure at all ages. ARDS is a diffuse pulmonary process that manifests as inflammation, alveolar edema, and hypoxemic respiratory failure after lung injury. Some causes of ARDS that are treated in EDs include sepsis, hypotension, pneumonia, aspiration of gastric contents, smoke or other inhalation injury, near drowning, and chest trauma with pulmonary contusion. Chest radiographs may show diffuse infiltrates that resemble left-sided congestive heart failure, but left atrial pressures must be normal for the diagnosis of

ARDS. According to the Pediatric Acute Lung Injury Consensus Conference (PALICC), the diagnostic criteria for pediatric ARDS are as follows:
- Acute onset, within 7 days of clinical insult
- Chest radiograph findings of new infiltrates consistent with parenchymal disease
- Respiratory failure not explained by cardiac failure or fluid overload
- Oxygen supplementation requirement: minimum continuous positive airway pressure of 5 cm H_2O or invasive mechanical ventilation

21. **Why are some patients who meet the definition for respiratory failure not intubated and mechanically ventilated to normalize their blood gases?**
    Children tolerate hypercarbia better than adults. If oxygenation is adequate and hypercarbia is likely to be reversed in the near future, some providers permit the hypercarbia to persist for a period of time. So-called *permissive hypercarbia* reduces barotrauma to the lungs that results from positive-pressure and mechanical ventilation. In patients with reactive airway disease or asthma, positive-pressure ventilation is fraught with risk of pneumomediastinum and pneumothorax. Because there are effective medications to reverse airway obstruction in a relatively short period of time, some patients can be closely monitored without endotracheal intubation and mechanical ventilation, despite levels of CO_2 that define respiratory failure.

22. **Is endotracheal intubation the only way to manage the airway when a child is in respiratory distress?**
    No. In fact, bag-valve-mask ventilation is adequate for most children with transient, reversible airway problems. Positioning the child with some extension of the neck and moving the mandible forward by lifting the angles of the jaw pulls the tongue off of the posterior pharynx, often relieving airway obstruction. Oral airways (for unconscious patients) and nasal airways can also be used to maintain the patency of the upper airway during bag-valve-mask ventilation. All children should be provided effective bag-valve-mask ventilation with 100% oxygen prior to intubation.

23. **What are the indications to perform endotracheal intubation in a child?**
    - Respiratory failure that is unlikely to be reversed quickly, especially if hypoxemia is present despite greater than 60% oxygen administration
    - Apnea, hypoventilation, or progressive respiratory exhaustion
    - Need for airway protection for children who have upper airway obstruction or an inability to protect their airway from aspiration
    - Desire to decrease the work of breathing for patients in shock (under normal circumstances, work of breathing requires less than 5% of the total energy expenditure, but with respiratory distress it can demand up to 50%; in a shock state, energy can be better utilized for other essential body functions)
    - Therapeutic interventions, such as tracheal administration of medications and suctioning for pulmonary toilet

---

KEY POINTS: INDICATIONS FOR ENDOTRACHEAL INTUBATION

1. Progressive respiratory exhaustion—unlikely to reverse quickly
2. Apnea and hypoventilation that require mechanical ventilation
3. Need for airway protection (upper airway obstruction, loss of protective airway reflexes)
4. Shock
5. Airway access for pulmonary toilet

---

24. **What are the steps for emergency endotracheal intubation of a child?**
    1. Preoxygenate with bag-valve-mask ventilation with 100% oxygen.
    2. Ensure accurate weight in kilograms. Prepare all equipment, including suction, endotracheal tubes, laryngo-scopes, capnometry, and tape or tube holder.
    3. Make certain there is vascular access that is functioning well.
    4. Rapid sequence Intubation is generally recommended in all emergent intubations as most patients are suspected to have "full stomachs."
       a. Consider atropine (for younger children and those receiving succinylcholine).
       b. Administer a sedative followed by a paralytic agent.
    5. Once paralysis is complete, perform direct or video laryngoscopy, and watch the endotracheal tube go through the vocal cords into the trachea.
    6. Auscultate for equal breath sounds and check for the presence of CO_2 by capnometry or end-tidal capnography. Observe symmetric chest expansion, misting in the tube with exhalation, and improvement in oxygen

saturation by pulse oximetry. If you hear gurgling over the stomach without improvement in oxygen saturation, this suggests an esophageal intubation.

7. Secure the tube with tape or a prefabricated endotracheal tube holder.
8. Evacuate the stomach with a nasogastric or orogastric tube.
9. Obtain a chest radiograph to check the position of the tube and adjust accordingly.

KEY POINTS: STEPS TO PERFORM ENDOTRACHEAL INTUBATION

1. Preoxygenate with 100% oxygen using bag-valve-mask device.
2. Prepare equipment (e.g., suction, endotracheal tubes, laryngoscopes, monitors—electrocardiogram, pulse oximeter, end-tidal CO_2 detector, or monitor).
3. Confirm functioning intravenous line.
4. Administer medications (atropine, sedative, paralytic agent).
5. Intubate the trachea, observing the tube pass through the vocal cords.
6. Verify proper placement—auscultate the chest, check for CO_2 by capnometry, chest radiograph.
7. Secure the endotracheal tube.
8. Evacuate the stomach with a nasogastric or orogastric tube.

Table 3.1 Conditions Found in Difficult Intubations

CONGENITAL	ACQUIRED
Micrognathia	Hoarseness/stridor/drooling
Macroglossia	Facial burns/singed facial hairs
Cleft or high-arched palate	Facial fractures/oral trauma
Protruding upper incisors	Foreign body
Small mouth	Excessive blood, secretions, or vomitus
Limited mobility of temporomandibular joint	

25. **Why is cricoid pressure (Sellick maneuver) no longer recommended?**
Cricoid pressure was recommended for rapid sequence intubation for many years as a means of preventing gaseous distention of the stomach from bag-valve-mask ventilation and passive regurgitation with aspiration during the intubation procedure. However, cricoid pressure can compress the trachea, making passage of the endotracheal tube more difficult. It often displaces the esophagus laterally, and there is little evidence that it decreases the risk of aspiration.

26. **Can a difficult endotracheal intubation be predicted?**
Not always. It is important to anticipate a difficult intubation and have people experienced with airway management available. The conditions found in Table 3.1 often result in difficult intubations.

27. **What should you consider if a patient deteriorates after endotracheal intubation?**
If an intubated patient's condition deteriorates after endotracheal intubation, consider the mnemonic, DOPE:
- **D**isplacement of the endotracheal tube—no longer in the trachea, or in the right main stem bronchus
- **O**bstruction of the tube—perhaps by blood, vomitus, or other secretions
- **P**neumothorax
- **E**quipment failure—perhaps the ventilator is malfunctioning, or perhaps you are not actually delivering 100% oxygen as you thought

BIBLIOGRAPHY

1. American Heart Association. 2020 Guidelines for cardiopulmonary resuscitation and emergency cardiovascular care. Part 4: Pediatric basic and advanced life support. *Circulation*. 2020;142(16):S469–S523.
2. Brown L, Dannenberg B. Pulse oximetry in discharge decision-making: a survey of emergency physicians. *Can J Emerg Med*. 2002;4(6):388–393.
3. Butler J, Sen A. Best evidence topic report. Cricoid pressure in emergency rapid sequence induction. *Emerg Med J*. 2005;22(11):815–816.

4. King C, Rappaport LD. Emergent endotracheal intubation. In: Henretig FM, King C, eds. *Textbook of Pediatric Emergency Procedures.* 2nd ed. Wolters Kluwer/Lippincott, Williams & Wilkins; 2008:146–190.

5. Lee WW, Mayberry K, Crapo R, et al. The accuracy of pulse oximetry in the emergency department. *Am J Emerg Med.* 2000;18:427.

6. Nelson K, Hirsch A, Nagler J. Pulmonary emergencies. In: Shaw KN, Bachur RG, eds. *Fleisher & Ludwig's Textbook of Pediatric Emergency Medicine.* 8th ed. Wolters Kluwer; 2021:936–964.

7. Pediatric Acute Lung Injury Consensus Conference Group Pediatric acute respiratory distress syndrome: consensus recommendations from the Pediatric Acute Lung Injury Consensus Conference. *Pediatr Crit Care Med.* 2015;16(5):428–439.

8. Urschitz MS, Wolf J, Von Einem V, et al. Reference values for nocturnal home pulse oximetry during sleep in primary school children. *Chest.* 2003;123(1):96–102.

CHAPTER 4

SHOCK

Samuel J. Prater and Suzanne Seo

1. **What defines shock in the pediatric patient?**
Shock exists when the patient's metabolic demand exceeds the body's ability to deliver oxygen and nutrients. This occurs most commonly when metabolic demand is normal or slightly elevated, but the delivery of oxygen and nutrients is dramatically reduced. Examples include excessive blood or volume loss, poor cardiac function, and sepsis. The shock state can, and often does, exist in the presence of a "normal" blood pressure. Shock is not defined by the blood pressure or by any other vital sign.

KEY POINTS: DEFINITION OF SHOCK

1. Shock is a condition in which the patient's metabolic requirements are unmet.
2. The shock state is a complex interplay between the physiologic insult and the host's response to that insult.
3. In its earliest phase, shock might be recognized only by abnormal results of laboratory tests that measure tissue acid-base status (e.g., serum lactate). Overt clinical signs are seen as the shock state progresses.

2. **How can shock be recognized clinically?**
The clinical manifestations of shock are those of **inadequate perfusion and compensation**. Inadequate perfusion of the brain results in an alteration in the child's level of consciousness. Inadequate perfusion of the kidneys results in decreased urine output.
   As perfusion decreases, compensatory changes occur. These changes improve the delivery of oxygen and nutrients and direct blood flow to vital organs. The first compensatory mechanism is usually an **increased heart rate; tachycardia out of proportion to the child's clinical picture (i.e., fever, distress) should be a red flag**. Since cardiac output is equal to the output is equal to the heart rate multiplied by the stroke volume, an increased rate can maintain cardiac output in the face of decreased stroke volume. Additionally, peripheral vasoconstriction helps to maintain blood flow to the central organs and to the brain. The patient therefore has pale, cool extremities and a delayed capillary refill time. This increased vascular tone also affects the measured blood pressure. The diastolic pressure is slightly elevated, so the difference between the systolic and diastolic pressures—the pulse pressure—is smaller. This is referred to as a "narrowed" pulse pressure.
   To compensate for both the decreased oxygen delivery and the acidosis created by underperfusion of peripheral tissues, the respiratory rate increases. The blood pressure eventually falls, but this is a late, ominous finding and may signal that the shock state is irreversible.

3. **Which laboratory values may indicate shock?**
Laboratory evidence of shock may include elevated lactate, an excessively negative base deficit, and a metabolic acidosis. Later, the patient may have evidence of end-organ dysfunction such as elevated blood urea nitrogen, creatinine, and transaminases.

4. **What is compensated shock?**
Various physiologic changes allow continued delivery of oxygen and nutrients to the vital organs in early shock. Tachycardia is usually the first compensatory mechanism. The increased heart rate helps to maintain cardiac output in the face of low blood volume, excessive vasodilation, or pump failure. Increased vasomotor tone shunts blood away from the skin and the extremities to more vital organs. In compensated shock, the patient is able to continue to meet his or her metabolic demand, even if only marginally.

5. **Are there exceptions to the compensatory mechanisms described above?**
Yes. In *septic shock* the patient sometimes develops so-called warm shock or warm distributive shock. In this state, the patient has flushed skin and bounding pulses associated with a hyperdynamic precordium. The capillary refill time can be normal or sometimes what is referred to as flash capillary refill. This state can be explained by the cascade of inflammatory mediators that is responsible for the condition called septic shock. Likewise, in *neurogenic shock*, loss of sympathetic tone can result in bradycardia in the face of profound hypotension.

6. **What is uncompensated shock?**

If the shock state progresses without intervention, the patient's compensatory mechanisms eventually fail. Hypoperfusion of organ systems causes acidosis and further release of inflammatory mediators. As blood flow to the brain decreases, the patient can become irritable or stuporous and may eventually slip into a coma. Likewise, decreased renal blood flow causes decreased urine output and finally results in anuria. The gastrointestinal tract is similarly affected, so the patient often has decreased bowel motility followed by distention and edema of the bowel wall. As tissue ischemia and acidosis progress, the inflammatory mediators cause diffuse vascular injury and capillary leakage. The pulmonary bed is especially sensitive to this type of injury. Damage to the pulmonary tissues exacerbates tissue hypoxemia. The ultimate result of progressive shock is multiorgan system failure and acute respiratory distress syndrome.

7. **Is the pathophysiology of shock really that simple?**

No, it is exceedingly complex. What we refer to as "shock" is the final common pathway for a variety of physiologic insults. Whether the process starts with acute blood loss or with an overwhelming infection, eventually the host mounts a response to the insult, and this response—at least in some cases—seems to contribute to the shock state.

8. **What are the types (or mechanisms) of shock?**

- **Distributive or vasodilatory shock:** This type of shock is the final common pathway of a variety of conditions that result in vasodilation. Neurogenic distributive shock is caused by a spinal cord injury that eliminates sympathetic innervation to the blood vessels, causing profound vasodilation and bradycardia. Accidental ingestion of vasodilating medications can also result in distributive shock. Anaphylaxis results in vasodilation, and although anaphylaxis has many other components, shock is a part of the clinical picture.
  - **Septic shock:** Septic shock is largely distributive in nature but is a complex process that requires disease-specific management. In septic shock, an infectious stimulus causes the formation of inflammatory mediators that result in profound vasodilation and shock. However, some of these mediators also directly depress myocardial activity; thus septic shock can have features of both distributive and cardiogenic shock.
  - **Anaphylactic shock:** Patients suffering from anaphylactic shock after an exposure to an allergen typically present with two-system involvement—classically an uriticarial rash which may be accompanied by stridor, wheezing, and/or vomiting.
  - **Toxic shock syndrome (TSS):** TSS is an illness characterized by fever, erythroderma, hypotension, and involvement of several organ systems. It is caused by strains of *Staphylococcus aureus* that produce exotoxins (TSST-1, enterotoxin B, and enterotoxin C). It is most often associated with prolonged use of tampons, but young children (boys and girls) with open skin wounds or minor abrasions can also develop TSS.
  - **Neurogenic shock:** In neurogenic shock, injury to the spinal cord results in decreased sympathetic input to the vascular system. This results in hypotension and bradycardia.
- **Hypovolemic shock:** Hypovolemia occurs with blood or volume loss in the setting of hemorrhage or gastroenteritis. Decreased volume leads to decreased perfusion to the tissues and leads to shock.
- **Cardiogenic shock:** Pump failure is the primary mechanism for cardiogenic shock. Decreased myocardial contractility makes adequate delivery of oxygen and nutrients impossible. Since children are very dependent on a normal heart rate to produce an adequate cardiac output, drugs and other conditions that cause bradycardia can also lead to shock. There will be evidence of congestive heart failure, such as rales on pulmonary auscultation, hepatomegaly, and peripheral edema. Viral myocarditis, hypertrophic cardiomyopathy, and certain myocardial depressant drugs can cause cardiogenic shock.
- **Obstructive shock:** As the name implies, obstructive shock occurs when blood flow from the heart (cardiac output) is diminished by a physical obstruction. A pulmonary embolism, cardiac tamponade, and tension pneumothorax can all cause obstruction of blood flow, leading to acquired obstructive shock. Infants born with congenital heart defects such as coarctation of the aorta, hypoplastic left heart syndrome, and other ductal-dependent lesions may present with shock during the first few weeks of life as the ductus arteriosus closes.

9. **What usually initiates septic shock?**

The most common and potent initiator of the inflammatory cascade called septic shock is exposure to **endotoxin**. Endotoxin is the lipopolysaccharide (LPS) coat of gramnegative bacteria. Other bacterial and viral agents can also start this process. Examples include certain viral proteins and teichoic acid. The presence of endotoxins leads to a response from the host. This response involves a cascade of inflammatory mediators, called cytokines, that are responsible for most of the symptoms of shock.

10. **Is gram-positive or gram-negative sepsis more severe?**

Gram-negative septic shock is more severe and accounts for mortality rates from 20% to 50%. Mortality rates from gram-positive septic shock are lower at 10% to 20%.

11. **Describe how the cascade of septic shock begins.**
Most commonly, endotoxin (LPS) is bound by a plasma protein called LPS-binding protein (LBP). The LPS-LBP complex then binds to the CD14 receptor on the surfaces of macrophages. This process stimulates the formation of both tumor necrosis factor and interleukin. These two cytokines begin the cascade that leads to septic shock.

12. **What is the most common cause of shock in children?**
Hypovolemia is the most common cause of shock in children. Acute blood loss, vomiting, and diarrhea are common causes of hypovolemia. Worldwide, diarrheal illness is the most common cause of hypovolemia. Millions of children die each year from hypovolemia caused by diarrhea.

13. **What are some ways in which trauma can cause shock?**
Traumatic injuries may contribute to various forms of shock. Most commonly, posttraumatic hemorrhage secondary to liver or spleen injury may cause hypovolemic shock.
Blunt chest trauma can result in a tension pneumothorax. Tension pneumothorax causes increased intrathoracic pressure, which in turn reduces venous return to the heart. Similarly, blunt chest trauma can result in pericardial tamponade. Both injuries may lead to an obstructive form of shock.
Finally, cervical spine injury, commonly from a motor vehicle crash, can result in neurogenic shock.

14. **How does isolated head trauma cause shock?**
In the absence of exsanguination from a large scalp laceration, it does not. If a patient has shock after what appears to be isolated head trauma without obvious exsanguination from a scalp wound, there must be another explanation for the shock.

KEY POINTS: ETIOLOGY OF SHOCK IN CHILDREN

1. Hypovolemia (not enough circulating volume to deliver oxygen and nutrients)
2. Impaired cardiac function (ineffective pumping of the circulating volume)
3. Inappropriate vasodilation (the circulating volume exists primarily in the venous capacitance system and is unavailable to deliver oxygen and nutrients)

15. **What are the classes of hemorrhage?**
   - **Class I hemorrhage:** The patient has lost up to 15% of the blood volume. Otherwise healthy patients are likely to have minimal tachycardia and no other symptoms. Unless there is ongoing hemorrhage, the patient should require no treatment.
   - **Class II hemorrhage:** The patient has lost 15% to 30% of the blood volume. Loss of this amount of blood stimulates the compensatory mechanisms usually associated with early, compensated shock. Tachycardia, increased respiratory rate, and narrowed pulse pressure are seen. Urine output is usually maintained, but the patient may have signs of early central nervous system impairment. Such signs may include fright or anxiety.
   - **Class III hemorrhage:** The patient has lost 30% to 40% of the blood volume. This amount of blood loss is clearly associated with signs of compensated shock but may also be associated with uncompensated shock. Even healthy individuals may have a drop in systolic blood pressure with this degree of blood loss. Urine output is likely to be decreased, and the patient may be very anxious or confused.
   - **Class IV hemorrhage:** This represents a loss of more than 40% of the circulating blood volume. This degree of hemorrhage is uniformly fatal if untreated. The shock state may, in some cases, be irreversible. The patient has a markedly decreased blood pressure. The patient can be expected to have complete peripheral vasoconstriction, extreme tachycardia, and little or no urinary output. Mental status is very depressed, and the patient may be unconscious.

16. **How can emergency physicians use point-of-care ultrasound (PoCUS) to make a presumptive diagnosis of cardiogenic shock?**
Recent studies have demonstrated that emergency physicians using bedside ultrasonography or PoCUS can correctly identify cardiac wall motion abnormalities as well as cardiac index. This technology makes it easy for the emergency physician to identify patients with abnormal cardiac function. Additionally, many patients with signs of early shock, such as tachycardia, are treated with fluid resuscitation. Emergency physicians should suspect cardiogenic shock in patients who deteriorate after fluid resuscitation, as giving too much fluid to a patient with cardiogenic shock can cause pulmonary edema and contribute to heart failure.

17. **How can hemorrhagic shock be distinguished from neurogenic shock?**
The patient with hemorrhagic shock has a rapid and possibly irregular pulse, while the patient with neurogenic shock has a slow and regular pulse due to the damaged innervation of the autonomic nervous system.

18. **In general, what is the initial treatment for shock?**
    There is no single treatment for shock: therapy is aimed at the cause. That being said, most types of shock respond well to fluid therapy; therefore if the cause cannot be identified, a single bolus of 20 mL/kg of a crystalloid solution may be helpful and is unlikely to cause serious harm. In patients who have had an obvious hemorrhage, as in the case of a trauma patient with significant bleeding from a noncompressible source (i.e., pelvic fracture hemorrhage, solid organ laceration), it is reasonable to start volume resuscitation with a balanced ratio of blood products. While there is no published evidence for this approach in pediatric patients, adult studies have shown favorable outcomes. Additionally, the patient should receive supplemental oxygen and may require assisted ventilation to ensure that oxygen delivery is maximized.

19. **Which treatments should be avoided?**
    The greatest error that you can make in the treatment of shock is to use pressor agents to treat hypovolemia. Even in cases of distributive shock, fluids should be used for initial treatment. Note that excessive fluid administration can be harmful in cardiogenic shock.

20. **Describe the benefits of the commonly used vasopressor agents—norepinephrine, epinephrine, dopamine, and dobutamine.**
    Norepinephrine is a potent central nervous system neurotransmitter that results in significant vasoconstriction and has minimal effect on inotropy or chronotropy. This is a good first agent to consider in warm shock or when a patient has significant vasodilation.
    Epinephrine is a natural hormone that results in increased inotropy and chronotropy. At lower doses, epinephrine results in vasodilation, whereas higher infusion rates (>0.3 µg/kg/minute) result in systemic and pulmonary vasoconstriction. Epinephrine is a common first-line pressor agent to manage patients in "cold shock."
    Dopamine is an endogenous catecholamine that results in increased inotropy (contractility), increased chronotropy (heart rate), and vasodilation at low doses. At higher doses, dopamine results in vasoconstriction. Some new adult data suggest increased mortality; thus it is used less commonly.
    Dobutamine is a synthetic catecholamine that results in increased inotropy and vasodilation (see Table 4.1).

21. **How should hypovolemic shock be treated?**
    Treat hypovolemia with volume. Initial therapy is usually crystalloids. Acceptable crystalloids are lactated Ringer solution, physiologic multielectrolyte solutions, and normal saline. Give boluses of 20 mL of fluid per kilogram of body weight over 5 to 10 minutes. Initial volume resuscitation can require 40 to 60 mL/kg or more before considering other etiologies causing shock. Vasoactive agents are not beneficial in hypovolemic shock and should be avoided.

22. **How should cardiogenic shock be treated?**
    Cardiogenic shock should be treated with afterload reduction coupled with inotropic support. This can be achieved with low-dose epinephrine (0.05-0.3 µg/kg/minute) and the inodilators, milrinone or amrinone.

23. **How should hemorrhagic shock be treated?**
    Compelling evidence exists in adult populations about massive transfusion protocols and balanced ratios of blood products in lieu of crystalloid resuscitation. Although little evidence exists in the pediatric literature, many trauma centers have adapted adult protocols to their pediatric patients. The tenets of these protocols involve minimizing crystalloid fluid and judicious transfusion of blood products in ratios that more closely mimic fresh whole blood. Undoubtedly, some patients with mild blood loss can be managed with crystalloid; however, patients with severe (class III and IV) hemorrhage will require blood replacement therapy.

24. **What is the treatment for neurogenic shock?**
    In neurogenic shock, injury to the spinal cord results in decreased sympathetic input to the vascular system. Most of the patient's blood supply is left in the venous or capacitance system. **Fluid therapy** is an appropriate initial

Table 4.1 Common Pressor Agents Used to Manage Shock				
	INOTROPE	**CHRONOTROPE**	**VASODILATION**	**VASOCONSTRICTION**
Norepinephrine				X
Epinephrine	X	X	Low dose	Higher doses
Dopamine	X	X	Low dose	Higher doses
Dobutamine	X		X	

treatment, but pressor agents may also be needed. **Norepinephrine and phenylephrine** are powerful α-agonists and are often recommended for neurogenic shock in the setting of normal heart rate and cardiac output. Due to its inotropic properties, **dopamine** is an excellent alternative to norepinephrine and phenylephrine when cardiac output and heart rate are inadequate. If the patient has profound bradycardia, **atropine** may be used to increase the heart rate and, therefore, the cardiac output.

25. Describe the first steps in the management of a patient with septic shock.
    Early recognition and aggressive resuscitation according to the 2020 Surviving Sepsis Guidelines are critical to improving outcomes. Immediately on recognition of septic shock and ideally within 5 minutes, two large-caliber intravenous (IV) lines should be inserted. At the minimum, obtain serum studies including blood culture, glucose, ionized calcium, and lactate.

    In an effort to avoid hypoxemia, give patients supplemental oxygen and/or more invasive airway support as indicated.

    Fluid therapy is paramount. Give patients 20 mL/kg of crystalloid over 5 to 10 minutes; this can be repeated to infuse up to 60 mL/kg in total.

    Interestingly, although antibiotics are needed to limit the infectious process, they alone are not sufficient treatment for septic shock. In certain cases, they may actually increase the antigen load in the system by destroying gram-negative organisms, which results in more LPS in the circulatory system. However, patients who do not receive adequate antibiotic therapy have a higher mortality than those receiving such therapy. Treatment with antibodies directed against the inflammatory mediators has not proven to be effective, but as our understanding of this complex process evolves, effective immunomodulator therapy may be developed.

    Occasionally, surgical control is required to eradicate the source in cases that are refractory to standard treatment modalities.

26. How should I choose an appropriate antibiotic for the patient in septic shock?
    Septic shock is a severe and life-threatening condition and should be treated promptly. It may, however, be impossible to identify the causative organism in a timely fashion. In most cases, it is prudent to choose broad-spectrum agents that are effective against a wide range of likely pathogens.

27. How should I select initial pressor agents for patients in septic shock?
    For patients who are hypotensive after fluid resuscitation, norepinephrine is the initial agent of choice when systemic vascular resistance (SVR) is low (warm shock), while "central doses" of epinephrine (<0.3 μg/kg/minute) and dopamine (<10 μg/kg/minute) are the agents of choice when SVR is elevated (cold shock). Recent adult data have suggested that dopamine may be associated with increased mortality; hence, this medication is less commonly used as an initial pressor.

28. Under what circumstances might the drug phenylephrine be useful in the management of shock?
    Phenylephrine causes vasoconstriction without causing excessive tachycardia. In the patient whose shock state is caused primarily by vasodilation, as in neurogenic shock, phenylephrine might be indicated.

29. What additional medications can be used for refractory shock?
    Administer hydrocortisone for fluid and vasopressor refractory shock in children with suspected or known adrenal insufficiency. Patients at risk for adrenal insufficiency include those with purpura fulminans, chronic treatment with corticosteroids, and adrenal or pituitary abnormalities. Stress-dose hydrocortisone, at a dose of 50 to 100 mg/m^2/day or approximately 2 to 4 mg/kg/day, should be given early in the course of resuscitation. If it is the first presentation of adrenal insufficiency, it is helpful to draw a cortisol level prior to the administration of steroids to aid with the diagnosis. Patients presenting with Addison's disease may also have hyperkalemia and hyponatremia.

30. What is early, goal-directed therapy?
    Early, goal-directed therapy is a management scheme that has been shown to be effective in the treatment of adult patients with sepsis and septic shock. There are four basic components of early, goal-directed therapy: (1) early recognition of the patient who is at risk for physiologic compromise using metabolic markers such as serum lactate; (2) correction of hypovolemia and cardiovascular function using predetermined goals or endpoints (e.g., fluid resuscitation until the central venous pressure has reached 8 to 12 mm Hg); (3) prevention of sudden cardiopulmonary dysfunction; and (4) interruption of the inflammatory cascade created by cellular hypoxemia.

31. How should anaphylactic shock be treated?
    Most manifestations of anaphylaxis, including hypotension, respond well to intramuscular epinephrine alone. Epinephrine has both α- and β-receptor agonist effects, so it can effectively treat bronchospasm and hypotension. Clinicians may consider adjuncts such as diphenhydramine, albuterol, intravascular fluids, and/or steroids.

32. **How do the exotoxins cause shock?**

TSST-1 and the other exotoxins are profound vasodilators, and their effect causes distributive shock. Additionally, vasodilation seems to cause rapid movement of fluids and serum proteins to the extravascular space, leading to intravascular volume depletion. Exotoxins also have a direct effect on the heart that results in decreased myocardial function. Finally, many patients with TSS experience vomiting or diarrhea, which leads to further volume depletion.

33. **Are there other forms of TSS?**

Yes, a clinical syndrome very similar to TSS has developed in association with group A streptococcal infections (*Streptococcus pyogenes*). Group A streptococci produce exotoxins very similar to those produced by staphylococci. These toxins are called streptococcal pyogenic exotoxins (SPEs). There are three of these: SPEs A, B, and C. SPE A has long been associated with the clinical features of scarlet fever. Exactly why these toxins have recently become more virulent is unknown.

34. **What is MIS-C?**

A new shock syndrome was recognized during the coronavirus disease 2019 (COVID-19) pandemic, called multisystem inflammatory syndrome in children (MIS-C). MIS-C is a rare complication of the severe acute respiratory syndrome coronavirus 2 (SARS-CoV-2) infection in children and typically presents in the month or so following the acute infection. It manifests as fever and multiorgan dysfunction, and patients have laboratory evidence of inflammation. It can be severe, leading to coronary artery aneurysms, ventricular dysfunction, hypotension, and shock. All children with the presumptive diagnosis of MIS-C should be admitted and/or transferred to a pediatric tertiary care center. Initial treatment includes judicious fluid resuscitation with a transition to vasoactive agents if evidence of pulmonary edema exists. Treatment for all patients with MIS-C includes IV immunoglobulin, and for those without contraindications (diabetes, hypertension, obesity), IV methylprednisolone should be administered as well. For patients with shock refractory to initial therapy, intensification therapy includes high-dose methylprednisolone or anakinra (interleukin-1 receptor antagonist).

KEY POINTS: SHOCK IN CHILDREN

1. The shock state can and often does exist in the presence of a "normal" blood pressure.
2. Hypovolemia is the most common cause of shock in children and is managed with aggressive volume resuscitation.
3. Early recognition and aggressive goal-directed resuscitation are critical to improving outcomes in children with septic shock.

BIBLIOGRAPHY

1. Chameides L, Samson RA, Scheznayder SM, et al. Hematologic system. *Pediatric Advanced Life Support: Provider Manual.* American Heart Association; 2016:190.
2. Chang R, Holcomb JB. Optimal fluid therapy for traumatic hemorrhagic shock. *Crit Care Clin.* 2017;33(1):15–36.
3. Dellinger RP, Levy MM, Rhodes AM, et al. Surviving Sepsis Campaign Guidelines Committee including the Pediatric Subgroup Surviving Sepsis Campaign. *Critical Care Medicine.* 2013;41(2):580–637.
4. Feldstein LR, Tenforde MW, Friedman KG, et al. Characteristics and outcomes of US children and adolescents with multisystem inflammatory syndrome in children (MIS-C) compared with severe acute COVID-19. *JAMA.* 2021;325(11):1074–1087.
5. Gupta A, Eckenswiller T. Point-of-care ultrasound in early diagnosis of cardiomyopathy in a child with viral myocarditis: a case report. *Clin Pract Cases Emerg Med.* 2021;5(2):186–189.
6. Henderson LA, Canna SW, Friedman KG, et al. American College of Rheumatology Clinical Guidance for multisystem inflammatory syndrome in children associated with SARS–CoV-2 and hyperinflammation in pediatric COVID-19: version 2. *Arthritis Rheumatol.* 2021;73:e13–e29.
7. Menon K, Schlapbach LJ, Akech S, et al. Criteria for pediatric sepsis-a systematic review and meta-analysis by the Pediatric Sepsis Definition Taskforce. *Crit Care Med.* 2022;50(1):21–36.
8. Mtaweh H, Trakas EV, Su E, et al. Advances in monitoring and management of shock. *Pediatr Clin North Am.* 2013;60(3):641–654.
9. Weiss SL, Peters MJ, Alhazzani W, et al. Surviving sepsis campaign international guidelines for the management of septic shock and sepsis-associated organ dysfunction in children. *Intensive Care Med.* 2020;46(suppl 1):10–67.

ABDOMINAL PAIN

Payal K. Gala

1. **Why is the evaluation of abdominal pain challenging in the pediatric patient?**
   Pediatric evaluations may be somewhat challenging for multiple reasons. First, depending on the age of the patient, histories may be provided secondhand from a parent or caregiver. Second, the physical examination may be difficult to obtain given stranger anxiety or generalized fear. Furthermore, infants with abdominal pain may present with nonspecific signs, such as irritability, poor feeding, and lethargy, making the etiology difficult to diagnose. Lastly, toddlers and young children may be able to report pain but are unable to provide further details, such as the quality, severity, or location of the pain.

2. **How can I organize my approach to the *stable* patient with abdominal pain?**
   The history and physical examination are the essential components of the evaluation, with judicious use of ancillary testing serving to aid in the diagnosis. Elicit the nature of the pain if possible, such as its onset, quality, severity, location, and duration, as well as the presence of any associated symptoms. The differential diagnosis of abdominal pain in children is extensive (Table 5.1). Understanding the most likely diagnoses per age group can be used in concert with the history and physical examination to narrow the differential and guide further diagnostic testing. Often, periods of observation on a stable and well-appearing patient followed by repeat assessments may be beneficial to determine the need for ongoing evaluation.

3. **How can I maximize the physical examination of the pediatric patient with abdominal pain?**
   In approaching any child with abdominal pain, one must take time to establish rapport. Essential information can be obtained before even touching the patient. Begin with observation, often best accomplished from outside the room. Notice the general appearance of the child. Is he lying still on the stretcher, suggesting peritonitis, or writhing with colicky pain? Is she running around the room playing with toys? Continue by examining the least threatening areas first and saving particularly invasive aspects of the examination for last (e.g., otoscopy). Distracting the child with a toy or by conversation will allow for a more reliable examination. Laying the child with his or her knees flexed may facilitate relaxation of the rectus muscles. The child's "help" can be elicited during the abdominal examination by allowing him to place his hands on top of the examiner's during palpation. Apply gentle pressure beginning in a location away from the area identified by the child as the most painful. To assess for peritoneal signs, ask the child to hop up and down; or ask parents to gently bounce a baby in their lap to elicit presence of pain. If a digital rectal examination is deemed necessary, insert a small finger into the rectal vault. Occasionally, when caring for a very challenging patient, the clinician may need to leave the examination room and return for a repeat abdominal examination during nap time or after the child has settled into their new environment.

4. **What are the life-threatening causes of abdominal pain?**
   - Appendicitis
   - Intussusception
   - Incarcerated hernia
   - Trauma (accidental or inflicted injury)
   - Tumors
   - Sepsis
   - Malrotation/volvulus
   - Ectopic pregnancy
   - Diabetic ketoacidosis
   - Intra-abdominal abscess (pelvic inflammatory disease, inflammatory bowel disease [IBD])
   - Hemolytic uremic syndrome
   - Intestinal obstruction
   - Pancreatitis
   - Megacolon
   - Metabolic acidosis/inborn error of metabolism
   - Aortic aneurysm
   - Toxic ingestion (iron, lead, aspirin)

Table 5.1 Differential Diagnosis for Acute Abdominal Pain

INFANTS (<2 YEARS OF AGE)	TODDLERS (2-5 YEARS OF AGE)	SCHOOL AGE (6-12 YEARS OF AGE)	ADOLESCENTS (>13 YEARS OF AGE)
Common			
Colic (age <3 mo), GERD, viral gastroenteritis, intussusception	Constipation, viral gastroenteritis, UTI, trauma	Constipation, viral gastroenteritis, trauma, appendicitis, UTI, functional abdominal pain	Constipation, viral gastroenteritis, gastritis, colitis, GERD, trauma, appendicitis, pelvic inflammatory disease, UTI, dysmenorrhea, mittelschmerz, lactose intolerance
Less Common			
Trauma (consider child abuse), incarcerated hernia, testicular torsion, milk protein allergy, appendicitis, malignancy (neuroblastoma, Wilms' tumor), sickle cell disease	Appendicitis, pneumonia, Meckel's diverticulum, Henoch-Schönlein purpura, intussusception, nephrotic syndrome, sickle cell disease	Pneumonia, inflammatory bowel disease, peptic ulcer disease, cholecystitis, pancreatitis, collagen vascular disease, testicular torsion, ovarian torsion, renal calculi, malignancy, sickle cell disease	Pneumonia, ectopic pregnancy, testicular torsion, epididymitis, ovarian cyst or torsion, imperforate hymen (hematocolpos), renal calculi, peptic ulcer disease, hepatitis, cholecystitis, pancreatitis, collagen vascular disease, inflammatory bowel disease, sickle cell disease

GERD, gastroesophageal reflux disease; UTI, urinary tract infection.

5. **What are some extra-abdominal causes of abdominal pain?**
   Pain originating at sites distant from the abdomen can manifest as abdominal pain. In processes such as lower lobe pneumonia, afferent nerves from the parietal pleura share central pathways with those that originate from the abdominal wall. Similarly, scrotal pain (e.g., testicular torsion) may be referred to the abdomen. Remember to always perform a testicular examination on all males with abdominal pain! Other illnesses that are associated with abdominal pain include streptococcal pharyngitis, diabetes mellitus, sickle cell disease with vaso-occlusive crisis, lead toxicity, and porphyria. Thorough history and physical examination may identify one of these diseases as the cause of abdominal pain.

6. **What historical "red flags" point toward an organic etiology of abdominal pain in children?**
   Historical findings including recent trauma, weight loss, inability to gain weight, severe vomiting especially if bilious or bloody, projectile vomiting, chronic severe diarrhea, hematochezia, fever, and family history of IBD may indicate abdominal pathology.

7. **What "red flags" on physical examination would indicate organic etiology of abdominal pain?**
   Findings of a tense abdomen, palpable mass, scrotal swelling, respiratory distress, vital sign abnormalities including fever, and focal tenderness may all point to a true abdominal emergency, and one should consider further workup with lab studies, imaging, and consultation as deemed necessary.

8. **Does the use of intravenous (IV) analgesia affect diagnostic accuracy in children with *acute abdominal pain of unknown cause?***
   No. Multiple studies with adults and children have shown that giving IV narcotics at adequate doses to decrease pain does not adversely affect the physical examination or diagnostic accuracy in patients with abdominal pain of unknown cause. In fact, pain control might facilitate localization of the origin of the pain, thereby improving the diagnostic accuracy of the physical examination. Therefore, avoid delaying administration of proper analgesia simply because the diagnosis is unknown or the child is awaiting examination by a consultant.

9. **Which blood tests may be useful in the evaluation of abdominal pain?**
Patients who have experienced persistent vomiting and appear dehydrated may have electrolyte abnormalities. In young infants, patients who will undergo surgery, or patients who are more severely ill, it may be more important to obtain blood studies to evaluate abdominal pain. The benefit of the complete blood count (CBC) remains controversial. Although an elevated white blood cell count is common in appendicitis, this finding is neither sensitive nor specific. The absolute neutrophil count and C-reactive protein (CRP) test may also be helpful in diagnosing appendicitis. The erythrocyte sedimentation rate may be helpful in the diagnosis of IBD. Measurement of liver aminotransferase values and bilirubin level is useful in patients with scleral icterus or right-upper-quadrant tenderness. An elevation of one or both serum amylase and lipase in the appropriate clinical context supports the diagnosis of pancreatitis.

10. **What other laboratory testing may be helpful in certain patients?**
A urinalysis can be helpful in diagnosing urinary tract infections and renal calculi but can be misleading if pyuria is due to cervicitis or bladder/ureteral irritation from an adjacent inflamed appendix. A urine pregnancy test is indicated in postpubertal females with abdominal pain. Additionally, include diagnostic testing for sexually transmitted infections when indicated.

11. **What are the two most common causes of acute abdominal emergencies in children?**
Appendicitis is the most common cause in the United States, followed by intussusception.

12. **What is the classical abdominal pain pattern associated with acute appendicitis?**
Classically, periumbilical abdominal pain precedes the onset of vomiting and is associated with low-grade fever, nausea/vomiting, and anorexia. As the inflammation of the appendix advances and touches the adjacent peritoneum, the pain localizes to the right lower quadrant at McBurney point. However, the clinical course often does not follow the "textbook" description, so the diagnosis can be difficult to make and the physician must maintain a high index of suspicion. Remember that history of abdominal pain that precedes vomiting is a clue to differentiate appendicitis from acute gastroenteritis.

13. **What are some of the pitfalls in diagnosing appendicitis?**
The presentation of a child with appendicitis is rarely "textbook." The absence of fever or anorexia, pain in an atypical location, the presence of diarrhea, prolonged symptoms, and normal laboratory values can occur in patients with appendicitis. An appendix that is located in the lateral gutter can cause flank pain and lateral abdominal tenderness; an appendix that lies toward the left may produce hypogastric tenderness; and a retrocecal appendix may cause back or pelvic pain or pain elicited only on deep palpation. Although vomiting occurs more commonly, diarrhea may result from direct sigmoid irritation from the adjacent low-lying pelvic appendix. Similarly, bladder or ureteral irritation may result in dysuria and pyuria, confusing the diagnosis for a urine infection.

14. **What are the benefits of ultrasound and computed tomography (CT) for the evaluation of children with suspected appendicitis?**
Ultrasonography is beneficial because it does not expose the child to ionizing radiation and therefore is typically used as the first imaging modality of choice. However, it is operator dependent and may have limited use in obese children or those patients with gas-filled bowels. If the study is equivocal or if the appendix is unable to be visualized, clinicians may consider additional imaging such as CT scan or magnetic resonance imaging (MRI) of the abdomen. CT and MRI are less operator dependent than ultrasonography, may provide several alternate diagnoses, and have excellent reported test characteristics in children.

15. **Is oral and IV contrast necessary in CT for the evaluation of children with suspected appendicitis?**
CT for appendicitis requires IV contrast to detect inflammation due to appendicitis or various other causes, but oral contrast is not necessary for the diagnosis of appendicitis. There is a high percentage of patients who do take oral contrast for whom the contrast does not even reach the point of interest, the terminal ileum, prior to the CT. In addition, delayed diagnostic evaluation, frequency of emesis after contrast bolus, and the need for a nasogastric tube to tolerate the bolus all limit the efficacy of oral contrast for CT in pediatric patients.

16. **Is MRI useful in the evaluation of children with suspected appendicitis?**
MRI is an alternative to CT in children suspected of appendicitis to avoid the detrimental effects of radiation. When readily available, the study can be completed quickly, does not typically require sedation, and provides similar test characteristics to CT scan diagnostics. It has been shown that the sensitivity of MRI without contrast in diagnosing appendicitis has been up to 100%, with a specificity of 96%, a positive predictive value of 88%, and a negative predictive value of 100%.

17. **Which patients are more likely to develop appendiceal perforation?**
    Young children, those with atypical presentations, and those who present late in their clinical course are at the highest risk.

18. **What is the "classic triad" of intussusception? Does it occur in most patients?**
    The classic triad of pain, currant jelly stool, and abdominal mass on palpation is present in only 20% to 25% of children with intussusception. Intussusception occurs when a portion of the bowel, usually the distal ileum, telescopes into an adjacent segment of the bowel. This effectively leads to intestinal obstruction followed by venous congestion and, finally, arterial insufficiency.

19. **What imaging modalities are commonly used in children to confirm or rule out intussusception?**
    - **Plain radiographs** are not the first-choice imaging modality for intussusception. They lack sensitivity and many false-negative results occur, so normal plain films should not exclude the diagnosis of intussusception. Later in the disease, they may show absence of air in the right upper and lower quadrants and evidence of soft tissue density. Plain radiographs do have a role in ruling out bowel perforation and may be considered prior to air contrast enema.
    - **Ultrasonography** is an important tool in diagnosing intussusception. It has the advantage of being relatively fast, noninvasive, and without exposure to ionizing radiation. Although it may be operator dependent, in experienced hands the sensitivity (98%-100%) and specificity (88%-100%) are high. It is important to note that if intussusception is detected on ultrasound, air or barium contrast enema under fluoroscopy is still indicated for treatment.
    - **Contrast enema** is beneficial in that it has both diagnostic and therapeutic values for intussusception. Despite this, it is rarely used as first-line imaging given the invasive nature and requirement of an attending radiologist to perform the procedure. Barium or air is introduced under pressure into the bowel via a tube in the rectum during fluoroscopy. Air is safer, cheaper, and more effective at reduction and poses less risk if there is bowel perforation. This procedure is quite uncomfortable and therefore pain management should be considered when preparing for the procedure.

20. **What abnormalities may appear on plain radiographs in children with abdominal pain?**
    The plain film should be assessed for "bones, stones, masses, and gas." An appendicolith is present in only about 5% to 15% of patients with appendicitis. Other findings in appendicitis may include sentinel loop, air-fluid levels, fecalith, mass in right lower quadrant, and indistinct psoas margins with scoliosis toward the right. Rarely, a perforated appendix may produce pneumoperitoneum. Some renal calculi can be visualized on plain radiographs of the abdomen. The invaginating bowel of intussusception may be apparent as an intraluminal density, but the more common finding is a paucity of air in the right upper and lower quadrants. Multiple stacked, dilated loops of bowel with air-fluid levels and the absence of distal air may signify intestinal obstruction. Abdominal radiographs may show evidence of constipation, previously unsuspected, or foreign bodies such as ingested magnets.

21. **Is ultrasound used to evaluate other abdominal pathologies?**
    In addition to appendicitis and intussusception, ultrasound is an integral component of the workup for pyloric stenosis, renal calculi, gall bladder disease, testicular torsion, and uterine/ovarian pathology.

22. **What imaging study would be used to detect intestinal malrotation?**
    An upper gastrointestinal series with small bowel follow-through is used to detect intestinal malrotation. Failure of the C-loop of the duodenum to cross the midline and an abnormal location of the cecum signify a malrotation is likely.

23. **What is Fitz-Hugh-Curtis syndrome and what type of abdominal pain is it associated with?**
    Fitz-Hugh-Curtis syndrome occurs in 5% to 10% of patients with chlamydial or gonococcal pelvic inflammatory disease and presents with focal right upper quadrant pain secondary to a perihepatitis. In affected women, the pelvic examination may be normal and cervical cultures may not isolate an organism. Hepatic aminotransferase values are normal or mildly elevated, though this is typically transient. In most cases, the diagnosis is inferred as the symptoms abate with antibiotic therapy. Definitive diagnosis can only be made laparoscopically.

24. **Describe the management of an acute abdominal emergency.**
    Begin immediate management with a careful assessment of the patient's airway, breathing, and circulation, particularly in an unstable patient. Obtain intravascular access and initiate fluid resuscitation with IV normal saline (20 mL/kg). Obtain and send laboratory studies during IV placement. Promptly administer broad-spectrum antibiotics, including anaerobic coverage, if there is a strong possibility of sepsis, and obtain surgical consultation

as early as possible if there is a suspicion of a surgical emergency. Communicate with the patient, family, and staff to maintain nothing by mouth status.

25. **What is the most common cause of recurrent abdominal pain?**
Although numerous organic causes are possible, up to 30% of patients will have functional pain with diagnoses such as irritable bowel syndrome and abdominal migraines. In the functional abdominal pain syndrome, the pain is generally episodic, is periumbilical, rarely occurs during sleep, and is rarely associated with eating or activities. There are no signs of systemic illness, such as fever, diarrhea, vomiting, rash, or joint pain. The child's growth and development are normal. The physical examination is usually unremarkable, with the exception of mild periumbilical abdominal tenderness without peritoneal signs.

KEY POINTS: ABDOMINAL EMERGENCIES

1. The pediatric abdominal examination begins with careful observation "from the door."
2. Children may not have "classic" features of appendicitis or intussusception.
3. CBC and CRP are not specific for appendicitis.
4. Analgesia should not be withheld from a child with abdominal pain of unknown cause simply for fear of delaying diagnosis or causing misdiagnosis.
5. Children are at particularly high risk of ruptured appendix, with the youngest children (<3 years old) possessing the highest risk.

26. **How should the diagnosis of functional abdominal pain be addressed in the emergency department (ED)?**
The diagnosis of functional abdominal pain is usually evident following the completion of the history and physical examination. Failure to mention this diagnosis early or obtaining unnecessary studies to appease an anxious family may only result in the parents feeling that "the right" diagnostic test has yet to be performed. Reassure the parents and child that stress-related abdominal pain is real pain and not due to the child's "faking it." Encourage children to continue their normal activities (e.g., school attendance) and seek psychological services. Finally, provide careful instructions on the symptoms that should prompt an immediate return to the ED and encourage follow-up with the child's primary care provider and/or a pediatric gastroenterologist.

Acknowledgment
The author wishes to thank Dr. Jill Posner for her contributions to this chapter in the previous edition.

BIBLIOGRAPHY

1. Anderson BA, Salem L, Flum DR. A systematic review of whether oral contrast is necessary for the computed tomography diagnosis of appendicitis in adults. *Am J Surg.* 2005;190:474–478.
2. Becker C, Kharbanda A. Acute appendicitis in pediatric patients: an evidence-based review. *Pediatr Emerg Med Pract.* 2019;16(9):1–20.
3. Craig S, Dalton S. Diagnosing appendicitis: what works, what does not and where to go from here? *J Paediatr Child Health.* 2016;52(2):168–173.
4. Edwards EA, et al. Intussusception: past, present and future. *Pediatr Radiol.* 2017;47(9):1101–1108.
5. Farrell CR, Bezinque AD, Tucker JM, et al. Acute appendicitis in childhood: oral contrast does not improve CT diagnosis. *Emerg Radiol.* 2018;25(3):257–263.
6. Kwan KY, Nager AL. Diagnosing pediatric appendicitis: usefulness of laboratory markers. *Am J Emerg Med.* 2010;28:1009–1015.
7. Lipsett SC, Bachur RG. Abdominal emergencies. In: Shaw KN, Bachur RG, eds.*Fleisher & Ludwig's Textbook of Pediatric Emergency Medicine.* 8th ed. Wolters Kluwer; 2021:1290–1312.
8. Marin JR, Alpern ER. Abdominal pain in children. *Emerg Med Clin North Am.* 2011;29(2):401–428.
9. Mustaq R, Desoky SM, Morello F, et al. First line diagnostic evaluation with MRI of children suspected of having acute appendicitis. *Radiology.* 2019;291:170–177.
10. Peter NG, Clark LR, Jaeger JR. Fitz-Hugh-Curtis syndrome: a diagnosis to consider in women with right upper quadrant pain. *Cleve Clin J Med.* 2004;71:233–239.
11. Smith J, Fox SM. Pediatric abdominal pain: an emergency medicine perspective. *Emerg Med Clin North Am.* 2016;34(2):341–361.

CHAPTER 6

ALTERED MENTAL STATUS

Eric W. Glissmeyer

1. **How can altered mental status (AMS) present in an infant?**
   It may present as a combination of excessive crying, irritability, poor feeding, or sleeping more or less than usual.

2. **Name the most life-threatening causes of AMS.**
   The list includes intracranial hemorrhage, cerebral edema, brain neoplasms, cerebral infarctions, cerebrospinal fluid (CSF) shunt malfunction, meningitis, encephalitis, toxic ingestions, carbon monoxide poisoning, hypotension, hypoxia, and sepsis.

3. **How can the breathing pattern of a child in coma help determine the cause for neurological dysfunction?**
   Slow breathing points to opiate or barbiturate intoxication. Deep, rapid breathing suggests acidosis or a pulmonary problem. Cheyne-Stokes respiration is likely due to increased intracranial pressure.

4. **How does the history related to onset of AMS help distinguish the etiology?**
   Coma that develops abruptly with no explanation suggests trauma, seizure, or intracranial hemorrhage. A vague or inconsistent history prompts suspicion for nonaccidental trauma (NAT). NAT must be considered in an infant with AMS. Unexplained AMS in a toddler or an older child suggests a toxic ingestion. These events are often unwitnessed. A history of preceding headache, nausea, or visual disturbance suggests increased intracranial pressure, perhaps a brain tumor that has suddenly bled. Gradual deterioration suggests an infection, a metabolic abnormality, or a slowly expanding intracranial mass. Inborn errors of metabolism may present with a slowly evolving coma or recurring episodic coma.

5. **An afebrile 3-year-old child looks acutely intoxicated yet has negative blood and urine toxicology screens and normal complete blood count (CBC), electrolytes, and brain computed tomography (CT). What is the likely diagnosis?**
   Toxic ingestion, despite the lack of a positive finding on toxicology screening. Many substances that affect the function of the central nervous system (CNS) are not detected on these screens, which focus on drugs of abuse. Those causing AMS with miosis include clonidine, organophosphates, and tetrahydrozoline. Mydriasis and AMS are found with other toxins: carbon monoxide, cyanide, methemoglobinemia, lysergic acid diethylamide (LSD), γ-hydroxybutyrate (GHB), and nicotine. Fentanyl and other synthetic opiates will not be positive on standard toxicological screens and their ingestion (unintentional and intentional) is recently increasing.

6. **Name some recreational drugs/therapeutic medications that are recently associated with increased pediatric visits to the emergency department (ED) for AMS.**
   Marijuana as edibles, vaping liquid, and other forms of tetrahydrocannabinol. These have become ubiquitous recently, and many children present with accidental ingestion of these substances. Effects can range from sleepiness or euphoria/irritability to more profound AMS, bradycardia, coma, and seizures. These can be detected on urine toxicology screens 1 to 4 hours after ingestion. In higher ingestions, seizures are common and generally respond to benzodiazepines.

7. **Which scales are in use to quantify AMS?**
   The level of consciousness of a neurologically impaired patient may initially be evaluated by using a simple AVPU scale, representing four major levels of alertness: alert (A), responsive to verbal stimuli (V), responsive to painful stimuli (P), and unresponsive (U).
   A more widely used measurement of consciousness is the Glasgow Coma Scale (GCS). Patients are graded on three areas of neurological function: eye opening, motor responses, and verbal responsiveness. These numeric scores are summed to determine the GCS score (minimum score of 3, maximum score of 15). Details of the scores assigned are listed, for children above 2 years of age and below, in Tables 6.1 and 6.2.

8. **Why should you assign a GCS score to every patient with AMS?**
   There are several good reasons to use a standard quantifiable mental status scale. It allows evaluation of a patient's changing neurological status over time and the recording of this information in the medical record. The effect of medical interventions may then be more easily assessed. The use of accepted scoring systems also facilitates communication with EMS (Emergency Medical Services) and consultants, such as neurologists and neurosurgeons.

Table 6.1 Glasgow Coma Scale

SCORE VALUE	EYE OPENING	BEST MOTOR RESPONSE	BEST VERBAL RESPONSE
6		Obeys command	
5		Localizes to pain	Oriented, converses
4	Spontaneous	Flexion withdrawal	Disoriented, confused
3	To command	Flexion posturing	Inappropriate words
2	To pain	Extension posturing	Incomprehensible sounds
1	None	None	None

Table 6.2 Pediatric Glasgow Coma Scale (Use for Patients Under 2 Years of Age)

SCORE VALUE	EYE OPENING	BEST MOTOR RESPONSE	BEST VERBAL RESPONSE
6		Normal spontaneous movement	
5		Withdraws to touch	Coos, babbles
4	Spontaneous	Withdraws to pain	Irritable, cries
3	To sound	Flexion posturing	Cries to pain
2	To pain	Extension posturing	Moans to pain
1	None	None	None

9. Can the GCS be used to guide your management of a child with AMS?
   Yes. When the "GCS is 8, it is time to intubate." When a child has significant AMS and the GCS is 8 or lower, the patient is usually unable to protect the airway and urgent endotracheal intubation is indicated.

10. What laboratory test should be considered first if the physical examination of a patient with AMS does not reveal the source of neurological disability?
    A rapid bedside test for glucose is the most important laboratory test to check first. It can be done by fingerstick to provide a value immediately. This is especially important for young infants who have limited glycogen stores. It is not advisable to wait 45 minutes to 1 hour for the laboratory to confirm that hypoglycemia is the cause of the infant's AMS. Low glucose levels should be immediately corrected with dextrose.

11. When should you consider obtaining a CT scan on a child with AMS?
    Consider CT if there is any history of trauma, any focal or lateralizing signs on physical examination, or any suspicion of physical abuse.

12. Why is CT usually performed first in a patient presenting with AMS when magnetic resonance imaging (MRI) provides a sharper, more detailed picture of the brain?
    MRI scans are more costly, take longer to obtain, and are generally more difficult to arrange than CT scans. CT images show most structural lesions that may present with AMS, such as tumors or hemorrhage. Young children may require sedation for MRI but not for a quick noncontrast head CT.

13. Can children presenting with AMS just be observed?
    The only common situation when a child with AMS can be observed is when they are in the postictal period from a recent seizure. Otherwise, children presenting with AMS due to trauma, illness, known toxic ingestions, or undefined reasons almost always need laboratory or radiographic studies. A large and impactful study by the Pediatric Emergency Care Applied Research Network identified children at low risk for clinically important traumatic brain injury (ciTBI), but children with GCS scores of 14 or less, or any other signs of AMS, were in the group at high risk of ciTBI, and CT scanning was recommended; other children can be observed for 4 hours from TBI and most of these do not need CT scan.

14. A teenager is brought to the ED by friends from a party. He arrives comatose and requires endotracheal intubation. He has a normal toxicology screen and head CT scan. Upon returning from CT scan, he sits up, rips the endotracheal tube out of his mouth, and wants to leave. Name the "club drug" most likely involved.

    At the party, he drank gamma-hydroxybutyrate (GHB), sometimes called liquid ecstasy. CNS effects of GHB include drowsiness, ataxia, confusion, hallucinations, amnesia, incontinence, seizures, and coma. Mydriasis and nystagmus may be present, accompanied by respiratory depression, bradycardia, and hypotension.

    Recovery from GHB intoxication is usually rapid, within several hours after ingestion. Routine toxicological screens miss the presence of this recreational drug. You might consider GHB and other "club drugs" in the differential diagnosis of all teens presenting with acutely altered, and rapidly normalizing, mental status.

15. A 16-year-old female is brought by emergency medical services (EMS) for respiratory depression and somnolence after hanging out with friends. The patient had miosis and respiratory depression. EMS administered naloxone 0.4 mg intranasally, and the patient awoke and denied taking anything. A urine drug screen is negative. What opioid was likely ingested?

    Fentanyl. This is a highly potent synthetic opioid that is very dangerous and not detected on typical urine drug screens. Though fentanyl is generally short acting, continuous intravenous naloxone infusion may be necessary to maintain normal respiratory drive when fentanyl is taken in overdose. Use of fentanyl has increased dramatically in recent years. Community availability and familiarity with naloxone have also increased in recent years, and rapid administration should be encouraged in patients with suspected fentanyl overdose. Reducing opiate prescriptions and safely discarding unused pills are key healthcare strategies to reducing opioid-related deaths.

16. An 11-year-old male born at 28 weeks' gestation with a history of cerebral palsy (CP) and shunt-dependent hydrocephalus is brought to the ED because of excessive somnolence and bradycardia. He has a CSF shunt and an intrathecal baclofen pump. How should this patient be evaluated to determine the cause of his AMS?

    Many infants born extremely prematurely have CP and live with implanted medical devices such as CSF shunts and intrathecal baclofen pumps. Any child with this technology and AMS has a shunt or pump problem until proven otherwise. Obtain a brain CT or fast MRI (if available) to determine if this patient's shunt is functioning. Query the patient's baclofen pump to look for a malfunction. Baclofen toxicity is a likely etiology for his AMS. Acute kidney injury may necessitate adjustment of baclofen dosing.

17. Describe the mostly likely cause of poor feeding and sleepiness in a 6-month-old infant brought in by her mother after being left alone with another caregiver.

    Nonaccidental head trauma is most likely. Subdural hematomas can occur bilaterally and are 5 to 10 times more common than epidural bleeding. Subdural hematomas may occur on a chronic basis in young, abused children and are associated with skull fractures in 30% of cases. Neuroimaging classically reveals crescent-shaped lesions between the brain and skull. Skeletal surveys performed on these children often show fractures in various stages of healing.

18. How can you elicit clues that a child's AMS may be due to psychogenic nonepileptic seizure (PNES) or a somatization disorder?

    Physical examination may give the answer. When you lift the patient's hand to a position directly over their face and let go, the patient will not hit himself, or herself, in the face unless there is a true alteration in mental status. Furthermore, patients with PNES often close their eyes tightly and resist opening during an event. In contrast, those with a true seizure often have their eyes open. PNES is a type of somatic symptom disorder, previously called pseudoseizure. These patients often have a psychiatric history or fall from "spells" without ever being injured. In unclear cases, it may be necessary to perform electroencephalography to rule out epileptiform activity.

19. A 3-year-old child presents with sleepiness and vomiting on a cold winter day. There is no history of head trauma or ingestion. She is drowsy but well appearing and has mild tachypnea and tachycardia. Oxygen saturation is 100% in room air. Of note, other family members report they have headache and dizziness today. What test comes back with abnormal results?

    The blood gas, which shows a carboxyhemoglobin level of 20%. This level indicates that the patient, and presumably her family, are being poisoned by carbon monoxide. This cause of AMS is seen most often in early winter, as families turn on their furnaces for the first time since the previous heating season, or in electrical blackouts with home generator use. Treatment usually consists of administering 100% oxygen. Severe cases may require hyperbaric oxygen. Those with exposure to superheated air from fire or with facial burns likely will require early endotracheal intubation. Pulse oximetry often reads 100%, as carboxyhemoglobin is misread as oxygenated hemoglobin.

20. **What subtle signs may represent seizure activity as the cause of AMS?**
Suspect seizure if the patient is dazed or confused and exhibits staring, swallowing, eye blinking, lip quivering/smacking, nystagmus, and automatisms (motor actions performed without conscious intent). The degree of neurological impairment can fluctuate over time.

21. **A 4-year-old boy presents with sleepiness, vomiting, and "not acting right." History is positive for birth at 30 weeks' gestation but is negative for head trauma, fever, toxic ingestion, or other signs of illness. He is afebrile, with a heart rate of 120 beats per minute, blood pressure (BP) of 170/100 mm Hg, and a respiratory rate of 36 breaths per minute. He is difficult to arouse and cries when awake. Lumbar puncture (LP) is not performed because of concerns of increased intracranial pressure. A CT scan shows subtle occipital abnormalities. What caused AMS in this patient?**
The patient has hypertensive encephalopathy. His BP is much greater than the 99th percentile for age. This is likely due to renal artery stenosis caused by an umbilical artery catheter used during his neonatal intensive care unit stay. Clinical findings may include AMS, seizures, headache, and vision changes. Appropriate treatment of hypertension results in resolution of neurological. BP values obtained in the ED setting are often falsely elevated, but in the setting of AMS or headache, they can be the root of the problem.

22. **A 12-year-old boy with a history of sinus and ear infections is brought to the ED by his parents, who are concerned by his diminished responsiveness. He recently complained of headache and felt warm to touch. He is somnolent with no focal neurological findings. What is the likely cause of his AMS?**
The patient has a subdural abscess from long-standing sinusitis. Intracranial complications of sinusitis are uncommon but possible in older children and teens. When pus-filled sinuses decompress into the cranial vault, minimal facial tenderness may be present. A high index of suspicion is needed in patients with a history or symptoms of sinus infections. Brain and sinus CT scans will reveal the cause of the patient's mental status.

23. **A 7-year-old girl with an unremarkable medical history is much sleepier than usual. Examination shows an afebrile, well-nourished, well-developed child who prefers to sleep. When awakened, she seems confused, and "not all there." CBC, electrolytes, blood gas, urinalysis, toxicological screen, and noncontrast head CT are all normal. What tests are indicated and what will they show?**
She needs an LP and an MRI to check for acute disseminated encephalomyelitis (ADEM). ADEM is an immune-mediated inflammatory process that may appear following a viral infection, after vaccination, or spontaneously. This autoimmune demyelination process produces AMS characterized by irritability, sleepiness, confusion, obtundation, seizures, and coma. CSF findings are variable but usually include moderate leukocytosis with a lymphocytic or monocytic predominance, although they can be normal in 20% of cases. MRI shows white matter lesions.

24. **An 8-year-old girl is brought to the ED from a rural area with agitation and confusion. She has had a low-grade fever and malaise for 48 hours. She has no history of head trauma or overseas travel, but she received a new puppy 3 months ago. CT scan is abnormal, with hypodensities in the basal ganglia bilaterally. What unusual illness would be of most concern in this patient?**
Rabies. Younger domestic animals are more susceptible to acquiring the disease from infected wild animal hosts (skunks, raccoons, ferrets, foxes, bats) via bites or inadvertent sharing of outdoor water bowls. Also consider the disease in a patient with a travel history to areas of the world, such as India, China, Ethiopia, and the Democratic Republic of the Congo, where the disease is endemic and still common in dogs.

KEY POINTS: WHEN TO SUSPECT TOXIC INGESTION IN A CHILD WITH AMS AND NO HISTORY OF INGESTION

1. No history or physical examination findings of head trauma
2. Sudden onset of symptoms
3. Large number of children, including visitors, in the home
4. Previous ingestions by the patient or their siblings
5. Presence in the home of illicit or recreational drugs or another person on multiple medications for behavior control or seizures

KEY POINTS: DRUGS THAT MOST COMMONLY CAUSE AMS IN TEENS

1. Cannabis (marijuana, "pot," "weed") and synthetic cannabinoids ("K2," "spice")
2. Prescription opioids ("oxy," "percs, "demmies") and synthetic opioids, especially fentanyl ("China white," "lollipop")
3. Prescription stimulants and amphetamines ("bennies," "crank," speed") and methamphetamine ("meth," "crystal")
4. "Club drugs" including GHB ("liquid ecstasy," "liquid X"), flunitrazepam (Rohypnol, "roofies"), ketamine ("vitamin K"), LSD ("acid"), and methylenedioxymethamphetamine ("ecstasy," "molly")

BIBLIOGRAPHY

1. Abdelal R, Banerjee AR, Carlberg-Racich S, et al. Real-world study of multiple naloxone administrations for opioid overdose reversal among emergency medical service providers. *Subst Abus.* 2022;43(1):1075–1084.
2. Anderson RC, Patel V, Sheikh-Bahaei N, et al. Posterior reversible encephalopathy syndrome (PRES): pathophysiology and neuro-imaging. *Front Neurol.* 2020;11:463.
3. Button K, Capraro A, Monuteaux M, Mannix R. Etiologies and yield of diagnostic testing in children presenting to the emergency department with altered mental status. *J Pediatr.* 2018;200:218–224.e2.
4. Glissmeyer EW, Nelson DS. Coma. In: Bachur RG, Shaw KN, Chamberlain J, Lavelle J, Nagler J, eds. *Fleisher & Ludwig's Textbook of Pediatric Emergency Medicine.* 8th ed. Lippincott Williams & Wilkins; 2020:99–108.
5. Kuppermann N, Homes JF, Dayan PS, et al. Identification of children at very low risk of clinically-important brain injuries after head trauma: a prospective cohort study. *Lancet.* 2009;374(9696):1160–1170.
6. Wilson N, Kariisa M, Seth P, Smith H, Davis NL. Drug and opioid-involved overdose deaths – United States, 2017-2018. *MMWR Morb Mortal Wkly Rep.* 2020;69(11):290–297.
7. Yeung MEM, Weaver CG, Hartmann R, Haines-Saah R, Lang E. Emergency department pediatric visits in Alberta for cannabis after legalization. *Pediatrics.* 2021;148(4):e2020045922.
8. Yildiz LA, Gultekingil A, Kesici S, Bayrakci B, Teksam O. Predictors of severe clinical course in children with carbon monoxide poisoning. *Pediatr Emerg Care.* 2021;37(6):308–311.

APNEA, SUDDEN INFANT DEATH SYNDROME, AND BRIEF RESOLVED UNEXPLAINED EVENTS

Andrew D. DePiero

1. **What is the definition of apnea?**

   Apnea is a pause in respiratory airflow. Apnea is usually defined by a respiratory pause greater than 20 seconds or a respiratory pause associated with bradycardia or oxygen desaturation. The 20-second threshold was established somewhat arbitrarily with the development of impedance monitoring and associated alarm settings. In some infants, bradycardia and cyanosis can occur within 5 seconds.

2. **What is the pathophysiology of apnea?**

   Apnea may occur secondary to a central or an obstructive mechanism. Central apnea is a dysfunction of the neurological centers that regulate breathing. During central apnea, all respiratory efforts cease. Obstructive apnea is related to an obstruction of the upper airway. Occasionally, both central and obstructive components are present. This is classified as mixed apnea.

3. **What is apnea of prematurity?**

   Apnea of prematurity is related to the underdeveloped respiratory and neurological systems of infants born prematurely. The incidence is inversely related to gestational age, and infants <28 weeks' gestation are at greatest risk. Apnea of prematurity spontaneously resolves. In most cases, apneic events cease by 37 weeks postmenstrual age (PMA) and events after 43 weeks PMA are extremely rare.

4. **How is apnea of prematurity treated?**

   Methylxanthines, in most cases caffeine, are the most common modality for the treatment of apnea. Other treatments include nasal continuous positive airway pressure and humidified high-flow nasal cannula. Blood transfusions provide a short-term decrease in the number of apneic events. Gastroesophageal reflux (GER) treatment has not proven to decrease apneic events.

5. **Does apnea occur in term babies?**

   Apnea can occur in term babies, even those with an uncomplicated pregnancy and perinatal course. Cases of apnea and cyanosis, as well as asystole, have been described as early as the first hours of life, including events associated with early skin-to-skin contact.

6. **What are some of the underlying causes of apnea in infants?**

   - **Central nervous system:** seizure activity, congenital anomalies
   - **Infection:** meningitis, bronchiolitis, sepsis, croup, influenza, infant botulism, pertussis
   - **Cardiac:** arrhythmia, congestive heart failure, congenital heart abnormalities
   - **Airway abnormalities:** upper and/or lower
   - **Gastrointestinal:** GER, aspiration syndromes
   - **Metabolic:** hypoglycemia, inborn errors of metabolism, toxin (ingestion)
   - **Trauma:** accidental or inflicted head or blunt abdominal injury
   - **Medical child abuse**
   - **Brief resolved unexplained events (BRUEs)**
   - **Idiopathic/unknown cause**

7. **What is periodic breathing?**

   Periodic breathing describes a pattern of a short respiratory pause followed by an increase in respiratory rate that is usually noted during quiet sleep. Periodic breathing occurs in cycles and is a normal pattern in infants. It is unusual for periodic breathing to occur during the first week of life; it occurs more commonly between 2 and 4 weeks, and it typically resolves by 6 months of age. During these episodes, babies are neither plethoric nor cyanotic.

8. **What is sudden infant death syndrome (SIDS)?**
   SIDS is defined as "the sudden death of an infant under 1 year that remains unexplained after a thorough case investigation, including performance of a complete autopsy, examination of the death scene, and review of the clinical history."

9. **What are the risk factors for SIDS?**
   Risk factors for SIDS can be grouped into maternal and infant/environmental risk factors. Maternal risk factors are young age, smoking during pregnancy, and late or no prenatal care. Infant and environmental factors include prematurity, low birth weight, prone sleeping position, sleeping on a soft surface, overheating, and smoking in the home.
   Prone and side sleep positions are associated with an increase in rebreathing of expired gases. Sleeping in the prone position can also increase the risk of overheating by decreasing the rate of heat loss. The prone sleep position is thought to alter the autonomic control of the infant's cardiovascular system during sleep. This can result in decreased cerebral oxygenation.

10. **What practices can minimize the risk of SIDS?**
    All newborns and infants should sleep on their backs. Babies should sleep in the parents' room but on a separate surface, ideally until the infant is 6 months old. Babies should sleep on a firm, flat sleep surface covered by a fitted sheet. Soft bedding (pillows, blankets, and bumper pads) and toys should be kept out of the sleep area. The baby's head should not be covered nor should the baby get overheated. The incidence of SIDS has declined in recent years, likely related to these practices.

11. **What is sudden unexpected infant death (SUID)?**
    "Sudden unexpected infant death" is a term used to describe all unexpected infant deaths. SUIDs are divided into those that are explained and those that are not explained. Unexplained infant deaths include cases of SIDS and other deaths that occur under unclear circumstances. Explained SUIDs would include, among other causes, ingestions, infections, and accidental suffocation.

12. **What is a BRUE?**
    - A BRUE is a sudden, brief, and now-resolved episode in an infant associated with one or more of the following:
      - Cyanosis or pallor
      - Absent, decreased, or irregular breathing
      - Marked change in tone (increase or decrease)
      - Altered level of consciousness
        With a BRUE, the infant is asymptomatic upon presentation and there is no explanation for the event after a complete history and physical examination.
        In 2016 the term BRUE was presented as a replacement for the term "apparent life-threatening event."

13. **How should the evaluation begin for an infant after a BRUE?**
    The evaluation should start with a cardiorespiratory assessment. The patient should be well-appearing. If there are additional findings such as abnormal vital signs, respiratory distress, or fever, the diagnosis of BRUE is no longer appropriate, and management should proceed accordingly.

14. **How should the history be obtained?**
    It is essential to question firsthand observers of the apneic event as objectively as possible. This can be challenging considering the stressful nature of the event. Focus initial questions on determining if the event meets criteria for a BRUE (color change, apnea or decreased/irregular breathing, change in tone, altered consciousness).

15. **Are there specific details that must be included in the history of a BRUE?**
    Yes. Ask these questions to ensure a thorough history:
    - Where did the event take place: in the infant's crib, in another bed, in a car seat?
    - How long did the episode last?
    - Was the infant awake or asleep?
    - Was there a change in the baby's color?
    - Was there a change in tone or posture, or were there abnormal movements?
    - Did the child require resuscitation, and, if so, how did he respond?
    - When was the infant last fed?

16. **Which other questions should be asked in the history of an infant with a BRUE?**
    - **History of present illness:** Prior to the event, was the child well? Are there symptoms of other illnesses, specifically changes in behavior, activity, or appetite? Has there been a recent illness, fever, cough, or cold? Has the infant recently received an immunization?
    - **Past medical history:** Have there been similar episodes in the past? Were there problems with pregnancy, labor, or delivery? What was the child's birth weight? Does the baby have GERD?

- **Family history:** Is there any family history of seizures, infant deaths, or serious illnesses in young family members?
- **Social history:** Who was watching the infant at the time of the episode? Are there medications or other toxins accessible to the child?

17. **What physical examination findings are consistent with the diagnosis of BRUE?**
The physical examination should be normal. As with the history, if there is any abnormality in the physical examination that suggests an etiology for the event, the diagnosis of BRUE should no longer be considered.

18. **Which physical findings indicate a specific cause for an apneic episode?**
Fever or hypothermia suggests the possibility of infection. Tachypnea may be the result of respiratory disease or metabolic acidosis. A young infant with cough or wheezing may have bronchiolitis. A child in shock may have sepsis or hypovolemia from an occult injury. Depressed mental status, bulging fontanel, and papilledema are consistent with central nervous system infection or injury. An infant with dysmorphic features may have an underlying congenital abnormality as the cause of apnea.

19. **What is the diagnostic evaluation for a child after a BRUE?**
There is no standard diagnostic evaluation for infants after a BRUE. The diagnostic evaluation is guided by the classification of the BRUE.
  If the history does not reveal any significant family history, respiratory, feeding, or social concerns and the physical examination is normal, infants meeting the following criteria can be considered low-risk BRUEs:
- Age >60 days
- Born ≥32 weeks' gestation and corrected gestational age >45 weeks
- No cardiopulmonary resuscitation (CPR) provided by a trained medical provider
- Duration <1 minute
- First event
  For those patients meeting low-risk criteria, consideration may be given to pertussis testing, obtaining an electrocardiogram and a period of cardiorespiratory monitoring. Additional diagnostic testing is not recommended. There are no guidelines regarding the appropriate diagnostic evaluation for patients not meeting low-risk criteria.

20. **Should all infants with a BRUE be admitted to the hospital?**
For infants meeting low-risk criteria noted above, admission to the hospital solely for monitoring is not recommended. Families should receive education and CPR training. There are no guidelines regarding admission for patients not meeting low-risk criteria.

21. **Should a home cardiorespiratory monitor be recommended for patients after a BRUE?**
Home cardiorespiratory monitoring is not routinely indicated after a BRUE. It is important to note that home monitoring has never been proven to prevent SIDS nor has the practice of home monitoring changed the incidence of SIDS.

22. **What is the relationship between respiratory syncytial virus (RSV) and apnea?**
RSV can lead to apnea due to respiratory failure from bronchiolitis or from RSV infection without bronchiolitis. The mechanism resulting in apnea is not clear. The incidence of apnea from RSV is difficult to quantify and ranges from 1.2% to 23.8%, depending on the study. Prematurity is the greatest risk factor. Most patients with apnea and RSV infection are younger than 2 months and have been ill for less than 5 days.

KEY POINTS: APNEA, SIDS AND BRUE

- The duration of the pause in respiration in the definition of apnea was not based on evidence, and cyanosis and bradycardia can occur more quickly than 20 seconds.
- Apnea of prematurity is related to underdevelopment of the respiratory and neurological systems and is expected to resolve.
- Apnea in infancy may have serious underlying causes.
- SIDS has decreased with the recommendation that babies sleep on their backs.
- Patients meeting criteria for a low-risk BRUE can be safely discharged home without admission for ongoing monitoring.
- Consider the risk of apnea in an infant less than 2 months old with an RSV infection.
- Home monitoring has not been associated with a decrease in SIDS cases.

Acknowledgment
The author wishes to thank Dr. Susan B. Torrey for her contributions to previous versions of this chapter.

BIBLIOGRAPHY

1. Colombo M, Katz ES, Bosco A, et al. Brief resolved unexplained events: retrospective validation of diagnostic criteria and risk stratification. *Pediatr Pulmonol*. 2019;54(1):61–65.
2. Eichenwald EC. Committee on Fetus and Newborn, American Academy of Pediatrics. Apnea of prematurity. *Pediatrics*. 2016;137(1).
3. Henderson-Smart DJ, De Paoli AG. Methylxanthine treatment for apnoea in preterm infants. *Cochrane Database Syst Rev*. 2010(12):CD000140.
4. Moon RY, Carlin RF, Hand I. Task Force on Sudden Infant Death Syndrome and The Committee on Fetus and Newborn. Evidence base for 2022 updated recommendations for a safe infant sleeping environment to reduce the risk of sleep-related infant deaths. *Pediatrics*. 2022;150(1):e2022057991.
5. Moon RY. Task Force on Sudden Infant Death Syndrome. SIDS and other sleep-related infant deaths: evidence base for 2016 updated recommendations for a safe infant sleeping environment. *Pediatrics*. 2016;138(5):e20162940.
6. Poets A, Steinfeldt R, Poets CF. Sudden deaths and severe apparent life-threatening events in term infants within 24 hours of birth. *Pediatrics*. 2011;127(4):e869–e873.
7. Ralston S, Hill V. Incidence of apnea in infants hospitalized with respiratory syncytial virus bronchiolitis: a systematic review. *J Pediatr*. 2009;155(5):728–733.
8. Shapiro-Mendoza CK, Palusci VJ, Hoffman B, et al. Half century since SIDS: a reappraisal of terminology. *Pediatrics*. 2021;148(4):e2021053746.
9. Tieder JS, Bonkowsky JL, Etzel RA, et al. Clinical practice guideline: brief resolved unexplained events (formerly apparent life-threatening events) and evaluation of lower-risk infants: executive summary. *Pediatrics*. 2016;137(5):e20160591.

CHAPTER 8

CHEST PAIN

Courtney E. Nelson and Steven M. Selbst

1. **How common is chest pain in children?**
   Chest pain is a common pediatric complaint. It is not nearly as frequent as abdominal pain or headache, but it is perhaps the third leading pain syndrome in children. Chest pain has been reported to occur in 0.3% to 0.6% of visits to a pediatric emergency department (ED). It affects children of all ages, and half of the children with chest pain are younger than 12 years of age.

2. **How does the cause of chest pain in children differ from that in adults?**
   Children with chest pain are far less likely to have a cardiac cause for their pain. Studies have found that only about 0.6% to 4% of children who present to a pediatric ED with chest pain have a cardiac cause for their pain, and some of those children were already known to have heart disease at the time of presentation. If a cardiac source of chest pain is identified, arrhythmia is the most common cause, followed by cardiac infections. Fortunately, most children with chest pain have a self-limited and "benign" cause, but the pain should always be taken seriously.

3. **Which diagnoses are most common in children who present to an ED with chest pain?**
   In many studies, up to 45% of cases of chest pain in children are labeled "idiopathic." That is, after a careful history and physical examination, the cause is still uncertain. When a diagnosis can be found, musculoskeletal injury is the most common. Costochondritis accounts for about 10% to 20% of cases of chest pain. This disorder produces tenderness over the costochondral junctions and is often bilateral. It is exaggerated by physical activity or breathing. Pain is often reproducible by palpation of the chest wall or by moving the arms and chest in a variety of positions. Table 8.1 lists the most common causes of pediatric chest pain.

4. **How is the cause of chest pain related to the child's age?**
   Young children are more likely to have chest pain related to a cardiorespiratory condition (cough, asthma, pneumonia, or heart disease). Children over the age of 12 years are more likely to have a psychogenic disturbance as the cause of their pain.

5. **What common gastrointestinal condition causes chest pain?**
   Gastroesophageal reflux, which is very common in children, accounts for at least 7% of instances of pediatric chest pain. The pain is usually worse in the recumbent position. History may reveal that the pain is "burning" in quality and may have developed after eating spicy foods. A trial of antacids is often diagnostic and therapeutic.

Table 8.1 Most Common Causes of Pediatric Chest Pain

Idiopathic Causes
Musculoskeletal conditions
Chest wall strain
Costochondritis
Direct trauma

Respiratory Conditions
Asthma
Cough
Pneumonia

Gastrointestinal Problems
Esophagitis
Esophageal foreign body

Psychogenic Causes (Stress Related)

Cardiac Disease
Myocarditis

KEY POINTS: MOST COMMON CAUSES OF CHILDHOOD CHEST PAIN

- Musculoskeletal pain
- Idiopathic cause
- Pulmonary conditions
- Psychological cause
- Trauma
- Gastrointestinal problems
- Cardiac disease
- Sickle cell disease

---

6. **What is precordial catch syndrome?**
   In 1955 Miller and Texidor described a syndrome of left-sided chest pain that is brief (less than a 5-minute duration) and sporadic. This pain may recur frequently for a few hours in some individuals and then remain absent for several months. The pain seems to be associated with a slouched posture or bending and is not related to exercise. It is usually relieved when the individual takes a few shallow breaths, or sometimes one deep breath, and assumes a straightened posture. It is believed that the pain arises from the parietal pleura or from pressure on an intercostal nerve, but the cause remains unclear. Some refer to this pain syndrome as "Texidor twinge" or a "stitch in the side."

7. **What is "slipping rib syndrome"?**
   This is a rare sprain disorder caused by trauma to the costal cartilage of the 8th, 9th, and 10th ribs, which do not attach to the sternum. Children with slipping rib syndrome report pain under the ribs or in the upper abdominal quadrants. They also hear a clicking or popping sound when they lift objects, flex the trunk, or even walk. It is believed that the pain is caused by one of the ribs hooking under the rib above and irritating the intercostal nerves. The pain can be duplicated, and the syndrome can be confirmed by performing the "hooking maneuver," whereby the affected rib margin is grasped and then pulled anteriorly. Intercostal block has been tried for pain relief. Surgery to resect the involved costal cartilage may provide long-term relief, though most patients are treated satisfactorily with oral analgesics.

8. **How can ingestion of medications in pill form lead to chest pain?**
   Patients can develop acute pill-induced esophagitis when swallowing medications, most commonly antibiotics such as tetracycline and doxycycline. The pain is especially likely if the patient takes the medication with a minimal amount of water and then lies down. A history of esophageal dysmotility or stricture makes the pain more likely. Because of the pH of the drug, doxycycline produces an acidic solution or gel as it dissolves, and thus it is caustic when it remains in the esophagus.

   The physical examination is generally unremarkable for these patients. Midesophageal ulcers are most common as the tablets are most likely to lodge in that location. Endoscopy can provide definitive diagnosis; however, discontinuing the inciting agent and treatment with sucralfate can be both diagnostic and therapeutic.

9. **When should a pneumothorax be suspected in a child with chest pain?**
   Suspect a pneumothorax if a child develops acute onset of sharp chest pain associated with some degree of respiratory distress. The pain is usually worsened by inspiration and may radiate to the shoulder, neck, or even abdomen. Children with this condition almost always present for care within 48 hours of developing the pneumothorax. The patient will usually have dyspnea, tachycardia, and, perhaps, decreased breath sounds on the affected side or even cyanosis. However, these signs and symptoms depend on the size of the pneumothorax and whether it is under tension (Fig. 8.1). A small pneumothorax may produce minimal findings on examination. History of trauma may increase your suspicion of pneumothorax, but many cases occur spontaneously or with exercise, cough, or just stretching. In those cases, a small, unrecognized subpleural bleb ruptures, leading to the air leak.

10. **What underlying conditions should be considered with a spontaneous pneumothorax in the absence of trauma?**
    Patients with asthma, cystic fibrosis, and Marfan syndrome are particularly prone to chest pain secondary to pneumothorax. Also, several cases have been reported in teenagers who smoke crack cocaine.

11. **How can anxiety or emotional stress lead to chest pain in children?**
    The relationship of pain to emotional stress is not quite clear. Studies have shown that stress (psychogenic pain) is the cause in about 10% of children with chest pain who present to pediatric ED. Possible stressors include poor success in school, recent death or illness in the family, recent loss of friends from moving to a new city or school, bullying, and school phobia. This should not always be a diagnosis of exclusion; if significant stress is temporally related to the pain, it is a reasonable diagnosis.

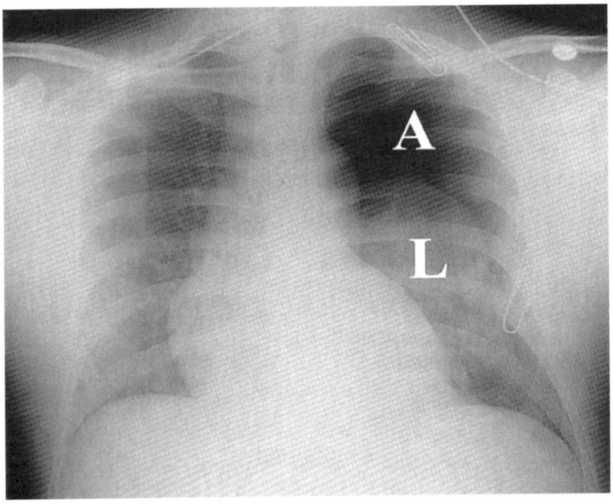

Fig. 8.1 Tension pneumothorax on a frontal chest radiograph. Note the thin, sharply defined visceral pleural "white" line between radiolucent lung (*L*) and radiolucent "black" free air (*A*) in the peripheral pleural space in addition to rightward mediastinal shift and inferior left hemidiaphragmatic shift due to the air under tension. (From Torigian DA, Miller WT Jr. Pleural diseases. In: Pretorius ES, Solomon JA, eds. *Radiology Secrets.* 2nd ed. Mosby; 2006:541.)

12. **Why do some adolescents who present with hyperventilation also have chest pain?**
    Hyperventilation may be associated with psychogenic chest pain and may lead to pain by producing a hypocapnic alkalosis. Prolonged hyperventilation can lead to coronary artery vasoconstriction and chest pain. Also, stomach distention due to concomitant aerophagia can occur with hyperventilation and produce chest pain.

13. **Which children with chest pain should receive an evaluation with an electrocardiogram (ECG) and chest radiograph?**
    - Those with worrisome historical features:
      - Acute onset of pain
      - Chest pain associated with exercise
      - Associated syncope, dizziness, palpitations
      - History of heart disease
      - History of a condition that can affect the heart or lungs—diabetes mellitus, Kawasaki disease, Marfan syndrome, asthma, anemia, systemic lupus erythematosus
      - History of sickle cell disease
      - Use of cocaine or vaping
      - Trauma
      - Foreign body ingestion
      - Fever
    - Those with abnormal findings on examination:
      - Respiratory distress
      - Decreased or abnormal breath sounds
      - Cardiac findings (murmur, rub, click, arrhythmia)
      - Fever
      - Trauma
      - Palpation of subcutaneous air

14. **Which children with chest pain do not need extensive evaluation with laboratory studies in the ED?**
    Those with chronic pain (and none of the worrisome features mentioned previously) do not require further evaluation. Management must be individualized, but most patients can be managed with analgesics, reassurance that cardiac disease is unlikely, and close follow-up.

15. **Why is chest pain of acute onset more worrisome?**
    Children with sudden onset of pain (within 48 hours of presentation) are more likely to have an organic cause for the pain. It is not necessarily a serious cause, but pneumonia, asthma, trauma, and pneumothorax are more likely.

16. **Why is fever associated with chest pain of concern?**

Fever is much more likely to be associated with an infectious source. Certainly, pneumonia must be considered, but also evaluate for myocarditis and pericarditis. Myocarditis is more common and usually presents with low-grade fever and dull substernal chest pain. There is often respiratory distress as the infection progresses, and there may be muffled heart sounds or a gallop rhythm heard. Tachypnea is common, and tachycardia out of proportion to the degree of fever is characteristic. Tachycardia and hypotension may be worse with standing, and this may not resolve after fluid resuscitation. A chest radiograph often reveals cardiomegaly (Fig. 8.2). Those with pericarditis may report a sharp, stabbing midsternal pain that is somewhat relieved when the patient sits up and leans forward. Distant heart sounds, neck vein distention, and a friction rub may be found. Endocarditis is a very rare condition in otherwise healthy adolescents but should also be considered. Also, consider COVID-19 infection (see Question 20).

KEY POINTS: FEVER AND CHEST PAIN

- Consider pneumonia, myocarditis, and pericarditis.
- Listen for decreased breath sounds (pneumonia).
- Listen for distant heart sounds (pericarditis, myocarditis).
- Obtain a chest radiograph.
- Consider an ECG if pneumonia is excluded.

17. **Which cardiac conditions can cause chest pain in children?**
- **Arrhythmia:** Supraventricular tachycardia (SVT) or ventricular tachycardia
- **Infection:** Myocarditis, pericarditis, or endocarditis
- **Structural abnormalities:** Hypertrophic cardiomyopathy, aortic valve stenosis, or anomalous coronary arteries
- **Coronary artery disease (CAD), ischemia, or infarction:** Kawasaki disease, long-standing diabetes mellitus, familial hypercholesterolemia, or lipidemia

18. **Which arrhythmias can possibly cause chest pain in children?**

Consider the possibility of an arrhythmia such as SVT as a cause of chest pain in an older child who reports having palpitations. Ventricular tachycardia and premature ventricular contractions are rare in children but may also cause sharp chest pain and an irregular cardiac rhythm. Arrhythmias may be found in children taking various medications or drugs such as cocaine.

19. **How helpful is the ECG or troponin level in the diagnosis of myocarditis or pericarditis?**

The ECG in patients with myocarditis is usually abnormal, but there is no specific rhythm associated with myocarditis. The most common ECG abnormality is sinus tachycardia. Troponin levels are elevated in roughly 80% of cases but can be normal and should not be used in isolation to exclude myocarditis. One study showed troponin has 100% sensitivity, 85% specificity, and 100% negative predictive value for myocarditis. Endomyocardial biopsy is the gold standard for diagnosing myocarditis, but it is an invasive test. Cardiac magnetic resonance imaging (CMRI) is increasingly used to confirm the diagnosis of myocarditis.

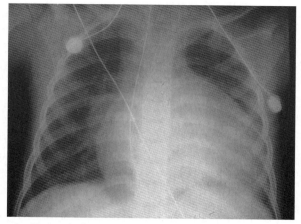

Fig. 8.2 Radiograph of large heart from myocarditis.

Patients with pericarditis go through several different ECG changes and can have a normal ECG at presentation. Similarly, troponin levels can be elevated but are not a negative predictive factor for pericarditis. Echocardiography can be helpful if a small effusion is seen, but the absence of a pericardial effusion does not exclude pericarditis. CMRI may be helpful in cases that are atypical or inconclusive.

20. **Can chest pain be related to coronavirus disease 2019 (COVID-19) infection?**
Yes. Acute COVID-19 infection has been associated with arrhythmias, pericarditis, and myocarditis. Likewise, following a COVID-19 infection, a rare complication known as multisystem inflammatory syndrome in children (MIS-C) can present with cardiac manifestations and, in the most severe cases, cardiogenic shock.

21. **Does the COVID-19 vaccine cause chest pain?**
Very rarely. Myocarditis after the COVID-19 mRNA vaccination is a very rare complication. Nearly all cases are seen 2 to 3 days after the second dose of the vaccine. Risk factors include male sex and age 16 to 24 years. Most patients present with chest pain. All patients have an elevated troponin level, and a majority of patients have abnormal ECG findings. Nearly all patients have complete resolution of symptoms regardless of treatment.

22. **When should I be concerned about ischemia or myocardial infarction (MI) in a pediatric patient with chest pain?**
Myocardial ischemia or infarction should be considered in any child with chest pain that is related to exercise or syncope. Some rare conditions may lead to ischemic myocardial dysfunction in children. For instance, hypertrophic cardiomyopathy can cause pain, especially with exercise. Aortic valve stenosis can also cause ischemia and chest pain, and those who had cardiac surgery for repair of transposition of the great vessels are at risk for subsequent MI. Finally, those with underlying problems with the coronary arteries may develop chest pain. This is not common in children, but some children with an anomalous left coronary artery, thrombophilia, familial hypercholesterolemia, and long-standing diabetes mellitus may have CAD, and children who had Kawasaki disease in the past may have persistent coronary artery aneurysms that can produce symptoms long after the initial illness.

KEY POINTS: CARDIAC CAUSES OF CHEST PAIN

- CAD: arteritis from Kawasaki disease, long-standing diabetes mellitus
- Arrhythmias: SVT, premature ventricular contractions, ventricular tachycardia
- Structural lesions: hypertrophic cardiomyopathy, aortic valve stenosis
- Infections: myocarditis, pericarditis, endocarditis

23. **Why is chest pain associated with exercise of concern?**
Young children with sudden deaths often had preceding chest pain with exercise. Pain related to serious conditions such as myocarditis, CAD, and hypertrophic cardiomyopathy is worsened by exertion. Consider obtaining troponin levels as well as an ECG and chest x-ray for these patients. Such patients should be told to avoid all physical activity until seen by a cardiologist for further testing, including echocardiography, Holter monitoring, or possibly exercise stress tests. Exercise-induced asthma is another condition in which chest pain is precipitated or worsened by exercise.

24. **What are the concerns of children with Marfan syndrome who report chest pain?**
These children may report chest pain due to the rupture of an aortic aneurysm, which can be fatal. They are also at risk for spontaneous pneumothorax. Consider this condition in a tall, thin patient with an upper extremity span that exceeds their height.

25. **Why do children with asthma report chest pain?**
Some possible causes include anxiety and overuse of chest wall muscles due to respiratory distress. Some have an associated pneumonia that could lead to diaphragmatic irritation. Others may develop a pneumothorax or pneumomediastinum.

26. **What cause should be considered in an afebrile, previously well toddler with no injury who reports sudden midsternal chest pain?**
Foreign body in the esophagus! Many young children ingest coins or button batteries, and most are asymptomatic. However, if the coin or battery lodges in the esophagus (especially in the upper esophagus), the child may report sudden chest pain. Dysphagia may also be present. A chest radiograph usually confirms the diagnosis.

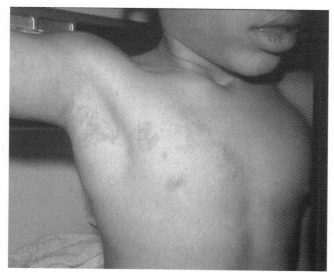

Fig. 8.3 Herpes zoster infection.

27. **When would you suspect hypertrophic cardiomyopathy in a child with chest pain?**
There may be a positive family history for this condition. It is generally inherited as an autosomal dominant disorder. A murmur may be heard best when the child is standing or performing a Valsalva maneuver. These positions and exercises may exaggerate the chest pain. Squatting or lying supine minimizes the obstruction and reduces the murmur. Shortness of breath is the most common symptom. This condition is concerning because it is among the leading causes of sudden death among young athletes.

28. **Name a cutaneous condition that is associated with chest pain.**
Herpes zoster infection (Fig. 8.3). Shingles is often associated with distressing chest pain when the lesions involve a chest wall dermatome. The chest pain can sometimes precede the vesicular rash by several days.

29. **What is the "devil's grip"?**
This unusual condition, also known as *pleurodynia*, is characterized by paroxysms of sharp pain in the abdomen or thorax. It is caused by coxsackievirus and may occur in mini-epidemics.

30. **What are the possible causes of chest pain in a teenage girl with systemic lupus erythematosus?**
These patients are at risk for pericarditis, myocarditis, endocarditis, pneumonia, pleural effusion, and myocardial ischemia if they have renal disease and hypertension.

31. **Should pulmonary embolism (PE) be considered as a cause of chest pain in a child?**
PE is a rare problem in children. Consider it in a patient with minor trauma to a lower extremity (usually a male) or any patient with increased likelihood of clotting or a hypercoagulable state (e.g., nephrotic syndrome). It is very rarely reported in teenage girls who are obese (body mass index > 25 kg/m^2), have deep vein thrombosis, systemic lupus erythematosus, or use oral contraceptives, and in those who have recently had an elective abortion. A patient with a PE usually has accompanying shortness of breath, pleuritic chest pain, fever, cough, and hemoptysis. The finding of a swollen, tender lower extremity on physical examination increases concern about venous thrombosis and a PE.

32. **Is a D-dimer diagnostic for PE in children?**
D-Dimer is a protein fragment present in the blood after a clot is degraded. It is often used in adult medicine as part of the workup for thrombosis. Unfortunately, some studies show D-dimer levels are neither sensitive nor specific for PE in pediatric patients. Similarly, the Wells criteria and Pulmonary Embolism Rule-out Criteria are not predictive of PE in children. One recent study showed D-dimer to be a very useful test to diagnose or exclude PE in adolescent patients who have the risk factors noted above. The diagnostic sensitivity was 89% and specificity was 54%. This suggests that, in patients with low clinical probability, a normal D-dimer can safely exclude PE

in children. If there is persistent concern for a PE in a pediatric patient, advanced imaging such as a computed tomography angiogram or ventilation-perfusion scan is necessary.

33. **What are the likely causes of chest pain in children with sickle cell disease?**
Vaso-occlusive crisis may be the cause of pain. However, consider acute chest syndrome in these patients. Pneumonia due to an encapsulated organism is also of concern. Though rarer, patients with sickle cell disease are at an increased risk for PE and testing for PE should be considered in the appropriate clinical setting. Finally, ischemia due to a heart weakened by chronic anemia is possible. All such patients should receive a chest radiograph and perhaps an ECG as part of their evaluation.

34. **Chest pain associated with a "crunching" sound on chest examination is found in which condition?**
Pneumomediasnum. This results in free mediastinal air and subcutaneous emphysema. It can be spontaneous or caused due to asthma exacerbation or trauma. Some children with this finding have associated dyspnea and cough. Crepitation is often noted in the suprasternal notch and may extend to the neck, axilla, and face. A chest radiograph confirms the diagnosis. The condition usually has a good outcome and resolves within a few days. Hospital admission and treatment of the underlying cause are recommended.

35. **Can drug use cause chest pain?**
Yes. Patients who abuse cocaine may complain of "chest tightness," "palpitations," and "pressure," and they may have associated nausea, vomiting, and anxiety. Physical examination may reveal tachycardia, tachypnea, and hypertension. Cocaine can also cause coronary artery vasospasm. The incidence of MI with cocaine abuse is as high as 6% in adults, but the incidence in adolescents is unknown. Some adolescents who snort cocaine may develop a pneumothorax or pneumomediastinum.
      Similarly, methamphetamines can also cause chest pain. Consider screening for illicit drugs in all teens with chest pain. An ECG may show ischemia or arrhythmia. Serum cardiac enzymes (troponins) may be elevated, indicating evidence of an MI.

36. **Can E-cigarette use cause chest pain?**
E-cigarettes are now the most common tobacco product used by US teens. Vaping solution can contain varying levels of nicotine, tetrahydrocannabinol, flavorings, and other additives. There are several cases of spontaneous pneumothorax related to vaping. A chest x-ray is indicated for any pediatric patient with chest pain and history of vaping.

37. **When should a referral to a cardiologist be considered for a child with chest pain?**
Chest pain associated with exercise (during or immediately after) or syncope requires an evaluation by a cardiologist. If the pediatric patient has pain associated with dizziness or palpitations, evaluation by a cardiologist is also reasonable. Furthermore, if the child has a history of underlying heart disease or cardiac arrhythmia or has a previous condition that subjects them to heart disease (i.e., long-standing diabetes mellitus, Kawasaki disease, MIS-C), referral to a cardiologist is prudent. It is also recommended to have a cardiologist evaluate the child if there is a history of premature sudden death in the family or if the child has hypertension or features of Marfan syndrome.

BIBLIOGRAPHY

1. Agha BS, Sturm JJ, Simon HK, et al. Pulmonary embolism in the pediatric emergency department. *Pediatrics*. 2013;132:663–667.
2. Alsaied T, Tremoulet AH, Burns JC, et al. Review of cardiac involvement in multisystem inflammatory syndrome in children. *Circulation*. 2021;143(1):78–88.
3. Ashraf O, Nasrullah A, Karna R, Alhajhusain A. Vaping associated spontaneous pneumothorax – a case series of an enigmatic entity! *Respir Med Case Rep*. 2021;34:101535.
4. Barbut G, Needleman JP. Pediatric chest pain. *Pediatr Rev*. 2020;41:469–480.
5. Biss TT, Brandão LR, Kahr WH, et al. Clinical probability score and D-dimer estimation lack utility in the diagnosis of childhood pulmonary embolism. *J Thromb Haemost*. 2009;7(10):1633.
6. Brancato F, DeRosa G, Gambacorta A, et al. Role of troponin determination to diagnose chest pain in the pediatric emergency department. *Pediatr Emerg Care*. 2021;37:e1589–1592.
7. Brown JL, Mahle WT. Use of troponin as a screen for chest pain in the pediatric emergency department. *Pediatr Cardiol*. 2012;33:337–342.
8. Dalal A, Czosek RJ, Kovach J, et al. Clinical presentation of pediatric patients at risk for sudden cardiac arrest. *J Pediatr*. 2016;177:191–196.
9. Drossner DM, Hirsh DA, Sturm JJ, et al. Cardiac disease in pediatric patients presenting to a pediatric ED with chest pain. *Am J Emerg Med*. 2011;29:632–638.
10. Durani Y, Egan M, Baffa J, et al. Pediatric myocarditis presenting clinical characteristics. *Am J Emerg Med*. 2009;27:942–947.
11. Eliacik K, Bolot N, Kanik A, et al. Adolescents with unexplained chest pain reported depression and impaired emotional and social functioning. *Acta Paediatr*. 2020;109:1642–1648.
12. Foley CM, Sugimoto D, Mooney DP, et al. Diagnosis and treatment of slipping rib syndrome. *Clin J Sports Med*. 2019;29:18–23.

13. Friedman KG, Alexander ME. Chest pain and syncope in children: a practical approach to the diagnosis of cardiac disease. *J Pediatr.* 2013;163:896–901.
14. Gasser CRB, Pellaton R, Rochat CP. Pediatric spontaneous pneumomediastinum: narrative literature review. *Pediatr Emerg Care.* 2017;33:370–374.
15. Haynes Jr D, Younger BR, Mansour HM, et al. Precordial catch syndrome. *Pediatr Emerg Care.* 2016;32:104–106.
16. Hennelly KE, Baskin MN, Monuteaux MC, et al. Detection of pulmonary embolism in high-risk children. *J Pediatr.* 2016;178:214–218.e3.
17. Hsu BS, Guillot Mosher J, et al. Chest pain and elevated troponin in a teenager. *Pediatr Rev.* 2017;38:388–390.
18. Imazio M, Gaita F, LeWinter M. Evaluation and treatment of pericarditis. A systematic review. *JAMA.* 2015;314:1498–1506.
19. Jain SS, Steele JM, Fonseca B, et al. COVID-19 vaccination–associated myocarditis in adolescents. *Pediatrics.* 2021;148(5):e2021053427.
20. Jain S, Bakshi N, Krishnamurti L. Acute chest syndrome in children with sickle cell disease. *Pediatr Allergy Immunol Pulmonol.* 2017;30:191–201.
21. Kanis J, Hall CL, Pike J, et al. Diagnostic accuracy of the D-dimer in children. *Arch Dis Child.* 2018;103:832–834.
22. Kaslow JA, Rosas-Salazar C, Moore PE. E-cigarette and vaping product use-associated lung injury in the pediatric population: a critical review of the current literature. *Pediatr Pulmonol.* 2021;56(7):1857–1867.
23. Khairandish Z, Jamali L, Haghbin S. Role of anxiety and depression in adolescents with chest pain referred to a cardiology clinic. *Cardiol Young.* 2017;27:125–130.
24. Lee TM, Hsu DT, Lipshultz SE. Pediatric cardiomyopathies. *Circ Res.* 2017;121:855–873.
25. Mahle WT, Campbell RM, Favaloro-Sabatier J. Myocardial infarction in adolescents. *J Pediatr.* 2007;151:150–154.
26. Majerus CR, Tredway TL, Yun NK, Gerard JM. Utility of chest radiographs in childrenpresenting to a pediatric emergency department with acute asthma[Q6] exacerbation and chestpain. *Pediatr Emerg Care.* 2021;37(7):e372–e375.
27. Martinez-Villar M, Gran F, Sabate-Rotes A, et al. Acute myocarditis with infarct-like presentation in a pediatric population: role of cardiovascular magnetic resonance. *Pediatr Cardiol.* 2018;39:51–56.
28. McCrindle BW, Rowley AH, Newburger JW, et al. Diagnosis, treatment and long-term management of Kawasaki Disease: a scientific statement for health professionals from the American Heart Association. *Circulation.* 2017;135:e927.
29. McMahon LE. Slipping rib syndrome: a review of evaluation, diagnosis and treatment. *Semin Pediatr Surg.* 2018;27:183–188.
30. Mohan S, Nandi D, Stephens P, et al. Implementation of a clinical pathway for chest pain in a pediatric emergency department. *Pediatr Emerg Care.* 2018;34:778–782.
31. Pettit MA, Koyfman A, Foran M. Myocarditis. *Pediatr Emerg Care.* 2014;30(11):832–835.
32. Ramphul K, Mejias SG, Joynauth J. Cocaine, amphetamines and cannabis use increases the risk of acute myocardial infarction in teenagers. *Am J Cardiol.* 2019;123:354.
33. Saleeb SF, Li WYV, Warren SZ, et al. Effectiveness of screening for life-threatening chest pain in children. *Pediatrics.* 2011;128:e1062–e1068.
34. Sumski CA, Goot BH. Evaluating chest pain and heart murmurs in pediatric and adolescent patients. *Pediatr Clin North Am.* 2020;67:783–799.
35. Selbst SM, Ruddy RM, Clark BJ, et al. Pediatric chest pain: a prosp-ective study. *Pediatrics.* 1988;82:319–323.
36. Selbst SM. Approach to the child with chest pain. *Pediatr Clin North Am.* 2010;57(6):1221–1234.
37. Sharaf N, Sharaf VB, Mace SE, et al. D-Dimer in adolescent pulmonary embolism. *Acad Emerg Med.* 2018;25(11):1235–1241.
38. Sharma J, Fernandes N, Alvarez D, et al. Acute myopericarditis in an adolescent mimicking myocardial infarction. *Pediatr Emerg Care.* 2015;31:427–430.
39. Smith N, DelGrippo E, Selbst SM. Approach to the adolescent with chest pain. In: Goyal M, Rowlett J, Greydanus DE, eds. *AM: STARs Adolescent Medicine: State of the Art Reviews.* American Academy of Pediatrics; 2016:528–551.
40. Varney JA, Dong VS, Tsao T, et al. COVID-19 and arrhythmia: an overview. *J Cardiol.* 2022;79(4):468–475.
41. Yeh TK, Yeh J. Chest pain in pediatrics. *Pediatr Ann.* 2015;44:e274–e278.

CHAPTER 9

COUGH

Todd A. Florin

1. **Describe the cough reflex.**

   The cough reflex is designed to clear the airway. Mechanical (e.g., foreign body, dust), chemical (e.g., capsaicin, acetic acid), or inflammatory mediators (e.g., histamine, bradykinin, prostaglandin E_2) can induce the cough reflex. Such stimuli interact with cough receptors in the upper and lower airways that cause the production of mediators, such as tachykinins and neurokinin A. Stimulation of the cough receptors is transmitted via the vagus nerve to the "cough center" of the brainstem. Direct (central) stimulation of a cough center in the brain occurs more rarely. The efferent limb of the cough pathway is poorly understood but is known to include the spinal cord from C3 to S2, spinal nerves, and the recurrent laryngeal nerve (for glottic closure). Activation of the efferent pathway causes constriction of the expiratory muscles, which produces increased airway pressure against the closed glottis. The airway also narrows slightly. When the glottis is suddenly opened, air is expelled at a high velocity, clearing the airway of secretions and foreign material.

2. **How is a cough suppressed?**

   As with respiration, coughing is largely involuntary but can be suppressed voluntarily to a certain extent (cortical modulation). Opioids that suppress cough (e.g., morphine) are believed to produce this effect by acting centrally on the cough center. Inhalation of nebulized lidocaine can suppress cough by affecting cough receptors in the airway.

3. **Is the cough reflex mediated by the same pathway that produces bronchospasm?**

   There has been a widely held belief that airway hypersensitivity (asthma/bronchospasm) and cough are manifestations of the same physiologic mechanism. By this thinking, persistent coughing, like wheezing, is a common presentation of asthma. This view has led, in part, to the practice of diagnosing children with persistent coughing with "cough-variant" asthma, even when these patients have no other evidence of bronchospasm (dyspnea, exercise intolerance, abnormal spirometry findings). However, evidence suggests that although airway hypersensitivity and cough receptor sensitivity can be *triggered* by the same stimuli, this probably occurs via two *different* pathways. For most children, it appears that persistent coughing results solely from increased sensitivity of cough receptors in the upper and lower airways and does not represent true asthma/bronchospasm.

4. **How much coughing is normal?**

   When cough meters were used in healthy children with no symptoms of respiratory illness, the range of cough episodes over 24 hours was 1 to 34 in one study and 0 to 141 in another study. The frequency of coughing episodes thus varies widely, even among children without respiratory problems. This occurrence of cough in healthy children has been referred to as "expected cough," and the normal variability within the population should be kept in mind when evaluating a pediatric patient with cough.

5. **What is the most common cause of an acute cough?**

   Cough in children can be characterized based on duration as acute (<2 weeks), protracted acute (2-4 weeks), and chronic (>4 weeks). Although the differential diagnosis of acute cough in children is relatively broad (Table 9.1), the most common causes include upper respiratory infections, laryngotracheitis, bronchiolitis, bronchitis, pneumonia, rhinitis, and reactive airways disease. The most common cause is probably postviral or inflammatory cough, which has also been called *nonspecific cough, isolated cough,* or *cough illness.* Children who develop a viral upper respiratory tract infection may continue to cough long after other viral symptoms (e.g., rhinitis, fever) have subsided. Patients often have a persistent dry cough (particularly at night) but do not have symptoms of bronchospasm. When symptoms of a preceding upper respiratory illness are elicited in a child with a persistent dry cough and no other associated symptoms (chest pain, rhinitis, recurrent fevers), reassurance that the coughing will most likely subside spontaneously is generally appropriate. However, for children who continue to cough beyond 4 weeks, further evaluation or referral to a specialist may be warranted.

6. **What are the most common causes of chronic cough in children?**

   The three most common causes of chronic cough in children are asthma, protracted bacterial bronchitis (PBB), and nonspecific cough. Importantly, the causes of chronic cough in children are different from those of adults; thus evaluating a child with chronic cough should use an age-specific approach. In fact, gastroesophageal

Table 9.1 Differential Diagnosis of Cough in Children

Infection
Upper respiratory infection
Sinusitis
Tonsillitis
Laryngitis
Laryngotracheitis (croup)
Tracheitis/tracheobronchitis
Bronchiolitis
Acute bronchitis
Pneumonia/empyema
Pleuritis/pleural effusion
Bronchiectasis/pulmonary abscess

Inflammation/Allergy
Allergic rhinitis
Laryngeal edema
Reactive airway disease
Chronic bronchitis
Cystic fibrosis
Vocal cord dysfunction

Mechanical or Chemical Irritation
Foreign body aspiration
Neck/chest trauma
Chemical fumes
Inhaled particulates
Smoking

Neoplasm
Pharyngeal or nasal polyp
Hemangioma of the larynx or trachea
Papilloma of the larynx or trachea
Lymphoma compresses the airway
Mediastinal tumors

Congenital Anomalies
Cleft palate
Laryngotracheomalacia
Laryngeal or tracheal webs
Tracheoesophageal fistula
Vascular ring
Pulmonary sequestration

Miscellaneous
Gastroesophageal reflux
Congestive heart failure
Swallowing dysfunction
Granulomatous diseases (e.g., pulmonary tuberculosis)
Vasculitis (e.g., granulomatosis with polyangiitis)
Psychogenic cough
Foreign body in otic canal
Medications (e.g., angiotensin-converting enzyme inhibitors)

reflux disease and postnasal drip, common causes of chronic cough in adults, are likely not common causes in children. In young children with failure to thrive or recurrent pulmonary infections, cystic fibrosis should be considered. Chronic cough with a history of recurrent pneumonias or chronic bronchitis can be suggestive of immunodeficiency or anatomic lesions.

7. **Is cough-variant asthma underdiagnosed?**
No. In fact, the opposite is more likely to be the case. In the past, children with persistent cough accompanied by the signs of true bronchospasm such as exercise intolerance, but without wheezing, were often not diagnosed with asthma. The syndrome of cough and acute exertional dyspnea was first identified in a series of adult patients in 1975, and the term *cough-variant asthma* was coined in 1979. Before that time, cough-variant asthma was certainly underdiagnosed. Now, however, the diagnosis of asthma in children with isolated cough has been widely embraced. In fact, some have suggested that recent increases in the prevalence of asthma are largely due to expanding the diagnostic criteria to include children with isolated cough. This has occurred despite evidence that many of these patients do not respond to conventional asthma therapy. It would appear that the pendulum has swung too far, and we are currently overdiagnosing and overtreating asthma in patients with other causes of cough.

8. **Do children with persistent cough respond to standard therapy for asthma?**
Given the caveats described in the previous question, it is safe to say that children with true cough-variant asthma should respond to treatment with bronchodilators or steroids within hours to a few days. However, these patients represent a relatively small percentage of the children presenting to the emergency department (ED) with a persistent cough. Most of them will have nonspecific cough that does *not* respond to conventional asthma therapy. Therefore unless a child with persistent cough has a history that suggests a true bronchospastic cause (severe cough and dyspnea occurring consistently with exertion), it is not generally wise to make a de novo diagnosis of cough-variant asthma and initiate bronchodilator or steroid treatment. Conversely, if a child has been receiving conventional asthma therapy for several days to weeks and coughing has not decreased, the patient is very unlikely to have cough-variant asthma, and the asthma treatments can be stopped.

9. **Does cough due to bronchitis respond to treatment with antibiotics?**
Most clinicians use the term *acute bronchitis* when referring to a patient who has a cough, with or without sputum production, without evidence of pneumonia. The diagnostic criteria for bronchitis are ambiguous, a situation that is exacerbated in children who tend to swallow rather than expectorate sputum. Some have used the term *wet* cough to identify a productive cough in children, and there is some evidence indicating that a chronic wet cough is more likely to be associated with a bacterial cause in pediatric patients. PBB is one of the most common causes of chronic cough in young children. The diagnostic criteria for PBB include a wet cough lasting more than 4 weeks with no symptoms of other causes and no evidence of an alternative diagnosis on radiography or spirometry. PBB generally responds after a 2-week course of antibiotics. Proper antibiotic treatment of PBB is important to prevent the development of bronchiectasis. It is important to recognize, however, that for the more common presentation of a child with "acute bronchitis" who has an isolated dry cough lasting days to a few weeks, antibiotics should not be prescribed.

10. **What is a staccato cough?**
A "staccato" cough is the classic finding in an infant with *Chlamydia trachomatis* pneumonia. It is a repetitive, dry, "rapid-fire" cough with inspiration between each single cough. Typically presenting as an insidious, afebrile pneumonitis syndrome in infants between the ages of about 3 weeks and 3 months, *C. trachomatis* pneumonia causes progressively worsening respiratory symptoms, with chest x-ray findings of bilateral pulmonary infiltrates and air-trapping. Diffuse crackles without wheezing are usually heard on chest auscultation. Conjunctivitis is present in about half of cases, and laboratory results may demonstrate peripheral eosinophilia. Very young infants can have more severe disease with episodes of apnea, but the overall prognosis of this condition in pediatric patients is good. In most cases, first-line antibiotic therapy for *C. trachomatis* pneumonia is oral erythromycin, but it should be remembered that this treatment has been associated with pyloric stenosis in infants younger than 4 to 6 weeks of age. Because the benefits of treatment outweigh the risks in this circumstance, caretakers should be apprised of the symptoms of pyloric stenosis and the need for reevaluation should these symptoms occur.

11. **What is a paroxysmal cough?**
A series of coughs that is difficult to stop is called a paroxysm. Pertussis (whooping cough) is characterized by violent coughing fits, or paroxysms of coughing, followed by an inspiratory "whoop" as well as posttussive emesis. There are four classic stages of clinical pertussis in children—the *incubation stage*, which is asymptomatic and lasts 7 to 10 days; the *catarrhal stage*, which resembles a viral upper respiratory infection and lasts 1 to 2 weeks; the *paroxysmal stage*, during which the coughing paroxysms and whoop occur and which lasts 1 to 6 weeks; and the *convalescent stage*, a period of gradual recovery with possible recurrent exacerbations lasting 2 to 12 weeks. The protracted course of pertussis has led to it being called the "hundred-day cough." Pertussis is highly contagious from the onset of the catarrhal stage through about 3 weeks into the paroxysmal stage. It is important to note that infants, the group at greatest risk for serious illness or even death, may not have paroxysmal cough (or any cough at all) and may instead present only with poor feeding, apnea, and bradycardia. Because of factors that include waning immunity from the vaccine (rarely lasting longer than 12 years) resulting in limited herd immunity, low immunization rates in some populations, and vulnerability of infants because of poor passive

immunity from mothers, pertussis is the only vaccine-preventable disease with increasing incidence and mortality risk in the United States. A presumptive diagnosis is made based on clinical findings and can be confirmed with laboratory testing. Although cultures and serologies were used in the past, polymerase chain reaction has become the current reference standard for diagnosis given its speed and sensitivity. Early treatment (before the catarrhal phase) with macrolide antibiotics may decrease symptoms, though treatment at any time within 21 days of the onset of cough will decrease transmission.

12. **What is a barking cough?**

A barking cough is common in young children with croup. It sounds "brassy" and caregivers often describe a seal-like barking cough. This type of cough suggests a tracheal process or airway malacia related to compression on the trachea, laryngotracheobronchitis, spasmodic croup, or, rarely, a foreign body. Clinicians should be certain to query the possibility of foreign body aspiration in patients with an acute-onset "barky" cough.

KEY POINTS: ETIOLOGY OF COUGH IN CHILDREN

1. Most children with persistent cough have a postviral or inflammatory cough that does not respond to any standard therapies but resolves spontaneously over a period of weeks.
2. Cough-variant asthma is very unlikely to be the appropriate diagnosis for a child with a persistent cough who does not have other signs of asthma (e.g., exertional dyspnea) and does not respond to an appropriate course of treatment for asthma.
3. Passive cigarette or cigar smoke aggravates coughing in children.
4. Persistent cough in a young child after a severe choking episode may represent the aspiration of a foreign body into a mainstem bronchus.
5. An infant with a "staccato" cough (repetitive, dry, "rapid-fire" with inspiration between each single cough) may have *C. trachomatis* pneumonia, especially when conjunctivitis is also present.
6. A child with violent coughing fits ("paroxysmal" cough) followed by an inspiratory "whoop" and posttussive emesis and a normal chest x-ray appearance can be clinically diagnosed as having pertussis.

13. **Do commonly used cough medications work?**

Most evidence indicates that the commonly used pediatric cough preparations are no more effective in suppressing cough than placebo. These medications include dextromethorphan, guaifenesin, and codeine. Furthermore, many of the pediatric cough preparations also contain potentially dangerous agents such as decongestants that, if used in excessive doses, can cause cardiac arrhythmias in children. In 2008 the US Food and Drug Administration issued a statement that strongly condemned the use of over-the-counter cough and cold medications in children under 4 years of age, and manufacturers voluntarily complied by adding "do not use" labeling for this population.

For parents seeking an intervention to help soothe their child's cough, honey (1 teaspoon, given only to children >12 months old due to botulism risk in infants) has been shown to be modestly more effective than placebo, dextromethorphan, or diphenhydramine to reduce cough frequency and severity.

KEY POINTS: MANAGEMENT OF COUGH IN CHILDREN

1. For most children with an isolated dry cough lasting less than 4 weeks who have no evidence of pneumonia, treatment with antibiotics is not indicated.
2. For children with a "wet cough" lasting longer than 4 weeks, a course of antibiotics (typically a macrolide) may be warranted.
3. Children with a cough lasting longer than 4 weeks may require referral to a specialist.
4. An appropriate course of bronchodilator may be prescribed if cough-variant asthma is suspected, but if the child does not respond, the treatment should be discontinued rather than escalated.
5. Honey has been shown to be more effective for symptomatic relief of cough than placebo and other cough suppressants (i.e., diphenhydramine, dextromethorphan) and can be used in children older than 12 months of age.

14. **What problem should come to mind if a toddler presents with a persistent, nagging cough after a severe choking spell?**

This is the classic history of foreign body aspiration. Caretakers of a young child who has ongoing episodes of moderate-to-severe coughing should be questioned about the occurrence of a choking spell. If the object is about the size of the trachea and cannot be expelled with coughing, the child will quickly develop signs of severe upper airway obstruction. Yet if the object is smaller than the diameter of one of the mainstem bronchi, it may lodge there so that the child recovers with only a persistent cough. A patient with normal lungs will have adequate oxygenation and ventilation despite even complete occlusion of one mainstem bronchus. Although expiratory or decubitus chest radiographs have traditionally been recommended imaging modalities (with decreased "deflation" of the affected lung), studies have shown limited clinical benefit of imaging, particularly in a history consistent with aspiration. Thus if the story is classic, it is wise to consult an otolaryngologist or pulmonologist (for possible bronchoscopy) even if the chest x-ray appearance is normal.

15. What is tic cough and somatic cough disorder (psychogenic cough)?
Tic cough (previously known as habit cough) is a cough with features similar to a vocal tic—characteristics include suppressibility, suggestibility, and distractibility. Somatic cough disorder, or psychogenic cough, is a diagnosis of exclusion after other causes of cough, including tic cough, are excluded in the setting of somatic symptoms. A psychogenic cough often begins after an upper respiratory infection. These two entities can be difficult to distinguish, but initial treatment is the same. Because symptoms are often persistent, the patient may undergo a series of extensive yet unrevealing medical evaluations. The cough tends to be short, single, loud, dry (tics), or honking ("like a Canada goose"). A hallmark is that cough is exacerbated during office visits and absent during sleep. Many children with this condition are required to stay out of school because the cough is so disruptive. The physical examination is normal, apart from the cough. Most cases of tic cough or somatic cough disorder occur in children older than 4 years old who have significant stress at home or school.

16. How is tic cough or somatic cough disorder managed in the ED?
Tic cough or somatic cough disorder cannot always be diagnosed definitively in the ED. It is generally a diagnosis of exclusion made after other possible conditions (e.g., pneumonia, bronchospasm) have been ruled out and may require additional outpatient testing by the primary pediatrician or specialist. If suspicion is high, it may be appropriate to have a preliminary discussion of this possibility with caretakers. Establishing rapport by demonstrating genuine concern for the overall well-being of the child while carefully avoiding any language that could be construed as pejorative is essential. Longer term treatment of these disorders consists of "suggestion therapy," where a distractor (e.g., sipping warm water) is used as an alternative to the cough, and explanation and reassurance.

17. What is one thing caretakers should always do if their child has a persistent cough?
If they are smokers, they should stop smoking and, in all cases, forbid others from smoking in the house where the child resides. Cessation of smoking by caretakers has been shown to be a successful therapy for children with chronic cough.

18. What is the strangest cause of persistent cough?
Although this is certainly open to debate, perhaps the oddest cause of persistent cough is an eyelash stuck in the child's ear. Curiously, stimulation of the auricular branch of the vagus nerve by an eyelash in the external auditory canal can repetitively provoke the cough reflex. Unlike other otic foreign bodies, an eyelash does not cause pain or diminish hearing and may therefore go undetected for an extended period of time. Furthermore, it may not be immediately obvious on otoscopy. Consequently, it is wise to carefully examine the ears of a child with persistent coughing in hopes of finding this elusive yet easily remedied cause of a troublesome symptom.

BIBLIOGRAPHY
1. Abuelgasim H, Albury C, Lee J. Effectiveness of honey for symptomatic relief in upper respiratory tract infections: a systematic review and meta-analysis. *BMJ Evid Based Med.* 2021;26(2):57–64.
2. Brown JC, Chapman T, Klein EJ, et al. The utility of adding expiratory or decubitus chest radiographs to the radiographic evaluation of suspected pediatric airway foreign bodies. *Ann Emerg Med.* 2013;61(1):19–26.
3. Chang AB, Upham JW, Masters IB, et al. Protracted bacterial bronchitis: the last decade and the road ahead. *Pediatr Pulmonol.* 2016;51(3):225–242.
4. Chang AB, Oppenheimer JJ, Irwin RS. CHEST Expert Cough Panel. Managing chronic cough as a symptom in children and management algorithms: CHEST guideline and expert panel report. *Chest.* 2020;158(1):303–329.
5. Chang AB, Oppenheimer JJ, Weinberger M, Grant CC, Rubin BK, Irwin RS. CHEST Expert Cough Panel. Etiologies of chronic cough in pediatric cohorts: CHEST guideline and expert panel report. *Chest.* 2017;152(3):607–617.
6. Decker MD, Edwards KM. Pertussis (Whooping Cough). *J Infect Dis.* 2021;224(12 Supp 2):S310–S320.
7. Haydour Q, Alahdab F, Farah M, et al. Management and diagnosis of psychogenic cough, habit cough, and tic cough: a systematic review. *Chest.* 2014;146(2):355–372.
8. Lougheed MD, Turcotte SE, Fisher T. Cough variant asthma: lessons learned from deep inspirations. *Lung.* 2012;190:17–22.
9. Malesker MA, Callahan-Lyon P, Ireland B, Irwin RS. CHEST Expert Cough Panel. Pharmacologic and nonpharmacologic treatment for acute cough associated with the common cold: CHEST Expert Panel report. *Chest.* 2017;152(5):1021–1037.
10. Morgan JR, Carey KM, Barlam TF, Christiansen CL, Drainoni ML. Inappropriate antibiotic prescribing for acute bronchitis in children and impact on subsequent episodes of care and treatment. *Pediatr Infect Dis J.* 2019;38(3):271–274.

11. Munyard P, Bush A. How much coughing is normal? *Arch Dis Child.* 1996;74(6):531–534.
12. Smith SM, Schroeder K, Fahey T. Over-the-counter (OTC) medications for acute cough in children and adults in community settings. *Cochrane Database Syst Rev.* 2014;2014(11):CD001831.
13. Tobias JD, Green TP, Coté CJ. Codeine: time to say "no". *Pediatrics.* 2016;138(4):e20162396.
14. Vertigan AE, Murad MH, Pringsheim T, et al. CHEST Expert Cough Panel. Somatic cough syndrome (previously referred to as psychogenic cough) and tic cough (previously referred to as habit cough) in adults and children: CHEST guideline and expert panel report. *Chest.* 2015;148(1):24–31.
15. Weinberger M, Lockshin B. When is cough functional, and how should it be treated? *Breathe.* 2017;13(1):22–30.

CRYING AND IRRITABILITY IN THE YOUNG CHILD

Laura L. Sells

CHAPTER 10

1. **Is there a "normal" amount of crying in a young infant?**
   Infants are known to cry more during the first 3 months of life than at any other age. Based on a meta-analysis, the mean duration of crying is approximately 2 hours per day in the first 6 weeks of life. The duration of inconsolable crying peaks at 3 to 6 weeks of age and most inconsolable crying occurs in the evening. After 12 weeks of age, the typical duration of crying decreases significantly.

   Creating a strict definition for "normal" versus "excessive" crying is difficult, but based on the same meta-analysis, the 95th percentile of crying duration was approximately 4 hours per day in the first 6 weeks of life.

2. **Why is an organized approach important to the evaluation of crying in an infant?**
   The cause of crying in the nonverbal and frequently uncooperative infant is often obscure. A well-organized approach is critical because the differential diagnosis is vast, ranging from a normal physiological or temperamental response, to a life-threatening medical or surgical emergency. Finding the right answer with reasonable utilization of resources is a big part of the "art" of pediatrics. Table 10.1 lists selected diagnoses by systems that can present with crying in infants.

3. **Are routine screening laboratory and radiological tests generally useful in the emergency department (ED) evaluation of the infant with a chief complaint of crying?**
   The short answer is "no." Routinely obtaining a panel of laboratory or x-ray studies as a diagnostic screen *seldom* adds to the evaluation (except for the expense). Generally, the diagnosis lies in a thoughtful history and a thorough physical examination.

4. **What is colic and what are its clinical features?**
   The classic definition of infantile colic (the Wessel criteria) describes otherwise healthy infants ≤3 months of age with episodes of crying lasting for ≥3 hours per day, occurring on ≥3 days per week and persisting for ≥3 weeks (the "rule of threes").

   Colic is widely thought to be related to gastrointestinal (GI) issues in young infants, though the exact cause is unknown. GI-related etiologies are thought to include overfeeding, air swallowing, and pain from lactose or cow's

Table 10.1 Select Diagnoses Associated With Crying in Infants

General	Colic, hunger, temperament
Cardiac	SVT, congestive heart failure, anomalous left coronary artery syndrome
Respiratory	Hypoxemia, pain from croup-like cough or agitation with nasal congestion
Infection	Otitis media, pharyngitis/coxsackie virus, UTI, meningitis, septic joint, retropharyngeal abscess
Trauma	Abusive injury, fracture, soft tissue injury (burns, bruises), hair tourniquet, corneal abrasion, eye foreign body, blunt abdominal injury
Surgical	Incarcerated hernia, intussusception, volvulus, appendicitis, ovarian or testicular torsion
Gastrointestinal	Constipation, anal fissure, GERD, esophageal foreign body, gastroenteritis
Neurological	Botulism, seizure activity, intracranial hemorrhage
Toxicological	Withdrawal, amphetamines, methamphetamine, pseudoephedrine, diphenhydramine
Skin	Diaper rash, urticaria

GERD, gastroesophageal reflux disease; SVT, supraventricular tachycardia; UTI, urinary tract infection.

milk protein intolerance. Non-GI factors, including environmental stimulation, family stress, maternal smoking, and nicotine exposure, may play a role in the prevalence of colic.

Clinically, colic presents with paroxysms of inconsolable crying. There often appears to be a relatively discrete onset and end to the episodes, and the description of the cry may be louder and with a different pitch than the infant's normal cry.

5. **Are there any effective treatments for colic?**
   - Providing education to parents and communicating empathy are crucial. Provide parents with accurate information on "normal" amounts of crying and reassure parents about the self-limited nature of colic and that their infants are not sick. Finally, acknowledge parental frustration. Assess their support system and recommend they get a babysitter at times or find some other respite from this stressful situation.
   - First-line therapy generally consists of soothing techniques including swaddling (allowing for hip flexion), pacifier use, and providing "white noise" for short periods of time. Some infants seem to have temporary relief when rocked, carried, or riding in a car. Feeding techniques such as the use of a collapsible bag in a bottle to limit air swallowing, frequent burping, and attention to the volume of feeds may help symptoms.
   - Changing infant formula is not helpful except in a small subset of patients with clinical features of allergy or cow's milk intolerance, including bloody stools, rash, and poor weight gain. In breastfed infants with symptoms of allergy a maternal hypoallergenic diet and decreasing maternal intake of milk may provide some benefit.
   - Medications including simethicone, probiotics, and herbal remedies including teas or gripe water are not recommended for the treatment of colic.

6. **What is a common GI problem in young infants that can mimic colic?**
   Gastroesophageal reflux disease (GERD) is common in young infants and can mimic colic. Some degree of GI reflux is present in many babies because of supine positioning and immaturity of the lower esophageal sphincter. Overfeeding may commonly add to symptoms. When babies have esophageal irritation/esophagitis from GERD, crying develops from pain and may lead to ED visits. In addition to crying, babies with esophageal irritation may arch and turn their head to the side (Sandifer syndrome) when experiencing pain from GERD. Babies with mild GERD have nonbilious vomiting, normal weight gain, and a normal physical examination.

   The most current recommendations for the treatment of GERD include parental education about overfeeding, upright positioning, and frequent burping. Thickening feeds and eliminating cow's milk protein may help. Medications including proton pump inhibitors are reserved for refractory cases.

7. **What are two life-threatening diagnoses in an infant that may present with excessive crying that should be considered in the differential diagnosis for all patients with crying episodes?**
   - Abusive head trauma (previously referred to as shaken baby syndrome) and physical abuse. Babies who have pain from soft tissue injuries or broken bones may cry excessively. Also, those with inflicted head trauma and subdural hemorrhages may present with crying, irritability, vomiting, and altered mental status.
   - Sepsis/meningitis. Young infants who have meningitis may present with inconsolability because any movement, even by known caregivers, can increase pain from meningeal irritation.

8. **Name three potential surgical diagnoses for the young infant who presents with excessive crying.**
   - Malrotation with midgut volvulus. Patients with malrotation alone may not be diagnosed until there is associated midgut volvulus and crying from pain associated with bowel infarction. Eighty percent of patients with malrotation and midgut volvulus present in the first month of life. Bilious emesis in early infancy is a red flag for this process and must be immediately addressed with surgical evaluation and upper GI imaging.
   - Ileocolic intussusception. The typical age range is 2 months to 2 years, with a peak at 9 months of age. The classic history is of a patient with episodes of inconsolable crying and drawing up their legs in pain. Episodes usually last several minutes up to an hour or more. As time goes on, patients typically have vomiting and are often described as listless or lethargic. This change in mental status may confuse the differential diagnosis, including processes such as ingestion, sepsis, and head trauma. The "currant-jelly" stool described in intussusception occurs with bowel infarction and is a late finding, though guaiac-positive stools may be present early in the presentation.
   - Incarcerated inguinal hernia. The "secret" here is that you have to look in the diaper area! Two-thirds of patients with incarcerated inguinal hernias present in the first year of life, and they are painful, leading to excessive crying.

9. **Are there any cardiac or pulmonary diagnoses that present with crying as a chief complaint?**
   - Supraventricular tachycardia (SVT) may present in young infants with excessive crying, as well as sweating, poor feeding, and irritability. Typically, the diagnosis is confirmed by identifying the elevated and nonvariable heart rate, often >220 beats per minute. Even if a patient is not in SVT at the time of evaluation, a 12-lead electrocardiogram may reveal a delta wave suggestive of the diagnosis.

- Patients with myocarditis or congestive heart failure from congenital heart lesions may be increasingly fussy, though a thorough history and physical examination should reveal other signs and symptoms including abnormal cardiac examination, hepatomegaly, vomiting, and a history of poor growth or feeding.
- Infants with an anomalous origin of the left coronary artery from the pulmonary artery (ALCAPA) may present with crying and sweating while feeding. These infants can be intermittently irritable (feeding increases myocardial demand) and the condition is misdiagnosed as GERD. In this syndrome, the infant has myocardial ischemia as the left ventricular myocardium is perfused with relatively desaturated blood under low pressure.
- In infants with primary respiratory complaints (bronchiolitis), excessive crying may be associated with underlying hypoxemia. Applying supplemental oxygen may ease an infant's work of breathing and restlessness.

KEY POINTS: ED EVALUATION OF THE CRYING INFANT

1. An organized approach and thoughtful history and physical examination of the crying infant are vital to making the appropriate diagnosis.
2. Knowledge of the natural history of crying and colic in infants can help distinguish what is "normal" from other clinical diagnoses.
3. Recognition of the clinical differences between colic and GERD is important, and familiarization with current treatment strategies will better help parents care for infants with crying associated with these processes.
4. Awareness of potentially life-threatening diagnoses that may present with crying in infancy, including abusive head trauma/physical abuse and sepsis/meningitis, is paramount.
5. Routine use of screening laboratory studies and radiographs, not guided by history and physical examination findings, is generally not helpful.

10. **Why is it important to look closely at the fingers and toes of an infant presenting with the acute onset of inconsolable crying?**

You might find a hair tourniquet. The hair tourniquet occurs when a hair (often from the mother or caregiver) causes constricting injury to an appendage. The vast majority of cases involve fingers or toes (Fig. 10.1). Rarely, the penis, clitoris, or even the uvula may be involved. The hair tourniquet syndrome is typically not an abusive injury.

Although easily diagnosed by meticulous physical examination, treatment of a hair tourniquet can be problematic. Options include grasping the loose end of the hair and "unwinding" it, placing a needle or scalpel under the hairs and incising them, or applying a chemical depilatory agent to dissolve disulfide bonds in hair. Depilatory agents may be applied to the affected area for no longer than 10 minutes total. These products should not be used on, or adjacent to, mucous membranes (glans penis or vulva) or skin that is macerated. If the hair tourniquet has penetrated into the soft tissues, or these methods are unsuccessful, skin incision or surgical consultation may be necessary.

Despite best efforts of the clinicians and consultants, sometimes all the encircling hairs cannot be completely removed. The patient's family must understand the importance of returning if there is increased swelling, discoloration, or persistent crying after discharge from the ED.

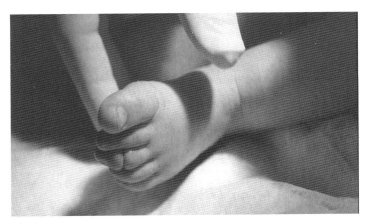

Fig. 10.1 Hair tourniquet.

11. **Is a corneal abrasion a real consideration for an infant with excessive crying?**
    Yes, but you should consider other diagnoses. Recent studies have cast doubt upon the true frequency of this diagnosis when crying is the chief complaint. Very young infants with sharp or irregular fingernails may injure their corneal surfaces by scratching themselves. Typically, young patients with corneal abrasions present with rubbing of the eyes, erythema of the skin around the eyes, and/or conjunctival infection, and ultimately the abrasion is seen using fluorescein testing. Application of a topical anesthetic drop during the examination should also temporarily resolve pain if corneal abrasion is the ultimate diagnosis.

12. **What about toxicological etiologies for crying?**
    Most unintentional ingestions occur in slightly older infants and toddlers who have developed a pincer grasp and are able to put objects in their mouth when they are walking and exploring their environment. However, unintentional ingestion or side effects from medication may cause crying and agitation even in young infants. Withdrawal symptoms from maternal opioid use can cause excessive crying. Diphenhydramine may cause a paradoxical reaction with agitation in an infant. Exposure to amphetamines (siblings with attention-deficit/hyperactivity disorder medications) or methamphetamine can cause tachycardia and agitation. Furthermore, corrosive substances such as household cleaners and hair-straightening preparations may cause crying and mouth pain, though most often patients have a history and physical examination findings to support the diagnosis.
    Finally, think about envenomation. Black widow spider bites may be associated with spasmodic muscle pain, abdominal cramping, and excessive crying. A thorough examination of the skin may reveal a bite mark.

13. **A 4-month-old male presents with the acute onset of inconsolable crying for the last 4 hours. There is no history of fever, vomiting or diarrhea, respiratory symptoms, or any known trauma. What diagnostic consideration must be included and which parts of the physical examination are crucial?**
    Abusive or inflicted injury should be considered. On physical examination, carefully evaluate the skin for any lesions from inflicted trauma (handprints, belt marks, burns), and unexplained ecchymoses. Consider the phrase "if you don't cruise, you don't bruise". (Babies who are not yet crawling, pulling to stand, and moving freely or "cruising" do not generally suffer injuries to the skin leaving bruises.) Palpate all bony surfaces for pain or edema. Examine the upper and lower frenulum in the mouth for injury. A frenulum injury is often due to jamming a bottle in the infant's mouth and may cause pain and crying. This is highly suspicious for child abuse in a young infant. The abdomen may be tender if there is blunt trauma resulting in liver or splenic injury.

14. **An 8-month-old girl presents to the ED with a history of crying, fever, and vomiting for 3 days. In the ED, she is awake and alert and has a reassuring and nonfocal physical examination. What is an important diagnosis to consider in your workup?**
    Remember to consider urinary tract infection (UTI). The presence of identifiable viral signs and symptoms makes the diagnosis of UTI less likely but does not exclude concomitant infection. Overall, the prevalence of UTI in febrile infants and children under age 2 is approximately 7%. White females have the highest likelihood of having UTI, but males under 3 months of age and uncircumcised males are also at increased risk. Obtaining a catheterized specimen of urine for urinalysis and culture should be strongly considered in these patients.

15. **A 3-month-old infant is brought to the ED with excessive crying. The mother reports the baby has been crying or whimpering all day and she describes the cry as "pathetic" and "weak." She states the baby is not feeding well and is "too weak to suck." The remainder of the history is only positive for lack of bowel movement for several days. There is no history of fever, cough, vomiting, or diarrhea. On examination, vital signs are normal. The baby is awake but hypotonic throughout with a weak cry when stimulated. There are no other abnormal examination findings. What is a likely diagnosis for this patient?**
    Infant botulism is likely. Sepsis is a consideration, but without fever or other infectious signs or symptoms, this is less likely. Poor suck, hypotonia, and constipation are common findings with infant botulism. However, the weak cry is often what the parents notice first and what precipitates a visit to the ED.

16. **An 11-month-old presents with crying and drooling for the last 3 hours. There is no history of illness. The mother reports hearing the child gag and vomit earlier today while she was in another room. The child is awake, crying, and refusing a bottle. The examination of the mouth and oropharynx is normal. What is a likely diagnosis?**
    Consider esophageal foreign body. At 11 months, an infant should have a well-developed pincer grasp and could pick a coin or other object up and swallow it. If the patient were ill or had supporting physical examination findings, pharyngitis, coxsackie virus infection, or stomatitis could be considered. Drooling and refusing oral input are often seen in patients with an esophageal obstruction caused by a foreign body.

17. **Any other "secrets" to consider?**

Despite your best attempts to reach a diagnosis with a careful history and physical examination, you may encounter infants in whom the ultimate cause of crying remains elusive. Hospitalization for ongoing observation and/or close follow-up with repeat examination is crucial for these patients.

BIBLIOGRAPHY

1. Bolte R, Dawn B. The crying child, part 1: potential causes. *Contemp Pediatr.* 2007;24(5):75–81.
2. O'Gorman A, Ratnapalan S. Hair tourniquet management. *Pediatr Emerg Care.* 2011;27(3):203–204.
3. Ismail J, Nallasamy K. Crying infant. *Indian J Pediatr.* 2017;84(10):777–781.
4. Khan A. An infant within consolable crying. *Am J Emerg Med.* 2022;55:227.
5. Pifko E, Price A, Sterner S. Infant botulism and indications for administration of botulism immune globulin. *Pediatr Emerg Care.* 2014;30(2):120–124.
6. Shaikh N, Morone NE, Bost JE, Farrell MH. Prevalence of urinary tract infection in childhood: a meta-analysis. *Pediatr Infect Dis J.* 2008;27(4):302.
7. Wessel MA, Cobb JC, Jackson EB, et al. Paroxysmal fussing in infancy, sometimes called colic. *Pediatrics.* 1954;14(5):421–435.
8. Wolke D, Bilgin A, Samara M. Systematic review and meta-analysis: fussing and crying durations and prevalence of colic in infants. *J Pediatr.* 2017;185:55–61.e4.

CHAPTER 11

DIARRHEA

Linda D. Arnold

1. **What is diarrhea?**
   Diarrhea is a decrease in stool consistency caused by a disturbance of the mechanisms regulating intestinal fluid and electrolyte transport. While "normal" stools may vary considerably between individuals, diarrhea "takes the shape of the container," often with an increase in frequency and/or volume of stool. The WHO defines diarrhea as the passage of three or more loose or watery stools per day. This is less well defined for infants and young children.

2. **How is diarrhea classified, based on duration?**
   - *Acute*: <2 weeks
   - *Persistent*: 2 to 4 weeks
   - *Chronic*: >4 weeks or recurrent episodes over time

3. **What are the major causes of acute diarrhea?**
   Acute diarrhea, in most cases, results from enteric infection by viral pathogens. Norovirus is responsible for most outbreaks and endemic cases of acute gastroenteritis. Rotavirus has become less common due to an effective vaccine. Other viruses, bacterial pathogens, food-borne toxins, and parasites also play a role. Extraintestinal infections, such as otitis media, urinary tract infections, and appendicitis can also cause acute diarrhea. Noninfectious causes include protein or carbohydrate intolerance, and the laxative effects of sugar substitutes (e.g., sucralose, sorbitol, and xylitol) used to sweeten a wide array of foods, beverages, and candies.

4. **Does coronavirus disease 2019 (COVID-19) infection cause diarrhea?**
   Since 2020 severe acute respiratory syndrome coronavirus 2 (SARS-CoV-2) has emerged as an important viral etiology for diarrhea in children. While most children with this infection have respiratory symptoms, fever and diarrhea can be the sole presenting symptoms in infants and children. One study, a meta-analysis of 32 articles, showed that while gastrointestinal symptoms are rare in adults with COVID-19, approximately 20% of children had diarrhea.

5. **When should I consider pseudomembranous colitis?**
   This is a serious disorder that should be considered in the differential diagnosis of acute watery diarrhea. Most children with this condition appear ill, have profuse diarrhea, crampy abdominal pain and distention, and, in the most serious cases, shock. It is caused by overgrowth of *Clostridium difficile* leading to destruction of normal gut flora. It usually occurs after treatment with clindamycin, but amoxicillin is another culprit. Occasional cases occur in children with no recent use of antibiotics.

6. **What causes persistent and chronic diarrhea?**
   - Persistent diarrhea in infants may be from infection, protein intolerance, malnutrition, anatomic anomalies, enzyme defects, or metabolic disorders such as cystic fibrosis.
   - In older infants and toddlers, common causes include protein intolerance, postinfectious diarrhea, and "toddler's diarrhea" from fruit juice, sugary drinks, and high-fructose corn syrup. Also consider *Giardia*, celiac disease, sucrase-isomaltase deficiency, and Hirschsprung enterocolitis.
   - For school-aged children and adolescents, think about giardiasis, celiac disease, irritable bowel, lactose intolerance, artificial sweeteners, and inflammatory bowel disease (IBD). Consider laxative abuse in teens.

7. **Name the common infectious causes of diarrhea.**
   - **Viral:** norovirus, rotavirus, enteric adenovirus, SARS-CoV-2, astrovirus
   - **Bacterial:** *Salmonella*, *Shigella*, *Campylobacter*, *Yersinia* spp., *Escherichia coli*, *C. difficile*
   - **Preformed bacterial toxins**: *Bacillus cereus*, *Clostridium perfringens*, *Staphylococcus aureus*
   - **Parasitic:** *Giardia* spp., *Cryptosporidium* spp., *Entamoeba histolytica*, *Strongyloides* spp., *Microsporidium* spp.

8. **Can specific signs or symptoms help identify a cause?**
   - Viral pathogens tend to target the proximal small intestine. Onset of illness is abrupt and duration is limited. Patients typically present with emesis and diarrhea, and respiratory symptoms are common.
   - Bacterial pathogens induce colonic inflammation, resulting in bloody or mucoid stools, cramping abdominal pain, fever, and tenesmus. Bacterial toxins may cause watery stool.

- Food poisoning is characterized by the abrupt onset of vomiting, as early as 30 minutes after a meal, followed by crampy abdominal pain and diarrhea. Norovirus causes half of all food poisoning; symptoms begin 12 to 48 hours after exposure and typically last 1 to 3 days. Bacteria or bacterial toxins are responsible in 40% of cases; symptoms appear up to 3 weeks after exposure, masking the etiology.
- Increased flatus, bloating, and loose stools are common with *Giardia* infection, lactose intolerance, and following consumption of "sugar-free" sweeteners.
- Irritable bowel syndrome is characterized by intermittent cramping pain and frequent, small-volume, liquid stools alternating with constipation.

9. **What are the key components of the history?**
   The initial history should focus on three things: (1) fluid status, (2) "red flags" for severe or complicated illness and risk factors (e.g., immunocompromised or underlying illness), and (3) potential exposures that provide clues to etiology. Quickly determine the number and volume of liquid stools to assess if the child needs urgent fluid resuscitation. Ask if the stools have mucous or blood indicating bacterial gastroenteritis. Confirm if there is associated vomiting and appropriate urine output.

10. **What else should I focus on when taking a history?**
    - Ask about the child's diet. Unpasteurized juices and dairy products, as well as improperly cooked meat, eggs, and poultry, may contain *E. coli*, *Salmonella*, *Campylobacter*, or parasites. One percent of healthy cows carry *E. coli* 0157:H7, while *Salmonella* is ubiquitous in chickens. Additionally, excessive ingestion of sugary drinks may lead to a noninfectious diarrhea, commonly known as toddler's diarrhea.
    - Ask about exposure to others who are ill. Children may become infected at daycare or in an institutionalized setting. A history of family members or close contacts with diarrhea may indicate a food-borne etiology.
    - Ask about recent antibiotic use and consider *C. difficile* colitis.
    - Ask about exposure to pets and animals. Children may develop diarrhea after visits to farms or petting zoos, or from contact with infected pets (usually due to *E. coli* 0157:H7). *Salmonella* can be acquired from backyard chickens, ducks, pet birds, frogs, turtles, lizards, iguanas, hamsters, and rodents fed to snakes. Many wild and domestic birds, farm animals, and young cats and dogs harbor *Campylobacter*.
    - Ask about recreational activities. *Giardia* is the leading cause of diarrhea from untreated drinking water or recreational waters contaminated with sewage or human or animal feces. *Cryptosporidium* is very chlorine resistant, and large outbreaks have been traced to swimming pools.

11. **Why is a good travel history so important?**
    Domestic travel involving hiking, camping, or visits to remote areas may expose children to pathogens (e.g., *Giardia*) in untreated drinking water. Among children traveling internationally, 28% develop diarrhea. Enterotoxigenic *E. coli* is a common cause. Children visiting foreign relatives, especially those traveling to disease-endemic areas or settings with inadequate sanitation are at greater risk of acquiring bacterial and parasitic infections from contaminated food or water. Ninety percent of diarrheal outbreaks on cruise ships are caused by norovirus, which is highly contagious, survives for long periods on many surfaces, and is resistant to alcohol-based disinfectants and many detergents. Enterotoxigenic *E. coli* is a less frequent cause.

12. **What "red flags" should I look for on physical examination?**
    Children with uncomplicated gastroenteritis tend to have mild diffuse abdominal tenderness and active bowel sounds. Localized or rebound tenderness and absent or high-pitched bowel sounds may indicate a possible surgical process or bowel obstruction. Palpation of a mass or a discrete loop of bowel suggests constipation, intussusception, or IBD. Children with IBD may also have perianal tags, fissures, or abscesses. Increased anal tone, abdominal distention and explosive stools raise concerns for Hirschsprung enterocolitis. Pallor and decreased urine output in the setting of bloody diarrhea are suggestive of hemolytic uremic syndrome (HUS). Children with protuberant abdomens and wasting of buttocks and extremities should be evaluated for giardiasis, celiac disease, and cystic fibrosis.

13. **How can I assess hydration status?**
    Detailed questions about type and duration of symptoms, weight loss, frequency of emesis, diarrhea and urination, and estimated oral intake will help determine the degree of dehydration. Decreased urine output is an early finding in dehydration; reliance on this symptom alone may lead to overdiagnosis of dehydration.
    Physical findings of dehydration are detectable when fluid deficit is equivalent to $\geq 3\%$ of body weight. Tachycardia, sunken eyes, decreased skin elasticity, and weight loss are important signs. A tired or fatigued general appearance, capillary refill longer than 2 seconds, dry mucous membranes, and reduced tears are also significantly associated with dehydration.

14. **When is it helpful to inspect the stool?**

Although the presence of blood or mucus in stool suggests an inflammatory process, stools described as "bloody" often contain visible remnants of red foods, rather than actual blood. Visual inspection and hemoccult testing can help confirm or exclude the presence of gross or occult blood.

Watery, explosive stools with a foul vinegar-like odor suggest carbohydrate malabsorption. Bulky, foul-smelling stools are seen in fat malabsorption. Consider celiac disease, cystic fibrosis, pancreatic insufficiency, and bile salt malabsorption in the presence of steatorrhea. Undigested cellulose particles are often visible in the loose stools of children with toddler's diarrhea.

15. **What foods can mimic hematochezia?**

Clinicians should use bedside hemoccult testing to assess red or black stool for the presence of blood. Children who have ingested red fruit juices, candies, gelatin, popsicles, Kool-Aid, tomatoes, beets, plums, watermelon, or cranberries may produce red stools that are highly suspicious for hematochezia. Tarry-looking stools may follow consumption of bismuth-containing antidiarrheal products, iron, black licorice, blueberries, spinach, purple grapes, chocolate, or grape juice. Red meat, cherries, tomato skin, and iron supplements can cause false-positive results on hemoccult testing.

16. **What method of rehydration is best for children with dehydration from diarrhea?**

Oral rehydration therapy (ORT) with an appropriate oral rehydration solution (ORS) is recommended for children with mild-to-moderate dehydration from gastroenteritis. Commercially available ORS such as Pedialyte and Enfalyte are similar to the ORS recommended by the WHO in 2002. They have more carbohydrate and less sodium than the WHO solution, but the differences are not clinically significant. In the emergency department (ED) setting, ORT is as effective as intravenous (IV) hydration, requires less staff time, is less invasive, has lower cost, and is preferred by families.

IV hydration is indicated for children with complicated illness, moderate-to-severe dehydration, shock, intractable vomiting or diarrhea, or mental status changes.

17. **Are antimotility or adsorbent agents safe for children?**

Pharmacological antimotility agents are not recommended for use in children because of insufficient testing and potential side effects. Bismuth-containing compounds pose a risk of salicylate absorption and toxicity at high doses, and bismuth encephalopathy has been reported in patients with renal insufficiency. Opiates, such as Lomotil, and synthetic opiates, such as Imodium (loperamide), both decrease intestinal motility, which may result in gastrointestinal ileus and the invasion of the bowel wall by infectious organisms. Loperamide may cause respiratory depression and arrhythmias in young children. Side effects of Lomotil, which combines an opioid with atropine, include central nervous system–induced sedation, respiratory depression, and anticholinergic toxicity. Dysentery is an absolute contraindication to the use of antimotility agents.

There is no evidence that adsorbents such as kaolin-pectin are effective in the management of acute gastroenteritis in children.

KEY POINTS: ORAL REHYDRATION THERAPY

1. Recommended for mild-to-moderate dehydration.
2. Use ORS that meets WHO guidelines for osmolality and electrolytes.[a]
3. Give frequent, small aliquots via 5-mL syringe.
4. Give 50 to 100 mL/kg body weight over 2 to 4 hours for rehydration.
5. Replace ongoing losses: 10 mL/kg per stool; 2 mL/kg per emesis.

[a]Osmolality 245 mmol/kg (200–260), Na Cl 75 mEq/L = 2.6 g/L, glucose 13.5 g/L

18. **Are probiotics useful to treat infectious diarrhea?**

A multicenter prospective study involving children 3 months to 4 years of age showed no benefit from probiotics. There was no difference in the frequency or duration of diarrhea and no difference in absenteeism from work or daycare in the group receiving probiotics versus the control group.

19. **When are antibiotics recommended for diarrhea?**

Viruses cause most infectious diarrhea; thus antibiotics are not indicated. Although antibiotics may be required to treat parasitic infections or prescribed for specific bacterial pathogens in selected populations, results of stool studies are seldom available at the time of ED evaluation. Empiric antibiotic treatment is not usually recommended for suspected bacterial enteritis, owing to its limited effectiveness in shortening the duration of illness, role in increasing antibiotic resistance, and controversy surrounding the potential for increased risk of HUS, resulting from acute toxin release following antibiotic-induced injury to bacterial cell membranes. As a rule, antibiotics should be administered only to children with signs of sepsis, bacteremia, or extraintestinal spread of infection. When *Salmonella* gastroenteritis is suspected or confirmed, antibiotics are indicated for infants, and for children who are toxic appearing, asplenic, immunocompromised, or malnourished. Empiric therapy and infectious disease consultation are warranted when the history and clinical presentation suggest typhoid fever, dysentery, or severe colitis, particularly among recent travelers.

KEY POINTS: ACUTE GASTROENTERITIS

1. Most cases of acute gastroenteritis are self-limited and require no specific therapy, other than early initiation of appropriate fluid replacement.
2. No high-quality evidence exists to support the use of probiotics.
3. Antidiarrheal agents are not recommended for use in children.
4. Dehydration is the major source of morbidity in children with diarrheal diseases.
5. Proper handwashing is extremely effective in preventing the transmission of enteric pathogens.

20. **Which complications of infectious diarrhea should I be concerned about?**
    Both *Shigella* spp. and *E. coli* can induce seizures via high fever or toxin elaboration. Also, up to 10% of infections with Shiga toxin–producing *E. coli*, such as *E. coli* 0157:H7, result in HUS or thrombotic thrombocytopenic purpura. *Salmonella* spp. cause bacteremia in approximately 6% of those infected, with rates of 11% to 45% reported in infants and neonates. Immunocompromised patients and those with hematological disorders are at increased risk of developing salmonella osteomyelitis.

21. **When is diarrhea a true emergency?**
    Urgent intervention is required when a surgical cause is suspected. Appendicitis can present with diarrhea secondary to cecal inflammation. Most children presenting to the ED with diarrhea will have mild dehydration, which can be easily treated with oral or IV fluids. Some children, however, present with hypernatremic dehydration; this must be managed carefully, as cerebral edema may develop with rapid rehydration. In addition, infants with infectious or allergic enteritis may present in compensated or uncompensated shock. Intussusception is a potentially life-threatening condition that can present with bloody diarrhea. Unlike infectious causes of diarrhea, which may have blood mixed in the stool, with intussusception there is often more blood than stool. The stool is classically described as looking like currant jelly. These patients also have severe episodic abdominal pain, lethargy, and often vomiting. Hirschsprung enterocolitis can also be life threatening; prompt decompression via rectal tube is imperative, pending definitive treatment.
    Fluids must be managed carefully in children with HUS, who frequently present with dehydration and acute renal failure, often complicated by hyperkalemia, hypertension, anemia, and thrombocytopenia. Although 85% of affected children recover fully, half require dialysis and mortality rates average 5%. Finally, neonates and immunocompromised hosts can have life-threatening complications, such as sepsis, from *Salmonella* gastroenteritis. *Salmonella* bacteremia and sepsis occur in 1% of patients with *Salmonella* gastroenteritis. These patients present with ill appearance and history of bloody diarrhea.

22. **When is testing indicated in children with diarrhea?**
    Most children with acute, nonbloody diarrhea and no risk factors for bacterial illness can be managed without diagnostic studies. Diarrhea that persists more than 5 days may warrant evaluation, as may cases with blood in the stool or exposure to contaminated food or water. A higher index of suspicion is required for infants, among whom sequelae are more common. Obtain a blood culture, complete blood count, and serum electrolytes for ill or toxic-appearing patients, and consider hypoglycemia when indicated. Children with persistent diarrhea or evidence of a noninfectious cause should be screened for conditions such as IBD, celiac disease, and carbohydrate intolerance. *Giardia* antigen or ova and parasite specimens should be sent and celiac antibody testing should be performed in children with persistent diarrhea and failure to thrive. Stool polymerase chain reaction is highly sensitive and useful in the ED to identify a pathogen when indicated. Testing for fecal leukocytes is not sensitive or specific and is not recommended.

23. **What instructions should parents be given about diet?**
    Breast milk and formula provide superior nutrition to clear liquids and should be offered throughout the course of an uncomplicated illness, if tolerated. When clear liquids are given for rehydration, families should be instructed to use one of the commercially available glucose electrolyte–containing solutions for children (e.g., Pedialyte, Enfalyte). This will avoid errors in mixing homemade solutions. Apple juice, soda, and sports beverages should be avoided; their hypertonicity and high carbohydrate load can cause diarrhea to worsen. The traditional BRAT diet (bananas, rice, applesauce, and toast) is well tolerated but fails to provide adequate calories, protein, fat, and fiber. Children should resume a regular diet, with age-appropriate foods and full-strength milk or formula, as soon as possible.

KEY POINTS: MANAGING FLUIDS AND NUTRITION WITH DIARRHEA

1. Mothers should be encouraged to continue breastfeeding.
2. Use of special or dilute infant formulas is generally not necessary.
3. Oral rehydration with hypotonic glucose electrolyte solutions is the therapy of choice for children with mild-to-moderate dehydration.
4. IV fluids are indicated in cases of moderate-to-severe dehydration or when oral fluids are not tolerated. Hypovolemic shock requires rapid administration of 20 mL/kg boluses of isotonic crystalloid, and frequent reassessments, until mental status and perfusion improve.
5. Rapid return to age-appropriate feeding patterns is indicated once children are rehydrated.

24. **What is the best way to prevent infectious diarrhea?**

Multiple studies, in multiple settings, have concluded that frequent handwashing is very effective in decreasing the frequency of diarrheal illness in children. Studies in daycare centers show decreases in episodes of diarrhea, up to 50%, following training and education of children and childcare providers. Alcohol-based hand sanitizers have little effect on norovirus; handwashing with soap is recommended.

BIBLIOGRAPHY

1. Crews JD, Koo HL, Jiang Z, Starke JR. A hospital based study of clinical characteristics of *Clostridium difficile* infection in children. *Pediatr Infect Dis J.* 2014;33(9):924–928.
2. Freedman SB, Williamson-Urquhart S, Farion KJ. Multicenter trial of a combination probiotic for children with gastroenteritis. *N Eng J Med.* 2018;379(21):2015–2026.
3. Mansourian M, Ghandi Y, Habibi D, Mehrabi S. Covid-19 infection in children: a systematic review and meta-analysis of clinical features and laboratory findings. *Arch Pediatr.* 2021;28(3):242–248.
4. Pereira F, Hsu DC. Diarrhea. In: Shaw KN, Bachur RG, eds. *Fleisher & Ludwig's Textbook of Pediatric Emergency Medicine.* 8th ed. Lippincott, Williams and Wilkins; 2021:152–156.
5. Schnadower D, O'Connell KJ, VanBuren JM, Vance C, et al. Association between diarrhea duration and severity and probiotic efficacy in children with acute gastroenteritis. *Am J Gastroenterol.* 2021;116(&):1523–1532.
6. Shane AI, Mody RK, Crump JA, Taarr PI. 2017 Infectious Diseases Society of America Clinical Practice Guidelines for the diagnosis and management of infectious diarrhea. *Clin Infect Dis.* 2017;65(12):e45–e80.
7. Vatandas NS, Yurdakok K, Yalcin SS, Celik M. Validity analysis on the findings of dehydration in 2-24 month old children with acute diarrhea. *Pediatr Emerg Care.* 2021;37(12):e1227–1232.

EAR PAIN

Shabana Yusuf and Joan E. Shook

CHAPTER 12

1. **What is the most common cause of ear pain in young children?**
Ear pain (otalgia) is a common complaint in the pediatric emergency department (ED). Although the differential diagnosis for otalgia is lengthy, the most common cause of ear pain is acute otitis media (AOM). Other otogenic causes include otitis externa and foreign bodies. Nonotogenic causes include dental caries or abscess, pharyngitis, cervical lymphadenitis, parotitis, sinusitis, and temporomandibular joint (TMJ) dysfunction.

   AOM is caused by an acute bacterial (or occasionally viral) infection resulting in inflammation of the middle ear that is usually associated with pain and fever. The peak age for AOM is 9 to 15 months of age but mostly occurs between 6 and 24 months of age.

2. **What are the diagnostic criteria for otitis media?**
   * Recent, usually abrupt onset of signs and symptoms of middle ear infection (such as pain, irritability, fever, otorrhea)
   * Presence of middle ear effusion
   * Signs of middle ear inflammation

3. **What are the most specific physical examination findings for otitis media?**
Bulging of the tympanic membrane (TM) is the most specific physical examination finding to suggest a bacterial pathogen in the middle ear. Impaired mobility of the TM with pneumatic otoscopy and the presence of cloudy middle ear fluid are strongly suggestive of a bacterial infection. A TM that is intensely erythematous is suggestive of AOM, but lesser degrees of erythema are not useful for diagnosis. Acute purulent otorrhea due to perforation of the TM also suggests a diagnosis of AOM (after otitis externa is ruled out). Examination of the ear is difficult, and pediatricians and otolaryngologists often vary in the identification of AOM.

4. **What are other presenting signs and symptoms of otitis media?**
New-onset ear pain is suggestive of otitis media. Other signs and symptoms of otitis are hearing loss, vertigo, tinnitus, postauricular swelling, facial paralysis, and conjunctivitis. The association between otitis media and conjunctivitis is referred to as the otitis-conjunctivitis syndrome. This is usually caused by nontypeable *Haemophilus influenzae*.

5. **What symptoms are not diagnostic of otitis media?**
Signs of concomitant viral infections such as fever, ear pulling, difficulty sleeping, or rhinorrhea are not indicative of otitis media. Only 50% of time does a child have otitis if parents suspect them of having one.

6. **What are the most common bacterial pathogens that cause otitis media?**
Streptococcus pneumoniae, nontypeable *H. influenzae*, and *Moraxella catarrhalis* are the most common bacterial organisms that cause otitis media. *Streptococcus pyogenes*, *Staphylococcus aureus*, *Mycoplasma pneumoniae*, and gram-negative bacilli are occasionally seen. The use of the conjugate pneumococcal vaccine has decreased the number of episodes from *S. pneumoniae*, but a proportionate increase in incidence from nontypeable *H. influenzae* and *M. catarrhalis* has been seen.

7. **Describe the initial management of AOM.**
The initial management of otitis media can be either observation with close follow-up or antibiotic treatment. The option of watchful waiting can be done in healthy children older than 6 months with unilateral otitis media with mild symptoms and without otorrhea. Many patients with otitis media will improve without antibiotics in 48 to 72 hours. Children younger than 6 months of age and children with severe otitis media (pain, fever greater than 39°C, toxic appearing) should be treated with antibiotics. Pain associated with the infection can be managed with either acetaminophen, or ibuprofen if older than 6 months.

8. **Which antibiotics best treat bacterial otitis media?**
The first-line drug in the treatment of otitis media is amoxicillin dosed at 80 to 90 mg/kg/day in two divided doses/day. Treatment is recommended for 10 days in children less than 2 years old and for 5 to 7 days in older children. The second-line drug for otitis media is amoxicillin-clavulanate. In patients who do not have type 1 allergic reaction to penicillin, alternates such as cefdinir, cefpodoxime, cefuroxime, or clindamycin can also be used. In patients with a history of type 1 allergic reaction to penicillin, it is recommended to treat with azithromycin,

clarithromycin, or trimethoprim-sulfamethoxazole. If the patient is vomiting or is noncompliant with medications, a single dose of intramuscular ceftriaxone (50 mg/kg) is also effective. A second dose of ceftriaxone can be given in 48 hours if symptoms have not resolved. Three doses of ceftriaxone may be needed for resistant *S. pneumoniae*. Infants younger than 4 weeks old are usually treated for otitis media with intravenous (IV) medications (ampicillin and gentamicin).

10. **What is a middle ear effusion and how is it treated?**
    A middle ear effusion is a collection of fluid in the middle ear without signs and symptoms of acute infection. On examination, bulging of the TM, limited or absent mobility of the TM with pneumatic otoscopy, air-fluid level behind the TM, or otorrhea is seen. Treatment with antibiotics is not recommended, as this condition is not related to a bacterial infection. Initial treatment is watchful waiting. If the effusion does not resolve in 6 months for one ear or 3 months for both ears, consider referral to an otolaryngologist for tympanostomy tubes. Steroids are not indicated.

11. **What is the role of vaccines in preventing otitis media?**
    General usage of the pneumococcal vaccine has resulted in a modest reduction in the frequency of AOM. It has reduced the incidence of children developing recurrent otitis media and the need for myringotomy tubes.

12. **What is the role of surgery in the management of otitis media?**
    The decision to place tympanostomy tubes depends largely on whether the child has associated symptoms such as hearing loss, thus placing the child at risk developmentally. Some otolaryngologists recommend myringotomy tubes if the child has more than three episodes of AOM in 6 months or more than four episodes in 12 months. The decision to place tubes is made on an individual basis. For initial surgery, myringotomy with tympanostomy without adenoidectomy is recommended unless nasal obstruction is present. Tonsillectomy is not recommended to treat otitis media with effusion.

13. **What are the complications of otitis media?**
    The complications of otitis media include perforation of the TM, cholesteatoma, adhesive otitis media, tympanosclerosis, mastoiditis, petrositis, labyrinthitis, subperiosteal abscess (Luc abscess), meningitis, facial paralysis, brain abscess, lateral sinus thrombosis, and suppurative complications of the brain. It can also cause hearing loss and speech delay.

14. **What is bullous myringitis? How is the diagnosis made?**
    Bullous myringitis is an infection of the TM with intensely painful bulla formation on the surface. The diagnosis is made easily by otoscopy. The cause is usually viral, but it can be caused by *S. pneumoniae, H. influenzae*, and *Mycoplasma*. Treatment is supportive with analgesics, and the same antibiotics are used as for otitis media without bullae.

15. **You are evaluating a patient who presents with ear pain. On taking the history, you learn that the illness began with itchiness of the ear canal, which has become increasingly severe and evolved into pain. What is the most likely diagnosis in this child?**
    This presentation is classic for otitis externa (swimmer's ear). Otitis externa is an inflammatory process affecting the external auditory canal. It can be localized or diffuse and is most commonly seen during the summer months. Other predisposing factors include moisture retention due to a tortuous narrow canal or obstructive cerumen, loss of acidic environment due to inadequate cerumen lavage, exposure to an alkaline substance, or interruption of the epithelial lining of the canal because of trauma or dermatitis.
    Physical examination of these patients is often revealing. There may be drainage from the ear. The pain can be elicited by pushing on the tragus or by traction of the pinna or moving the jaw from side to side. The most common causative organisms are *Pseudomonas* spp., *Staphylococcus*, and *Streptococcus*. *Proteus* spp. may also be seen in association with *Pseudomonas*.

16. **How is otitis externa treated?**
    Treatment includes avoidance of swimming, pain control with analgesics, ear drops with a combination of antibiotic-corticosteroid preparation (e.g., cortisporin), or antibiotic drops alone (e.g., ofloxacin otic solution 0.3%, a good choice because it covers *Pseudomonas* spp. well). A wick placed in the external auditory canal may be needed if severe edema of the canal is present. In severe infection, oral antibiotics may be necessary.

17. **What is malignant otitis externa?**
    This condition is a severe form of otitis externa that is not responsive to conventional therapy. It is caused by *P. aeruginosa* and involves the bone and marrow of the skull base, causing osteomyelitis. Malignant otitis externa may also result in chondritis and facial nerve paralysis. Other complications include stenosis of the canal and permanent hearing loss. It is rare in children but can be seen in patients with diabetes mellitus or those who

are immunocompromised. Both computed tomography (CT) scan and nuclear imaging are helpful in making the diagnosis. Treatment includes IV antibiotics and removal of granulation tissue.

18. **A toddler presents with bruising to the internal surface of the pinna. According to the mother, he is a very active child and falls frequently. What diagnosis should you consider?**
Bruising to the internal surface of the pinna may result from a direct blow (boxing) to the ear. You therefore must consider the possibility of child abuse. The unexplained presence of hemotympanum and the perforation of the TM may also suggest child abuse because they can result from a direct blow to the ear.

19. **Infections at the site of ear piercing are often extremely painful and cause some concern. What organisms should you consider covering when you choose an antibiotic?**
Cellulitis or perichondritis of the pinna can cause otalgia and is usually caused by *S. aureus* or *Pseudomonas* spp. High ear piercings are at greatest risk for this infection. These infections are managed first with removal of the piercing. Infection of the cartilage can be serious, so IV antibiotics are indicated and incision and drainage of abscesses may be needed.

20. **You are examining a child who came to the ED because of fever and ear pain. You notice that his ear is red and swollen and seems to be protruding from the side of his head. What diagnosis is most likely?**
This child likely has mastoiditis, a relatively uncommon complication of otitis media. On physical examination the posterior auricular area is erythematous and very tender. It is important to visualize the TM because severe otitis externa also can present with postauricular erythema, swelling, and protrusion of the pinna. With mastoiditis, the TM is erythematous and bulging, although with otitis externa, the TM is usually normal. CT can help differentiate between mastoiditis and severe otitis externa when a complete physical examination is not possible. Petrositis, which is an infection of the petrous part of the temporal bone, is rare. Gradenigo syndrome or petrositis presents as a triad of deep facial pain, otitis media, and ipsilateral abducens nerve paralysis.

21. **How is mastoiditis treated?**
Children with mastoiditis must be evaluated by an otolaryngologist and admitted to the hospital for IV antibiotics. Because the most common organisms in acute mastoiditis are *Staphylococcus* spp., *Streptococcus* spp., and *H. influenzae*, treat the patient with broad-spectrum antibiotics targeting these species. Operative intervention in the form of mastoidectomy may be required in children with complicated infection or evidence of abscess formation. Ear cultures either obtained from the ear canal, through tympanocentesis, or abscess drainage can help guide antibiotic therapy.

22. **What are the potential complications of mastoiditis?**
Complications of mastoiditis can be intratemporal or intracranial. Intratemporal complications include facial paralysis, labyrinthitis, and petrositis. Intracranial complications include meningitis, lateral sinus thrombosis, and epidural, subdural, or brain abscesses. In children less than 2 years of age, high white blood cell count $16.7 \times 10^9/L$) and C-reactive protein of more than 7.21 mg/dL were associated with complications.

23. **The presence of a foreign body in the external auditory canal can cause severe pain. What is the best method for removing the foreign body?**
Occasionally, a child places a foreign body in the external canal and presents with symptoms such as hearing loss or a sensation of fullness, as well as ear pain. Symptoms at presentation vary depending on the nature of the foreign material and the length of time that it has been present. Objects can be removed by using alligator forceps, curettes, right-angle hooks, balloon-tip catheters, Baron suction devices, or irrigation with warm water. If the foreign body is a bean or other vegetable material, do not irrigate with water as the foreign body may swell. A foreign object that is lodged tightly in the canal may require removal with sedation or even general anesthesia using an operating microscope.

Limit attempts at removal and be sure to have proper equipment and lighting before attempted removal. Consider sedation for some patients.

Canal wall lacerations are present 50% of the time after a foreign-body removal. It is recommended that after the object is recovered, the patient be treated with topical antibiotic or steroid drops to prevent the development of otitis externa.

24. **When should you NOT try to remove a foreign body from the ear canal?**
If the foreign body is up against the TM, removal may be difficult and painful. Sedation may be needed to successfully remove the foreign body. If the child is in severe pain or there is bleeding from the ear canal, consider referral to an otolaryngologist.

25. You have just examined a child who has a hearing aid battery in her external auditory canal. You have not been successful in your attempts to remove it with forceps. What should your next step be?

    Hearing aid batteries (or button batteries) can cause extensive caustic skin and bony damage in a short period of time. Removal of this foreign object is an otologic emergency and should be performed as soon as possible after detection. If you are unable to remove the battery, call an otolaryngologist for urgent removal in the operating room.

26. A child presents with severe ear pain of sudden onset. You determine there is a live insect, most likely a roach, moving in the ear canal. How should you manage this patient to relieve pain quickly?

    Before attempting to remove the insect, immediately place mineral oil, 2% lidocaine, or viscous lidocaine in the ear canal. This thick viscous solution will "paralyze" the insect and relieve pain promptly. The foreign body can then be removed with an ear curette or by flushing the canal with water.

27. What is middle ear barotrauma?

    This is an injury to the TM from a sudden change in pressure due to diving, flying, or blast injuries, and it can cause severe ear pain. On physical examination, the TM appears swollen and blue. Treatment for this condition is supportive with analgesics. Refer to an otolaryngologist if the patient has dizziness or hearing loss, which may indicate a perilymphatic fistula.

28. You are confronted with a patient who reports ear pain, and yet examination of the ear is normal. How can this phenomenon be explained?

    Otalgia can be the result of referred pain from distant sites secondary to inflammatory processes, tumors, or trauma. Nonotogenic otalgia is most often of dental origin. Pain can also be psychogenic when no other cause is found.

29. Name some nonotogenic causes of pain in the ear and the nerve that carries the sensation.

    - **Cranial nerve V:** Disturbances in the oral cavity, including stomatitis, gingivitis, lymphadenitis, parotiditis, trauma, and infections of the tongue; dental conditions, including eruption, impaction, trauma, caries, and abscess
    - **Cranial nerve VI:** Bell palsy, herpes zoster, tumors
    - **Cranial nerve IX:** Tonsillitis and retropharyngeal abscess, adenotonsillectomy, nasopharyngeal or oropharyngeal tumors
    - **Cranial nerve X:** Lesions at the base of the tongue, trachea, larynx, and esophagus; otalgia can be a manifestation of gastroesophageal reflux in infants and children
    - **Upper cervical nerves:** Cervical spine injuries, arthritis, or disk disease

30. What is Ramsay Hunt syndrome?

    This is the eponym applied to herpes zoster otitis or viral polycranial neuropathy affecting the ear. It presents with severe otalgia, facial palsy, and vesicles on the pinna, external auditory canal, and TM. All cranial nerves can be affected, and other symptoms include hearing loss, vertigo, nausea, vomiting, and dizziness. Treatment is with acyclovir, systemic steroids, and analgesics.

31. TMJ dysfunction is among the most common causes of referred otalgia. How can I confirm this as a source of ear pain?

    To confirm the diagnosis of TMJ dysfunction, carefully palpate the TMJ externally by placing the fingers just anterior to the tragus and having the patient open and close the mouth. The patient with this condition will report otalgia during attempted occlusion. The pain may be caused by nerve irritation, muscle spasm, or degenerative change in the joint. TMJ dysfunction can occur in children who have bruxism, frequently clench their teeth, indulge in frequent gum chewing, or have malocclusion. Tympanometry in these patients is normal. Treatment is directed at reducing the inflammation and pain with heat therapy, soft diet, analgesia, physiotherapy, occlusal splints, and rarely surgery.

32. What is a preauricular pit? Can this lead to ear pain?

    A preauricular pit is a small indentation located anterior to the helix and superior to the tragus of the external ear. These are common congenital anomalies and may be associated with hearing loss. Occasionally, these pits become infected, and the child may present with pain, erythema, swelling, and discharge from the area of the pit. Antibiotic treatment is recommended. Surgical management with excision of the pit may be required if the pit repeatedly becomes infected.

KEY POINTS: EAR PAIN

1. Ear pain in the child is most commonly due to AOM.
2. AOM is diagnosed when there is bulging of the tympanic membrane or impaired mobility and the presence of fluid in the middle ear, as found with pneumatic otoscopy.
3. If the examination of the ear is normal, consider secondary (referred) causes of otalgia, including TMJ syndrome, dental disease, pharyngitis, sinusitis, and gastroesophageal reflux.
4. Hemotympanum is a rare finding that can result from a basilar skull fracture, barotrauma from scuba diving, a turbulent airplane flight, or a direct blow to the ear. In the absence of such a history, consider child abuse.
5. A button battery lodged in the ear canal must be removed promptly.

BIBLIOGRAPHY

1. Gaddy HL, Wright MT, Nelson TN. Otitis media: rapid evidence review. *Am Fam Phys*. 2019;100(6):350–356.
2. Garcia C, Salgueiro AB, Luís C, Correia P, Brito MJ. Acute mastoiditis in children: middle ear cultures may help in reducing use of broad spectrum antibiotics. *Int J Pediatr Otorhinolaryngol*. 2017;92:32–37.
3. Hudgins JD, Lee GS. ENT emergencies. In: Shaw KN, Bachur RG, Chamberlain JM, Lavelle J, Nagler J, Shook JE, eds. *Fleisher & Ludwig's Textbook of Pediatric Emergency Medicine*. 8th ed. Lippincott Williams & Wilkins; 2021:1319–1332. Ch 118.
4. Joffe MD. Pain: Earache. In: Shaw KN, Bachur RG, Chamberlain JM, Lavelle J, Nagler J, Shook JE, eds. *Fleisher & Ludwig's Textbook of Pediatric Emergency Medicine*. 8th ed. Lippincott Williams & Wilkins; 2021:389–393.
5. Lieberthal AS, Carroll AE, Chonmaitree T, et al. Clinical practice guideline: the diagnosis and management of acute otitis media. *Pediatrics*. 2013;131:e964–e999.
6. Loh R, Phua M, Shaw CKL. Management of paediatric acute mastoiditis: systematic review. *J Laryngol Otol*. 2018;132(2):96–104.
7. Otteson T. Otitis media and tympanostomy tubes. *Pediatr Clin North Am*. 2022;69(2):203–219.
8. Oyama LC. Foreign bodies of the ear, nose and throat. *Emerg Med Clin North Am*. 2019;37(1):121–130.
9. Shaffer AD, Jacobs IN, Derkay CS, et al. Management and outcomes of button batteries in the aerodigestive tract: a multi-institutional study. *Laryngoscope*. 2021;131(1):E298–E306.

CHAPTER 13

FEVER

Jeffrey R. Avner

1. **What percentage of visits to the emergency department (ED) is for the evaluation of fever?**
   Fever is one of the most common presenting symptoms to the pediatric ED, representing 15% to 30% of all visits. During the first 2 years of life, a child typically has four to six episodes of febrile illness.

2. **What temperature is considered normal?**
   There is no single value that represents a "normal" temperature, since normal body temperature varies with age, time of day, physical activity, and environmental conditions. This variability limits the application of mean body temperature values derived from population studies. Thus no single temperature should be used as the upper limit of normal. Rather, normal temperature is best described as a range of values for each individual. Although only a rough guide, some consider abnormal temperature to be higher than 38.0°C to 38.2°C (rectally) in an infant and higher than 37.2°C to 37.7°C (orally) in an older child or adult.

3. **Who is credited with the first systematic measurement of body temperature?**
   In the 1860s German physician Carl Wunderlich used foot-long thermometers to record over 1 million axillary temperature readings from 25,000 patients. He identified 37.0°C (98.6°F) as the mean temperature of healthy adults.

4. **What are the differences in measurement among rectal, oral, tympanic, axillary, and skin temperature readings?**
   The core body temperature is best measured with an esophageal or nasopharyngeal probe, but this is difficult in the setting of an ED. Therefore rectal temperature is used as the standard measurement to measure core body temperature. Digital axillary and oral thermometry tend to underestimate rectal temperature by about 0.5°C to 1.0°C. Infrared tympanic and temporal thermometry are popular methods used in EDs, and studies show that, at least in older children and adults, the results are reasonably accurate, achieving high specificity. It should be noted that there are inherent limitations in temperature measurement and that the specific temperature determination by peripheral thermometry should be complemented by additional clinical elements (e.g., history, vital signs, physical examination findings) when assessing children.

5. **Can parents detect fever subjectively?**
   Touch is usually the first method parents use to detect fever. The forehead is the most common site used, and there is no difference in detection when multiple sites are palpated. Parents are usually able to detect if their child is "burning up" with fever. In general, parents are both moderately sensitive (75%-93%) and specific (48%-86%) in detecting the presence of fever subjectively in children. However, because the positive predictive value of "fever to touch" is 52% to 76%, maternal report of fever should always be confirmed by thermometry. A child noted to be afebrile subjectively by the parent is very likely to be afebrile, especially in the primary care setting. Additionally, parents may not be as accurate in estimating the height of fever. In young infants (less than 2 months old), when the height of the fever is crucial for determining management, always obtain a rectal temperature.

6. **Does body temperature vary during the day?**
   The variation of body temperature in the typical circadian rhythm becomes established by 2 years of age. Peak temperature typically occurs in the late afternoon (5:00-7:00 PM), and the trough occurs in the early morning (2:00-6:00 AM). Daily temperature variation ranges from 0.1°C to 1.3°C.

7. **How does the body produce fever?**
   With infection, exogenous pyrogens (microbial products such as endotoxins) produced by various infectious organisms act on host inflammatory cells (especially monocytes and macrophages) to produce numerous cytokines, including endogenous pyrogens (interleukin, tumor necrosis factor, and interferon). These circulating pyrogens act on the preoptic area of the anterior hypothalamus, which produces prostaglandin E_2 and causes fever.

8. **Where is the core body temperature set?**
   Core body temperature is set in the anterior hypothalamus. Variation in the body temperature is detected by thermosensitive neurons in the preoptic nucleus, which then directs autonomic changes in sweat glands, blood vessels, somatic neurons, and skeletal muscles.

9. **How does the body regulate temperature?**
Thermoregulation is controlled by a variety of physiologic and behavioral mechanisms under the direction of the hypothalamus. Elevation of body temperature occurs primarily through metabolic activity associated with increased cell metabolism, increased muscle activity, and involuntary shivering. Body temperature is decreased primarily through vasodilatation, which thereby increases heat loss by conduction, convection, or radiation through the skin. In addition, sweating and cold preference behaviors (e.g., removing clothes) help dissipate the heat.

10. **Is fever beneficial or harmful?**
Whether fever is a friend or foe is a question for all ages. Fever has some physiologic benefits for the host, including an enhancement of both cellular and humoral immune responses as well as direct antimicrobial activity. On the other hand, fever makes the child uncomfortable and can lead to a significant increase in metabolic activity, which increases oxygen consumption, carbon dioxide production, and insensible water loss. Whether the benefits outweigh the metabolic costs is debatable. Regardless, the presence of fever alerts the parents and clinicians that the child is in the process of fighting disease and, as such, can serve as an invaluable diagnostic aid.

11. **What is "fever phobia"?**
Barton Schmitt coined the term in the early 1980s in reference to parents' excessive concern about low-grade fever. Nowadays, the term *fever phobia* is often used to describe heightened anxiety about the presence of fever in a child that can lead to aggressive antipyretic use, unnecessary ED visits, laboratory testing, or empiric antibiotic treatment. Of note, both parents and providers may have "fever phobia."

12. **Does bundling cause fever in infants?**
Overbundling of young infants (<3 months old), especially during the summer months, is known to increase skin temperature but has less effect on rectal temperature. Thus these infants may feel warm to touch (tactile fever) but not have an elevation in their core temperature. If an infant is heavily bundled or in a particularly hot environment, a 30- to 60-minute period of equilibration should be followed by a repeat temperature determination. Overbundling should never be considered the cause of a temperature >38.5°C (taken by any method) or an explanation as to why an infant may be ill-appearing.

13. **Who started the belief that a high fever caused death?**
Dr. Claude Bernard, the father of human physiology, heated animals in a makeshift oven and found that sustained temperatures over 106°F (41.1°C) were fatal. This report published in 1876 in *Lecons sur la Chaleur Animale* (Lessons from Animal Heat) began the erroneous concern that high fever is inherently dangerous. Of note, his findings were the result of hyperthermia, *not* fever due to the elevation of the hypothalamic set point.

14. **Does high fever cause brain damage?**
Although this concern is a cornerstone of "fever phobia" among parents, this fear is unfounded. There is no evidence that otherwise healthy children with fever, *as opposed to hyperthermia*, are at increased risk of serious sequelae. Deleterious effects of temperatures higher than 41°C are based on in vitro effects on enzyme systems and not clinical studies. When brain damage does occur in association with fever, it is usually due to sequelae of the underlying disease (such as meningitis) rather than the fever itself.

15. **What is the difference between fever and hyperthermia?**
Fever is caused by a rise in the hypothalamic set point, which is usually the result of the triggering of several pyrogenic cytokines. *Hyperthermia* is often used to describe a condition in which the thermoregulatory system is either dysfunctional or simply overwhelmed by a variety of internal or external factors. Hyperthermia may result from disorders of excessive heat production (exertional heatstroke, thyrotoxicosis, cocaine intoxication), disorders of diminished heat dissipation (classic heatstroke, severe dehydration, autonomic dysfunction), or disorders of hypothalamic function (cerebrovascular accidents, trauma). Unlike fever, management of *hyperthermia* usually involves aggressive attempts at cooling.

16. **Does fever trigger seizures?**
Fever lowers the seizure threshold in children with an underlying seizure disorder and may precipitate a seizure in children (6 months to 6 years old) who are susceptible to simple febrile seizures.

17. **Does teething cause fever?**
Although some studies show a mild temperature elevation associated with teething, significant fever (temperature >38°C) has never been shown to be associated with tooth emergence.

18. **Are sponging or alcohol baths recommended for fever management?**
    No. Sponging (even with tepid water) and alcohol baths may cause excessive vasoconstriction and shivering, limiting the child's ability to dissipate heat. In addition, isopropyl alcohol can be toxic through skin absorption.

19. **Does fever reduction decrease the sequelae from a febrile illness, including febrile seizures?**
    No. There is no evidence that reducing fever, in an otherwise healthy child, reduces the morbidity or mortality risks of a febrile illness. In fact, there is some evidence that antipyresis may prolong the underlying infection, albeit at the expense of child discomfort. However, for children who are chronically ill or have limited metabolic reserve, the additional metabolic demand of the febrile state might be poorly tolerated. There is also no evidence that antipyretic therapy decreases the recurrence of febrile seizures.

20. **Does the response of a fever to an antipyretic predict a more benign illness?**
    No. Fever response to antipyretics is not clinically useful in differentiating children with serious bacterial illness from those with a more benign cause. Most children, regardless of the underlying cause of their fever, experience some temperature decline with antipyretics, although rarely do they become afebrile. However, a child who has a serious illness often continues to appear ill after fever is reduced, whereas the appearance of a child who has a benign illness usually improves. The decision to perform additional diagnostic tests should be determined based on clinical grounds and not the degree of defervescence.

21. **Does the height of the fever indicate serious bacterial illness?**
    Most studies show limited usefulness of the height of fever as a predictor of serious bacterial illness. Even temperatures higher than 39°C have relatively low sensitivity and predictive value for serious illness in otherwise healthy infants over 6 months and limited usefulness in infants 3 to 6 months. Other clinical signs such as age, appearance, and peripheral perfusion are better predictors. Thus it appears that the presence or absence of fever is what is most important. This does not mean that a thorough evaluation of a child with high fever is unnecessary; rather, *any child with fever, regardless of the height of the temperature, should receive a thorough evaluation.*

22. **What are the normal increases in heart rate and respiratory rate with each degree rise in body temperature?**
    Fever is associated with an increase in heart rate of about 10 to 15 beats per minute and an increase in respiratory rate of about 5 to 7 breaths per minute for each rise of a Celsius degree.

23. **Is alternating acetaminophen and ibuprofen more effective for fever reduction?**
    Although a common practice among practitioners, there is currently limited scientific evidence that this combination of antipyretics has greater efficacy than either agent used alone. Although there is some evidence that the antipyretic combination results in slightly lower temperatures at 4 to 6 hours, there is no evidence in overall improvement in other clinical outcomes. Furthermore, this practice may, in fact, increase fever phobia and potential toxicity from incorrect dosing. Therefore most guidelines discourage this practice, although one permits alternating use if discomfort persists after the administration of one antipyretic.

24. **What are the risk factors to consider in evaluating a febrile child?**
    Children who have either an immature or specific impairment of immunologic function are at higher risk of bacteremia and serious bacterial illness. Therefore, very young infants (less than 2 months), children with immune compromise (e.g., human immunodeficiency virus infection, neutropenia, sickle cell disease), and children receiving immunosuppressive medication (such as chemotherapy and steroids) may require a blood culture and empiric antibiotic treatment as part of their management.

25. **Why do we treat infants less than 2 months old with fever differently than older child?**
    There are three main reasons: (1) the risk of serious bacterial illness in this age group is relatively high (approximately 10%), (2) young infants have immature immune responses that may not be able to contain infection, and (3) clinical appearance is difficult to interpret. At this age, the ability of a child to interact in an interpretable social manner is inconsistent. For example, a social smile is inconsistent, if not absent, in a 1-month-old.

26. **What are the common pathogens that cause serious bacterial illness in febrile infants?**
    In infants less than 2 months old, maternal organisms, acquired perinatally, predominate: gram-negative enteric organisms (*Escherichia coli*), group B streptococcus (GBS), *Staphylococcus aureus*, and *Listeria*. *E. coli* is now the most common cause of not just urinary tract infections (UTIs) at this age but also of bacteremia, likely due to improved screening and treatment of maternal GBS. GBS remains the most common cause of meningitis in most studies.

Table 13.1 Management Options for Well-Appearing Febrile Young Infants

AGE	8-21 DAYS	22-28 DAYS	29-60 DAYS
Urine	Yes	Yes	Yes
Blood culture	Yes	Yes	Yes
Inflammatory markers	Optional	Yes	Yes
CSF	Yes	Maybe	Maybe
Antibiotics	Yes	Maybe	Maybe
Disposition	Hospitalize	Hospital vs home	Hospital vs home

CSF, cerebrospinal fluid.
Adapted with permission from Pantell RH, Roberts KB, Adams WG, et al., Subcommittee on Febrile Infants. Evaluation and management of well-appearing febrile infants 8 to 60 days old. *Pediatrics*. 2021;148(2):e2021052228. https://doi.org/10.1542/peds.2021-052228. Epub 2021 Jul 19. Erratum in: *Pediatrics*. 2021;148(5). PMID: 34281996.

27. **What are the low-risk criteria for the management of febrile infants?**
   In an attempt to avoid routine hospitalization of all febrile young infants, many investigators have sought to devise clinical and laboratory criteria that would identify a subset of febrile infants at "low risk" of having bacterial disease as a cause of their fever. Recently, the American Academy of Pediatrics (AAP) developed evidence-based guidelines to help clinicians develop a strategy for the evaluation and management of these infants. These guidelines apply to well-appearing febrile (temperature $\geq$38.0°C) infants 8 to 60 days old and are stratified by age into three categories: 8 to 21 days, 22 to 28 days, and 28 to 60 days.

28. **What is a "sepsis workup"?**
   A "sepsis workup" is typically considered an evaluation of certain body fluids for bacterial infection. It usually includes a complete blood count (CBC), urinalysis, lumbar puncture, and cultures of blood, urine, and spinal fluid. A "*septic*" workup is a test performed with a dirty needle.

29. **Which inflammatory markers are used in risk stratification of febrile young infants?**
   The AAP guidelines use the following for risk stratification: temperature >38.5°C, procalcitonin >0.5 ng/mL, C-reactive protein (CRP) >20 mg/L, and absolute neutrophil count (ANC) <4000 or >5200 mm³. Other prediction rules included white blood cell (WBC) count and band-to-neutrophil ratio.

30. **Do all febrile infants need a sepsis workup and admission?**
   Although there is no absolute consensus, most agree that all febrile infants younger than 21 days who are evaluated in the ED require an evaluation for sepsis and hospitalization pending culture results. Many also feel that the same evaluation applies to infants 22 to 28 days old. Evaluation of febrile infants aged 29 to 60 days is more variable and depends on clinical judgment, benefit-harm assessment, and shared decision-making (Table 13.1). Selected low-risk infants can be managed as outpatients with close observation and follow-up within 24 hours.

31. **When should you consider herpes syncytial virus (HSV) in the evaluation of febrile young infants?**
   HSV should be considered in the evaluation of febrile infants, especially those less than 3 weeks old, if the infant appears ill, has seizures, has vesicles, or cerebrospinal fluid pleocytosis (with a negative Gram stain). While maternal history of genital HSV lesions or fever 48 hours before or after delivery is an important factor, most infants with HSV are born to women with no history of genital HSV infection. Other suggestive findings include hypothermia, mucous membrane ulcers, leukopenia, thrombocytopenia, or elevated alanine aminotransferase levels. Because of the high morbidity and mortality associated with HSV, acyclovir should be started empirically if HSV is considered.

32. **Do young febrile infants with a documented viral infection need a sepsis workup?**
   A recent multicenter study of almost 3000 infants with viral testing found that viral infection in febrile infants <60 days of age was associated with a decreased, but not negligible, serious bacterial infection (SBI) risk compared with nonviral-infected febrile infants. These findings suggest that at a minimum, an evaluation for UTI should be strongly considered regardless of viral status and that clinicians need to exercise caution, especially in the first month of life, regarding the comprehensiveness of the evaluation, including performance of lumbar punctures, regardless of virus infection status.

KEY POINTS: THE FEBRILE INFANT

1. Febrile infants <21 days of age who are evaluated in the ED require an evaluation for sepsis and hospitalization pending culture results.
2. Viral infection in febrile infants <60 days of age was associated with a decreased, but not negligible, SBI risk compared with non viral-infected febrile infants; at a minimum, an evaluation for UTI should be strongly considered regardless of viral status, and clinicians need to exercise caution, especially in the first month of life, regarding the comprehensiveness of the evaluation.
3. UTI is the most common bacterial infection in febrile infants less than 2 months old.
4. For well-appearing febrile infants 4 to 8 weeks old, a variety of testing and management strategies are available.

33. **Has universal pneumococcal vaccine (PCV) use affected the incidence of invasive pneumococcal disease (IPD)?**
Pneumococcal disease was the most common cause of unsuspected (occult) bacteremia in a subset of febrile children (usually 3-36 months old) who are well-appearing and have no focus of infection but, nevertheless, have bacteremia. Since the introduction of PCV7 in 2000 and PCV13 in 2010, there has been a precipitous decline in IPD. From 1998 through 2019, overall, IPD rates among children less than 5 years old decreased by 93% (from 95 cases per 100,000 population in 1998 to 7 cases per 100,000 in 2018).

34. **Are febrile young children still at risk for occult bacteremia?**
While the decline in IPD has increased the relative importance of other etiologies of bacteremia (e.g., *E. coli*, *Salmonella*, *S. aureus*), the incidence of bacteremia in otherwise well-appearing febrile toddlers without a source *who are completely immunized* is a relatively rare event. However, children who are unimmunized or incompletely immunized may still have substantial risk, similar to that of the pre-PCV era. Thus many would recommend some assessment of inflammatory markers (WBC, ANC, procalcitonin) and blood culture as well as urinary studies. Of course, children who are *ill-appearing* need immediate evaluation for sepsis and other serious infections.

35. **Are biomarkers useful for predicting serious bacterial illness in otherwise healthy febrile children?**
Peripheral WBC count, ANC, and CRP are often used as nonspecific inflammatory markers, but they provide limited diagnostic value in identifying serious illness in children. Procalcitonin, at a threshold level of about 0.5 ng/mL, is most predictive of invasive bacterial infection (meningitis, bacteremia, and sepsis) in children with fever and no source of infection. Of note, all inflammatory markers are less valuable when used closer to the start of the fever.

36. **In older children, should the decision on whether to perform a lumbar puncture be guided by the height of the fever or the peripheral WBC count?**
No! Neither of these measures alone is sensitive enough at any threshold to predict meningitis. The criteria for lumbar puncture should be based on history and physical examination findings rather than nonspecific laboratory tests.

37. **How should a febrile child with coronavirus disease 2019 (COVID-19) be managed?**
Fever is one of the most common symptoms of acute COVID-19 in children (along with cough, dyspnea, headache, and myalgias), although it is important to remember that many children may be asymptomatic. Fortunately, most cases of COVID-19 in healthy infants and children are similar to more common viral illnesses. In young infants (<90 days) who present with fever but are well-appearing, there is a decreased chance of SBI if the infant is COVID-19 positive. Similar to other concomitant viral infections in this age, an evaluation for UTI should be strongly considered, and until more data are available for infants younger than 1 month, most recommend a sepsis workup. In older infants and children, evaluation and management should be based on symptoms.

38. **When should the diagnosis of multisystem inflammatory syndrome in children (MIS-C) be considered in the evaluation of a febrile child?**
MIS-C is a relatively uncommon postinfectious inflammatory response to severe acute respiratory syndrome coronavirus 2 (SARS-CoV-2) occurring about 2 to 6 weeks after COVID-19. MIS-C should be considered in a child with persistent fever that is temporally related to recent COVID-19 who has some of the clinical features of MIS-C (abdominal pain, vomiting, diarrhea, skin rash, mucocutaneous lesions, neurocognitive findings) and no plausible alternative diagnosis. In comparison to other febrile illnesses commonly seen in the ED, children with MIS-C tend to have higher fever and longer duration of fever on presentation. MIS-C shares many of the presenting symptoms as Kawasaki disease. The child's age, inflammatory markers, and recent SARS-CoV-2 infection can help differentiate these diseases.

Table 13.2 Tiered Approach to Multisystem Inflammatory Syndrome in Children Evaluation

	TIER 1	TIER 2	AS INDICATED
Labs	CBC with differential Serum chemistries Liver function tests CRP, ESR Respiratory viral panel SARS-CoV-2 PCR SARS-CoV-2 antibody	Procalcitonin Ferritin, D-dimer PT/PTT Troponin, BNP Urinalysis Cytokine panel Blood culture	
Imaging		ECG Echocardiogram	CXR Chest CT Abdominal CT Abdominal ultrasound
Consults		Infectious diseases Cardiology Rheumatology	Hematology Nephrology

BNP, B-type natriuretic peptide; CBC, complete blood count; CRP, C-reactive protein; CT, computed tomography; CXR, chest x-ray; ECG, electrocardiogram; ESR, erythrocyte sedimentation rate; PCR, polymerase chain reaction; PT, prothrombin time; PTT, partial thromboplastin time; SARS-CoV-2, severe acute respiratory syndrome coronavirus 2.
Adapted with permission from Henderson LA, Canna SW, Friedman KG, et al. American College of Rheumatology Clinical Guidance for multisystem inflammatory syndrome in children associated with SARS-CoV-2 and hyperinflammation in pediatric COVID-19: version 3. *Arthritis Rheumatol.* 2022;74(4):e1–e20.

39. **If MIS-C is suspected, what workup should be done?**
    Management of a child with suspected MIS-C in the ED generally consists of a tiered approach to testing (Table 13.2). Tier 1 studies are for suspected mild cases. Tier 2 studies are for more moderate-to-severe cases, as well as those with elevated inflammatory markers. Of course, as continued evidence and experience with COVID-19 evolve, these recommendations may change.

40. **Why is the presence of a petechial rash in a febrile child of concern?**
    A petechial rash, especially if associated with fever, may be an early sign of infection with an invasive bacterial organism, especially *Neisseria meningitidis.* Early identification of a child with meningococcemia is essential, because the disease can progress rapidly and has a high morbidity rate. Other bacterial causes for fever and petechiae include *Streptococcus pneumoniae*, group A streptococcus, *S. aureus, E. coli*, and *Rickettsia.* The incidence of invasive bacterial disease has been estimated to be as high as 20% in children who are hospitalized but much lower for patients presenting to the ED.

KEY POINTS: THE FEBRILE CHILD

1. Clinical signs such as age, appearance, and peripheral perfusion are better predictors of serious illness than the height of fever.
2. The presence or absence of fever, rather than a specific value, is what is most important for determining a management strategy.
3. A child who has a serious illness often continues to appear ill after the fever is reduced, whereas the appearance of a child who has a benign illness usually improves.
4. The incidence of occult bacteremia in otherwise well-appearing febrile toddlers who are *completely immunized* is relatively rare.

41. **What evaluation is necessary in managing the child with fever and petechiae?**
    If the child is ill-appearing or immunocompromised, an evaluation for sepsis is necessary. Hospitalization and empiric antibiotics are essential. For children who are well-appearing and have no clear cause for the petechiae, a CBC and blood culture should be considered, as well as a rapid streptococcal antigen test if there is pharyngitis. Additional studies, such as coagulation tests and lumbar puncture, hospitalization, and need for empiric antibiotics, are somewhat controversial. Management must be individualized. Most physicians admit and treat

with parenteral antibiotics any child who is young (<12 months), has an elevated (or low) WBC count, or has an abnormal CRP. For children who have normal laboratory tests, outpatient management with close follow-up is an option.

42. **How long must fever be present to be considered a fever of unknown origin (FUO)?**
    FUO is generally applied to any febrile illness with an unexplained, persistent (daily) temperature higher than 38.5°C for at least 8 days.

43. **What is the leading cause of FUO?**
    In pediatrics, almost half of the cases of FUO are due to infectious diseases (usually respiratory tract infections, followed by infections of the urinary tract, skeleton, and central nervous system). Malignancy (e.g., leukemia) should also be considered.

44. **How often does FUO have no diagnosis or resolve spontaneously?**
    Almost 25% of children with FUO are either undiagnosed or have spontaneous resolution.

45. **What kind of fever is associated with bizarre movements in response to disco music?**
    Saturday Night Fever was first identified in the 1970s by a group of adolescents wearing unbuttoned silk shirts, flared pants, and platform shoes.

BIBLIOGRAPHY

1. Carlin RF, Fischer AM, Pitkowsky Z, Abel D, Sewell TB, Landau EG, Caddle S, Robbins-Milne L, Boneparth A, Milner JD, Cheung EW, Zachariah P, Stockwell MS, Anderson BR, Gorelik M. Discriminating multisystem inflammatory syndrome in children requiring treatment from common febrile conditions in outpatient settings. *J Pediatr.* 2021;229:26–32.e2.
2. Chiappini E, Bortone B, Galli L, de Martino M. Guidelines for the symptomatic management of fever in children: systematic review of the literature and quality appraisal with AGREE II. *BMJ Open.* 2017;7(7):e015404.
3. Edwards G, Fleming S, Verbakel JY, et al. Accuracy of parents' subjective assessment of paediatric fever with thermometer measured fever in a primary care setting. *BMC Prim Care.* 2022;23(1):30.
4. Hubert-Dibon G, Danjou L, Feildel-Fournial C, Vrignaud B, Masson D, Launay E, Gras-Le Guen C. Procalcitonin and C-reactive protein may help to detect invasive bacterial infections in children who have fever without source. *Acta Paediatr.* 2018;107(7):1262–1269.
5. Greenhow TL, Hung YY, Herz A. Bacteremia in children 3 to 36 months old after introduction of conjugated pneumococcal vaccines. *Pediatrics.* 2017;139(4):e20162098. https://doi.org/10.1542/peds.2016-2098. Epub 2017 Mar 10.
6. Lyons TW, Garro AC, Cruz AT, et al. Performance of the modified Boston and Philadelphia criteria for invasive bacterial infections. *Pediatrics.* 2020;145(4):e20193538.
7. Mahajan P, Browne LR, Levine DA, et al. Risk of bacterial coinfections in febrile infants 60 days old and younger with documented viral infections. *J Pediatr.* 2018;203:86–91.e2.
8. Pantell RH, Roberts KB, Adams WG, et al. Evaluation and management of well-appearing febrile infants 8 to 60 days old. *Pediatrics.* 2021;148(2):e2021052228.
9. Payson A, Etinger V, Napky P, Montarroyos S, Ruiz-Castaneda A, Mestre M. Risk of serious bacterial infections in young febrile infants with COVID-19. *Pediatr Emerg Care.* 2021;37(4):232–236.
10. Pecoraro V, Petri D, Costantino G, Squizzato A, Moja L, Virgili G, Lucenteforte E. The diagnostic accuracy of digital, infrared and mercury-in-glass thermometers in measuring body temperature: a systematic review and network meta-analysis. *Intern Emerg Med.* 2021;16(4):1071–1083.
11. Kimberlin DW, Barnett ED, Lynfield R, Sawyer MH. Committee on Infectious Diseases, American Academy of Pediatrics *Red Book: 2021–2024 Report of the Committee on Infectious Diseases.* 32nd ed. American Academy of Pediatrics; 2021.
12. Section on Clinical Pharmacology and Therapeutics; Committee on Drugs Sullivan JE, Farrar HC. Fever and antipyretic use in children. *Pediatrics.* 2011;127(3):580–587.
13. Vicens-Blanes F, Miró-Bonet R, Molina-Mula J. Analysis of nurses' and physicians' attitudes, knowledge, and perceptions toward fever in children: a systematic review with meta-analysis. *Int J Environ Res Public Health.* 2021;18(23):12444.
14. Waterfield T, Maney JA, Fairley D, et al. Validating clinical practice guidelines for the management of children with non-blanching rashes in the UK (PiC): a prospective, multicentre cohort study. *Lancet Infect Dis.* 2021;21(4):569–577.
15. *Centers for Disease Control and Prevention.* Surveillance and reporting. <https://www.cdc.gov/pneumococcal/surveillance.html> Accessed 01.06.22

FOREIGN BODIES IN CHILDREN

Sydney Ryan

CHAPTER 14

1. **Where are foreign bodies most commonly found?**
   During normal play and exploration, children place objects anywhere they will fit. The nose is the most common site for a retained foreign body. The mouth is a common portal allowing for potential ingestion or aspiration. Ears complete the common location list, and rarely, objects are placed in the vagina, rectum, or urethra. Seventy-five percent of foreign body ingestions are in children younger than 5 years of age due largely to normal developmental exploration.

2. **What are common symptoms of a retained esophageal foreign body?**
   With impacted esophageal foreign bodies, many infants and children will not have significant symptoms at the time of presentation. Common symptoms of acute ingestion for infants and young children include drooling, gagging, unexplained crying, and decreased oral intake, vomiting, or inability to take fluids or solids. In older children, they might describe chest pain or pain or difficulty with swallowing. Less commonly, a foreign body in the esophagus can present with respiratory symptoms such as stridor or respiratory distress due to pressure on the airway. If an object has been retained more chronically, symptoms can include weight loss, food refusal, fever, blood in the stool, vomiting, or persistent pain.

3. **Where do objects impact the esophagus?**
   Impaction at the level of the cricopharyngeus muscle is most common, followed by the lower esophageal sphincter and, less likely, the level of the aortic arch. Patients with a history of congenital esophageal abnormalities or acquired strictures are at risk of retained foreign bodies at the site of anatomic narrowing. While a foreign body that has passed into the stomach is less likely to become impacted, some objects may become stuck at the pylorus or ileocecal valve.

4. **What are common esophageal foreign bodies?**
   Coins, which make up >50% of ingested foreign bodies, are the most commonly impacted foreign body. Pennies are more commonly ingested than other coins and quarters are more likely to become lodged in the esophagus (Fig. 14.1). Other foreign bodies include toys/toy parts, jewelry, batteries, nails/screws/tacks, household supplies, and pieces of food.

5. **What is the expected outcomes of ingested foreign bodies?**
   Overall, between 80% and 90% of foreign bodies pass through naturally, 10% to 20% require endoscopic removal and only 1% will need surgical intervention. Spontaneous passage of coins depends on size and location: coins with diameters >2.3 cm are at risk for esophageal retention. Disc/button batteries can cause erosion and mucosal damage and, thus, must be evaluated and removed quickly. Sharp objects, such as safety pins, are at higher risk of complications including perforations. The size of an object may limit passage through the pylorus. In young children, objects larger than 1 cm × 3 cm are unlikely to pass through the pylorus. For older children, objects measuring greater than 2 cm × 5 cm may be more difficult to pass.

6. **How are ingested foreign bodies evaluated?**
   Radiographs including neck soft tissue, chest, and abdomen can be used to assess mouth to the anus for radiopaque foreign bodies which account for about two-thirds of cases. For radiolucent objects, such as aluminum, plastic, food boluses, and thin objects, computed tomography (CT), fluoroscopic studies, or other imaging modalities can be considered.

7. **How should esophageal foreign bodies be removed?**
   Due to the variability of each foreign body case (age, object, location, patient size, etc.), management can range from urgent removal to closely observed follow-up. In the case of symptomatic foreign bodies of the esophagus, they are commonly removed endoscopically. Other high-risk objects, such as sharp or large objects, may also be removed endoscopically. For blunt, smaller esophageal objects, removal can be accomplished with a balloon catheter or bougie. With the balloon catheter method, the balloon is dilated distal to the object, then inflated and pulled back so that the object finds its way back to the mouth. With the bougienage method, the dilator is used to push the object into the stomach. With low-risk objects that have passed the stomach, close follow-up and strict return precautions can often be provided to the family.

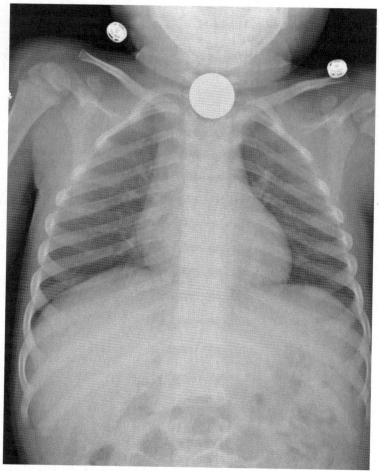

Fig. 14.1 This radiograph shows the typical location of an impacted esophageal coin at the thoracic inlet.

8. **How can one determine if a round, metallic impacted esophageal foreign body is a coin or a disc/button battery?**
   Disc/button batteries will display a double ring near the outer border (Fig. 14.2). Over the past several decades, lithium batteries have become more common due to longer shelf life, lighter weight, and increased voltage. Due to increased availability, lithium composition and size, button batteries have resulted in an increase in morbidity and mortality.

9. **How do batteries cause injury so quickly when impacted?**
   Mucosal damage can occur very quickly if the disc battery becomes lodged in the esophageal tissue through different mechanisms including tissue breakdown from the electrical current and the rapid increase in pH after the production of hydroxide radicals, which can cause mucosal breakdown similar to caustic lye ingestion (liquefaction necrosis). Animal studies have shown this effect on the lamina propria can occur within 30 minutes. If tissue damage occurs, this can lead to esophageal stricture, perforation, fistulas, hemorrhage, and recurrent laryngeal nerve injury.

10. **How are button batteries managed?**
    The management is dependent on the location, size, and time since ingestion as well as the age of the child. Emergent endoscopic removal is necessary for an esophageal button battery. Due to the basic pH environment

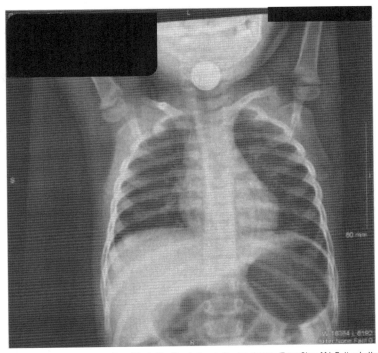

Fig. 14.2 This radiograph shows the double ring of the button/disc battery in the esophagus. (From Ohns MJ. Button battery ingestion: a case report. *J Pediatr Health Care*. 2022;36(5):465–469.)

that is created, new neutralization/mitigation strategies have been introduced if removal is delayed (patient coming from home, transported from another facility, etc.). These interventions include the administration of honey and sucralfate. If the button battery is noted in the stomach or more distal to the stomach, consider outpatient management with close radiological follow-up. For larger button batteries in a younger child, endoscopic removal may be considered. The majority of serious outcomes from button battery ingestion are from batteries measuring more than 20 mm.

11. **Why is there great concern when a child ingests more than one magnet?**
When two or more magnets are ingested, they can align in different portions of the gastrointestinal tract and cause ulceration, perforation, or fistula formation. Deaths from magnet ingestions have been reported. Over the past couple of decades, "rare earth magnets" have become popular. These magnets tend to contain neodymium, which has a greater attractive force than traditional magnets. In order to assess the number and location, two-view radiographs of the chest and abdomen are indicated, recognizing that coupled magnets may appear as one on a single view. If the magnets are in the esophagus or stomach, endoscopic removal is needed. If the magnets are beyond the stomach, management can include immediate removal or serial radiographs with removal for failure of the magnets to progress or if symptoms develop (Fig. 14.3).

12. **What are some other high-risk gastrointestinal foreign bodies?**
Sharp objects (e.g., safety pins, tacks, staples) are known to cause perforation, extraluminal migration, peritonitis, and fistula formation. Initial radiographs can be helpful in diagnosis, but for radiopaque objects, consider CT or other imaging modalities. Removal is indicated if the sharp foreign body is in the esophagus. The treatment for sharp objects in the stomach or beyond ranges from close observation with serial radiographs to surgical removal.

13. **Why are children at risk for aspiration?**
Over 75% of airway foreign bodies evaluated in hospitals occur in children less than 3 years of age. Toddlers are at higher risk for aspiration because of a natural desire to explore the environment using their mouth and easy distractibility during meal time. Additionally, while incisors are present for the biting of food pieces, molars

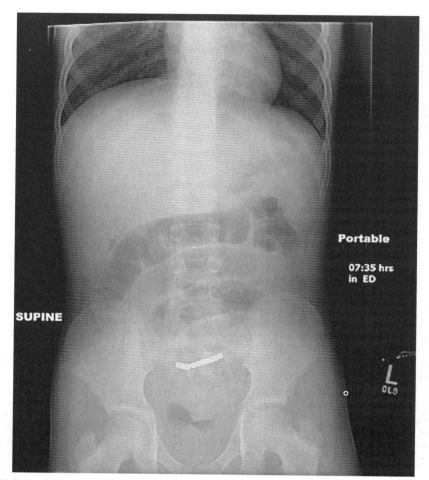

Fig. 14.3 Magnets in the intestines.

required for grinding food are not seen until about 1.5 to 2 years of age. Even with the presence of the molars, the development of proper mastication is not completed until early childhood. Children with developmental delays are also at higher risk for aspiration events.

14. **Why is there high morbidity and mortality with aspirated foreign bodies in children?**
As we know from Poiseuille's law, flow is inversely related to the radius of a tube, to the fourth power. In the case of aspiration, the diameter of airways in children is smaller than that of adults and creates significantly less airflow when obstructed. Young children are not always able to generate a cough with enough force to dislodge foreign bodies as well, which makes clearing foreign bodies naturally more difficult. A few items associated with mortality include latex balloons, hot dogs, round candy, and peanuts that can cause complete occlusion of the airway.

15. **What foreign bodies do children usually aspirate?**
The majority of aspirated foreign bodies are found to be food items and can vary by region. Overall, the most common food items include nuts, seeds, legumes, grapes, candy, popcorn, apples, and hot dogs. Common nonfood items include toys, plastic pieces, pin/nail, balls or beads, coins, and paper/foam products.

16. **What are the signs and symptoms of an aspirated foreign body?**

The signs and symptoms are largely based on the location and size of the aspirated object. The classic triad of cough, wheezing, and diminished breath sounds is not always seen at the time of presentation. Common acute signs and symptoms include the following:

- Cough
- Choking
- Dyspnea
- Wheezing
- Asymmetric breath sounds
- Fever
- Stridor
- Foreign-body sensation

Some children present without signs and symptoms and the object may be found incidentally if imaging is obtained for other reasons. With delayed diagnosis of a foreign body, the child can present with pneumonia, chronic cough, hemoptysis, failure to thrive, or more severe pulmonary conditions.

17. **Do the signs of an aspirated foreign body differ those of other respiratory conditions?**

Unfortunately, there is considerable overlap in both signs and symptoms with very common conditions such as upper respiratory infection, bronchiolitis, asthma, and pneumonia. Always inquire about the possibility of aspiration or a recent choking episode when confronted with a child with acute or chronic respiratory symptoms. Ask specifically about high-risk foods (e.g., nuts, apples, seeds, popcorn). A history of choking followed by coughing is the most common presentation in patients with aspirated foreign body.

18. **How good is a plain film at screening for an aspirated foreign body?**

In the uncommon instances of an aspirated radiopaque foreign body, the radiograph is an excellent test. However, radiopaque foreign bodies only make up about 10% of aspirated objects (Fig. 14.4). The majority of aspirated foreign bodies may have a negative initial anterior-posterior (AP) radiograph. Inspiratory and expiratory views improve sensitivity and may demonstrate air trapping, secondary to a ball-and-valve mechanism, as indirect evidence of an aspirated foreign body (Fig. 14.5). Right and left lateral decubitus views (Fig. 14.6A and B) also provide an alternative, especially in the younger child. Both views are performed during inspiration, and normally the dependent (downside) lung will be relatively deflated. Failure of the dependent lung to show deflation suggests a retained foreign body (Fig. 14.6B). Given the overall lack of sensitivity of plain films, when the history suggests an aspiration event, consider alternative diagnostic testing such as fluoroscopy, CT, or bronchoscopy along with specialty consultation (Fig. 14.7).

19. **Are there other imaging alternatives to detect aspirated foreign bodies?**

Some CT studies have shown a sensitivity of 91% with a specificity of 100% and have decreased the number of negative bronchoscopy rates. While practices vary throughout institutions, bronchoscopy can be both diagnostic and therapeutic. Fluoroscopy can be used but may prove to be more difficult in an uncooperative patient.

20. **What is the appropriate management of a child with an aspirated foreign body?**

Make the patient NPO (nil per os or "nothing by mouth"), and admit them to a hospital where appropriate expertise and age-appropriate equipment are available for the removal of the foreign body. A bronchoscopy (flexible or rigid) is generally used for the removal of the foreign body. In some circumstances, there is the potential for loss of the airway with bronchoscopy, and there have been successful outcomes using extracorporeal membrane oxygenation in conjunction with bronchoscopy.

21. **A teenage boy presents to the emergency department (ED) after a choking episode while drinking beer. He reports that he removed the pull tab of a beer can and placed it inside the can. He believes he may have then swallowed or aspirated the pull tab while gulping beer. What study is best to determine the location of the pull tab?**

CT of the chest may be needed in this case. Plain radiographs have lower sensitivity for aluminum pull tabs of a beer or soda can.

22. **What foreign bodies end up in the ear or nose?**

Just about anything that will fit in the nose could end up there, including food (beans, seeds, nuts, popcorn kernels), small toys, beads, pebbles, magnets, batteries, and rubber/sponge material. If there is a concern for magnets or a battery in the ear or nose, urgent removal is necessary. Foreign bodies in the ear include beads, popcorn kernels, paper or tissue paper, jewelry, toys, and desk supplies. There are case reports of insects, including moths, ants, and cockroaches, found in the ear canal as well.

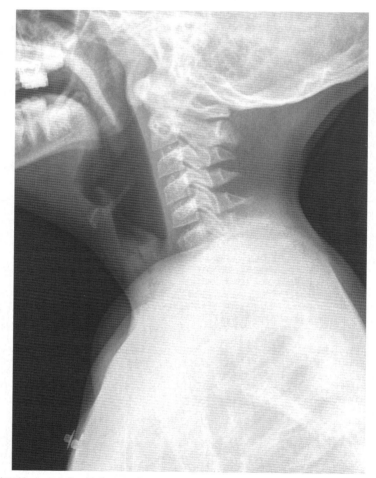

Fig. 14.4 Aspirated foreign body (Lego) in the upper airway.

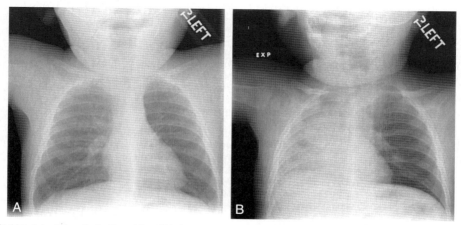

Fig. 14.5 A, Inspiratory chest radiograph in a child who choked on popcorn. **B,** Expiratory chest radiograph of the same child seen in **A** who choked on popcorn. The left lung fails to deflate with expiration, providing indirect evidence of a retained foreign body.

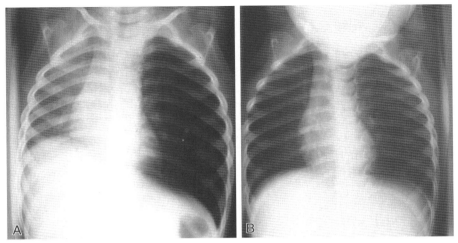

Fig. 14.6 A, Right lateral decubitus chest radiograph. Normal relative deflation of dependent lung (*right*). **B,** Left lateral decubitus chest radiograph. Left lung does not show typical deflation of the dependent lung. Foreign body is on the left side.

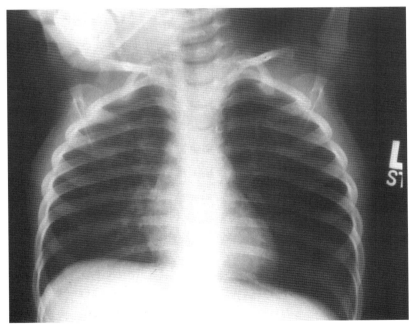

Fig. 14.7 Inspiratory chest radiograph of the same patient shown in Fig. 14.6A and B.

23. **What are the signs and symptoms of children with a nasal foreign body?**
    Up to 80% of the children are asymptomatic and present because of a witnessed insertion, an admission from the child or a nasal foreign body was seen (or smelled) by a caregiver or primary provider. If the patient is symptomatic, most have epistaxis, nasal drainage, or pain. Complications can include infection, necrosis, or septal perforation.

24. **Can a "kiss" help get a foreign body out of the nose?**

Yes. In the ED, instruct the parent to give the child a quick, well-sealed, mouth-to-mouth breath (short and sharp puff) while occluding the unaffected nostril to help advance the foreign body out of the nose. This step may need to be repeated. The literature refers to this as a "mother's kiss" or "parent's kiss" and has been noted to be successful 60% of the time. Other low-tech methods for removal of a foreign body include encouraging the child (if old enough) to blow out through the nose while the unaffected nostril is occluded.

25. **What is the best method for nasal foreign body removal?**

There is no best method because the location and nature of the foreign body, the age and compliance of the child, the skill and comfort of the provider, and available equipment all play a role. Positive pressure technique: While occluding the uninvolved nostril, squeeze the bag mask to increase the pressure and expel the foreign body from the nose, similar to the "kiss technique" described earlier. This positive pressure technique has been shown to have a first-pass success rate of about 50%. Nasal balloon tip catheters (extractors) and Foley catheters have up to a 95% first-past success rate. This involves passing the uninflated balloon on the tip of the catheter past the foreign body, then inflating it before pulling the catheter back out of the nostril. Direct visualization and removal with curettes, forceps (alligator, straight, or bayonet), or hemostats can be used. Hooks and right-angle probes can be used for solid or spherical objects. A cotton swab can be used, adding tissue adhesive to the end but might be more uncomfortable for the patient due to the removal of nasal hair as well. The use of a vasoconstrictor may enhance the success of all nasal foreign-body removal methods.

26. **What are the clinical pearls regarding the removal of foreign bodies from the ear?**

Use of alligator forceps, right-angle hooks, or curved Rosen picks under direct visualization or microscopy is effective in removing foreign bodies from the ear canal. Irrigation is a useful technique, but do not irrigate if (1) the foreign object could expand with liquid (e.g., peas, beans, or a sponge-like material), (2) the tympanic membrane is perforated, or (3) the foreign body is a battery. Ear foreign body removal is a more delicate procedure (the inner portion of the external canal is very sensitive) than the removal of nasal foreign bodies, so sedation should be considered. The suction technique can also be considered, as well as the cotton swab with tissue adhesive technique described previously for nasal foreign bodies.

For a live bug in the ear canal, it is best to immediately drown the insect with something inert like mineral oil, olive oil, or viscous lidocaine and then remove it. Another possible option is to spray 1% lidocaine into the canal to hasten the insect's exit.

27. **Should a child be sedated for the removal of a foreign body from the ear or nose?**

This choice depends on your level of comfort, but in general, nasal foreign bodies can be removed without sedation. However, the inner one-third of the external auditory canal is exquisitely sensitive, and sedation may be needed for difficult foreign bodies in the ear.

28. **Which patients with an ear foreign body should be referred?**

Refer patients to a specialist if there is swelling or a macerated canal (from previous removal attempts), a very tight foreign body, a foreign body against the tympanic membrane, concern for damage to the tympanic membrane, or a disc/button battery in the ear canal or when adequate equipment and lighting are not available.

KEY POINTS: FOREIGN BODIES

1. Remove disc/button batteries impacted in the esophagus emergently and from the ear/nose urgently.
2. Ingestion of multiple magnets poses a significant risk of intestinal complications, including perforation.
3. Many children with retained esophageal foreign bodies are asymptomatic.
4. Signs and symptoms often fail to diagnose an aspirated foreign body; place increased emphasis on a history of choking.
5. Further studies or workup is indicated for a child with a history and examination that is suspicious for an aspirated foreign body.

BIBLIOGRAPHY

1. Ahmed OG, Guillerman RP, Giannoni CM. Protocol incorporating airway CT decreases negative bronchoscopy rates for suspected foreign bodies in pediatric patients. *Int J Pediatr Otorhinolaryngol*. 2018;109:133–137. https://doi.org/10.1016/j.ijporl.2018.03.016. Epub 2018 Mar 19. PMID: 29728167.

2. Ayotunde O, Burkard DJ, Kolacki C, Zamarripa A, Ouellette L, Hamilton M, Jones JS. Nasal foreign body removal: success rates for techniques and devices. *Am J Emerg Med*. 2021;56:384–385. https://doi.org/10.1016/j.ajem.2021.11.027. Epub ahead of print. PMID: 34840003.

3. Baranowski K, Al Aaraj MS, Sinha V. *Nasal foreign body. 2021 Dec 17. StatPearls [Internet]*. StatPearls Publishing; 2022. PMID: 29083647.

4. Berdan EA, Sato TT. Pediatric airway and esophageal foreign bodies. *Surg Clin North Am*. 2017;97(1):85–91. PMID: 27894434. https://doi.org/10.1016/j.suc.2016.08.006.

5. Committee on Injury, Violence, and Poison Prevention Prevention of choking among children. *Pediatrics*. 2010;125(3):601–607. https://doi.org/10.1542/peds.2009-2862. Epub 2010 Feb 22. PMID: 20176668.

6. Conners GP, Mohseni M. *Pediatric foreign body ingestion. 2021 Jul 18. StatPearls [Internet]*. StatPearls Publishing; 2022. PMID: 28613665.

7. Cook S, Burton M, Glasziou P. Efficacy and safety of the "mother's kiss" technique: a systematic review of case reports and case series. *CMAJ*. 2012;184(17):E904–912. https://doi.org/10.1503/cmaj.111864. Epub 2012 Oct 15. PMID: 23071371; PMCID: PMC3503923..

8. Cramer N, Jabbour N, Tavarez MM, Taylor RS. *Foreign body aspiration. 2021 Aug 3. StatPearls [Internet]*. StatPearls Publishing; 2022. PMID: 30285375.

9. Dann L, Doody J, Howard R, Blackburn C, Russell J, Barrett M. Nasal foreign bodies in the paediatric emergency department. *Ir J Med Sci*. 2019;188(4):1401–1405. https://doi.org/10.1007/s11845-019-02000-z. Epub 2019 Mar 11. PMID: 30859417.

10. Dipasquale V, Romano C, Iannelli M, Tortora A, Melita G, Ventimiglia M, Pallio S. Managing pediatric foreign body ingestions: a 10-year experience. *Pediatr Emerg Care*. 2022;38(1):e268–e271. https://doi.org/10.1097/PEC.0000000000002245. PMID: 32970025.

11. Dray X, Cattan P. Foreign bodies and caustic lesions. *Best Pract Res Clin Gastroenterol*. 2013;27(5):679–689. https://doi.org/10.1016/j.bpg.2013.08.009. Epub 2013 Sep 5. PMID: 24160927.

12. Foltran F, Ballali S, Passali FM, Kern E, Morra B, Passali GC, Berchialla P, Lauriello M, Gregori D. Foreign bodies in the airways: a meta-analysis of published papers. *Int J Pediatr Otorhinolaryngol*. 2012;76(Suppl 1):S12–19. https://doi.org/10.1016/j.ijporl.2012.02.004. Epub 2012 Feb 12. PMID: 22333317.

13. Gibbons AT, Casar Berazaluce AM, Hanke RE, McNinch NL, Person A, Mehlman T, Rubin M, Ponsky TA. Avoiding unnecessary bronchoscopy in children with suspected foreign body aspiration using computed tomography. *J Pediatr Surg*. 2020;55(1):176–181. https://doi.org/10.1016/j.jpedsurg.2019.09.045. Epub 2019 Oct 25. PMID: 31706607.

14. Grigg S, Grigg C. Removal of ear, nose and throat foreign bodies: a review. *Aust J Gen Pract*. 2018;47(10):682–685. https://doi.org/10.31128/AJGP-02-18-4503. PMID: 31195771.

15. Huankang Z, Kuanlin X, Xiaolin H, Witt D. Comparison between tracheal foreign body and bronchial foreign body: a review of 1,007 cases. *Int J Pediatr Otorhinolaryngol*. 2012;76(12):1719–1725. https://doi.org/10.1016/j.ijporl.2012.08.008. Epub 2012 Sep 1. PMID: 22944360.

16. Kramer RE, Lerner DG, Lin T, Manfredi M, Shah M, Stephen TC, Gibbons TE, Pall H, Sahn B, McOmber M, Zacur G, Friedlander J, Quiros AJ, Fishman DS, Mamula P. North American Society for Pediatric Gastroenterology, Hepatology, and Nutrition Endoscopy Committee. Management of ingested foreign bodies in children: a clinical report of the NASPGHAN Endoscopy Committee. *J Pediatr Gastroenterol Nutr*. 2015;60(4):562–574. PMID: 25611037. https://doi.org/10.1097/MPG.0000000000000729.

17. Laya BF, Restrepo R, Lee EY. Practical imaging evaluation of foreign bodies in children: an update. *Radiol Clin North Am*. 2017;55(4):845–867. https://doi.org/10.1016/j.rcl.2017.02.012. PMID: 28601182.

18. Leinwand K, Brumbaugh DE, Kramer RE. Button battery ingestion in children: a paradigm for management of severe pediatric foreign body ingestions. *Gastrointest Endosc Clin N Am*. 2016;26(1):99–118. https://doi.org/10.1016/j.giec.2015.08.003.

19. Lotterman S, Sohal M. *Ear foreign body removal. 2021 Dec 4. StatPearls [Internet]*. StatPearls Publishing; 2022. PMID: 29083719.

20. Orsagh-Yentis D, McAdams RJ, Roberts KJ, McKenzie LB. Foreign-body ingestions of young children treated in US Emergency Departments: 1995-2015. *Pediatrics*. 2019;143(5):e20181988. Epub 2019 Apr 12. PMID: 30979810. https://doi.org/10.1542/peds.2018-1988.

21. Park AH, Tunkel DE, Park E, Barnhart D, Liu E, Lee J, Black R. Management of complicated airway foreign body aspiration using extracorporeal membrane oxygenation (ECMO). *Int J Pediatr Otorhinolaryngol*. 2014;78(12):2319–2321. https://doi.org/10.1016/j.ijporl.2014.10.021. Epub 2014 Oct 24. PMID: 25465455.

22. Sethia R, Gibbs H, Jacobs IN, Reilly JS, Rhoades K, Jatana KR. Current management of button battery injuries. *Laryngoscope Investig Otolaryngol*. 2021;6(3):549–563. https://doi.org/10.1002/lio2.535. PMID: 34195377; PMCID: PMC8223456.

23. Valente JH, Lemke T, Ridlen M, Ritter D, Clyne B, Reinert SE. Aluminum foreign bodies: do they show up on x-ray? *Emerg Radiol*. 2005;12(1–2):30–33. https://doi.org/10.1007/s10140-005-0437-9. Epub 2005 Dec 2. PMID: 16322976.

24. Wright CC, Closson FT. Updates in pediatric gastrointestinal foreign bodies. *Pediatr Clin North Am*. 2013;60(5):1221–1239. https://doi.org/10.1016/j.pcl.2013.06.007. Epub 2013 Jul 13. PMID: 24093905.

25. Xiao CC, Kshirsagar RS, Rivero A. Pediatric foreign bodies of the ear: a 10-year national analysis. *Int J Pediatr Otorhinolaryngol*. 2020;138:110354. https://doi.org/10.1016/j.ijporl.2020.110354. Epub 2020 Sep 1. PMID: 33152957.

26. Zavdy O, Viner I, London N, Menzely T, Hod R, Raveh E, Gilony D. Intranasal foreign bodies: a 10-year analysis of a large cohort, in a tertiary medical center. *Am J Emerg Med*. 2021;50:356–359. https://doi.org/10.1016/j.ajem.2021.08.045. Epub 2021 Aug 21. PMID: 34454399.

CHAPTER 15

HEADACHE

Robert D. Schremmer and Joan Elizabeth Giovanni

1. **How common are migraine headaches in children?**

   Migraine is one of the most common causes of headache in children. The reported prevalence is 1% to 3% in children 3 to 7 years of age, and 8% to 23% in adolescence. The variation in prevalence between studies is due primarily to differences in diagnostic criteria used and the age range of children studied. Males tend to have more migraines in their prepubertal years, while females report more frequent headaches after puberty.

2. **List the criteria for pediatric migraine without aura.**

   1. Headache has at least two of the following characteristics:
      a. Bilateral (frontal/temporal) or unilateral location
      b. Pulsatile quality
      c. Intensity described as moderate or severe
      d. Aggravation by or causing avoidance of routine physical activity
   2. At least five attacks fulfilling the above characteristics:
   3. Attacks have a duration of 2 to 72 hours; either untreated or unsuccessfully treated
   4. During the headache at least one of the following:
      a. Nausea and/or vomiting
      b. Photophobia and/or phonophobia
   5. Not better accounted for by another international classification of headache disorders-3 (ICHD-3) diagnosis

3. **Describe atypical migraine variants in children.**

   - Cyclic vomiting syndrome. This condition typically begins between the ages of 5 and 9 and usually resolves around puberty. There is typically a strong family history of migraines, and symptoms often improve with interventions that are used for migraine headaches for symptom resolution.
   - Abdominal migraine. This variant is typically seen between 3 and 12 years of age and presents with frequent episodes of pain with intervals of pain-free periods. There is a strong association between abdominal migraines with a family history of migraine headaches. This condition of abdominal migraines can often transform into migraine headaches without abdominal pain after puberty. Migraine prophylaxis medications often help recurrent bouts of abdominal migraine.
   - Hemiplegic migraine. This is described as hemiplegia or hemiparesis followed by a headache on the contralateral side. Familial cases have been described. Symptoms can last up to 72 hours. Although other workup is needed, antiepileptics have been used to prevent further occurrences.
   - Confusional migraine. This can occur with a variety of migraines and is described as a headache associated with confusion, agitation, and aggressive behaviors. Symptoms typically resolve in 4 to 6 hours.
   - Alice in Wonderland syndrome. This migraine variant is described as bizarre visual hallucinations and spatial distortions. The child may appear confused or can otherwise be completely lucid in describing symptoms. Other differential diagnoses should be considered prior to this diagnosis.

4. **List some common triggers for migraine in children.**

   Stress, lack of sleep, changes in normal eating patterns, weather changes, and some medications (including asthma treatments and stimulants) are common triggers. Certain foods containing nitrates, caffeine, tyramine, glutamate, or salt are potential dietary triggers. Eye strain, cold foods, and high altitude are less common.

5. **How common are tension-type headaches (TTH) in children?**

   TTH are very common in children. Their prevalence ranges from 10% to 25%, but one study reported a prevalence of 73% in Brazilian children and adolescents aged 10 to 18 years. The ICHD-3 lists three subtypes of TTH: (1) infrequent episodic (headaches on <1 day per month), (2) frequent episodic (headaches on 1-14 days per month), and (3) chronic (headaches on ≥15 days per month). These headaches are characterized by mild-to-moderate pressing or tightening pain that is nonpulsatile and typically last 4 to 6 hours. The pain is usually bilateral and not aggravated by routine activity. Nausea and vomiting do not occur, but phonophobia or photophobia may be present. Clinical features are the same in children and adults. It is common for children to continue with their normal activities despite the headache.

6. Do psychological stress factors contribute to TTH in children?

Anxiety and stress factors are often present in children and adolescents with TTH. Divorced parents, fewer peer relations, being a victim of bullying, and an unhappy family atmosphere or child abuse are all associated with childhood TTH. Children with episodic TTH are more likely to report other somatic complaints as well as family problems than children who do not suffer from headaches. TTH often start in the afternoon while at school and may be absent during extended school vacations. Pediatric patients with chronic diseases and who experience stressful family events have an increased risk for chronic TTH. In fact, over 50% of children with chronic TTH have had predisposing physical or emotional stress factors.

7. Can children suffer from both migraines and TTH?

Distinguishing between migraine and TTH in children can be challenging due to frequent overlapping symptoms and the inherent difficulties with history and physical examination in younger children. Up to 30% of children may have difficulty describing their pain to differentiate between headache types. Some researchers have postulated that episodic TTH and migraine may fall along the same continuum of disorder. Long-term outpatient follow-up studies have also reported that TTH may develop into a migraine over time and vice versa. However, there seems to be a smaller genetic effect on TTH than migraine in other studies, which may suggest they are distinct conditions and not a continuum.

8. How will I recognize a child with a brain tumor headache?

Although headache is the most frequent presenting symptom of a new brain tumor, rarely will a child with a headache have a neoplasm. Even so, brain tumors are commonly feared as the cause of a child's headache. Certain features can help to distinguish a headache that is caused by a tumor or other intracranial mass.

- Headaches associated with neurologic signs or symptoms
- Headaches associated with blurry vision, diplopia, or papilledema
- Headaches that awaken the child from sleep or are worse in the morning and improve upon rising
- Headaches that worsen with body movement, especially bending forward
- Headaches associated with Valsalva maneuver (straining, coughing, and sneezing)
- Acute headache following strenuous exercise
- Headaches accompanied by vomiting (except migraine headaches)
- Headache that is progressive or changes in frequency, severity, or other characteristics
- New or changed headache, especially in an oncology patient
- Headaches associated with new educational or behavioral problems
- Age <6 years old

KEY POINTS: BRAIN TUMOR HEADACHES

1. Accompanied by neurologic signs or symptoms
2. Worse in the early morning or awakens child from sleep
3. Progressive or change in character over time
4. Worse with straining, coughing, sneezing, or bending forward
5. Accompanied by vomiting (except with migraine headache)

9. How common are chronic daily headaches (CDHs) in children?

CDH encompasses a group of headache disorders that manifest headaches at least 15 days per month. Although studied much more frequently in adults, estimates of lifetime prevalence for pediatric CDH are 1% to 4.5%. CDH primarily refers to three types of headaches with substantial phenotypic overlap among them:

- **Chronic migraine:** At least half of headache days involve symptoms of migraine with or without aura (pounding or throbbing, moderate to severe pain, difficulty tolerating normal physical activity, sensitivity to light and/or sound, and nausea/vomiting)
- **Chronic TTH:** Absence of migraine symptoms during headache episodes
- **New daily persistent headache (NDPH):** Clearly remembered onset of a daily continuous headache lasting at least 3 months

Risk factors for developing CDH include female sex, transition to adolescence, acute stress, development of obesity, and history of recurring headaches (especially migraines). Comorbid mental health conditions, particularly symptoms of anxiety and depression, are common. There also seems to be an association with attention deficit hyperactivity disorder.

10. What is an NDPH?

NDPH is a rare primary headache disorder characterized by a persistent headache with a clearly remembered onset. Prevalence is higher in pediatric patients (21%-28% vs 1.7%-10.8%). A distinct and clearly remembered onset is necessary for diagnosis, but other characteristics are more nonspecific. The headache is typically bilateral, constant, can be anywhere from mild to severe in intensity, and lacks any special characteristic features. Some patients display typical migraine characteristics of pulsating quality, photophobia, phonophobia, worsening with movement, nausea, and vomiting. Some precipitating factors have been identified, but most patients do not have any. The most common precipitating event is an infection or flu-like illness. Others include stressful life events, minor head injury, surgical procedures with intubation, menarche, syncope, hormone therapy, postpartum state, and thyroid disease. Diagnosis of NDPH is based on typical history; physical examination and neuroimaging are unremarkable. Unfortunately, NDPH is highly resistant to treatment. In the emergency department (ED), patients can be treated according to their symptoms and referred to a headache specialist. Inpatient admission may be necessary for those who experience little or no relief.

11. **When should you worry about idiopathic intracranial hypertension as a cause of headache?**
Consider idiopathic intracranial hypertension (previously called pseudotumor cerebri) when an adolescent female with obesity presents with severe persistent headache that is gradually worsening. Etiology of this condition is often unknown, though some medications (e.g., tetracycline and vitamin A derivatives, such as isotretinoin) have been implicated. Fundoscopic examination usually reveals papilledema. These patients are often misdiagnosed as migraine, sinusitis, or psychogenic headaches. It is very important to recognize this condition because there may be excessive pressure on the optic nerves, which can result in permanent blindness if untreated. Neuroimaging is indicated and a lumbar puncture will reveal an elevated opening pressure, greater than 25 cm.

12. **Describe the most important aspects of the physical examination for children with headaches**
Pay special attention to vital signs such as heart rate and blood pressure, weight and height, and, if appropriate, head circumference. The neurologic examination should focus on mental status, speech, strength, sensation, gait, coordination, cranial nerve function (especially II, III, IV, and VI), and fundoscopic examination. Look for signs of trauma and examine the skin for evidence of a neurocutaneous disease. Multiple café-au-lait lesions suggest neurofibromatosis and possible intracranial tumor. The presence of a ventriculoperitoneal or other shunt can also suggest potential cause of headache.

13. **What is the role of emergent neuroimaging in children with headache?**
Although most headaches in children are benign, the use of neuroimaging for the evaluation of headaches in the ED is not uncommon. Several studies have shown that 6% to 44% of children presenting to the ED with headache receive a computed tomography (CT) or magnetic resonance imaging (MRI) of the brain. Neuroimaging is useful in identifying patients with space-occupying or surgical lesions. An important concern is brain tumor, which, although rare, represents the largest group of solid neoplasms in children. Indications for neuroimaging are as follows:
- Headache associated with abnormal neurologic findings, especially papilledema, nystagmus, mental status changes, or gait or motor disturbances
- Seizures
- Persistent headaches not associated with a family history of migraine
- Headaches that awaken a child from sleep or are present immediately upon awakening
- Persistent headaches associated with episodes of confusion, disorientation, or vomiting
- New severe headache or worsening of a previously stable headache
- Family history or medical history of disorders predisposing one to central nervous system (CNS) lesions (such as neurofibromatosis)
- Clinical or laboratory findings suggestive of CNS involvement

A practice parameter on the evaluation of pediatric patients with recurrent headaches written by the American Academy of Neurology discusses the issues of neuroimaging in clinic patients. The parameter concludes that routine neuroimaging should be avoided in children with a normal neurologic examination. It should be considered, however, in patients with headache who have a history of seizures, an abnormal neurologic examination, a recent change in type of headache experienced, or characteristics implying neurologic dysfunction. The evaluating physician must weigh the risks of each modality when deciding on neuroimaging—the ionizing radiation of CT versus the potential need for sedation or anesthesia for MRI.

14. **What pharmacologic treatments are available for acute headache management in the ED?**
Medications are most effective in aborting an acute headache episode when they are administered early after headache onset or when the pain is still mild. Often patients present to the ED, however, with prolonged pain or unsuccessful attempts for relief at home. Even so, most headaches in children respond to hydration and the over-the-counter analgesics of acetaminophen and nonsteroidal anti-inflammatory drugs (NSAIDs) such as ibuprofen. Triptans are often second-line medications used at home for migraines and can be considered in the ED. Rizatriptan has been approved for children aged 6 and over; almotriptan, sumatriptan, and sumatriptan/naproxen can be used in adolescents. Unfortunately, early administration is usually necessary for them to be effective, so their utility in the ED may be limited. Intravenous medications such as prochlorperazine, metoclopramide, ketorolac, valproic acid, divalproex sodium, and dihydroergotamine can all be considered. Generally, the first line

of management for severe headaches in the ED is prochlorperazine and intravenous fluids if the over-the-counter analgesics have already been attempted. Due to the rare potential for dystonic reactions, many physicians choose to concomitantly administer diphenhydramine which has the added benefit of drowsiness for the patient. If the headache remains refractory, second-line medications include ketorolac and valproic acid. Dihydroergotamine may only improve headache pain after several doses, so it is less likely to be useful acutely unless the patient is to be admitted to the hospital. Premedication with an antiemetic is also required since nausea is a common side effect. Narcotic analgesics should be avoided. Patients with persistent significant headaches following treatment may require hospital admission.

15. **What lifestyle changes can be made to prevent headaches?**
    Adequate sleep, avoiding the use of electronics in the bedroom at night, a regular bedtime schedule, routine exercise, and eating well-balanced and healthy meals (including breakfast) can help reduce frequency of headaches. Adequate hydration is also essential in the prevention of headaches. Water should be emphasized over juices and soda, and caffeine should be limited to less than three servings per week. Identifying, avoiding, and managing triggers and stressors are also important.

16. **Is there any benefit to acupuncture in the treatment of headache in children?**
    There is not much validation for alternative treatments for headache in the scientific literature, but there is more evidence for acupuncture than any other alternative therapy. Acupuncture has been used to effectively treat a variety of painful conditions for both adults and children in the ED, including headaches. The mechanism of action is unclear, but there are several theories that support its success. Traditional body acupuncture and battlefield auricular (BFA) acupuncture have been proposed as techniques to relieve headache pain. There are multiple traditional body acupuncture techniques that can be used; BFA consists of five specific acupuncture points on both ears (Fig. 15.1). Side effects of both traditional body acupuncture and BFA are mild and may include pain at the needle site, bleeding, and syncope. One challenge is the availability of trained acupuncturists in the ED (Fig. 15.2).

17. **Describe the management of posttraumatic headaches.**
    Patients with concussion frequently experience headache, imbalance, cognitive impairment, fatigue, and sleepiness. Most children will recover and return to baseline functioning within a month of the injury. About a third of patients still have symptoms a month after the injury, 14% are symptomatic at 3 months, and 2% of patients are still symptomatic at 1 year after a mild traumatic brain injury. Risk factors for experiencing prolonged symptoms include adolescent

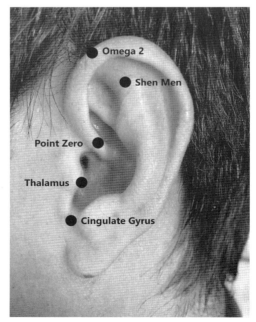

Fig. 15.1 Battlefield auricular acupuncture sites.

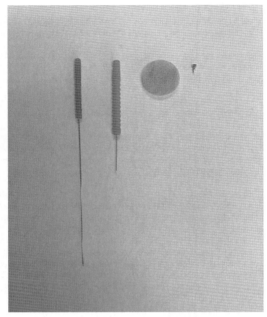

Fig. 15.2 Typical acupuncture needles that can be used for pain management in the emergency department. From left to right: Serin, Detox 5, Pyonex, Gold ASP.

age, female sex, high symptom burden at the time of the injury, history of migraine headache diagnosis, prior concussions, and preinjury mental health diagnosis. Providing education about the expected symptom course can improve outcomes for patients in the ED. Ibuprofen or other NSAIDs can be recommended once structural brain injury has been excluded. Migrainous posttraumatic headache can be managed in the same way as preinjury migraine headache. Patients should be cautioned about the possibility of medication-induced headaches and should not continue NSAIDs past 7 days without talking to their physician. Regular sleep schedule, good hydration and nutrition, avoidance of further head injury, minimizing caffeine intake, and avoidance of drugs and alcohol are thought to help minimize posttraumatic symptoms. The role of rest following a concussion has evolved over time. Instead of strict rest for a defined period, patients should gradually increase physical and cognitive activity as they are able to tolerate it. Multidisciplinary care is helpful for patients with persistent symptoms.

KEY POINTS: HEADACHES

The International Headache Society has published criteria for the definition of adult headache types that includes some concessions for children, but inadequacies remain.
1. Avoid routine neuroimaging in children who suffer from headaches; specific "red flags" in the patient's history and physical examination should prompt CT or MRI evaluation.
2. Acute headache pain is usually relieved by hydration, rest, and over-the-counter analgesics. Antiemetics and triptans may be useful in select cases resistant to those measures.
3. Management of frequent and persistent headache should include a multidisciplinary approach utilizing both pharmacologic and nonpharmacologic therapies and is best accomplished by a headache specialist.

Acknowledgment
The authors wish to acknowledge the work of Dr. Jane F. Knapp as an author of previous versions of this article.

BIBLIOGRAPHY
1. Blume HK. Childhood headache: a brief review. *Pediatr Ann.* 2017;46:e155–e165.
2. Blume HK. Posttraumatic headache in pediatrics: an update and review. *Curr Opin Pediatr.* 2018;30:755–763.
3. Bougea A, Spantideas N, Chrousos GP. Stress management for headaches in children and adolescents: a review and practical recommendations for health promotion programs and well-being. *J Child Health Care.* 2018;22(1):19–33.

4. Cain MR, Arkilo D, Linabery AM, Kharbanda AB. Emergency department use of neuroimaging in children and adolescents presenting with headache. *J Pediatr*. 2018;201:196–201.

5. Connelly M, Sekhon S. Current perspectives on the development and treatment of chronic daily headache in children and adolescents. *Pain Manag*. 2019;9:175–189.

6. Dao JM, Qubty W. Headache diagnosis in children and adolescents. *Curr Pain Headache Rep*. 2018;22:17.

7. Gelfand AA. Pediatric and adolescent headache. *Continuum (Minneap, Minn)*. 2018;24:1108–1136.

8. Graff DM, McDonald MJ. Auricular acupuncture for the treatment of pediatric migraines in the emergency department. *Pediatr Emerg Care*. 2018;34:258–262.

9. Hadidchi S, Surento W, Lemer A, Liu C-SJ, Gibbs WN, Kim PE, Shiroishi MS. Headache and brain tumors. *Neuroimag Clin N Am*. 2019;29:291–300.

10. Headache Classification Committee of the International Headache Society (HIS). The International Classification of Headache Disorders, 3rd edition. *Cephalgia*. 2018;38:1–211.

11. Kelly M, Strelzik J, Langdon R, DiSabella M. Pediatric headache: overview. *Curr Opin Pediatr*. 2018;30:748–754.

12. Langdon R, DiSabella MT. Pediatric headache: an overview. *Curr Probl Pediatr Adolesc Health Care*. 2017;47:44–65.

13. Oskoul M, Pringsheim T, Holler-Managan Y, Potrebic S, Billinghurst L, Gloss D, et al. Practice guideline update summary: acute treatment of migraine in children and adolescents. *Neurology*. 2019;93:487–499.

14. Rausa VC, Anderson V, Babl FE, Takagi M. Predicting concussion recovery in children and adolescents in the emergency department. *Curr Neurol Neurosci Rep*. 2018;18:78.

15. Rothner A. Migraine variants in children. *Pediatr Ann*. 2018;47(2):e50–e54.

16. Tsai S, Reynoso E, Shin DW, Tsung JW. Acupuncture as a nonpharmacologic treatment for pain in a pediatric emergency department. *Pediatr Emerg Care*. 2021;37:e360–e366.

17. Yamani N, Olesen J. New daily persistent headache: a systematic review on an enigmatic disorder. *J Headache Pain*. 2019;20:80.

CHAPTER 16

HEMATURIA AND DYSURIA

Erica Y. Popovsky and Sandra H. Schwab

1. **What is the definition of hematuria?**
   Hematuria is the presence of red blood cells (RBCs) in the urine. Hematuria can be categorized as gross or microscopic. Gross hematuria is defined as pink to brown discoloration of the urine with confirmation of RBCs by microscopy. Microscopic hematuria is normal-appearing urine that, when centrifuged, has more than five RBCs per high-power field (HPF) on microscopy.

2. **What else, besides RBCs, can cause urine to appear red or brown?**
   Reddish or brownish discoloration of the urine from some compound other than blood is common. Myoglobinuria and porphyrinuria present with red- or tea-colored urine. Many dyes, drugs, pigments, and metabolites also discolor the urine. Common substances that turn urine red include red food dye, beets, blackberries, bile pigments, rifampin, phenazopyridine (Pyridium), ibuprofen, salicylates, and deferoxamine. Infants may have precipitation of urate crystals that make their urine appear red or orange in the diaper.

3. **What can cause a "false-positive" urine dipstick?**
   You may encounter a urine dipstick positive for blood, but on microscopic examination no RBCs are seen. The dipstick is sensitive to any heme compound and will be positive for intact RBCs as well as hemoglobin from hemolyzed RBCs and myoglobin from rhabdomyolysis. Dehydration, strenuous exercise, and oxidizing compounds, such as bleach or microbial peroxidase, can turn the dipstick spuriously positive. Delayed reading of the dipstick may also produce a false-positive result.

4. **Is there a way to determine glomerular versus nonglomerular blood in the urine?**
   Yes. Determination of the origin of blood is important in directing further evaluation and testing. If the RBCs come from glomeruli, the acidic nature of the urine may change hemoglobin to hematin, causing the urine to appear brownish, tea-colored, or cola-colored. Blood from the lower collecting system frequently appears pink or red. Microscopic examination of the urine will give more specific information, including identifying the presence of urine casts or RBC dysmorphology if blood is from the glomeruli (Table 16.1).

5. **What is the differential diagnosis of hematuria in a child?**
   The differential diagnosis of hematuria in a child is in Table 16.2.

6. **What is the most likely diagnosis of a child presenting to the emergency department (ED) with hematuria?**
   The causes of gross hematuria and microscopic hematuria are very different. In general, the majority of children who visit an ED for hematuria are diagnosed with urinary tract infections (UTIs) or cystitis. Other common causes of gross hematuria include glomerulonephropathies, trauma (with or without underlying anatomic abnormality), nephrolithiasis, hypercalciuria, bleeding disorders, and nutcracker syndrome (left renal vein entrapment) (see Question 9).
   Most children with asymptomatic microscopic hematuria have a benign condition that is self-limited.
   Even though parents or patients may assume that blood in the diaper or toilet is from urine, it may be from several other sources: vaginal bleeding (menses, foreign body, infection, trauma), rectal bleeding (fissure, hemorrhoid, trauma), urate crystals in infants, or urethral prolapse.

Table 16.1 Glomerular Versus Nonglomerular Blood in the Urine

GLOMERULAR	NONGLOMERULAR
Brown- or tea-colored urine	Bright red or pink urine
RBC casts	Blood clots
Dysmorphic RBCs	Normal RBC morphological appearance
Proteinuria	Blood at initiation or termination of urination

RBC, red blood cell.

Table 16.2 Differential Diagnosis of Hematuria in Children

GLOMERULAR	NONGLOMERULAR
Benign familial hematuria	Chemical cystitis
Cystic renal disease	Coagulopathy or hemoglobinopathy
Glomerulonephritis	Exercise
Henoch-Schönlein purpura	Hypercalciuria
IgA nephropathy	Malignancy
Membranoproliferative GN	Leukemia
Membranous nephropathy	Nephroblastoma
Polyarteritis nodosa	Neuroblastoma
Poststreptococcal GN	Rhabdomyosarcoma
Rapidly progressive GN	Wilms tumor
Systemic lupus erythematosus	Medications
Wegener granulomatosis	Nutcracker syndrome
Goodpasture disease	Structural anomalies
Hemolytic uremic syndrome	Trauma
Hereditary nephritis (Alport syndrome)	Urinary tract infection
Interstitial nephritis	Urolithiasis
Renal vein thrombosis	Vascular malformation

IgA, immunoglobulin A; GN, glomerulonephritis.
Adapted from Yap HK, Lau PYW. Hematuria and proteinuria. In: Geary DF, Schaefer F, eds. *Comprehensive Pediatric Nephrology.* Mosby Elsevier; 2008:180.

7. **What are important physical examination findings to look for in a child with hematuria?**
   Measure the child's blood pressure. Hypertension is often found in patients with hematuria, and this combination may indicate a renal emergency. If noted, consider glomerulonephritis, obstructive uropathy, polycystic kidney disease, hemolytic uremic syndrome, systemic lupus erythematosus, and Wilms tumor. A thorough abdominal examination is important, as Wilms tumor may present with a palpable abdominal mass. Between 12% and 25% of patients with Wilms tumor have hematuria at the time of presentation, and 25% have hypertension. Edema is another important finding and is suggestive of protein loss or fluid overload. Key places to check for edema include the periorbital region, the scrotum in males and the lower extremities. Rapid weight gain may also be suggestive of fluid overload, and current weight should be compared to recent weights if available.

8. **What signs and symptoms associated with hematuria require urgent/emergent evaluation?**
   Children with hematuria should be evaluated with a full history, family history, and physical examination, which will allow a directed workup of the cause. In general, gross hematuria requires emergent evaluation for significant renal trauma, tumor, congenital abnormality, or bleeding disorder. Hematuria accompanied by proteinuria or systemic symptoms such as edema, oliguria, hypertension, or headache may portend glomerular renal disease that requires emergent evaluation. Additional signs and symptoms such as fever, dysuria, flank pain, abdominal pain, bloody diarrhea, rash, recent sore throat, or respiratory illness are important signs and symptoms to consider. Asymptomatic isolated microscopic hematuria is found at one time or another in 1% to 4% of children and, in most cases, is benign. This is a diagnosis of exclusion, and referral for outpatient evaluation is indicated.

9. **What is nutcracker syndrome?**
   Nutcracker syndrome refers to compression of the left renal vein between the aorta and the superior mesenteric artery before the renal vein joins the inferior vena cava. Children usually present with unilateral flank pain and intermittent gross or microscopic hematuria. Some experts believe this is an underrecognized cause of hematuria, and diagnosis is increasing with improved diagnostic testing such as ultrasound and magnetic resonance imaging.

10. **When is a renal and bladder ultrasound indicated in the workup of hematuria?**

Ultrasound is a noninvasive test without exposure to radiation, so it should be considered early in the evaluation of gross hematuria or persistent microscopic hematuria. Children who present with gross hematuria in the absence of proteinuria or RBC casts should have an ultrasound to evaluate for malignancy or cystic renal disease. Ultrasound is helpful to rule out anatomic abnormalities, obstruction, and nutcracker syndrome.

11. **Which laboratory tests are helpful in the evaluation of hematuria?**

All patients with signs or findings of hematuria should have a urine dipstick and microscopic urinalysis. Depending on the history and physical examination, further blood tests may be indicated. Hematuria with fever, flank pain, urgency, and dysuria usually indicates a UTI and should be evaluated with a urine Gram stain and culture. Complete blood count, blood urea nitrogen, and serum creatinine may be helpful, except in cases of isolated microscopic hematuria or obvious UTI. If the child has sustained or suspected trauma, liver function tests, amylase, and lipase are also recommended. Prothrombin time and partial thromboplastin time will help diagnose any bleeding disorder, particularly in the setting of petechial or purpuric rashes. If the clinical picture indicates nephritis, then electrolytes, complement levels (C3 and C4), antistreptolysin O or streptozyme test, antinuclear antibody titer, hepatitis screen, and erythrocyte sedimentation rate may be helpful.

A patient with a positive dipstick without evidence of RBCs on urine microscopic examination should be evaluated with plasma creatine kinase and urinary myoglobin concentration for rhabdomyolysis and a bilirubin level for signs of hemolysis.

12. **Why is it important to ask about a history of recent infections in children with gross hematuria?**

A common cause of macroscopic hematuria in children is postinfectious glomerulonephritis (PIGN). Poststreptococcal glomerulonephritis is most common and follows streptococcal infections of the throat by 1 to 2 weeks, versus a period of 3 to 5 weeks for skin infections such as impetigo. PIGN can also be caused by other pathogens including viruses, parasites, and other bacteria. PIGN is characterized by hematuria with the majority presenting with gross hematuria that is "cola" colored and may have associated edema and hypertension. Obtain laboratory studies to look for decreased renal function, proteinuria, RBC casts, decreased C3, and positive streptococcal antibody testing (antistreptolysin or anti-DNase B).

13. **Describe the causes of nephrolithiasis in children.**

Nephrolithiasis is an increasing problem in children in the United States. Stone formation results from environmental and hereditary factors. Hypercalciuria is the most common cause of pediatric urinary stones and has many causes. Genetic syndromes, such as familial idiopathic hypercalciuria, as well as other diseases such as Bartter syndrome and distal renal tubular acidosis, lead to increased urinary calcium excretion and stone formation. Iatrogenic causes include treatment with loop diuretics and prednisone.

Other causes of stone formation include infection with urease-producing organisms (struvite or "staghorn" calculi); cystinuria; hyperoxaluria; medications such as protease inhibitors; and high-protein, low-carbohydrate diets (ketogenic diet).

14. **How do you diagnose urinary stones in children?**

Evaluation should begin with a complete history and physical examination, including a history of urinary infections, current medications, and a detailed family history. Most children present with flank or abdominal pain. Obtain a urinalysis and urine culture. Microscopic hematuria is present in more than 90% of children with urinary stones. Infection is commonly seen with stones, so evidence of UTI does not exclude stones.

A nonenhanced helical CT scan is the most sensitive imaging method for diagnosis. Very small stones throughout the entire urinary tract can be identified. Renal ultrasound is the first-line imaging modality in stable pediatric patients; however, it may fail to identify stones in >40% of cases. Ultrasound sensitivity and specificity vary based on the location and size of the stone and are also operator dependent. Even if the stone is not visualized, it can be helpful to detect hydroureter or hydronephrosis caused by obstructing stones. Plain radiographs will detect large, radiopaque stones but have limited sensitivity, so they are not routinely recommended.

15. **Why are children at more risk than adults for renal injury after blunt trauma?**

In children, the kidneys are situated lower, are less protected by the ribs and abdominal wall, and are proportionally larger and more mobile than in adults. Fetal lobations of the kidney may persist, which allows for easier tissue damage. Children usually have less protective perirenal fat and musculature. All of these factors make them more susceptible to renal injury.

16. **How would you evaluate a child with blunt abdominal trauma for renal injury?**

Children who are hemodynamically unstable following abdominal trauma require immediate evaluation for significant renal injury. A computed tomography (CT) scan with intravenous (IV) contrast agent is the standard imaging study of choice.

Children with focal examination findings or significant mechanisms of injury (rapid deceleration, direct flank trauma, falls from heights) should also be evaluated further, regardless of the presence of hematuria. Using urinalysis as a screening test for significant injury is helpful, but it should be interpreted with caution. Most experts agree that children with macrohematuria (>50 RBC/HPF on microscopy) or gross hematuria should undergo a CT scan. In clinically stable children with concern for genitourinary trauma, the gold-standard imaging is a CT scan with contrast and delayed images. Children with microscopic hematuria may instead be able to be monitored with reliable follow-up in order to reduce exposure to radiation.

A focused assessment by sonography for trauma ultrasound is not sensitive enough to rule out renal injuries in pediatric trauma compared to CT.

17. **What findings in an injured child should make you suspicious of a lower genitourinary tract injury?**
Children with any of the following: a pelvic fracture, blood at the urethral meatus, perineal hematoma, high-riding prostate or inability to void have concerning injuries for a lower genitourinary tract injury and may require a CT cystourethrogram. Most children with bladder injuries will have hematuria and dysuria, with almost all having gross hematuria in bladder rupture. Blunt trauma is the most common cause of urethral injuries and is usually related to motor vehicle accidents, straddle injuries, and high-velocity falls.

KEY POINTS: HEMATURIA

1. UTIs are the most common cause of hematuria in children.
2. Distinguishing between glomerular and nonglomerular hematuria can help narrow the differential diagnosis and lead to a diagnosis.
3. Any child with gross hematuria requires emergent evaluation.
4. Any child with hematuria should have a urine dipstick, microscopic urinalysis, and blood pressure measurement.
5. Asymptomatic microscopic hematuria without proteinuria is usually benign and self-limited.
6. Children with posttraumatic gross hematuria require emergent imaging.

18. **What are the most common causes of dysuria in children?**
Dysuria (painful urination) is usually caused by irritation of the bladder or urethra. Common causes of this symptom include infectious cystitis (viral or bacterial), urethritis (infectious, chemical, or traumatic), vaginitis, and balanitis. Bacterial cystitis will demonstrate an abnormal urinalysis that is positive for at least one of the following: leukocyte esterase, nitrites, or more than five white blood cells from a catheterized specimen and a urine culture with bacterial growth of >50 to 100,000 CFU/mL depending on the method of urine collection. Sexually transmitted infections such as gonorrhea or chlamydia are important considerations for sexually active adolescents. Young children may report or exhibit perineal discomfort, and parents may interpret this discomfort as dysuria in the case of pruritus from pinworms (*Enterobius vermicularis*) or in cases of sexual abuse.

19. **Which systemic diseases may present with dysuria?**
Urethritis, producing dysuria, is associated with several serious systemic diseases, such as Stevens-Johnson syndrome, Reiter syndrome, and Behçet syndrome. Crohn's disease can predispose patients to fistula formation and subsequent dysuria.

20. **Name some common causes of urethritis in children.**
Infectious urethritis in adolescents is most commonly due to *Neisseria gonorrhoeae* and *Chlamydia trachomatis*. Bubble baths, detergents, fabric softeners, and perfumed soaps are often the cause for cases of chemical urethritis in younger children.

21. **Can labial adhesions cause dysuria?**
Painful urination may be related to labial adhesions in a prepubertal girl. It is important to examine the genitalia for this condition. It is also important to consider a urinary tract infection, which is sometimes related to the adhesions. Labial adhesions can be treated with topical estrogen and/or steroid cream. Most girls with labial adhesions are asymptomatic.

22. **What parasitic infection should be considered in a traveler or recent immigrant presenting with hematuria or dysuria?**
Urinary schistosomiasis, caused by *Schistosoma haematobium*, is a common cause of hematuria and dysuria worldwide. This worm is found mostly in sub-Saharan Africa and enters through the skin after contact with fresh water that harbors the larval form. The worms eventually migrate to the bladder mucosa, where eggs are produced and secreted in the urine. Diagnosis can be made by examination of the urine for eggs. Praziquantel is the mainstay of treatment and is curative in most cases.

23. **What symptomatic treatment should be recommended for dysuria while urine cultures are pending?**
    When a diagnosis is pending, symptomatic treatment of dysuria includes warm water sitz baths for young girls with urethritis or vulvovagintis. For children older than age 6, consider prescribing phenazopyridine for up to 2 days. Recommend increased fluid intake as dilute urine may cause less discomfort than concentrated urine.

KEY POINTS: DYSURIA

1. The most common causes of dysuria in children are UTIs and urethritis.
2. Chemical urethritis is a common cause of dysuria in young children.
3. Consider diagnoses such as pinworms, systemic illness, or sexual abuse in children presenting with dysuria.

BIBLIOGRAPHY

1. Bacon GL, Romano ME, Quint EH. Clinical recommendations: labial adhesions. *Pediatr Adolesc Gynecol*. 2015;28(5):405–409.
2. Brown DD, Reidy KJ. Approach to the child with hematuria. *Pediatr Clin North Am*. 2019;66(1):15–30.
3. Bryngil J, Corboy JB, Lopez P. Pain—dysuria. In: Shaw K, Bachur R, eds. *Textbook of Pediatric Emergency Medicine*. 8th ed. Wolters Kluwer; 2021:383–388.
4. Flores FX. Clinical evaluation of the child with hematuria. In: Kleigman RM, ed. *Nelson Textbook of Pediatrics*. 21st ed. WB Saunders Elsevier; 2020:2718–2720.
5. Kovell R, Tasian G, Belfer R. Genitourinary trauma. In: Shaw K, Bachur R, eds. *Textbook of Pediatric Emergency Medicine*. 8th ed. Wolters Kluwer; 2021:1131–1142.
6. Liebelt EA, Davis V. Hematuria. In: Shaw KN, Bachur RG, eds. *Textbook of Pediatric Emergency Medicine*. 8th ed. Wolters Kluwer; 2021:235–239.
7. Meyer J, Rother U, Stehr M, Meyer A. Nutcracker syndrome in children: appearance, diagnostics, and treatment: a systematic review. *J Pediatr Surg*. 2022;57(11):716–722.
8. Melek E, Kilicbay F, Sarikas NG, Bayazit AK. Labial adhesions and urinary tract problems: the importance of a genital exam. *J Pediatr Urol*. 2016;12(2):111.
9. Miah T, Kamat D. Pediatric nephrolithiasis: a review. *Pediatr Ann*. 2017;46(6):e242–244.
10. Rabinowicz S, Leshem E, Schwartz E. Acute schistosomiasis in paediatric travelers and comparison with their companion adults. *J Travel Med*. 2021;28(6):taaa238.

CHAPTER 17

HYPERTENSION

Laura Mercurio and Susan J. Duffy

1. **What is considered high blood pressure or hypertension in a child?**
   There's elevated blood pressure, and then there's hypertension. Aligning with adult American Heart Association's guidelines, children can be classified into *stage 1* and *stage 2* hypertension. These classifications by age, sex, and height were initially established by the Task Force on Blood Pressure Control in Children and revised in 2017 by a new task force sponsored by the American Academy of Pediatrics. A key update involved accounting for known elevations in blood pressure among obese children and for children >13 years mirroring adult guidelines, the following values were determined using data from normal-weight children:

   Children aged 1 to 12 years
   - Normal BP: Both systolic and diastolic BP <95th percentile
   - Stage 1 hypertension: Systolic BP and/or diastolic BP ≥95th percentile to <95th percentile + 12 mm Hg or 130/80 to 139/89 mm Hg (whichever is lower)
   - Stage 2 hypertension: Systolic BP and/or diastolic BP ≥95th percentile + 12 mm Hg or ≥140/90 mm Hg (whichever is lower)

   Children aged 13 years and older
   - Normal BP: <120/<80 mm Hg
   - Stage 1 hypertension: BP between 130/80 and 139/89 mm Hg
   - Stage 2 hypertension: BP ≥140/90 mm Hg

2. **What is the difference between hypertensive urgency and a hypertensive emergency?**
   The distinction is not absolute and depends somewhat on clinical judgment. *Hypertensive urgency* refers to severely elevated blood pressure without evidence of end-organ damage. The child with this condition may be asymptomatic or may have symptoms such as headache, nausea, or vomiting with *normal* mental status. A *hypertensive emergency* occurs when a child's blood pressure is severely elevated and the child shows evidence of end-organ damage, with or without life-threatening conditions such as seizure, intracranial hemorrhage, or congestive heart failure. Left ventricular hypertrophy (LVH) is an example of chronic end-organ damage. Although relatively uncommon in children as compared to adults, hypertensive urgencies and emergencies are known to cause significant health problems and even death.

KEY POINTS: CLASSIFICATION OF HYPERTENSION BASED ON AGE, HEIGHT, AND SEX

1. Hypertension definitions are now divided into age categories 1 to 12 and ≥13 years of age (see above).
2. Hypertensive definitions among children ≥13 years of age mirror the adult guidelines.
3. Hypertensive urgency is an acute severe blood pressure elevation *without* evidence of end-organ damage.
4. Hypertensive emergency is an acute severe blood pressure elevation *with* evidence of end-organ damage.

---

3. **If high blood pressure is found incidentally by the triage nurse, what two questions should you ask before you get too worried?**
   - **"What size cuff was used?"** Inappropriate cuff size can give spuriously high or low blood pressure readings. They will be falsely elevated if the cuff is too small, and low if the cuff is too big. The width of the cuff bladder should be about 40% of the circumference of the arm measured at the midpoint between the shoulder and the elbow (technically, between the acromion and the olecranon). The cuff should encircle 80% to 100% of the circumference of the upper arm and be about two-thirds of its length.
   - **"Will you please repeat it?"** Nonpathological elevations in blood pressure can be caused by patient response to white coats, pain, recent activity, heat, and agitation. Ideally, a child's blood pressure should be measured after a few minutes of inactivity, as he or she sits calmly in a parent's lap. The most accurate reading may occur after the child adapts to their new environment, but don't forget to repeat it!

4. **Which emergency department (ED) patients need evaluation and treatment in the ED, and which patients can follow up with their primary care physician (PCP)?**
   - **Evaluation and treatment:** Patients with symptomatic hypertensive emergencies as described below, should be treated in the ED with the initial focus on airway, breathing, and circulation (ABCs) and rapidly establishing intravenous (IV) access.

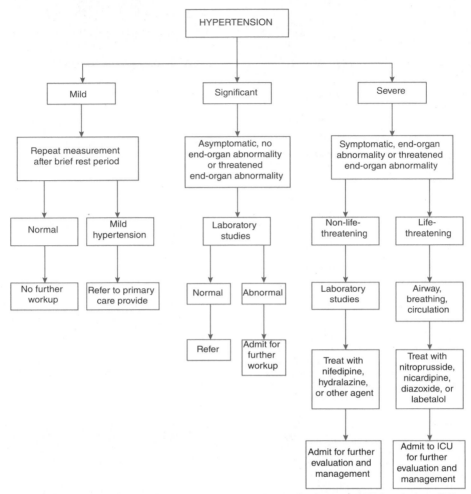

Fig. 17.1 Approach to the initial emergency department triage and stabilization of the hypertensive child. ICU, intensive care unit. (From Linakis JG. Hypertension. In: Fleisher GR, Ludwig S, eds. *Textbook of Pediatric Emergency Medicine.* 5th ed. Wolters Kluwer; 2006, used with permission.)

- **Evaluation only:** For asymptomatic patients with *stage 2* elevated blood pressure readings, perform a thorough history and physical examination and some screening laboratory tests. If there are no signs of underlying medical conditions in this workup, the patient can be discharged with close follow-up. Unlike for adults, there are no recommendations for home blood pressure monitoring in children.
- **Discharge without evaluation:** Patients being evaluated for other medical concerns, who were incidentally found to have *stage 1* hypertension and are asymptomatic, can be discharged to the care of their PCP. Ideally, the doctor should record several readings in a series of visits before confirming the diagnosis of hypertension (Fig. 17.1).

KEY POINTS: APPROACH TO THE HYPERTENSIVE CHILD

1. Evaluate, treat, and admit patients with hypertensive emergencies.
2. Evaluate asymptomatic patients with *stage 2* hypertension; discharge those who have normal screening laboratory test results.
3. Discharge *with follow-up* patients with incidentally found *stage 1* hypertension.

5. **Name the causes of pathological hypertension. Discuss likely causes in babies, small children, and older children.**
   In general, as the age of a child increases, the likelihood of finding a secondary cause for hypertension decreases. A newborn infant with hypertension is most likely to have either a congenital renal anomaly or a vascular problem (e.g., a renal artery or venous thrombosis or stenosis, or coarctation of the aorta). Small children may present with these vascular or congenital causes but become more likely to have renal parenchymal diseases such as pyelonephritis, glomerulonephritis, or reflux nephropathy. In general, low birth weight and prematurity have been associated with elevated blood pressure in childhood. Older children and teenagers are more likely to have essential hypertension (including obesity), though they may still present with parenchymal disease. The mnemonic HYPERTENSION may help you recall some of the major causes of high blood pressure:
   - **H:** Hyperthyroidism (and other autoimmune diseases)
   - **Y:** Why? Cause unknown—primary hypertension
   - **P:** Pheochromocytoma
   - **E:** Eats too much—obesity (or other unhealthy habits—alcohol, tobacco)
   - **R:** Renal parenchymal disease
   - **T:** Thrombosis (renal artery, particularly if the umbilical catheter was used as neonate)
   - **E:** Endocrine disorder (*congenital adrenal hyperplasia*, primary aldosteronism, hyperparathyroidism)
   - **N:** Neurological disorder (increased intracranial pressure, Guillain-Barré syndrome, neurofibromatosis)
   - **S:** Stenosis (renal artery stenosis or coarctation of the aorta, supravalvular aortic stenosis with Williams syndrome)
   - **I:** Ingestion (cocaine, sympathomimetics, birth control pills, steroids, decongestants, sudden withdrawal, or chemotherapy)
   - **O:** Obstetric cause (eclampsia)
   - **N:** Neuroblastoma

6. **How might a child present with hypertension?**
   Often hypertension is silent and picked up on routine physical examination. If a child does present with symptoms, they may be as vague as irritability and headache or as significant as seizure and coma. Other possible symptoms include visual disturbances, personality changes, dizziness, nausea and vomiting, weight loss, polyuria and polydipsia, and facial nerve palsy.

7. **What historical questions are important to ask the parent of a hypertensive child?**
   - Does the child have a history of recurrent urinary tract infections? Prior genitourinary surgery? Unexplained fever? Hematuria? Frequency? Dysuria? Any recent illness? Sore throat? Chest pain? Shortness of breath?
   - Was your child born prematurely? Low birth weight? Did the child have an umbilical artery catheter as a neonate?
   - Does he or she have intermittent sweating, flushing, and palpitations?
   - Has the child been growing well?
   - Has the child suffered any recent head trauma?
   - Is there a family history of hypertension, renal disease, or deafness?
   - Has the child ingested anything? Decongestants? Birth control pills? Steroids? Cocaine or PCP? Psychoactive medications?

8. **What physical examination findings are important with a hypertensive child?**
   Carefully examine the child for evidence of end-organ damage from hypertension. Look for clinical features that may suggest the possible causes of hypertension:
   - **General:** dysmorphism (e.g., elfin facies of Williams syndrome), cushingoid features, over/underweight
   - **Head, ears, eyes, nose, throat:** evidence of head trauma, decreased visual acuity, papilledema, retinal infarcts, abnormal pupillary reflex
   - **Neck:** webbed neck, thyroid enlargement
   - **Lungs:** crackles (evidence of ventricular failure), increased work of breathing
   - **Heart:** displaced point of maximal impulse (suggestive of LVH), murmurs
   - **Abdomen:** bruits, hepatomegaly, abdominal masses
   - **Renal:** flank pain
   - **Back:** signs of spina bifida
   - **Extremities:** decreased femoral pulses, discrepant four-extremity blood pressure, edema
   - **Skin:** café-au-lait spots or skinfold freckling (neurofibromatosis), xanthomas (hyperlipidemia), hirsutism, purpuric rash on lower extremities
   - **Neurological:** headache, seizures, altered mental status, encephalopathy, cranial nerve palsies, sensorimotor asymmetry, hyperreflexia

9. **What diagnostic tests should you obtain in the initial workup of a patient with hypertension?**
Relatively few laboratory tests are needed. Usually, a set of electrolytes with a blood urea nitrogen and creatinine, a complete blood count, and a urine dipstick test are enough to get started in the asymptomatic patient. A lipid profile may be helpful in obese children, while a urine culture would be recommended in all children with known renal disease. In symptomatic patients, electrocardiography and chest radiography may help you determine the presence and severity of end-organ damage by demonstrating LVH and signs of heart failure, respectively. It is important to note that many children with aortic coarctation or chronic hypertension with LVH are asymptomatic. In addition to a thyroid stimulating hormone, providers should carefully review symptomatic patients' medications, supplements, and use of recreational substances, and obtain relevant blood and urine analysis. Renal ultrasonography can be particularly helpful in identifying underlying renal pathology in an infant with hypertension.

KEY POINTS: DIAGNOSTIC WORKUP FOR A HYPERTENSIVE CHILD

1. Targeted history, physical examination, vital signs including four-extremity blood pressure.
2. Urine dipstick test (and culture if indicated).
3. Electrolytes, blood urea nitrogen, creatinine, with or without lipid profile if asymptomatic, thyroid-stimulating hormone, renin, serum metanephrines, 24-hour urine catecholamines and metanephrines if symptomatic and if glomerular disease suspected complement, strep antigen testing, 24-hour protein to creatine ratio.
4. Electrocardiography and chest radiograph if the patient is symptomatic.
5. Renal ultrasonography if available.

10. **What is hypertensive encephalopathy?**
This is a hypertensive emergency that results in increased intracranial pressure. The patient may have seizures, confusion, focal neurological deficits (such as facial nerve palsy) or visual changes, or even blindness. Papilledema may be noted on the examination. The diagnosis is clinical, and the condition is likely to improve when the blood pressure is controlled. If left untreated, coma and death may result.

11. **If a child has dangerously high blood pressure, should it be lowered to normal as quickly as possible?**
Well, sort of. It is important to normalize blood pressure to below the 95th percentile to prevent further end-organ damage, but doing so too rapidly can be harmful to those same organs, specifically the brain. Cerebral autoregulation maintains a relatively constant cerebral blood flow with variations in peripheral pressures. When peripheral blood pressure increases, cerebral vessels constrict. When peripheral pressure drops, those vessels dilate. There are points, however, at extremes of blood pressure, at which this system is exhausted. When the cerebral vessels are maximally constricted or dilated, the brain can no longer autoregulate. In the setting of a hypertensive emergency, it is key to remember that autoregulation ceases at a *higher blood pressure* than normal (i.e., maximal cerebral vasodilatation occurs at a higher blood pressure). Lowering the blood pressure below this "new" setpoint can lead to cerebral ischemia. For this reason, elevated blood pressure should be normalized gradually, ideally over days rather than minutes. When treating hypertensive emergencies, the mean arterial pressure should be lowered to *no more than 25% of the initial value* in the first hour, and a gradual reduction should be obtained over the next 24 to 48 hours.

12. **Which medications would you use to treat hypertension in the ED?**
The medicines you choose will depend on the patient's current medications, the suspected cause of hypertension, your comfort with particular medicines, and whether the child's life is in danger. For hypertensive urgencies, nicardipine and hydralazine are generally safe and effective choices. They begin to work about 2 to 10 minutes after administration and can last for several hours. Nicardipine is a calcium channel blocker that acts quickly to reduce peripheral vascular resistance. Another alternative is labetalol, which has rapid effects on both α- and β-adrenergic receptors; is a bit more difficult to titrate; and is contraindicated in patients with asthma, heart block, heart failure, and pheochromocytoma. Hydralazine acts to relax arteriolar smooth muscle, but the exact mechanism of action is unknown; hydralazine can be given intramuscularly if immediate blood pressure management is required and IV access cannot be established. Enalapril, clonidine, minoxidil, and furosemide are other reasonable choices, particularly for targeted causes of hypertension (Table 17.1). For immediate results in hypertensive emergencies, a nitroprusside infusion can give dose-related effects that will cease within minutes of stopping the infusion. Esmolol is a beta-blocker that can be easily titrated but is contraindicated in amphetamine-like ingestions. Alternatives for specific clinical indications include fenoldopam, phentolamine, and others (see Table 17.1).

Table 17.1 Medications for Management of Hypertensive Emergency and Urgency in Children

MEDICATION	TYPE	ROUTE	ONSET/ DURATION	MECHANISM OF ACTION	COMMON INDICATIONS	CONTRAINDICATION/ CONCERNS
Hypertensive Emergencies						
Nicardipine	Calcium channel blocker	IV (titrate to effect)	Onset 1-10 min/ duration 2-4 hr	Arterial vasodilator promotes cerebral and coronary dilation, decreases SVR	Acute severe HTN; perioperative HTN, stroke or ICH-related HTN, acute renal failure; sympathetic crisis	Hypovolemia may cause reflex tachycardia, headache Use with caution in hepatic dysfunction
Labetalol	Alpha and beta-blocker	IV (titrate to effect)	Onset 2-10 min/ duration 2-12 hr	Decreases SVR	Acute severe HTN; stroke or ICH-related HTN	Asthma, CHF, insulin-dependent diabetes
Hydralazine	Vasodilator	IV/IM (bolus dosing)	Onset 10-20 min IV, 20-30 min IM/duration 1-4 hr	Direct arterial vasodilator	No IV access, IM bolus dosing, preeclampsia	Heart disease may overshoot desired BP due to bolus dosing Can trigger hypersensitivity reactions; associated with drug-induced lupus
Esmolol	Beta-blocker	IV (titrate to effect)	Onset 2-10 min/ duration 10-30 min	Reduction in CO (through contractility and HR)	Acute aortic dissection; perioperative HTN (primarily OR/ICU) Counteracts reflex tachycardia	Asthma, CHF, cocaine or amphetamine toxicity, bradycardia
Sodium nitroprusside	Vasodilator	IV (titrate to effect)	Onset <2-10 min/ duration 1- 10 min	Direct venous and arterial vasodilator	Acute severe HTN; CHF pulmonary edema	Intracranial hypertension may cause cyanide toxicity
Fenoldopam	Dopamine D1 receptor agonist	IV	Onset 5-20 min/ duration 30-60 min	Increases renal blood flow/natriuresis and urine output	Acute renal failure; sympathetic crisis; perioperative HTN	Anaphylaxis in patients with sulfite sensitivity, glaucoma
Phentolamine	α-Adrenergic blocker	IV	Onset <1 min/ duration 15-30 min	Antagonism of circulating epinephrine and norepinephrine, inotropic and chronotropic effects on heart	Pheochromocytoma, cocaine, pseudoephedrine, amphetamine toxicity	Myocardial infarction or coronary artery disease

			duration 6-8 hr	sympathetic output	hemodialysis; HTN from pain, anxiety, drug withdrawal	
	α_2-agonist					
Nifedipine	Calcium channel blocker	PO/SL	Onset 20-30 min/ duration 3-8 hr	Coronary vasodilatation reduces peripheral vascular resistance	When IV therapy is delayed	Cardiogenic shock, myocardial infarction
Isradipine	Calcium channel blocker	PO	Onset 60 min/ duration 3-8 hr	Coronary vasodilatation reduces peripheral vascular resistance		Can cause hypotension when combined with azole antifungals
Furosemide	Rapid-acting diuretic	IV/PO	Onset minutes/ duration 4-6 hr	Diuretic, inhibits NaCl and water reabsorption	HTN with fluid overload, in addition to antihypertensives	Gout

From Raina R, Mahajan Z, Sharma A, Chakraborty R, Mahajan S, Sethi SK, Kapur G, Kaelber D. Hypertensive crisis in pediatric patients: an overview. *Front Pediatr.* 2020;8:588911. https://doi.org/10.3389/fped.2020.588911. Figure 3: Characteristics of medications for management of hypertensive crises. PMID: 33194923; PMCID: PMC7606848.
BP, blood pressure; CHF, congestive heart failure; CO, cardiac output; HR, heart rate; HTN, hypertension; ICH, intracranial hemorrhage; ICU, intensive care unit; IM, intramuscular; IV, intravenous; NaCl, sodium chloride; OR, operating room; PO, per os (taken orally); SL, sublingual; SVR, systemic vascular resistance.

1. Focus treatment on the specific cause of hypertension.
2. Nonlife-threatening: Use nifedipine or hydralazine or other condition-appropriate medication (see Table 17.1).
3. Life-threatening: Use nicardipine, nitroprusside, or similar intravenous titratable agents (see Table 17.1).

13. **Name some other classes of medications that might be useful in the treatment of a hypertensive emergency.**
    Depending on the type of end-organ damage, treatment of complications associated with severely elevated blood pressure may be necessary. For example, lorazepam for seizures, diuretics for heart failure, and appropriate intubation medications should be available when treating a child with a hypertensive emergency. For rapid sequence intubation of the trachea, consider using etomidate instead of ketamine. Be sure to premedicate with a benzodiazepine.

14. **An adolescent boy is brought to the ED at 5:00 AM after a night out dancing. He is euphoric and diaphoretic and has a dry mouth. He is tachycardic and hypertensive. You consider giving him a beta-blocker but think better of it. Why?**
    The patient has probably ingested an amphetamine-related compound, such as 3,4-methylenedioxymethamphetamine (ecstasy). The cardiovascular effects of phenylethylamines are due to both α- and β-adrenergic stimulation. A beta-blocker would leave α-adrenergic effects unopposed and result in vasospasm and paradoxical hypertension. Instead, consider treating him with nicardipine or nitroprusside.

15. **A school-aged child is in your ED being evaluated for an upper respiratory tract infection. You notice he is hypertensive >95th percentile for age on repeated measurements with an appropriately sized cuff. He is an otherwise healthy child. When asked, he admits to some leg pain after playing soccer. He has a systolic ejection murmur. His radial pulses are bounding, but you have trouble feeling his dorsalis pedis pulses. What might be the cause of his hypertension?**
    Coarctation of the aorta can present after infancy, with hypertension as the presenting sign. Claudication symptoms and a heart murmur may or may not be present. It is important to feel for differential upper- and lower-extremity pulses in patients with hypertension of all ages and to check four-extremity blood pressure if there is any concern about coarctation of the aorta. In normal patients, lower-extremity blood pressures are higher than upper-extremity pressures by 10 to 20 mm Hg. In patients with coarctation of the aorta, the blood pressure in the legs is lower than that in the arms.

16. **A 15-year-old male with body mass index >40 kg/m^2 presents with recurrent headaches for "at least 2 years." He is noted in the ED to have tachycardia to 110 beats per minute and an elevated blood pressure of 142/92 obtained with an appropriately sized cuff. His mother reports that this is a very similar blood pressure to the one he had at his last doctor's appointment 6 months ago. He does not take any medications daily. His electrocardiogram (EKG) demonstrates repolarization abnormalities in V6 and V7 (flipped T-waves). What is his most likely diagnosis, and what do his EKG findings represent?**
    This patient most likely has chronic, idiopathic, stage II hypertension in the setting of obesity. His EKG changes suggest left ventricular hypertrophic changes in response to his hypertension and will likely be confirmed on follow-up echocardiography. Renal disease is the most common cause of secondary hypertension in children, including renal parenchymal disease (e.g., polycystic kidney disease, chronic nephritis), or renal vascular malformation. His differential diagnosis also includes thyroid disease (though he does not have secondary signs), adverse drug reactions (no daily medications), or aortic coarctation.

17. **A teenager presents with "dark-colored urine" and is found to be hypertensive. What is the most likely diagnosis?**
    Poststreptococcal glomerulonephritis. Gross hematuria is present in about 30% to 50% of patients with this condition. The urine may appear smoky and/or tea- or cola-colored. Hypertension is present in 50% to 90% of patients with this condition and varies from mild to severe. It is primarily caused by fluid retention. Hypertensive encephalopathy is an uncommon but serious complication. These patients require emergent intervention. Generalized edema is present in about two-thirds of patients with acute glomerulonephritis due to sodium and water retention. In severe cases, fluid overload leads to respiratory distress due to pulmonary edema. A chest radiograph may show cardiomegaly and signs of heart failure.

18. A 6-year-old boy complains of abdominal pain and is found to be hypertensive. When you get him undressed, you notice multiple purpuric lesions on his buttocks and lower extremities. What is the most likely diagnosis?

Henoch-Schönlein purpura. Although hypertension is unusual in this condition, it is still important to measure the child's blood pressure in all cases. Hypertension may justify admission to the hospital for further observation and management.

BIBLIOGRAPHY

1. Flynn JT, Kaelber DC, Baker-Smith CM, et al. Clinical practice guideline for screening and management of high blood pressure in children and adolescents. *Pediatrics.* 2017;140(3):e20171904.
2. Flynn JT, Tullus K. Severe hypertension in children and adolescents: pathophysiology and treatment. *Pediatr Nephrol.* 2009;24(6):1101–1112. Epub 2008 Oct 7. Erratum in *Pediatr Nephrol.* 2012;27(3):503–504. Dosage article in article text. PMID: 18839219. https://doi.org/10.1007/s00467-008-1000-1.
3. Genisca AE, Merritt C. Hypertension. In: Shaw KN, Fleisher GR, Ludwig S, eds. *Textbook of Pediatric Emergency Medicine.* 8th ed. Wolters Kluwer/Lippincott Williams & Wilkins; 2021:240–247.
4. Grinsell MM, Norwood VF. At the bottom of the differential diagnosis list: unusual causes of pediatric hypertension. *Pediatr Nephrol.* 2009;24(11):2137–2146. https://doi.org/10.1007/s00467-008-0744-y. PMID: 18320238; PMCID: PMC2755748.
5. Kaelber DC, Liu W, Ross M, et al. Diagnosis and medication treatment of pediatric hypertension: a retrospective cohort study. *Pediatrics.* 2016;138(6):e20162195.
6. National High Blood Pressure Education Program Working Group on Hypertension Control in Children and Adolescents: The fourth report on the diagnosis, evaluation, and treatment of high blood pressure in children and adolescents. *Pediatrics.* 2004;114:555–576.
7. Raina R, Mahajan Z, Sharma A, Chakraborty R, Mahajan S, Sethi SK, Kapur G, Kaelber D. Hypertensive crisis in pediatric patients: an overview. *Front Pediatr.* 2020;8:588911. Figure 3: Characteristics of medications for management of hypertensive crises in. PMID: 33194923; PMCID: PMC7606848. PMC760684810.3389/fped.2020.588911.
8. Vieux R, Gerard M, Roussel A, et al. Kidneys in 5-year-old preterm-born children: a longitudinal cohort monitoring of renal function. *Pediatr Res.* 2017;82(6):979–998.

CHAPTER 18

JAUNDICE

James M. Callahan

1. **What is jaundice?**
   Jaundice, or icterus, is a yellow or green-yellow discoloration of the skin, mucous membranes, sclerae, and body fluids caused by increased levels of circulating bilirubin. Jaundice is usually noticeable at serum bilirubin levels of 5 mg/dL.

2. **Where does bilirubin come from?**
   The major source of bilirubin is the breakdown of heme pigment released from senescent erythrocytes by the liver, spleen, and bone marrow. Bilirubin is bound to albumin and then is usually cleared from circulation by the liver, where it is conjugated and excreted in bile. Hemolysis that exceeds the liver's capacity to conjugate bilirubin or processes that impair the excretion of bile cause increased levels of bilirubin.

3. **Is jaundice always pathological?**
   More than 80% of newborns develop visible jaundice at some point in the first few weeks of life. Most of these infants have "physiological," "breastfeeding," or "breast milk" jaundice and not a pathological process. Potentially harmful causes must be excluded before deciding that these benign conditions are present. In children above 3 months, jaundice is almost always associated with a pathological process.

4. **What is physiological jaundice?**
   A mildly elevated bilirubin level in the first few days after birth is known as physiological jaundice. This is seen in healthy newborns without underlying or associated diseases. Total bilirubin levels rarely exceed 12 mg/dL (205 μmol/L). The breakdown of the large red cell mass present in utero, relatively low levels of conjugating enzyme activity in the liver at birth, reabsorption of some bilirubin monoglucuronides from the intestine, and the lack of intestinal bacterial flora that will later breakdown some bilirubin in the gut lead to increased bilirubin. Physiological jaundice is rarely seen in the first 24 hours of life and is usually noted between the second and fourth days of life. Bilirubin levels usually peak by day 5 and decrease by the end of the second week.

   Physiological jaundice is a diagnosis of exclusion. Although extensive testing other than measurement of total and direct (or conjugated) bilirubin may not be needed in well, full-term infants with jaundice, any findings not consistent with what is usually seen with physiological jaundice should prompt further investigation. Specific investigations and therapy are guided by the infant's clinical condition and the results of preliminary investigations.

5. **How do you begin the evaluation of a patient with jaundice?**
   In newborns, the total serum bilirubin level (TSB) and the age of the child help determine the likelihood that jaundice is pathological. Then, whether the patient is a newborn or an older child, it should be determined whether the jaundice is due to conjugated or unconjugated hyperbilirubinemia by obtaining total and direct (or conjugated) bilirubin levels. *Conjugated* hyperbilirubinemia is defined as jaundice in which direct bilirubin level is higher than 2 mg/dL or accounts for more than 20% of the total bilirubin. *Unconjugated* hyperbilirubinemia (high indirect bilirubin level) is usually due to hemolytic processes or defects in conjugation. Conjugated hyperbilirubinemia is pathological at any age and is usually associated with cholestatic processes due to a hepatic disease or anatomic obstruction to bile flow. Further workup and treatment are guided by the determination of the type of hyperbilirubinemia. The approach also varies depending on the age of the patient (newborn vs. older infant/child).

6. **What are the causes of unconjugated hyperbilirubinemia in a newborn?**
   - Placental dysfunction
   - Diabetes in the mother
   - Swallowing maternal blood
   - Cephalohematoma or extensive bruising
   - Sepsis
   - Upper gastrointestinal obstruction (pyloric stenosis, duodenal web, or atresia)
   - Red blood cell (RBC) defects
   - ABO, Rh, and minor blood group incompatibility
   - Crigler-Najjar syndrome (defect in bilirubin conjugation)
   - Lucey-Driscoll syndrome (familial benign unconjugated hyperbilirubinemia)
   - Trisomy 21
   - Breastfeeding jaundice

- Breast milk jaundice
- Physiological jaundice

6. **What are acute bilirubin encephalopathy (ABE) and kernicterus?**
At high levels, unconjugated bilirubin may cross the blood-brain barrier and cause lethargy, hypotonia, poor feeding, fever, seizures, and signs of increased intracranial pressure in the days and weeks following birth. The American Academy of Pediatrics uses the term *acute bilirubin encephalopathy* to describe this constellation of signs and symptoms. Untreated, unrecognized, and severe cases of ABE in which treatment was instituted but not effective may lead to severe cognitive delays, cerebral palsy, and sensorineural hearing loss. These chronic and irreversible manifestations of bilirubin toxicity are termed kernicterus.

7. **Which infants are at increased risk of developing significant hyperbilirubinemia?**
   - Infants born before 40 weeks' gestation (risk increases with each additional week <40 weeks)
   - Infants who develop visible jaundice in the first 24 hours of life, who had TSB or transcutaneous bilirubin levels near the threshold for phototherapy, or who required phototherapy before discharge from the hospital
   - Infants with hemolysis from any cause including isoimmune hemolytic disease, enzymatic defects (i.e., glucose-6-phosphatase [G6PD] deficiency), and disorders of increased RBC fragility
   - Infants where there is a family history of need for phototherapy or exchange transfusion or a family history of inherited RBC disorders
   - Infants who have scalp hematomas or other significant bruising
   - Infants with Trisomy 21
   - Macrosomic infants of diabetic mothers
   - Exclusively breastfed infants with suboptimal intake

8. **Why do breastfed infants have higher bilirubin levels?**
Breastfed infants are about three times as likely as formula-fed babies to have high bilirubin levels in the first week of life. In the first few days of life, this is probably due to decreased fluid and caloric intake (until their mother's milk is fully in) and decreased passage of meconium stools. This has been termed *breastfeeding jaundice*. Later in the first week of life and after, it has been proposed that lipase and nonesterified long-chain fatty acids in breast milk inhibit hepatic conjugation and excretion of bilirubin and the β-glucuronidase in breast milk increases enterohepatic circulation of bilirubin. This is known as *breast milk jaundice*. Children with breast milk jaundice often have the onset of jaundice (or continued increases in levels of unconjugated bilirubin) late in the first week of life and elevated bilirubin levels may last up to 3 months. Healthy infants with breast milk jaundice do not show signs of dehydration, have appropriate weight gain after the first week of life, and do not have conjugated or direct hyperbilirubinemia.

9. **Which children are at risk for ABE and kernicterus?**
Neonates with jaundice associated with coexisting serious conditions are most likely to develop kernicterus. Children with sepsis, hypoxia or hypercarbia, brisk hemolysis (e.g., that seen with Rh incompatibility), hypoglycemia, or prematurity are most at risk. In healthy, full-term infants, kernicterus is almost never seen at unconjugated bilirubin levels lower than 25 mg/dL. Infants with type I Crigler-Jajjar syndrome often have severe, indirect hyperbilirubinemia in the absence of hemolysis. This often develops in the first few hours after birth and can be difficult to treat. These children are at high risk of developing kernicterus. Premature infants and those with intercurrent illnesses may experience kernicterus at lower bilirubin levels. Kernicterus, though rare, still occurs, even in otherwise healthy children born at or near term.

10. **What indicates that jaundice is *not* physiological and therefore should prompt further investigation in newborns?**
   - Jaundice on the first day of life
   - Bilirubin level that increases more than 5 mg/dL per day or more than 0.3 mg/dL per hour on the first day of life or more than 0.2 mg/dL per hour on day 2 or beyond
   - Conjugated bilirubin levels higher than 1.5 mg/dL or higher than 10% of total bilirubin.
   - Jaundice beyond the first week of life
   - Jaundice with hepatosplenomegaly and anemia
   - Jaundice in ill-appearing infants

11. **What other laboratory tests are indicated in neonates with unconjugated hyperbilirubinemia?**
For most infants, no other laboratory tests are needed. In children meeting the preceding criteria and in all children who appear ill or dehydrated, consider pathological causes of jaundice. In children at risk of hemolysis based on the maternal blood type, obtain a complete blood count (CBC) with a differential examination of the blood smear, a reticulocyte count, and a direct Coombs test.

Anemia or reticulocytosis suggests blood loss or ongoing hemolysis. If the Coombs test result is positive, isoimmunization has probably occurred (because of Rh, ABO, or minor blood group incompatibility). Determine maternal and neonatal blood types (this may be known at the hospital of delivery). Hemolysis in the absence of isoimmunization suggests an RBC defect in this age group, and a G6PD assay as well as fragility testing should be obtained.

Ill-appearing children and children with fever or hypothermia may have an underlying infection. Obtain a CBC for these children as well. The white blood cell count and differential may indicate an infectious process. Unconjugated hyperbilirubinemia in the absence of hemolysis may be seen with infections (although conjugated hyperbilirubinemia is more commonly seen), and a urinalysis, Gram stain, and culture may be helpful.

12. **When is treatment indicated, and what treatment is helpful in neonates with unconjugated hyperbilirubinemia?**
The American Academy of Pediatrics recently published an updated Clinical Practice Guideline for the management of hyperbilirubinemia in newborns who are at least 35 weeks of gestational age. Nomograms based on the age of the child and risk stratification based on gestational age and other risk factors are provided to guide the use of phototherapy, escalation of therapy, and exchange transfusions. Preterm infants or infants with other risk factors for developing ABE and kernicterus are treated with phototherapy at lower bilirubin levels than healthy, full-term infants. The bilirubin level at which phototherapy is started also increases with the age of the infant. In healthy, full-term infants, the recommended levels for starting phototherapy have increased from previous guidelines. Although temporary interruption of breastfeeding may lead to a rapid and sustained decrease in bilirubin levels in infants with breast milk jaundice, one should thoroughly consider the risks, benefits, and likelihood of need for escalating therapy before deciding to interrupt breastfeeding.

In lethargic infants and infants who are not nursing well, once concerns for pathological causes of jaundice have been addressed, additional feedings with expressed breast milk or formula may be helpful. In some infants with dehydration, intravenous (IV) fluids may be needed.

13. **What should you do if bilirubin levels reach the threshold for exchange transfusion?**
In infants whose bilirubin levels approach the level where exchange transfusion is recommended, escalation of therapy is indicated. The Guideline calls for consultation with a neonatologist, admission to a neonatal intensive care unit (NICU), additional laboratory testing, frequent TSB measurements, preparation for exchange transfusion (type and cross-match blood and blood bank notification), maximum intensity phototherapy, and for children with isoimmunization, intravenous immunoglobulin (IVIG) therapy.

If despite these efforts, bilirubin levels reach the exchange transfusion threshold, cross-matched, washed-packed RBCs mixed with fresh-frozen plasma is needed, so that the resulting hematocrit of the transfused blood is approximately 40%, which is recommended. Exchange transfusion thresholds are lower in full-term infants who are ill (those with hemolysis, sepsis, hypoglycemia, acidosis, or hypoxia) and preterm infants. Exchange transfusions are usually performed in NICUs. Policies and procedures for rapid admission or transfer of infants potentially requiring these therapies to such units should be in place.

14. **Is treatment for unconjugated hyperbilirubinemia an emergency?**
Yes, when the level is very high. An outside laboratory or a visiting home nurse often does a bilirubin test, and the abnormal result prompts the emergency department (ED) visit. Thus the report may be several hours old by the time the infant presents to the ED. The bilirubin level can sometimes rise quickly to a dangerous level. Avoid unnecessary delays in evaluation and management. When the unconjugated or indirect bilirubin approaches a dangerous level, start phototherapy promptly, even before the ED TSB result is known. This is sometimes difficult to do in an ED setting. Institution of a clinical pathway for the treatment of neonates with jaundice in the ED can lead to marked improvements in time to phototherapy and a decreased ED length of stay.

15. **List the causes of conjugated hyperbilirubinemia in neonates.**
   - Sepsis
   - TORCH infections (toxoplasmosis, other agents, rubella, cytomegalovirus, and herpes simplex)
   - Idiopathic neonatal hepatitis
   - Alagille syndrome (arteriohepatic dysplasia)
   - α_1-Antitrypsin deficiency
   - Inborn errors of metabolism (e.g., galactosemia, tyrosinosis)
   - Urinary tract infections
   - Hypopituitarism
   - Postshock or postasphyxia biliary sludging
   - Cholestasis associated with total parenteral nutrition
   - Cystic fibrosis
   - Biliary atresia
   - Gestational alloimmune liver disease (GALD)
   - Anatomic obstruction (e.g., choledochal cyst)

16. **Which laboratory tests are helpful in determining the cause of conjugated hyperbilirubinemia in neonates?**
    Obtain a CBC with differential, urinalysis, Gram stain, blood culture, and urine culture to look for signs of sepsis or urinary tract infection. A urinalysis with increased reducing substances other than glucose suggests galactosemia, especially in a patient with hypoglycemia. Viral and toxoplasmosis titers may help establish the diagnosis of a TORCH infection. Any vesicular lesions of the skin or mucous membranes can be tested with immunofluorescence assays and cultured for herpes simplex virus. Hepatic aminotransferase levels that are markedly elevated suggest hepatitis. Sweat chloride testing (to rule out cystic fibrosis), α_1-antitrypsin phenotyping, and repeated thyroid hormone testing may be needed in some infants. Albumin and clotting studies will reflect the synthetic capabilities of the liver. Closely monitor serum glucose because infants with hepatic disease may be at risk for hypoglycemia.

17. **What imaging studies are helpful?**
    Abdominal ultrasonography can evaluate the extrahepatic biliary tract, looking for choledochal cysts as well as other signs of obstruction. Abdominal ultrasonography should be performed emergently. Early diagnosis of biliary atresia (BA), the most common cause of cholestasis in neonates, is imperative to preserve hepatic function. The absence of the gallbladder or the presence of an echogenic cord of fibrous tissue in the hilar region is often seen. Some patients with BA may have small or atretic gallbladders. If there is continued concern for BA, a liver biopsy or laparotomy with intraoperative cholangiogram may be needed. These advanced studies and procedures are generally obtained after admission rather than in the ED.

18. **What treatment is required for neonates with conjugated hyperbilirubinemia?**
    Because conjugated hyperbilirubinemia always indicates a pathological process, admit all infants with conjugated hyperbilirubinemia and consult with a gastroenterologist. While diagnostic testing is in progress, supportive therapy may be required, including IV fluids and dextrose; antibiotics or antivirals if indicated (e.g., acyclovir for neonatal herpes infection); vitamin K; and clotting factor replacement. Specific therapy is based on the outcome of the diagnostic evaluation and does not usually occur in the ED. In children with GALD, IVIG has been associated with decreased mortality in some reports. Phototherapy is not helpful unless there is also a markedly elevated indirect bilirubin level.

19. **In older infants and children, can anything else be mistaken for jaundice?**
    Yes. Children who eat large amounts of yellow, orange, or red vegetables can develop yellow discoloration of their skin. Carotene-containing vegetables can produce carotodermia, and red vegetables (e.g., tomatoes) can produce lycopenemia. Unlike jaundice, this discoloration does not affect the sclerae, and the child with carotodermia will be thriving and well-appearing.

20. **What are the causes of unconjugated hyperbilirubinemia in older infants and children?**
    Unconjugated hyperbilirubinemia after the neonatal period is due to either hemolysis or decreases in the hepatic conjugation of bilirubin. Hemolysis is seen in children with hemoglobinopathies (e.g., sickle cell disease), RBC defects (e.g., G6PD deficiency after exposure to oxidant stress or children with hereditary spherocytosis or elliptocytosis), autoimmune hemolytic anemia, or Wilson disease. Unconjugated hyperbilirubinemia in the absence of hemolysis is seen in Gilbert disease or Crigler-Najjar syndrome.

21. **What is the diagnostic approach to children with unconjugated hyperbilirubinemia?**
    Obtain a CBC with an examination of the smear, reticulocyte count, and direct Coombs test. In the absence of hemolysis, there is probably a defect in hepatic uptake of albumin-bound bilirubin, as seen with Gilbert disease and Crigler-Najjar syndrome. Seek a gastroenterology consultation.
    If hemolysis is present, findings of sickle cells, spherocytes, or elliptocytes on the CBC smear may be diagnostic. Hemoglobin electrophoresis or osmotic fragility tests may confirm these diagnoses. If the Coombs test result is positive, the patient is probably experiencing autoimmune-mediated hemolysis. Hemolysis without a suggestive RBC morphological appearance and a negative Coombs test result may be seen in patients with G6PD deficiency (usually after exposure to salicylates, sulfonamides, naphthalene, etc.) or Wilson disease (usually accompanied by psychiatric problems and physical or laboratory signs of hepatic disease).

22. **List the causes of conjugated hyperbilirubinemia in older infants and children.**
    - Viral infections (hepatitis A, B, and C; cytomegalovirus; Epstein-Barr virus, and other viruses)
    - Bacterial infections (sepsis, pneumonia, hepatic abscess)
    - Toxins (*Amanita* mushrooms, carbon tetrachloride and solvents, drugs)
    - Total parenteral nutrition
    - Biliary tract disease (cholelithiasis, cholecystitis, choledochal cyst, cholangitis)
    - Inflammatory disease (autoimmune chronic active hepatitis, primary sclerosing cholangitis)
    - Genetic diseases (Wilson disease, α_1-antitrypsin deficiency, cystic fibrosis)
    - Hemochromatosis

23. **What medications can cause cholestasis, leading to conjugated hyperbilirubinemia?**
Anticonvulsants (phenobarbital, phenytoin, carbamazepine, and valproic acid); antibiotics (estolate preparations of erythromycin, penicillin-based antibiotics, tetracycline, sulfonamides, nitrofurantoin, isoniazid, rifampin, ketoconazole, and griseofulvin); anabolic steroids; corticosteroids; oral contraceptives; acetaminophen; salicylates; chlorpromazine; prochlorperazine; terbinafine; sulindac; tolbutamide; cimetidine; and immunosuppressants (cyclosporine, azathioprine, and methotrexate) have all been associated with cholestasis.

24. **What is the diagnostic approach to *older* children with conjugated hyperbilirubinemia?**
Consider biliary tract disease in patients with a predisposition to hemolysis (e.g., sickle cell disease) and in patients with severe right-upper-quadrant pain and vomiting. Cholelithiasis and other entities causing biliary tract obstruction are more likely in these patients, although there seems to be an increasing incidence of biliary tract disease in children, even in the absence of underlying hemolytic disease. Always obtain abdominal ultrasonography.
   If the onset of jaundice is acute, consider toxic and infectious causes. Hepatic aminotransferase levels are usually increased in these patients. Seek a history of medication use or toxic exposures. A prodrome of nonspecific symptoms and fever is more often seen with infections. Obtain viral serological tests.
   A less acute onset and jaundice associated with signs of chronic, systemic disease should prompt investigations of possible genetic or autoimmune causes (e.g., Pi typing to rule out α_1-antitrypsin deficiency or a sweat test to exclude cystic fibrosis).

25. **When does a child with jaundice require admission to the hospital?**
Admit children to the hospital for dehydration, hypoglycemia, signs or laboratory findings of active biliary tract disease, severe bacterial infections, ongoing hemolysis, or signs of systemic disease or a change in mental status. Also, admit any patient with indications of hepatic failure and monitor them closely. When the underlying diagnosis is uncertain, admission for continued diagnostic investigations is often warranted.
   Children without signs of hepatic failure who can maintain oral hydration and who have laboratory evidence of intact hepatic synthetic function (normal albumin, normal prothrombin time) can often be safely discharged. Many of these patients will have viral hepatitis. If discharged, obtain serological tests and ensure close follow-up.

26. **What are the complications of severe hepatic disease (i.e., hepatic failure)?**
Abnormal bleeding and a decreased level of consciousness are the most worrisome complications of severe hepatic disease. Decreased hepatic synthetic function leads to decreased levels of coagulation proteins and prolonged bleeding. The prothrombin time is elevated. Spontaneous hemorrhages, including intracerebral hemorrhages, may occur. Increased plasma ammonia levels and cerebral edema are associated with hepatic encephalopathy.

27. **Are adenovirus infections associated with hepatic failure in healthy children?**
Reports from the United Kingdom, Europe, Israel, and the United States have highlighted a high prevalence of adenovirus type 41 infections in previously healthy children with temporally related episodes of hepatic failure. Adenovirus has been associated with liver failure in immunocompromised individuals. Although many of these children were found to have adenovirus 41, there is not yet a causal link between these infections and the episodes of hepatic failure. Histological evidence of hepatocellular infection with adenovirus has not been found in these cases, and the overall incidence of liver failure in children in the United States has not been increasing. Adenovirus infections are common in children. It has been suggested that registries and clinical studies of acute hepatitis and liver failure in children are needed.

28. **What treatment is required for an older infant or child with jaundice?**
The main goal is to determine the cause of the patient's jaundice so that specific therapies can be started. While the diagnostic evaluation is proceeding, supportive treatment may involve the administration of IV fluids, vitamin K, or clotting factors as necessary, lactulose and neomycin for the treatment of hepatic encephalopathy, and possible endotracheal intubation and ventilatory support in patients with a decreased level of consciousness.

KEY POINTS: JAUNDICE IN INFANTS AND CHILDREN

1. Jaundice is very common in healthy, term newborn infants, and although it is usually benign and self-limited, physiological jaundice is a diagnosis of exclusion.
2. In infants and children with pathological jaundice, determine if there is indirect or direct (conjugated) hyperbilirubinemia. This will guide further investigations and help establish underlying etiologies and ultimate therapy.
3. In newborns with pathologically elevated indirect bilirubin levels, phototherapy, escalation therapy, and exchange transfusions guided by clinical practice guidelines may prevent or minimize morbidity associated with

ABE and kernicterus. Preterm infants and infants with associated illnesses (e.g., sepsis or other infections or isoimmunization) are at increased risk of developing ABE and kernicterus.
4. In infants, conjugated hyperbilirubinemia is always due to a pathological process and requires emergent diagnostic workup (including imaging studies to rule out biliary obstruction) and hospital admission.
5. In patients of all ages with jaundice, be sure there are no signs of hepatic failure. Abnormal albumin, prothrombin time, and ammonia levels indicate hepatic failure and warrant admission (often to an intensive care setting), close observation, and supportive care, including treatment with vitamin K (fresh-frozen plasma if there is active hemorrhage).

BIBLIOGRAPHY

1. Brumbaugh D, Mack C. Conjugated hyperbilirubinemia in children. *Pediatr Rev.* 2012;33:291–302.
2. Clemente MG, Schwarz K. Hepatitis: general principles. *Pediatr Rev.* 2011;32:333–340.
3. Devictor D, Tissieres P, Afanetti M, Debray D. Acute liver failure in children. *Clin Res Hepatol Gastroenterol.* 2011;35:430–437.
4. Guiterrez Sanchez LH, Shiau H, Baker JM, et al. A case series of children with acute hepatitis and human adenovirus in children. *New Engl J Med.* 2022 https://doi.org/10.1056/NEJMoa2206294.
5. Kambhampati AK, Burke RM, Dietz S, et al. Trends in acute hepatitis of unspecified etiology and adenovirus stool testing in children – United States, 2017-2022. *Morbid Mortal Weekly Rep.* 2022;71(24):797–802.
6. Karpen SJ. Acute hepatitis in children in 2022 – human adenovirus 41? *New Engl J Med.* 2022;387:656–657. https://doi.org/10.1056/NEJMe2208409.
7. Kemper AR, Newman TB, Slaughter JL, et al. Clinical practice guideline revision: management of hyperbilirubinemia in the newborn infant 35 or more weeks of gestation. *Pediatrics.* 2022;150(3):e2022058859.
8. Pan DH, Rivas Y. Jaundice: newborn to age 2 months. *Pediatr Rev.* 2017;38(11):499–510.
9. Schwartz HP, Haerman BE, Ruddy RM. Hyperbilirubinemia: current guidelines and emerging therapies. *Pediatr Emerg Care.* 2011;27:884–889.
10. Wolff M, Schinasi DA, Lavelle J, et al. Management of neonates with hyperbilirubinemia: improving timeliness of care using a clinical pathway. *Pediatrics.* 2012;130:e1688–e1694.

CHAPTER 19

LIMP

Monique Devens

1. What is the most common cause of limp in children?

   Trauma is the most common cause of limp in all ages. This can be either due to an acute injury or repetitive microtrauma, such as a stress fracture. Soft tissue injury can also cause a child to limp. Young children are more likely to have a fracture than a sprain, but sprains and strains are possible in all ages. Older children can usually describe the mechanism of injury and they can localize the pain. Toddlers present a diagnostic challenge because they cannot give a good history and may not cooperate fully for the examination.

2. What is the most common cause of a nontraumatic acute limp in children?

   Transient synovitis, formerly known as toxic synovitis, is the most common nontraumatic cause of limp in children, affecting up to 3% of the pediatric population. Transient synovitis is believed to be a postinfectious reactive arthritis, occurring most commonly in the hip, but occasionally in the knee or ankle. It is usually preceded by or concurrent with a viral respiratory or gastrointestinal illness.

3. Describe a classic case of transient synovitis.

   A classic patient with transient synovitis is a White boy (male-female ratio, 2:1) between 3 and 10 years old (incidence peaks at age 6) with a 1- to 2-day history of limp, reporting unilateral pain in the hip, thigh, or knee. His past medical history will include viral symptoms within the past 1 to 2 weeks in over half the cases. He will have little or no fever and will appear well (unlike septic arthritis). His examination will be remarkable for a painful hip on passive range of motion, and he will prefer to hold the hip abducted and externally rotated. Transient synovitis typically causes a lesser degree of pain and limitation of motion than septic arthritis.

4. If you had to choose one clinical feature and one laboratory test to distinguish transient synovitis from septic arthritis, what would be most helpful?

   Ability to bear weight and C-reactive protein (CRP). White blood cell (WBC) counts are normal (<15,000 cells/mL) in the majority of patients with both conditions. Erythrocyte sedimentation rate (ESR) is elevated (>20 mm/hour) in most patients with septic arthritis and about half of patients with transient synovitis. Fluid in the joint space on plain radiographs and ultrasound is common in both conditions. A review of over 300 children with hip pain and effusion found that patients with both inability to bear weight and a CRP higher than 2.0 mg/dL had a 74% probability of septic arthritis, and those patients with neither feature had less than 1% probability. Elevated CRP was the best independent predictor of septic arthritis, with an odds ratio of 82.

5. A 5-year-old boy presents in the Northeastern United States (NE US) with limp. Examination reveals a warm knee with moderate effusion, but the patient can range the knee and bear weight. What is the suspected diagnosis? Describe the workup and treatment.

   Arthritis is a late-stage manifestation of Lyme disease. It commonly presents more than 2 months after a tick bite. In an endemic region (most commonly, the NE US) Lyme arthritis should be considered especially in those who present with monoarticular arthritis of the knee that is not particularly painful. Workup should include serum antibody testing that when positive is confirmed by western blot. All patients with Lyme arthritis will have positive immunoglobulin G antibodies to *Borrelia burgdorferi*. The mainstay of treatment is a 28-day course of either oral amoxicillin or doxycycline.

6. Describe the common presentations of the following hip diseases of children: developmental dysplasia of the hip, Legg-Calvé-Perthes disease, and slipped capital femoral epiphysis (SCFE).

   The common presentations of hip disorders in children can be seen in Fig. 19.1A and B and Table 19.1.

7. Which underlying conditions are associated with SCFE?

   SCFE is most associated with obesity. Endocrinopathies including hypothyroidism and, more rarely, acromegaly, excess growth hormone, hypopituitarism, and hypogonadism are also associated with SCFE. Hypothyroidism is especially important to consider if the SCFE occurs in a patient under the age of 10. SCFE is also associated with trisomy 21. SCFE is more likely to be bilateral in patients who are under 12 or who have these underlying endocrinopathies.

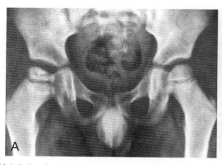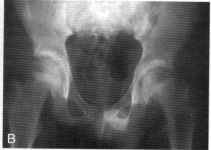

Fig. 19.1 **A**, Aseptic necrosis of the femoral head (right hip) in Legg-Calvé-Perthes disease. **B**, Slipped capital femoral epiphysis, more prominent on the left hip ("ice cream slipping off the cone").

Table 19.1 Common Presentations of Hip Disorders in Children

VARIABLE	DDH	LCP	SCFE
Typical patient	Newborn-toddler; more common in breech positioning; female-male ratio, 9:1	Early school age; male-female ratio, 5:1	Early adolescence; obese; more common in African-Americans; male-female ratio, 3:2
Pathologic features	Spectrum of acetabular dysplasia, hip subluxation, and hip dislocation	Avascular necrosis of the femoral head; cause unknown; associated with delayed bone age	Weakness of the femoral head physis; cause unknown; associated with endocrinopathies
Clinical presentation	Positive result on Barlow test in a newborn; painless limp with hip contracture in a toddler; "waddling" gait if bilateral	Hip or knee pain; insidious limp, with limitation of flexion and internal hip rotation	Can be acute (sudden severe hip or knee pain) or chronic (gradually worsening, mildly antalgic, externally rotated limp)
Best imaging test	Ultrasonography of the hips	MRI of the hips (early); plain radiography later	Plain radiographs (anteroposterior and frog-leg lateral)

DDH, developmental dysplasia of the hip; LCP, Legg-Calvé-Perthes disease; MRI, magnetic resonance imaging; SCFE, slipped capital femoral epiphysis.
Adapted from Brancati DS, Jewell J, Omori M. Evaluation of the child with a limp. *Pediatr Emerg Med Rep.* 2004;9:25–36.

8 Explain the importance of the modified Klein line in diagnosing SCFE.
The Klein line is a line drawn along the superior border of the femoral neck on an anteroposterior (AP) radiograph of the hip. This line would normally pass through a portion of the femoral head (Fig. 19.2). If not, SCFE is diagnosed. If we measure the width of the epiphysis lateral to the Klein line, diagnostic sensitivity improves from 40% to 79% (a difference of 2 mm between hips is indicative of SCFE). This modified Klein line more than doubled the detection of SCFE in a retrospective review of 55 patients (from 39% to 87%); however, 100% of the cases were identified on frog-leg lateral radiographs; thus, both AP and frog-leg lateral views should be obtained when SCFE is suspected.

9 What is the best test for distinguishing Legg-Calvé-Perthes disease (avascular necrosis of the hip) from transient synovitis?
Tincture of time. The typical duration of transient synovitis is 1 to 2 weeks. Legg-Calvé-Perthes disease is chronic, with a typical course of 18 to 24 months. Radiographs of the hips may be helpful later in the course of the disease. Changes are best seen in the frog-leg lateral position and begin with a small, dense epiphysis and widening of the medial joint space due to cartilage hypertrophy. Later, a subchondral fracture (crescent sign) or fragmentation may be seen. As the disease progresses, reossification and healing result in deformity of the proximal femur.

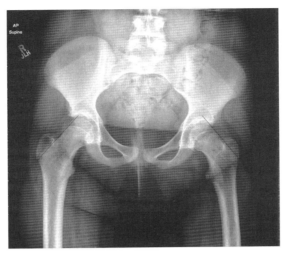

Fig. 19.2 Klein line. AP, anteroposterior.

10. A 4-year-old girl comes to the emergency department (ED) at 3:00 AM for vague leg pain, worse now but present intermittently for 3 weeks. No fever, rash, or trauma is reported. Her primary care provider had previously suspected growing pains and considered early juvenile idiopathic arthritis (JIA). What test should you perform?

You should order a complete blood count. This clinical scenario is very concerning for the possibility of acute lymphoblastic leukemia (ALL). A review of 277 children referred to a rheumatology clinic for nonspecific limb pain found the combination of low WBC count, mild thrombocytopenia, and nighttime limb pain had a high likelihood of ALL. Seventy-five percent of the 71 patients found to have ALL did not have blast cells on peripheral smear. A similar study found that limb pain and thrombocytopenia were significant independent variables for differentiating ALL from JIA, with odds ratios of 553 for limb pain and 754 for thrombocytopenia.

Growing pains should be a diagnosis of exclusion. Pain in this condition occurs in the evening hours and should be better in the morning. The pain is bilateral, and the examination is normal.

11. A 3-year-old female presents with fever, limp, and fleeting rash. What historical clues would help aid your diagnosis of systemic JIA (sJIA)?

Systemic JIA often presents with high fever in a quotidian pattern (daily spiking fever $\geq 38.5°C$ with return to normal temperature between). Patients typically have difficulty with walking that is more pronounced in the morning or "morning stiffness." If a rash is present, it would be worse with fever. Arthralgias are common but arthritis is not always seen. Commonly affected joints are knees, wrists, and ankles. sJIA is a diagnosis made after other infectious or inflammatory causes have been ruled out. There is no specific diagnostic laboratory test for sJIA. Elevated WBC count, thrombocytosis, and elevation of ferritin, ESR, and/or CRP are all suggestive of sJIA. Anemia is commonly present but not profound.

12. A 4-year-old girl presents with limping secondary to knee pain, fever, and a rash. Match the following rashes to the underlying disease.

1. Purpuric rash primarily on the lower extremities	A. Lyme disease
2. Salmon-pink evanescent diffuse maculopapular rash	B. Erythema multiforme
3. Multiple large oval papules, some with central clearing	C. Henoch-Schönlein purpura
4. Symmetrical papulovesicular rash with target lesions	D. JIA

Answers:

1. C
2. D
3. A
4. B

13. A well-appearing toddler is refusing to bear weight. Parents deny trauma and your examination is nonfocal. Is your x-ray study made from the hips down or from the knees down?

Tibial films may be sufficient as an initial screen. Results of a retrospective case-control study looking at 261 patients aged 9 months to 4 years presenting with this clinical picture found an unsuspected fracture in 40 patients—39 of the 40 fractures were located in the tibia and 1 in a metatarsal bone. No patient in the "hips down" group had a pelvic or femur fracture, Legg-Calvé-Perthes disease, or developmental dysplasia of the hip. Tibial films spared radiation to the pelvis and saved $500 per patient compared to total lower extremity films. One patient in the "hips down" group was later found to have diskitis with epidural abscess (initial films negative), emphasizing the need for good follow-up care if no cause is found with initial evaluation.

14. A 2-year-old child refuses to walk after jumping off a toy box. He is tender over the distal portion of his left tibia. Plain radiographs of the lower leg are negative. What is the most likely explanation for his pain?

The most likely reason for his pain is a nondisplaced spiral (single helix) fracture of the tibia, also known as a toddler's fracture. This type of fracture may be seen in children from the age of walking up to 5 or 6 years. Although radiographically subtle, the fracture is usually seen on the AP view, rarely on the lateral. Additional views, particularly the internal oblique, may demonstrate the fracture if it is not apparent on the AP view. Even with normal radiographs, if clinical suspicion is high, presumptive treatment with follow-up films in 10 to 14 days is indicated.

15. An oblique view of the tibia in the previously described case reveals a subtle spiral fracture. The resident wants to consult child protective services given the spiral fracture with minimal trauma. What do you recommend?

Unlike spiral fractures of other long bones, even with a history of minor or unobserved trauma, toddler's fractures in an ambulatory child generally do not indicate abuse, and a report is not warranted. Conversely, transverse or metaphyseal fractures of the tibia are concerning for the possibility of inflicted trauma.

16. A teenager with upper leg pain and a limp for 2 weeks is found to have a lesion in the proximal femur on a plain radiograph. What are the most common benign and malignant bone tumors, and how do you tell the difference?

Adolescence is the peak age of incidence for both benign and malignant bone tumors. Benign tumors are more common but their prevalence is unknown as they are frequently asymptomatic and discovered incidentally. Common benign tumors are bone cysts (unicameral and aneurysmal), osteochondromas, and osteoid osteomas. Cysts and chondromas do not typically hurt unless they lead to a pathologic fracture. Osteoid osteomas can be painful and are treated with nonsteroidal anti-inflammatory medications. The most common malignant pediatric bone tumor is osteosarcoma, followed by Ewing sarcoma.

Clues to radiographic distinction between benign and malignant bone tumors are outlined in Table 19.2.

Table 19.2 Radiographic Distinction Between Benign and Malignant Bone Tumors

BENIGN FEATURES	MALIGNANT FEATURES	EXAMPLES
Well-defined or sclerotic border	Poor definition	Osteoid osteoma (benign, small, sclerotic)
Small or multiple lesions	Large	Langerhans cell histiocytosis (multiple lytic lesions, benign)
Lack of cortical destruction	Cortex spiculated or extensive periosteal reaction	Osteosarcoma (spiculated "sunburst" cortical pattern, malignant); Ewing sarcoma (layered "onion skin" periosteal reaction, malignant)
Confined to bone	Extension into soft tissue	Metaphyseal bone cysts (benign, may expand bone, does not invade soft tissue)

17. Match the following potential causes of limp with the location of pain.

1. Sever disease	A. Patella
2. Sinding-Larsen-Johansson syndrome	B. Calcaneus
3. Osgood-Schlatter disease	C. Proximal tibia
4. Kohler disease	D. Metatarsal
5. Freiberg disease	E. Navicular

These osteochondroses are a group of lesions that occur in the lower extremity in growing bones, with a clinical picture of localized pain and limp. They are presumed to be related to repetitive stress. Radiographic changes include irregularity, increase in density, and decrease in size of the affected bone.

Answers:
1. B. Sever disease: insertion of the Achilles tendon on the calcaneus
2. A. Sinding-Larsen-Johansson syndrome: the attachment of the patellar tendon to the inferior patellar pole
3. C. Osgood-Schlatter disease: insertion of the patellar tendon on the proximal tibial tuberosity
4. E. Kohler disease: the tarsal navicular
5. D. Freiberg disease: usually the second metatarsal head, less often in the third and fourth

18. What else should you consider in a young child with limp or refusal to walk, when there is no obvious pathology of the legs?
If there is no tenderness or other signs of pain or injury of the legs, a neurologic problem may be the cause of limp. Assess for weakness of the lower extremity, which suggests a neurologic condition. For example, Guillain-Barre syndrome is an acquired peripheral neuropathy to consider. Also, the pathology may be in the spine rather than the lower extremities. Consider discitis, an uncommon, inflammatory condition that usually involves a lumbar or lower thoracic disc space. The etiology is poorly understood, however, *Staphylococcus aureus* is sometimes isolated from a disc space aspirate and occasionally from blood in these patients. Young children with discitis present with vague symptoms. The child may limp or refuse to walk. They are usually afebrile, unlike patients with vertebral osteomyelitis. Physical examination may show a normal range of motion of the hips, but a careful examination often reveals tenderness over the involved disc space.

KEY POINTS: EVALUATION OF A CHILD WITH A LIMP

1. SCFE is an orthopedic emergency (and may present with referred knee or thigh pain).
2. Limp may be the acute presentation of a more chronic problem, abdominal or back problems, or even systemic illness.
3. Normal laboratory studies do not exclude the possibility of septic arthritis or osteomyelitis.
4. Plain radiography is often the first step in workup of a limp but follows historical clues to determine the need for laboratory studies or advanced imaging.

BIBLIOGRAPHY

1. Baron CM, Seekins J, Hernanz-Schulman M, et al. Utility of total lower extremity radiography investigation of nonweight bearing in the young child. *Pediatrics.* 2008;121(4):e817–e820.
2. Joffe M, Loiselle J. Musculoskeletal emergencies. In: Shaw K, Bachur R, eds. *Fleisher and Ludwig's Textbook of Pediatric Emergency Medicine.* 8th ed. Wolters Kluwer; 2020:1358–1381.
3. Kost S, Thompson A. Limp. In: Shaw K, Bachur R, eds. *Fleisher and Ludwig's Textbook of Pediatric Emergency Medicine.* 8th ed. Wolters Kluwer; 2020:301–306.
4. Lantos P, Rumbaugh J, Bockenstedt L, et al. Clinical practice guidelines by the Infectious Diseases Society of America (IDSA), American Academy of Neurology (AAN), and American College of Rheumatology (ACR): 2020 guidelines for the prevention, diagnosis and treatment of Lyme disease. *Clin Infect Dis.* 2021;72(1):e1–e48.
5. Pinkowsky GJ, Hennrikus WL. Klein line on the anteroposterior radiograph is not a sensitive diagnostic radiologic test for slipped capital femoral epiphysis. *J Pediatr.* 2013;162(4):804–807.
6. Singhal R, Perry DC, Khan FN, et al. The use of CRP within a clinical prediction algorithm for the differentiation of septic arthritis and transient synovitis of the hip in children. *J Bone Joint Surg Br.* 2011;93(11):1556–1561.
7. Tamashiro MS, Aikawa NE, Campos LMA, et al. Discrimination of ALL from systemic-onset JIA at disease onset. *Clinics (Sao Paulo).* 2011;66(10):1665–1669.

CHAPTER 20

NECK MASSES

Magdy W. Attia

1. **What are the important components of the medical history of a child with a neck mass?**
   - Onset
   - Duration of symptoms
   - Rapidity of growth with changes in size or position
   - Pain
   - History of recent infection or trauma
   - Generalized symptoms, such as fever, weight loss, poor appetite, night sweats, or fatigue
   - History of exposure to communicable diseases
   - Pet exposure
   - Travel history

2. **What are the important components of the physical examination of a child with a neck mass?**
   - **Observe** the general appearance of the child. Screen rapidly for true emergencies.
   - **Inspect** the patient in a neutral position to discern subtle swellings on one side compared to the other.
   - **Palpate** the neck from behind with the patient seated or with the child on the caregiver's lap. Examine all masses to determine location, size, multiplicity, consistency, mobility, color, and temperature. Note other characteristics, such as tenderness, compressibility, and mobility with swallowing and tongue protrusion. Pay special attention to associated systems, such as the chest, abdomen, and lymphatic system, to ensure a complete examination.

3. **Which true emergencies are associated with neck masses?**
   True emergencies involving a neck mass relate to direct compression on vital structures leading to respiratory distress, vascular compromise, and cervical spinal cord compression.

4. **Describe an initial focused evaluation of a child with a neck mass.**
   Address the airway, breathing, and circulation (ABCs) appropriately. Immediately note the child's level of consciousness and work of breathing. Obtain a focused and pertinent history. Evaluate for subcutaneous emphysema stridor, hoarseness, dysphagia, and drooling. These are ominous indications of airway compromise. Perform a neurological examination.

5. **List the etiological classifications of neck lesions/masses.**
   See Table 20.1.

Table 20.1 Etiological Classifications of Neck Lesions and Masses

CONGENITAL	INFECTIOUS	NEOPLASTIC	TRAUMATIC
Hemangiomas	Lymphadenitis	Lymphomas	Subcutaneous emphysema
Cystic hygromas	Soft tissue abscess	Thyroid neoplasms	Hematoma
Preauricular pits, sinuses, and cysts	Infected cysts (i.e., thyroglossal duct, branchial cleft, dermoid)	Teratoma	Cervical spine trauma
Thyroglossal duct cysts		Rhabdomyosarcoma	
		Neuroblastoma	
Sternocleidomastoid mass			
Cervical ribs			
Dermoid cysts			
Brachial cleft abnormalities			

Table 20.2 Anatomic Classifications of a Neck Mass, With the Most Common Masses in Each Category

MIDLINE	LATERAL
Thyroglossal duct cyst	Lymphadenopathy
Lymphadenopathy	Cystic hygroma
Dermoid cyst	Branchial cleft cyst
Epidermoid cyst	Sternocleidomastoid mass
Ectopic thyroid tissue	Sialadenitis
Parotitis	Thyroid gland tumors

6. **List the anatomical classifications of a neck mass, with the most common masses in each category.**
   See Table 20.2.

7. **How is the workup of a child with a neck mass conducted?**
   Generally, a thorough history and physical examination lead to a provisional diagnosis and initiation of either therapy or watchful waiting. The lack of rapid resolution or the presence of worrisome clinical findings should trigger the workup. The choice of the best study depends on the type of mass (solid vs. cystic, benign vs. malignant) and the location and extent of the lesion. Initially, ultrasonography is a good screening study; if further anatomic details are needed, contrast-enhanced computed tomography (CT) or magnetic resonance imaging (MRI) is then indicated. MRI is more advantageous than CT in delineating soft tissue infection; however, it may delay diagnosis if sedation is required. If signs of malignancy are present (i.e., a painless, firm, slow-growing mass in the upper third of the neck, or lymph nodes fixed to underlying tissue) or the lesion does not resolve, then surgical referral and biopsy are warranted. Consider a complete blood count, erythrocyte sedimentation rate (ESR), chest radiography, and purified protein derivative test in the early workup.

8. **What are cystic hygromas? When do they usually appear?**
   Cystic hygromas or cystic lymphatic malformations are believed to be formed from congenital failure of the lymphatic primordial buds to establish drainage into the venous system. This leads to the accumulation of lymphatic fluid and cyst formation and a large neck mass. They are discrete, soft, mobile, and nontender masses most commonly found in the posterior triangle of the neck. They may be transilluminated and usually grow in proportion to the child.
   Cystic hygromas usually appear by the end of the second year of life (80%-90% of cases) during the period of active lymphatic growth; they appear less commonly at birth (10%-20% of cases).

9. **What are the most common locations of cystic hygromas?**
   They develop in close proximity to large veins and lymphatic ducts:
   - Lateral neck (75%)
   - Axilla (20%)
   - Mediastinum (5%)
   - Retroperitoneum (5%)
   - Pelvis (5%)
   - Groin (5%)

10. **What is the most serious complication of cystic hygroma? What are the treatments for this condition?**
    Respiratory compromise is seen when a large mass extrinsically compresses the airway. The treatment is usually surgical excision of the lesion; however, sclerotherapy, repeated aspiration, incision and drainage, radiation therapy, and intralesional injections are other treatment modalities that have been recently recommended.

11. **What is a thymic mass? What are the clinical features and treatment?**
    Thymic cysts result from faulty implantation of thymic tissue in the neck during embryological descent into the chest. They are present in a midline position but they can be present anywhere between the angle of the mandible and the midline of the neck. Thymic cysts are managed with surgical excision.

12. **What is the most common head and neck congenital lesion identified in infancy?**
    Hemangioma. These are most noticeable after the first month of life. Females are affected three times more commonly than males.

13. **How do hemangiomas appear on physical examination?**
    These masses are soft, mobile, and nontender and have a bluish or fiery red hue. Regressing hemangiomas are gray. The most common locations of hemangiomas are on the scalp, lips, nose, eyelids, and ears.

14. **List some of the complications of hemangiomas.**
    - Hemorrhage
    - Ulceration
    - Infection
    - Necrosis
    - Thrombocytopenia and coagulopathies: due to platelet trapping; Kasabach-Merritt syndrome
    - Airway compromise—the child may have stridor
    - Congestive heart failure
    - Visual impairment in some periorbital hemangiomas

15. **What are the treatments for hemangiomas?**
    The treatment of hemangiomas is observation; most hemangiomas resolve spontaneously. Other treatment modalities include topical or systemic beta-blockers such as propranolol, steroids, chemotherapy, radiation therapy, and laser therapy. Surgical excision is reserved for rapidly growing lesions compromising vision, hearing, or the airway.

16. **What is the origin of branchial cleft cysts?**
    These develop due to malformations of the branchial arches (first through fourth). Most of them arise from the second branchial cleft.

17. **How does a child with a branchial cleft sinus or cyst present?**
    Generally, the child presents with a single, painless, cystic lesion deep to the anterior, upper one-third of the sternocleidomastoid. The lesion is movable, smooth, tense, and nontranslucent, and occasionally has clear mucoid drainage from a small opening along the anterior border of the sternocleidomastoid muscle (lateral to midline). Sometimes the tract is palpable.

18. **What is the most common complication of branchial cysts?**
    Infection is the most common complication, and this usually responds well to antibiotics and warm soaks. The definitive treatment is a complete excision of the cyst and tract.

KEY POINTS: BRANCHIAL CLEFT CYSTS

1. Usually a single painless cystic lesion.
2. May become infected, thus appearing red and tender.
3. Found on the lateral neck, at the anterior upper third of sternocleidomastoid.
4. Treat infection with antibiotics and surgical excision.

---

19. **Compare dermoid and epidermoid cysts.**
    See Table 20.3.

Table 20.3 Comparison Between Dermoid and Epidermoid Cysts

FEATURES	DERMOID CYST	EPIDERMOID CYST
Origins	Congenital. Inclusion of embryonic epidermis within embryonal fusion planes.	Traumatic or inflammatory. Follicular infundibulum of the hair shaft.
Contents	Lined by epithelium and contain sebaceous glands, hair follicles, connective tissues, and papillae.	Lined by epithelium, does not contain cutaneous appendages but rather keratinized cellular debris.
Location	Head and neck: lateral to the supraorbital palpebral ridge, midline face, especially nasal bridge or neck.	Head and neck: lateral to the supraorbital palpebral ridge, midline face, especially nasal bridge and neck.
Treatment	Surgical excision.	Surgical excision.

20. How is radiological imaging helpful in the management of a dermoid cyst?
Either MRI or CT may be used to evaluate a dermoid cyst prior to complete excision because dermoid cysts occasionally have intracranial extension.

21. What is a thyroglossal duct cyst?
This common congenital neck mass is due to a ductal ectodermal remnant that is never obliterated. Remember, a thyroglossal duct cyst has no external opening because the tract does not reach the skin surface.

22. How does a thyroglossal duct cyst present clinically?
This is commonly noted in a child 2 to 10 years old, as a midline cystic structure, immediately adjacent to the hyoid bone, at or about the level of the thyroid cartilage. Some may be sublingual (3%) or suprasternal (7%). A thyroglossal duct cyst is a soft, smooth, nontender (unless infected) mass that elevates when the child swallows or with tongue protrusion.

23. Describe the workup of a child with a thyroglossal duct cyst
The diagnosis is often made on clinical grounds alone. Ultrasonography, CT, or MRI may be indicated in unusual clinical presentations. CT provides better visualization of lesions adjacent to the hyoid bone. Radioisotope scanning is used for detecting ectopic thyroid tissue within thyroglossal ducts. Postoperative thyroid function tests may be indicated to determine whether thyroid replacement therapy is needed.

KEY POINTS: THYROGLOSSAL DUCT CYSTS

1. Midline swelling, usually near the thyroid cartilage.
2. Moves (elevates) when the child swallows or protrudes the tongue.
3. Diagnosis is made clinically.

24. Is cervical lymphadenopathy common in childhood?
Yes, cervical lymphadenopathy is common during the middle years of childhood but is seldom pathological. Children usually present with an indolent, nontender, dominant node in the jugular chain that persists over several months. Systemic symptoms are rare. Although laboratory studies are not usually indicated, most children have a normal blood count and normal chest radiograph, and if the node is biopsied it shows reactive hyperplasia.

25. Is a supraclavicular lymph node more concerning?
Yes. Supraclavicular adenopathy in any age group should be considered pathological until proven otherwise. Swelling of these nodes may be the first sign of occult thoracic or abdominal pathology, such as malignancy (lymphoma). Initiate a workup including a chest x-ray and consultation with a surgeon immediately.

26. What is the most common cause of acute cervical lymph node enlargement?
- **Viral infections**: Severe viral pharyngitis can cause cervical lymph nodes to enlarge acutely, usually bilaterally. Infections of the upper respiratory tract can lead to lymph node enlargement. Agents most commonly implicated are Epstein-Barr virus and adenovirus. Also, consider HIV infection.
- **Bacterial infections:** Acute suppurative cervical lymphadenitis secondary to bacterial infection is another cause of cervical lymph node enlargement. Common bacterial pathogens include *Staphylococcus aureus*, group A β-hemolytic streptococci, *Streptococcus pneumoniae* (rarely), anaerobes from mouth flora, and *Bartonella henselae* (cat-scratch disease).

27. How does a child with acute suppurative cervical lymphadenitis present?
Acute suppurative cervical lymphadenitis often presents after upper respiratory tract infection, pharyngitis, or tonsillitis, with rapid, *unilateral* enlargement of multiple adjacent lymph nodes. Marked tenderness, warmth, and erythema are often seen. Fever, irritability, and toxic appearance are more common in younger child. Spontaneous purulent drainage may occur if the infection is untreated. Occasionally, the infected cervical lymph nodes herald a retropharyngeal abscess. This entity should be considered in the differential diagnosis of cervical adenitis.

28. How is acute suppurative cervical lymphadenitis best treated?
The initial treatment consists of oral antibiotics and warm soaks for the neck. If the child is young and toxic, admission is warranted for IV antibiotic therapy and close observation. The initial antimicrobial therapy should be directed at the common organisms listed. Methicillin-resistant *Staphylococcus aureus* should be suspected if

initial therapy is ineffective. When fluctuance is identified, drainage by surgical incision or ultrasonography-guided needle aspiration is recommended for both therapeutic and diagnostic purposes.

29. **What is the differential diagnosis of subacute or chronic cervical lymphadenitis?**
This condition refers to a child with a large, minimally tender, mildly inflamed, and nonfluctuant cervical lymph node that appears slowly over several weeks with no associated prodrome or systemic illness. Elements of the differential diagnosis are the following:
   - Reactive response to a nonspecific infection (bacterial or viral)
   - Cat-scratch disease
   - Infectious mononucleosis
   - *Mycobacterium tuberculosis:* typical or atypical
   - Toxoplasmosis
   - Cytomegalovirus
   - HIV infection
   - Sarcoidosis
   - Histoplasmosis
   - Actinomycosis
   - Malignancy

30. **What is the workup for a child with subacute or chronic cervical lymphadenitis?**
   - Perform a complete history and physical examination. Note the child's overall general appearance. Assess the number, size, and location of lymph nodes. Palpate for any organomegaly. Consider laboratory studies, including complete blood count with differential, ESR, chest x-ray, and a purified protein derivative test. Begin antibiotics to cover *Staphylococcus* and *Streptococcus*.
   - Arrange for the patient to be followed closely by his or her primary care physician.

31. **When should a child with chronic lymphadenopathy be referred for biopsy?**
Referral is warranted if the condition does not respond to treatment or a lymph node persists or enlarges despite adequate antibiotic therapy (of a few week's duration).

32. **Describe the clinical picture of cat-scratch disease.**
Children with cat-scratch disease may give a history of a scratch by a kitten or only exposure to a kitten. Cat-scratch disease is a common infectious disease in all age groups. Kittens, in particular, are the reservoir for the pathogen. Although most children do not recall the scratch, a papule at the primary inoculation "scratch site" and regional lymphadenopathy usually develop in 1 to 2 weeks. A positive result on a cat-scratch disease antigen skin test (not recommended) or demonstration of microorganism (*B. henselae*) by silver stain from an aspirated node is confirmatory. If cat-scratch disease is suspected, the best initial test is the *B. henselae* IgM enzyme immunoassay. If the test result is negative, consider polymerase chain reaction (PCR) for *Bartonella* by using the biopsy tissue.

33. **Should I test for cat-scratch disease?**
The diagnosis can be easily established clinically in most cases. There are a number of confirmatory tests:
   - Serology: Can be helpful; however, there are considerable limitations due to both suboptimal sensitivity and false positive rates. Indirect fluorescence assay titers of immunoglobulin G >1:256 (rises 10-14 days after infection) and positive immunoglobulin M (IgM) (rises early and briefly) tests strongly suggest either active or recent cat-scratch disease. The serological diagnosis of acute infection can be elusive due to the timing of the rise of these titers.
   - Blood and tissue culture: Growing *B. henselae* requires specific laboratory conditions for optimal growth, rendering it impractical. Histopathological examination of the initial entry site and the involved gland can be supportive of the diagnosis in the presence of other criteria. Not routinely performed.
   - PCR: Though highly specific, the sensitivity remains a significant limitation.

34. **What is the treatment for cat-scratch disease?**
Cat-scratch disease is self-limited; resolution is expected in 6 to 8 weeks. Initial treatment may consist of warm compresses and analgesics. Treatment should be reserved for those with systemic symptoms or severe local reactions. However, many physicians start antibiotics, such as trimethoprim-sulfamethoxazole or azithromycin, upon clinical suspicion.

KEY POINTS: CAT-SCRATCH DISEASE

1. Most patients do not recall a cat scratch.
2. Kittens are usually the reservoir.
3. Lymphadenopathy develops 1 to 2 weeks after the scratch.
4. *B. henselae* IgM enzyme immunoassay is the best test during the acute phase.
5. Treat with observation or trimethoprim-sulfamethoxazole or azithromycin.

35. **What OTHER conditions should be considered in the differential diagnosis of a unilateral neck mass?**
    A unilateral neck mass of nontender, 1.5 cm or larger cervical lymph node associated with fever should raise the possibility of Kawasaki disease. This disease is associated with severe vasculitis of medium-sized blood vessels with a predilection for the coronary arteries.
    The acronym **FRAME** is a way to remember the other typical findings of Kawasaki disease:
    - **Fever** 39° C or higher for more than 5 days.
    - **Rash** of various forms and desquamation of the skin of hand, feet, and occasionally perianal area.
    - **Adenopathy** (as described above).
    - **Mucositis** involving the bulbar conjunctivae, oral mucosa, lips, and external urethral meatus.
    - **Edema** and redness of the hands and feet. Other findings include irritability and fatigue.
    Early diagnosis is suspected clinically and confirmed by elevated sedimentation rate and platelet counts. Mild normocytic anemia, sterile pyuria, and abnormal lipid profile. An emergent echocardiogram for the early detection of coronary aneurysms is a must. Initiate therapy with aspirin and intravenous immunoglobulin infusion to avoid the development of coronary artery aneurysms, myocardial ischemia, or infarction.

36. **Describe the most common neoplasm of the neck based on age.**
    - In preschool-aged children: neuroblastoma, non-Hodgkin lymphoma, rhabdomyosarcoma, and Hodgkin lymphoma are most common.
    - In school-aged children: lymphomas, either non-Hodgkin or Hodgkin, thyroid carcinoma, and rhabdomyosarcoma are more likely.
    - In adolescents: Hodgkin lymphoma predominates.

37. **When should a neoplastic lesion in the neck be suspected? What evaluation is necessary?**
    A neoplastic lesion presents as a painless, firm, fixed cervical mass. Supraclavicular location is also concerning (see Question 25). Other presenting signs and symptoms are unilateral ptosis, nasal obstruction, or otorrhea. A detailed history and physical examination, complete blood count with differential, renal and liver profiles, chest x-ray, or CT/MRI are sometimes obtained in the emergency department. An urgent referral to a surgeon or oncologist is recommended for further studies, such as a bone marrow examination.

38. **Name a life-threatening dental infection that can cause neck swelling?**
    Ludwig angina is a very rare life-threatening infection of the floor of the mouth that follows a dental procedure or trauma. It is more likely to occur in those who are immunocompromised or have poor dentition. Patients appear very ill or toxic. In addition to induration of the floor of the mouth, submandibular swelling is noted. Trismus is a late finding. Rapid airway compromise is possible. If this diagnosis is considered, emergently consult anesthesia and otolaryngology and arrange for admission to the intensive care unit for treatment with broad-spectrum antibiotics that cover anaerobic oral flora.

39. **When should you consider a goiter?**
    A goiter is a large midline neck mass due to diffuse enlargement of the thyroid gland. Patients with goiter may have signs of excess thyroid hormone, such as tachycardia, systolic hypertension, bounding pulses, and exophthalmos. Some have signs of thyroid deficiency. Most are asymptomatic and euthyroid. Children with large goiters may have compressive symptoms such as shortness of breath, cough, and dysphonia. In the United States, Hashimoto thyroiditis (chronic autoimmune thyroiditis) is the most common cause of goiter. When a thyroid mass is suspected, obtain serum thyroid hormone and thyroid-stimulating hormone levels.

BIBLIOGRAPHY

1. Abdulkader F, Mukhtar NEE. Evaluation of pediatric head and neck masses. In: Al-Qahtani A, Haidar H, Larem A, eds. *Textbook of Clinical Otolaryngology*. Springer; 2021. https://doi.org/10.1007/978-3-030-54088-3-58.
2. Bilal M. Cystic hygroma: an overview. *J Cutan Aesthet Surg*. 2010;3(3):139–144. https://doi.org/10.4103/0974-2077.74488.

3. Bridwell R, Gottlieb M, Koyfman A, Long B. Diagnosis and management of Ludwig's angina: an evidence-based review. *Am J Emerg Med*. 2021;41:1–5.

4. Brouchard C, Peacock ZS, Troulis MJ, Maria J. Pediatric vascular tumors of the head and neck. *Oral Maxillofac Surg Clin North Am*. 2016;28(1):105–113.

5. Gorelik M, Chung SA, Ardalan K, et al. 2021 American College of Rheumatology/Vasculitis Foundation guidelines for the management of Kawasaki disease. *Arthritis Rheumatol*. 2022;74(4):586–596.

6. Nurminen J, Velhonoja J, Heikkinen J, et al. Emergency neck MRI: feasibility and diagnostic accuracy in cases of neck infection. *Acta Radiol*. 2021;62(6):735–742.

7. Khan L. Thyroid disease in children and adolescents. *Pediatr Ann*. 2021;50(4):e143–e147.

8. Ho M-L. Pediatric neck masses: imaging guidelines and recommendations. *Radiol Clin North Am*. 2022;60(1):1–14.

9. Pruden CM, McAneney CM. Neck mass. In: Bachur RG, Shaw KN, Chamberlain J, Lavelle J, Nagler J, eds. *Fleisher & Ludwig's Textbook of Pediatric Emergency Medicine*. 8th ed. Wolters Kluwer; 2021:317–323.

10. Sturm JJ, Dedhia K, Chi DH. Diagnosis and management of cervical thymic cysts in children. *Cureus*. 2017;9(1):e973. Published online. https://doi.org/10.7759/cureus.973.

CHAPTER 21

PEDIATRIC RASHES

Rebecca J. Hart and Kerry S. Caperell

1. **Name five bioterrorism agents that may have skin manifestations.**
   Smallpox, anthrax, tularemia, plague, and viral hemorrhagic fever. See Table 21.1 for descriptions of skin manifestations.

2. **What are four skin findings associated with syphilis?**
   Chancre, rash, condyloma lata, and gumma. See Table 21.2 for the rash description.

3. **How does perianal streptococcal dermatitis manifest?**
   Perianal streptococcal infection usually occurs in children between 6 months and 10 years of age. It presents as sharply circumscribed superficial perianal erythema. In some patients, the rash is bright red with a wet surface, while in others it is dry and pink. Fever is generally absent. Delays in culturing, diagnosing, and initiating therapy are common.

4. **An atopic child with chronic eczema suddenly develops a painful vesicular eruption in previous areas of eczema. What is the most likely diagnosis?**
   Eczema herpeticum, caused by the herpes simplex virus (HSV), is a vesicular eruption concentrated in areas of eczematous skin. Children with eczema herpeticum often become seriously ill with high fever because the disease can be complicated by secondary bacterial infections and viremia, leading to multiple organ involvement with meningitis and encephalitis. Treatment with intravenous (IV) acyclovir is necessary for children with extensive or rapidly progressing involvement (Fig. 21.1).

5. **What are the clinical features of measles?**
   Measles, caused by an RNA virus in the paramyxovirus family, had almost been eradicated in the United States as of the year 2000. Unfortunately, increasing number of cases have occurred over the last decade, linked to

Table 21.1 Bioterrorism Agents That May Have Skin Manifestations

AGENT	SKIN FINDINGS
Smallpox	Maculopapular rash on face, forearms, and mucus membranes that becomes vesicular/pustular within 48 hr
Anthrax	Painless pruritic papules on skin that develop into a painless ulcerated black eschar within a few days
Tularemia	Painful maculopapular lesion that ulcerates; associated with painful inflamed regional lymph nodes
Plague	Acutely swollen lymph nodes called buboes, typically situated in the groin, axilla, or neck that may be tender, firm to the touch, and may drain pus
Viral hemorrhagic fever	Maculopapular rash on trunk followed by mucosal bleeding

Table 21.2 Skin Findings Associated With Syphilis

FINDING	DESCRIPTION
Chancre	Painless ulcer of skin and mucous membranes at the site of inoculation
Rash	Maculopapular rash of secondary syphilis frequently involving palms and soles
Condylomata lata	Cauliflower-appearing warts on penis, labia, or rectum
Gumma	Painless pink to dusky red nodules of various sizes that may necrose or ulcerate

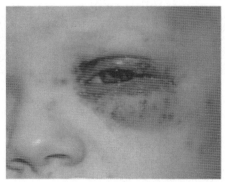

Fig. 21.1 A neonate with eczema herpeticum presenting as clusters of crusted vesicles and papules around the eye.

importation from countries where the spread is endemic and subsequent spread among unimmunized individuals, including intentionally unimmunized children. Large-scale outbreaks in the United States have occurred as recently as 2019, when more than 1200 cases were confirmed in 31 states.

Measles is an acute disease characterized by fever, cough, coryza, conjunctivitis, and an erythematous maculopapular rash that begins on the forehead and behind the ears, spreading to the face, neck, torso, and extremities. Koplik spots, bright red punctae with central white flecks on the buccal mucosa near the second molars, are seen early in the disease course and are pathognomonic for measles. Complications such as otitis media, pneumonia, croup, and diarrhea are common in young children and immunocompromised individuals. A less common, but feared complication is subacute sclerosing panencephalitis, which affects up to 1 in 1000 children infected with measles. Infants are more likely to be afflicted.

6. **How can one differentiate between erythema multiforme (EM), Stevens-Johnson syndrome (SJS), and toxic epidermal necrolysis (TEN)?**
EM classically consists of an erythematous maculopapular rash, characterized by target lesions that may coalesce and develop annular or serpiginous borders with clear or dusky centers in a primarily acral distribution. It typically manifests over a period of 12 to 24 hours and resolves within 2 weeks, although it may recur. EM is commonly associated with viral illnesses (including HSV and Epstein-Barr virus [EBV]) and *Mycoplasma pneumoniae* infection, and as such may be preceded by prodromal upper respiratory tract symptoms. It can also be precipitated by certain drug exposures, although this is now felt to be less common.

SJS and TEN represent a spectrum of diseases that is now thought to be separate from EM. Medications are a leading trigger, with phenobarbital, carbamazepine, lamotrigine, and sulfonamide antibiotics leading causes in children; *M. pneumoniae* is also a common infectious trigger. SJS is characterized by fever and significant involvement of the mucosa of the mouth and oropharynx, conjunctivae, as well as a diffuse rash of discrete dark red macules, often with a necrotic center. There may be sloughing of skin, with <10% body surface area affected. TEN is the more severe version of the disease, with extensive loss of epidermis (>30% body surface area, or BSA) due to necrosis. There is some SJS/TEN overlap in patients with 10% to 30% BSA skin detachment. Mortality rates for SJS can range up to 10%, and up to 30% to 50% with TEN.

7. **How does the rash of Rocky Mountain spotted fever (RMSF) change over time?**
RMSF is a potentially lethal tick-borne disease caused by *Rickettsia rickettsii* infection. Despite its name, RMSF cases occur throughout the United States, but most commonly in the Midwest and Southeast. The rash is initially erythematous and macular, although it frequently progresses to papules and petechiae. The rash first appears on the wrists and ankles, spreading centrally within hours to involve the proximal extremities and trunk. The palms and soles are usually involved. While testing is available via tick-borne illness panels, treatment with doxycycline should typically be initiated if there is any suspicion of illness, especially in high-spread areas.

8. **A child helps his mother cut limes before going outside to play and then returns with inflamed hands that quickly develop hyperpigmentation. What is the name of the rash and the causative agent?**
This condition is a type of toxic photoreaction called phytophotodermatitis. It is caused when the skin comes into contact with psoralen, a photosensitizing agent, and then immediately with sunlight. Psoralen can be found in some perfumes, plants, grasses, fruits, and vegetables. Limes, celery, and parsley are examples of foods containing psoralen.

9. **What are the typical features of pityriasis rosea?**
   Seen primarily in adolescents, pityriasis rosea begins in 80% of patients with a large, oval, solitary lesion known as a *herald patch* somewhere on the trunk or upper thighs. This is followed by an eruption of smaller, oval, and slightly raised papules that are pink to brown and have peripheral scales. The lesions are described as having a Christmas tree pattern on the back and involve mostly the truncal areas (Fig. 21.2), usually sparing the face, scalp, and distal extremities. The eruption is prolonged and can last 4 to 8 weeks.

10. **List key features that help differentiate the purpuric rash of Henoch-Schönlein purpura (HSP) from more serious infectious purpuric rashes, such as purpura fulminans.**
    See Table 21.3 for features that help differentiate HSP from purpura fulminans.

11. **Describe the typical presentation and skin findings seen in immune thrombocytopenia (ITP), and how you might distinguish this from other more serious causes of similar findings.**
    ITP can present in children at any age, although it peaks in incidence between 2 and 5 years. Affected children are often asymptomatic but can frequently present with sudden bruising, purpura/petechiae, and/or mucosal bleeding (e.g., gums bleeding after brushing teeth). Children are usually otherwise healthy appearing and without other symptoms. Laboratory studies reveal a platelet count of typically <100,000. Importantly, other cell lines (including white blood cells and hemoglobin) are not affected.

    By comparison, other autoimmune-mediated cytopenias, such as Evans syndrome, will typically demonstrate suppression of other cell lines, with findings suggestive of hemolytic anemia (low hemoglobin, elevated bilirubin) or leukopenia. Oncologic processes such as leukemia can also present with bruising and thrombocytopenia, but again will typically involve derangements of other cell lines and are often accompanied by other symptoms, such as fever, fatigue, night sweats, or weight loss.

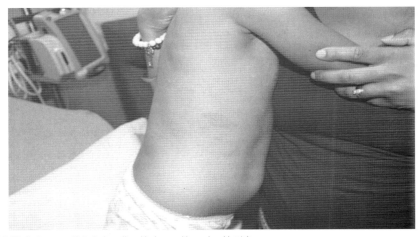

Fig. 21.2 Pityriasis rosea with typical small oval lesions and larger herald patch.

Table 21.3 Henoch-Schönlein Purpura Versus Purpura Fulminans

HENOCH-SCHÖNLEIN PURPURA	PURPURA FULMINANS
Distribution is usually limited to extremities, appearing most commonly on lower legs, buttocks, and occasionally upper extremities. In infants, facial involvement may be seen.	Distribution of purpura is widespread.
Associated features include athralgias, abdominal pain, and hematuria.	Associated features include lethargy, hypoventilation, and shock.
Children appear well except for painful joints and abdominal pain.	Children appear ill, with varying degrees of toxicity.
Platelet count and results of other coagulation tests are normal.	Thrombocytopenia is present, and coagulation test results are abnormal.

12. **What are five skin manifestations that may be seen in Kawasaki disease?**
    1. Dry, cracked, erythematous lips
    2. Erythematous polymorphic truncal rash that may be scarlatiniform or morbilliform
    3. Red, swollen hands and feet

Table 21.4 Common Mimics Versus Findings Concerning for Child Abuse

COMMON "MIMICS" OF CHILD ABUSE		FINDINGS CONCERNING FOR CHILD ABUSE	
FINDING	**DESCRIPTION**	**FINDING**	**DESCRIPTION**
Lichen sclerosis	Indurated and shiny atrophic plaques in vulvar and perianal areas.	Inflicted bruising	Although accidental bruising is extremely common in active children, inflicted bruising is the most common physical sign of abuse. The TEN-4 mnemonic can help recall "red flags" for inflicted bruising: bruising over the torso (including genitals and buttocks), ears, or neck in children under age 4 years, or ANY bruising on a child under age 4 months, should raise suspicion for abuse.
Congenital dermal melanocytosis (formerly known as Mongolian spots)	Irregularly shaped hyperpigmented areas that may appear blue/gray/purple in color, commonly seen over sacrum in neonatal period.	Patterned bruising	Any bruise that reflects the shape of any object (such as hand, paddle, belt, electrical cord, or similar).
Coining	Asian folk remedy of rubbing coin or spoon on back/trunk, which may result in annular red areas or bruise-like appearance.	Bite marks	Human bites are typically superficial and maybe more clearly visualized 2-3 days after injury. Adult-inflicted marks demonstrate intercanine distance of >3 cm.
Accidental ecchymoses	Normal childhood bruises—commonly found over bony prominences, such as shins, knees, forearms, elbows, foreheads, and chins.	Burns	Accidental burns are common; the presence of a "stocking glove" distribution or "zebra stripes" should raise suspicion for forcible immersion in hot water. Small (7-10 mm) round burns with well-demarcated edges and deep central crater should raise suspicion for cigarette burns.
ITP	Diffuse bruising, may include petechiae and purpura, in otherwise healthy child. Plt <100,000.		
Congenital cutaneous tumors	Hemangiomas and other vascular malformations grow quickly in the first months of low, followed by slow growth and eventual involution. Well-demarcated and present in neonatal period, but may appear as bruising or ulceration during the involution phase.		

ITP, immune thrombocytopenia; Plt, platelet.

4. Peeling around nails and fingers (typically a late finding, usually when the patient is otherwise in the recovery phase of illness)
5. Desquamating perineal rash (also a late finding in the recovery phase)

13. **What are some skin findings that may be mistaken for child abuse? How are these different from findings that are concerning for child abuse?**
    See Table 21.4 for skin findings that are common "mimics" of child abuse versus findings that are typically concerning for abuse.

14. **How does scabies manifest in infants?**
    Scabies in infants and young toddlers may cause more intense and persistent nodular reactions to the mite, rather than the classic linear, scaly papules with pinpoint vesicles that are commonly seen in older patients. The distribution of lesions also differs in infants and toddlers, with the head, neck, trunk, palms, soles, dorsal and lateral/instep portions of the feet, and lateral aspect of the wrists being more prominently involved. Because infants are not able to scratch the intensely pruritic lesions, they may become irritable and sleep poorly (see Fig. 21.3).

15. **What are the cutaneous manifestations of disseminated gonococcemia?**
    The skin lesions associated with disseminated gonococcemia are often located on the extremities and may overlie the involved joints. Small macules appear initially and progress to papules. These tender lesions may develop a small vesicle and then a gray umbilicated center. A diagnosis can be established with a Gram stain or culture of the skin lesion.

16. **Describe the rash seen in poison ivy and its effective treatments.**
    Poison ivy rash is a type IV hypersensitivity reaction that commonly presents with extreme pruritus. The rash consists of erythematous papules which may form large, weeping vesicles or bullae, often with surrounding erythema and swelling. It may occur in a linear or patchy fashion wherever the plant touches the skin. While sometimes believed to be contagious, this is a misconception—once the skin, clothes, and fingernails are cleaned of the sap from the poison ivy plant, the rash will not spread beyond the areas already exposed.
    Unfortunately, good studies have shown that topical hydrocortisone and topical antihistamine creams have no more effect than bland, soothing lotions, such as calamine. To be effective, use steroid creams and ointments that are at least of moderate potency. Supportive care includes baths, cool compresses, and calamine lotion for mild cases. Systemic oral steroids (often with a prolonged taper) almost always bring the dermatitis under control and are appropriate for moderate to severe cases. Oral antihistamines may also be helpful.

17. **What is a pyogenic granuloma?**
    A pyogenic granuloma is a rapidly growing vascular proliferation that develops at the site of an obvious or unnoticed trauma (Fig. 21.4). Despite its name, this lesion is not infectious. Patients usually present to the emergency department with spontaneous bleeding or after local minor trauma. Acute bleeding can be controlled with prolonged pressure or silver nitrate sticks. Ultimately, treatment consists of electrodesiccation and curettage.

18. **Describe key features that differentiate common newborn rashes erythema toxicum, transient pustular melanosis, milia, and acne neonatorum.**
    See Table 21.5 for descriptions of the common rashes listed.

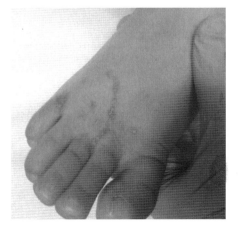

Fig. 21.3 Scabies in a toddler with pruritic, nodular, and linear rash.

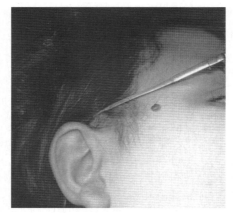

Fig. 21.4 Pyogenic granuloma. (From Morelli JG. Vascular neoplasms. In: Fitzpatrick JE, Morelli JG, eds. *Dermatology Secrets in Color.* 3rd ed. Elsevier; 2006.)

Table 21.5 Descriptions and Comparison of Common Newborn Rashes

FINDING	DESCRIPTION
Acne neonatorum	Small red or white bumps primarily on face, upper chest, and back. It usually starts around 3 weeks of age and last for up to 4 months, with resolution by 6 months of age.
Erythema toxicum	Self-limited eruption usually appears in the first 3-4 days of life, sometimes as late as day 10. Lesions begin as blotchy erythema that develops into pale yellow or white papules or pustules with a surrounding erythematous base. Individual lesions last an average of 2 days, and cytologic examination, if needed to differentiate from other rashes, reveals clusters of eosinophils and neutrophils without bacteria.
Milia	Benign and transient dermal cysts of keratin that present as small, firm white papules. Most common on the face, although they can also be present on the upper trunk, extremities, and genitals. Typically present at birth and self-resolve within a couple of weeks. May be seen in up to 50% of healthy full-term neonates.
Transient pustular melanosis	Benign rash consisting of superficial vesiculopustular lesions that are present at birth. Lesions rupture easily with the first bath, leaving a collarette of fine, white scales and brown, hyperpigmented macules. Lesions fade within several weeks to months and are asymptomatic.

19. **What is the appropriate treatment for a herpetic whitlow?**
A herpetic whitlow is a localized HSV infection consisting of a single or multiple vesicular lesions on the distal fingers or toes (Fig. 21.5). The first episode may accompany herpetic gingivostomatitis. Treatment consists of local care for mild cases, and those with severe lesions may benefit from oral acyclovir. Avoid incision and drainage, which can prolong recovery and worsen the condition.

20. **What condition is associated with recurrent pustules on the feet of infants?**
Infantile acropustulosis consists of 7- to 10-day episodes of pruritic pustules and papulovesicles on the hands and feet of infants. The age of onset is usually between 2 and 10 months, and the condition resolves by 2 to 3 years of age. Treatment with mid to high-potency topical corticosteroids is effective.

21. **A diaper rash consisting of diffuse papular, scaly, and fissuring eruptions does not respond to anti-inflammatory or antifungal agents. What is the potential serious cause?**
This rash may be one of the skin manifestations of histiocytosis X, which is a disorder characterized by the proliferation of Langerhans histiocytes in the skin and other organ systems. Consider a biopsy to confirm the diagnosis or absence of histiocytosis X when a difficult-to-treat diaper rash does not improve with standard therapy.

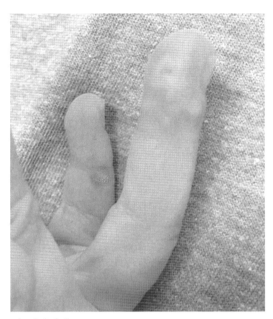

Fig. 21.5 Digit with erythema and vesicular lesions.

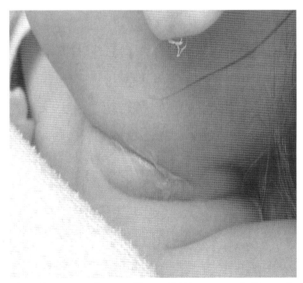

Fig. 21.6 Nikolsky sign: gentle traction causes peeling away of the superficial layers, as seen in this case of scalded skin syndrome.

22. **What is Nikolsky sign?**

    Nikolsky sign is a vulnerability of the skin such that apparently normal epidermis can be rubbed off with slight trauma. It may be seen in epidermal blistering diseases, such as scalded skin syndrome and pemphigus vulgaris (Fig. 21.6).

23. **How long do patients with erythema infectiosum (fifth disease) need isolation?**
This infection is caused by parvovirus B19. For most patients with the typical presentation of a "slapped cheek" and a lacelike rash on the arms and legs, no isolation is needed at the time of diagnosis. By the time the rash becomes clinically obvious, these patients are unlikely to be infectious. The rash usually resolves within 3 to 5 days of onset.

24. **What are the similarities and differences between granuloma annulare and tinea corporis?**
Both are characterized by circular plaques consisting of a ring of papules around a depressed center. Granuloma annulare is a ring of *nonscaling* skin-colored or red papules that are most commonly seen on the dorsal surface of the hands and feet. They are asymptomatic and resolve spontaneously after a few months to a year. Tinea corporis is a common, superficial fungal infection consisting of lesions with *scaly* inflammatory borders that appear anywhere on the body. There may be multiple lesions. Tinea corporis can be treated with topical antifungals. When the same virus affects the scalp (known as Tinea capitis), it may present similarly but can also cause areas of hair loss/alopecia. Tinea capitis cannot be treated topically due to the need to infiltrate the hair follicle; as such, prolonged courses of oral antifungals, most commonly Griseofulvin, must be used.

25. **What causes roseola? What are the usual features?**
Roseola infantum (exanthem subitem) is an acute febrile illness that primarily affects young children between the ages of 6 and 36 months. Most cases are now thought to be caused by human herpesvirus 6 and human herpesvirus 7. After 3 or more days of high fever, the patient abruptly defervesces and an erythematous, morbilliform rash with discrete rose-pink macules appears. The rash begins first on the trunk and then spreads rapidly to the extremities, neck, and face. By this time, the rash is bothering the parents more than the patient.

26. **What is Gianotti-Crosti syndrome?**
This self-limiting condition is characterized by symmetrical erythematous papules that are primarily found on the extremities but often involve the cheeks and buttocks. Also known as papular acrodermatitis, the rash may last 2 to 8 weeks and may become recurrent. Although first identified in Europe in children with hepatitis B virus, it is seen in the United States primarily in association with other viruses, including EBV, cytomegalovirus, and coxsackievirus A16. In extremely young infants or children with risk factors for hepatitis B infection, testing may be appropriate; otherwise, viral testing is typically not recommended.

27. **A toddler presents with several small, round, erythematous, and inflamed macules in a straight column down the middle of his chest and abdomen. What is the most likely cause?**
This is likely to be a contact dermatitis related to an allergy to nickel. Infants commonly present with skin lesions corresponding to the location of snaps on their pajamas or other garments. Avoidance of the offending object, by using an undershirt or nonsnap clothes, and application of a mild topical steroid will solve the problem.

28. **Which organisms cause bullous and nonbullous impetigo?**
Bullous impetigo involves vesicles that may enlarge to form flaccid bullae; ruptured bullae may leave a thin brown crust. It frequently affects the trunk and intertriginous areas more than the extremities, with relatively few lesions. It is usually caused by toxin-producing strains of *Staphylococcus aureus* and can often be treated topically with mupirocin or similar antibiotics. Oral antibiotics can be used with extensive lesions or when topical therapy is impractical. Due to the local nature of the infection, it is important to know that otherwise well-appearing neonates with bullous impetigo can still be treated topically and do not require evaluation for systemic bacterial infection or broad-spectrum IV antibiotics.

Nonbullous impetigo consists of small vesicles or pustules that rupture and then develop honey-colored, crusting lesions. These are particularly common on the face (near the mouth and nose) but can involve the extremities. Multiple lesions may develop but tend to remain well-localized. It is most commonly caused by group A streptococcus and can also be treated topically with mupirocin unless there are extensive lesions.

29. **What are the dermal manifestations of zinc deficiency?**
Dietary deficiency or inadequate absorption of zinc leads to acrodermatitis enteropathica. It is characterized by erythema, crusting, and fissuring of the perioral skin and cheeks. The diaper area may develop a diffusely erythematous rash with a sharply marginated border on the abdomen. Psoriasiform lesions may develop around the anus and on the buttocks and feet. Treatment with dietary zinc supplementation provides dramatic resolution for all dermal and systemic symptoms.

30. **Compare and contrast smallpox with chickenpox.**
Smallpox and chickenpox are compared in Table 21.6.

31. **Describe the skin findings associated with Lyme disease.**
Erythema chronicum migrans develops 4 to 20 days after a tick bite in 60% to 70% of patients who have contracted Lyme disease (Fig. 21.7). The first sign may be a red papule at the site of the tick bite. An annular ring

Table 21.6 Smallpox Versus Chickenpox

CHARACTERISTIC	SMALLPOX	CHICKENPOX
History	Febrile with systemic symptoms for several days prior to the rash	Mild fever with minimal symptoms for 1-2 days prior to rash
Severity	Very ill from the onset	Not severely ill unless complications develop
Lesions	Hard circumscribed pustules	Vesicles on an erythematous base (dewdrop on a rose petal)
Distribution	Face and distal extremities, involving palms and soles	Face and trunk, with no involvement of palms or soles
Lesion development	Slow, with all lesions at the same stage of development	Rapid, with lesions at different stages

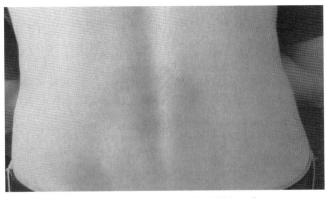

Fig. 21.7 Classic annular and erythematous rash with central clearing associated with Lyme disease.

with a flat border slowly grows while clearing develops in the center, leading to the development of a "target" appearance. Some patients develop multiple secondary annular rings days after the primary lesion appears.

32. **What is the typical skin finding following a bite from the brown recluse spider?**
Loxosceles recluse spiders are often found in old buildings and produce a number of toxins in their venom. A painful hemorrhagic blister may initially appear. Over several days a dry, gangrenous eschar will develop. Treatment is typically with local wound care, tetanus prophylaxis as indicated, and pain management. Most lesions stop extending within 10 days and heal by secondary intention; severe bites may require skin grafting to repair the ulceration. Antibiotics are only indicated if there are signs of infection. Rarely, patients may also experience life-threatening systemic effects (called *Loxoscelism*) with angioedema, hemolytic anemia, disseminated intravascular coagulopathy, rhabdomyolysis, renal failure, and even death.

33. **What are the major examination findings that differentiate cellulitis, erysipelas, and lymphangitis?**
Cellulitis is a common soft tissue infection in children, manifesting with erythema, edema, and warmth. It develops due to bacterial entry via breaches in the skin barrier. Typically unilateral, the lower extremities are the most common sites of involvement—bilateral involvement should prompt consideration of alternative causes. Cellulitis may ultimately progress to the development of an abscess with a collection of pus in the dermis or subcutaneous space, which typically requires incision and drainage to resolve. Patients may have fever and localized pain, but other systemic symptoms are uncommon.

Whereas cellulitis involves the deeper dermis and subcutaneous fat, erysipelas involves only the upper dermis and is always nonpurulent. Classically, erysipelas is identified by the raised, clearly demarcated border between affected and normal tissue. Patients with erysipelas more commonly have systemic symptoms such as fever, malaise, and headache. While cellulitis is commonly caused by beta-hemolytic streptococci and

Staphylococcus aureus, erysipelas is somewhat more likely to be caused by group A streptococcus. Both can be treated with oral antibiotics. Consider hospital admission and parenteral antibiotics for those with systemic symptoms, such as fever.

Lymphangitis can occur when local skin infection spreads to the draining lymphatic tissue, resulting in spreading, streaking erythema that progresses proximally from the site of the initial infection. Due to the (often) rapid progression of this disease, it is commonly treated with IV antibiotics.

34. **A 7-year-old child presents with four café-au-lait spots that are 2 to 4 mm in diameter. Does this child have neurofibromatosis?**
    Probably not. The diagnostic criteria for neurofibromatosis type 1 include six or more care-au-lait spots (see Fig. 21.8) greater than 5 mm in diameter in prepubertal children and greater than 15 mm in older children.

35. **What common skin features are present in children with scarlet fever?**
    - Flushed face with perioral pallor
    - Diffuse, blanching, erythematous rash that has a sandpaper consistency, with accentuation in the axillae and groin
    - Pastia lines in the flexural surface of the elbows
    - Desquamation as the acute phase of the illness resolves

36. **How can you distinguish irritant contact diaper rash from candida diaper dermatitis?**
    Generic diaper rash is caused by contact of the skin with urine or feces in the moist, closed environment created by a diaper. Red papules or patches appear on the prominent surfaces of the diapered areas, especially in areas of overlapping skinfolds and skin directly adjacent to the plastic parts of the diaper or elastic.

    Candidal diaper dermatitis comes from the gut flora *Candida albicans*. Features of this infectious rash consist of perianal erythema and maceration spreading to produce moist, bright red, confluent plaques in the diaper area, especially in the intertriginous folds. Satellite lesions are common.

37. **Name five cutaneous manifestations of lupus erythematosus.**
    1. Erythematous maculopapular eruption on cheeks and nose in a butterfly distribution
    2. Discoid lesions-chronic persistent skin changes that progress to scarring and pigmentary changes
    3. Transient annular papulosquamous lesions in sun-exposed areas of skin
    4. Erythema on the palms and pulps of the fingers and diffuse erythematous scaly macules on the dorsum of the fingers
    5. Pallor and cyanosis of the digits when exposed to cold (Raynaud phenomenon)

38. **What are the two main types of epidermolysis bullosa (EB)?**
    Epidermolysis bullosa is used to describe a group of inherited conditions that result in blisters after mild trauma (Fig. 21.9, no change). There are two main categories:
    a. Nonscarring types (EB simplex and junctional type EB)
    b. Scarring or dystrophic forms of EB

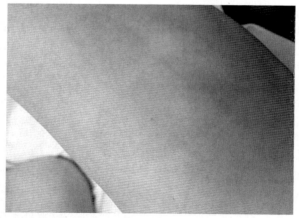

Fig. 21.8 Hyperpigmented lesion on extremity consistent with café-au-lait spot.

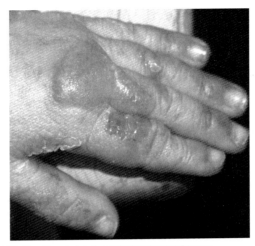

Fig. 21.9 Blistering rash on a child with epidermolysis bullosa following minor hand trauma.

39. A 2-year-old child presents with a chief complaint of fever, rhinorrhea, and malaise and is refusing to take any food or drink by mouth. What findings would lead you to conclude that the most likely diagnosis is hand, foot, and mouth disease (HFMD)?

   HFMD is a common childhood viral illness linked to Coxsackievirus A serotypes. It frequently spreads in large outbreaks in daycare and childcare settings, typically in summer and early autumn. HFMD typically presents with complaints of mouth or throat pain (in verbal children) or refusal to eat/drink (in nonverbal children). Low-grade fever can be present, along with fussiness, abdominal pain, vomiting, and diarrhea (although these are not universal). The pathognomonic rash consists of macular, maculopapular, or vesicular lesions on the palms or soles that typically resolve in 3 to 4 days; lesions are also commonly found on the buttocks and upper thighs. Oral lesions start as erythematous macules and progress to vesicles surrounded by a thin halo of erythema. These are seen anterior to the tonsillar pillars, frequently on the tongue and buccal mucosa, and less commonly on the palate or tonsils. In the weeks following the resolution of the illness, patients may experience desquamation of the distal fingers/toes and can sometimes lose fingers or toenails. A related illness, herpangina, results in similar oral lesions but is not typically associated with any skin findings. Treatment is supportive, but refusal to drink fluids may result in the need for IV fluid resuscitation.

KEY POINTS: PEDIATRIC EMERGENCY DERMATOLOGIC CONDITIONS

1. Children with eczema herpeticum can become seriously ill with high fever; the condition can be complicated by secondary bacterial infections and viremia.
2. SJS and TEN represent a spectrum of disease separate from EM; medications are a leading trigger in children. (Phenobarbital, carbamazepine, lamotrigine, and sulfonamide antibiotics are the leading causes.)
3. The rash of RMSF is initially erythematous and macular, and frequently progresses to papules and petechiae. The rash first appears on the wrists and ankles, spreading to the proximal extremities and trunk. The palms and soles are usually involved.
4. Children with ITP present with sudden bruising, purpura/petechiae, and/or mucosal bleeding (e.g., gums bleeding after brushing teeth). They are usually otherwise healthy appearing and without other symptoms.
5. The skin lesions associated with disseminated gonococcemia are often located on the extremities and may overlie the involved joints. Small macules appear initially and progress to papules.
6. A pyogenic granuloma is a rapidly growing vascular proliferation. Despite its name, this lesion is not infectious; patients present with spontaneous bleeding.
7. Treatment of herpetic whitlow consists of local care for mild cases; severe lesions may benefit from oral acyclovir. Avoid incision and drainage, which can prolong recovery and worsen the condition.
8. The rash of Lyme disease is an annular ring with a flat border that clears in the center as it grows, leading to a "target" appearance. Some patients develop multiple lesions.

BIBLIOGRAPHY

1. Pickering LK, Baker CJ, Kimberlin DW, et al., eds. *Red Book: 2021 Report of the Committee on Infectious Diseases.* 32nd ed. American Academy of Pediatrics; 2021: 489–4499, 539–541
2. Beatrous S, Grisoli S, Riahi R, et al. Cutaneous manifestations of disseminated gonococcemia. *Dermatol Online J.* 2017;23(1): 13030/qt33b24006.
3. Block SL. Perianal dermatitis: much more than just a diaper rash. *Pediatr Ann.* 2013;42(1):12–14.
4. Çakmak SK, Tamer E, Karadağ AS, Waugh M. Syphilis: a great imitator. *Clin Dermatol.* 2019;37(3):182–191. https://doi.org/10.1016/j.clindermatol.2019.01.007.
5. Chumpitazi CE, Tran JQ. Images in emergency medicine. Child with diarrhea and rash. Acrodermatitis enteropathica. *Ann Emerg Med* . 2013;62(4):303–318.
6. Cohen B, Davis H, Gehris R. Dermatology. In: Zitelli B, McIntire S, Nowalk A, eds.*Zitelli and Davis' Atlas of Pediatric Physical Diagnosis.* 6th ed. Elsevier; 2012.
7. Ferrandiz-Pulido C, Garcia-Patos V. A review of causes of Stevens-Johnson syndrome and toxic epidermal necrolysis in children. *Arch Dis Child.* 2013;98:998.
8. Gottlieb M, Long B, Koyfman A. The evaluation and management of Rocky Mountain spotted fever in the emergency department: a review of the literature. *J Emerg Med.* 2018;55(1):42–50.
9. Grunning K, Pippitt K, Kiraly B, et al. Pediculosis and scabies: treatment update. *Am Fam Physician.* 2012;15:535–554.
10. Hafsi W, Badri T.*Erythema multiforme [Updated August 7, 2021]. StatPearls [Internet].* StatPearls Publishing; 2022. Available from: https://www.ncbi.nlm.nih.gov/books/NBK470259/.
11. Hankinson A, Lloyd B, Alweis R. Lime-induced phytophotodermatitis. *J Community Hosp Intern Med Perspect.* 2014;4(4).
12. Herpetic whitlow. Painful grouped red-blue vesicles on the middle finger of a child. Available from: http://www.medicinenet.com/image-collection/herpetic_whitlow_picture/picture.htm
13. Ianelli V. Poison ivy pictures. Available from: http://pediatrics.about.com/od/poisonivy/ig/Poison-Ivy-Pictures/Poison-Ivy-Rash.-PF.htm
14. Jen M, Chang MW. Eczema herpeticum and eczema vaccinatum in children. *Pediatr Ann.* 2010;39(10):658–664.
15. Johnston R, ed. Viral diseases. In: *Weedon's Skin Pathology Essentials.* 2nd ed. Elsevier Limited; 2017:467–486.
16. *Mayo Foundation for Medical Education and Research.* Nickel allergy. Available from http://www.mayoclinic.com/health/medical/IM00384
17. Nunley KS, Gao F, Albers AC, et al. Predictive value of café au lait macules at initial consultation in the diagnosis of neurofibromatosis type 1. *Arch Dermatol.* 2009;145(8):883.
18. Patel B, Butterfield R. Common Skin and bleeding disorders that can potentially masquerade as child abuse. *Am J Med Genet.* 2015;169(4):328–336.
19. Patel M, Lee A, Clemmons N, Redd S, et al. National update on measles cases and outbreaks – United States, January 1-October 1, 2019. *MMWR Morb Mortal Wkly Rep.* 2019;68:893–896.
20. Pennycook KM, McCready TA.*Perianal Streptococcal Dermatitis. StatPearls.* StatPearls Publishing; 2022.
21. Raff AB, Kroshinsky D. Cellulitis: a review. *JAMA.* 2016;316:325.
22. Ravanfar P, Wallace JS, Pace NC. Diaper dermatitis: a review and update. *Curr Opin Pediatr.* 2012;24(4):472–479.
23. Rodegherio F, Stasi R, Gernsheimer T, et al. Standardization of terminology, definitions, and outcome criteria in immune thrombocytopenic purpura of adults and children: report from an international working group. *Blood.* 2009;113:2386.
24. Romero J. Hand, foot, and mouth disease and herpangina. In: Edwards M, Drutz J, Torchia M, eds. *UpToDate* [Retrieved March 3, 2022]. Available from: https://www.uptodate.com/contents/hand-foot-and-mouth-disease-and-herpangina
25. Stein S, Paller A, Haut P. Langerhans cell histiocytosis presenting in the neonatal period: a retrospective case series. *Arch Pediatr Adolesc Med.* 2001;155(7):778–783.
26. Swanson DL, Vetter RS. Bites of brown recluse spiders and suspected necrotic arachnidism. *N Engl J Med.* 2005;352:700–707.
27. Weston WI.. Lane AJ, Morelli JG.*Color Textbook of Pediatric Dermatology.* 4th ed. Mosby; 2007: 25–38, 51–55, 113–147, 149–180, 343–364, 381–411.
28. Wormser G. Lyme disease. In: Goldman L, Schafer AI, eds.*Goldman-Cecil Medicine.* 26th ed. Elsevier; 2020:1991–1996. Chapter 305.
29. Wu IB, Shchwartz RA. Herpetic whitlow. *Cutis.* 2007;79:193–196.

SCROTAL PAIN

Elysha Pifko

CHAPTER 22

1. **What exactly is a testicular torsion?**
   Testicular torsion is a twisting of the spermatic cord and its contents. Undiagnosed testicular torsion may lead to testicular ischemia with subsequent infarction and necrosis. Torsion can either occur extravaginally or intravaginally depending on whether the twisting occurs within the tunica vaginalis or not. Patients with a bell-clapper deformity have an increased risk of testicular torsion. This deformity occurs when the entire testis, epididymis, and spermatic cord are surrounded by the tunica vaginalis, which prevents the posterior attachment of the testis to the gubernaculum. The loss of this anchor predisposes the testicle to twist.

2. **When does testicular torsion typically occur?**
   Testicular torsion has a bimodal distribution. Typically, extravaginal torsion occurs during the antenatal or early neonatal period. These babies are often born with a hard, discolored, and non-tender scrotal mass. Intravaginal torsion most commonly occurs near the time of puberty in the second decade of life. Nevertheless, boys of any age with acute scrotal pain and swelling require prompt attention, likely radiological evaluation, and possible surgical evaluation.

3. **How does testicular torsion present?**
   Testicular torsion has distinct features that can be elucidated with a thorough history and physical examination.
   a. Key historical features include the following:
      - Rapid onset of unilateral scrotal pain
      - Persistent unrelenting pain
      - Nausea/vomiting
      - Change in position of the testicle within the scrotal sac
   b. Key physical examination features include the following:
      - Unilateral testicular tenderness
      - A "high-riding" or elevated testicle within the scrotal sac
      - Transverse testicular orientation
      - Absent cremasteric reflex
      - Palpation of the epididymis anteriorly

      Important notes: Boys may report that they had similar scrotal pain on prior occasions, but that does not rule out acute testicular torsion. Fever and painful voiding are uncommon. A history of trauma does not preclude and can even predispose the patient to torsion. Many patients report lower abdominal or groin pain rather than scrotal pain. Always perform a genital examination on the male patient reporting abdominal pain!

4. **How much time is there to save the testicle when it is torsed?**
   Ischemic changes of the testis start within the first few hours of torsion. The likelihood that a testicle can be salvaged after a testicular torsion is directly related to how quickly blood flow can be restored after the onset of symptoms. The salvage rate of a testicle repaired within the first 6 hours of the onset of symptoms is 90% to 100%. After 12 hours since symptom onset, salvage rate decreases from 20% to 50%. At 24 hours after symptom onset, the salvage rate decreases to 10%. Sperm count decreases in patients who must undergo an orchidectomy and in those who have any testicular atrophy.

5. **What is a TWIST score?**
   The TWIST (i.e., Testicular Workup for Ischemia and Suspected Torsion) score is a validated scoring system based on five signs and symptoms of testicular torsion that help to predict the likelihood of testicular torsion. Table 22.1 shows how to calculate the TWIST score.

   Researchers were able to achieve 100% positive predictive value with a score ≥ 5 and 100% negative predictive value with a score ≤ 2.

6. **What are the next steps if you are suspicious of testicular torsion based on your history and physical examination?**
   The next step in the evaluation and management of testicular torsion is based on your degree of suspicion. In patients for whom there is a high suspicion of testicular torsion (e.g., in those patients with a TWIST score ≥ 5), prompt urological consultation for surgical exploration is recommended. Any imaging or further testing will only delay repair and decrease the likelihood that the testicle is salvaged.

Table 22.1 TWIST Score	
SIGN/SYMPTOM	**POINTS**
Testicular swelling	2
Hard testicle	2
Absent cremasteric reflex	1
Nausea/vomiting	1
High-riding testis	1

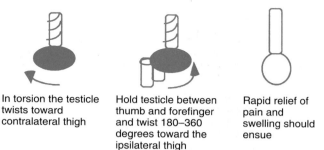

In torsion the testicle twists toward contralateral thigh

Hold testicle between thumb and forefinger and twist 180–360 degrees toward the ipsilateral thigh

Rapid relief of pain and swelling should ensue

Fig. 22.1 Technique for manual detorsion of the testicle.

If there is a low or moderate level of suspicion for testicular torsion (e.g., in patients with a TWIST score <5), Doppler ultrasound is the best imaging modality if available. Decreased or absent blood flow to the testicle on ultrasound is concerning for testicular torsion and warrants a urological evaluation.

7. Should you attempt to manually detorse the testicle?
Recent studies have shown lower rates of orchiectomy in patients who undergo a successful manual detorsion. Manual detorsion does not involve a lot of technical skill so it would be reasonable to attempt the procedure prior to surgical exploration. Testicles typically torse in a medial direction. Therefore to manually detorse the testicles they should be rotated in a lateral direction. The technique is often described as a similar motion to "opening a book (Fig. 22.1)."
Confirmation with a Doppler ultrasound is needed after manual detorsion. When this procedure is successful, bedside ultrasound may reveal increased blood flow to the testicle, but surgical correction (bilateral orchiopexy) is still necessary after this maneuver. It is important to get urology involved promptly.

8. Can you always rely on physical examination or ultrasound to diagnose testicular torsion?
Unfortunately, no. Physical examination findings vary, and a high index of suspicion is needed in all cases of scrotal pain. A high-riding testicle is associated with torsion, and the presence of a cremasteric reflex is usually reassuring that torsion is not present. Most patients with testicular torsion do not have a cremasteric reflex on the affected side. However, this reflex remains present in a significant number of patients (8%-20%) with torsion, and it alone cannot be relied upon to make the diagnosis or rule out torsion.
Some of these cases are just too close to call clinically. While color Doppler ultrasound is considered the best test to assess perfusion and exclude testicular torsion, false-negative results are possible. No diagnostic study is completely reliable, and in some cases when the examination is worrisome, urological consultation and surgical exploration of the scrotum are still warranted regardless of what the study shows.

9. Why do emergency physicians sometimes fail to diagnose testicular torsion?
   • It may not be suspected/considered in an infant.
   • The chief complaint may be abdominal pain rather than scrotal pain.
   • History of trauma may confuse the diagnosis.

- Physical examination findings can be inconsistent.
- Examination of the genitalia is sometimes omitted.
- A diagnostic study such as an ultrasound is trusted rather than physical examination findings.
- A urologist is not consulted even though the history or examination is worrisome.

Failure to diagnose and/or promptly manage testicular torsion is one of the most common reasons for malpractice lawsuits in pediatric emergency medicine.

10. **What is a torsed appendix testis?**
A torsed appendix testis is the most common source of scrotal pain in children. It typically occurs in boys aged 7 to 14 years old. It can present similarly to testicular torsion with pain, nausea, and vomiting but often has a more gradual onset. The examination is significant for tenderness localized to the anterior testis. A "blue dot" may be seen on examination, which indicates an infarcted testicular appendix. A Doppler ultrasound often shows normal or increased flow to the testis and possibly a hypoechogenic focus. Management of a torsed appendix testis is typically conservative with nonsteroidal anti-inflammatory drugs (NSAIDs), rest, ice, scrotal support (tight underwear), and elevation. Pain may persist for several weeks before resolution.

11. **What is epididymitis, and how do I tell it apart from testicular torsion?**
Epididymitis is inflammation of the epididymis. It often also involves inflammation of the testes, which is called epididymo-orchitis. Just like testicular torsion, epididymitis also presents with acute testicular pain and swelling but is often more gradual in presentation, occurring over 1 to 2 days. Epididymitis may also present with concurrent fever, dysuria, hematuria, and pain that radiates to the lower abdomen. Conversely, testicular torsion is more likely to present with nausea and vomiting and has more of a sudden onset of pain. On physical examination, the testicle typically has a normal position in the epididymitis as opposed to the high-riding testicle often seen in testicular torsion. The cremasteric reflex also remains intact in epididymitis and pain is also often relieved with elevation of the scrotum.

12. **How do I treat epididymitis?**
In prepubertal males, the treatment is largely supportive care, which includes NSAIDs and scrotal elevation. In the rare instance that midstream urine is positive for an infection, antibiotics should be started. In sexually active males with acute epididymitis, prophylactic treatment with intramuscular ceftriaxone and oral doxycycline is recommended since the most likely etiology in this population is from *Chlamydia trachomatis* or *Neisseria gonorrhea*.

13. **What can happen when a male is hit in the scrotum?**
While relatively uncommon, blunt trauma injuries to the scrotum can lead to decreased fertility, hypogonadism, and chronic testicular pain if not treated appropriately. These injuries most often occur during sporting events but can also be found after motor vehicle accidents, physical assaults, and straddle injuries. Blunt scrotal trauma can cause testicular rupture, dislocation, intratesticular hematomas, and hematoceles. Patients will often present with scrotal pain and associated swelling. A scrotal ultrasound is useful to evaluate and characterize the extent of any injury. Indications for immediate surgical repair include a testicular rupture, which is a disruption of the tunica albuginea or extrusion of the seminiferous tubules, an expanding intratesticular hematoma or hematocele that is three times the size of the contralateral testicle, and a dislocated testicle that cannot be manually repositioned.

14. **Help! What should I do when I am worried my patient has an incarcerated inguinal hernia?**
Inguinal hernias often present as an intermittent painless "bulge" seen in the inguinal area or scrotum, especially during times when there is increased abdominal pressure, such as while crying or having a bowel movement. When the hernia becomes incarcerated, the bulge is often painful and associated with vomiting and abdominal distension. There may also be a change in the color of the skin covering the hernia.

Attempt manual reduction when there is a concern for an incarcerated hernia. Prior to the procedure, lift the buttocks of the patient so that gravity can help reduce the hernia. Ice packs can be applied to reduce scrotal swelling. Provide analgesia or sedation to decrease patient discomfort. The hernia can be then reduced with constant slow pressure applied to its distal end. Surgical reduction should be performed if a manual reduction is not completely successful. Patients with a successful reduction are at an increased risk for reincarceration, and strict return criteria should be provided to families.

15. **What else can cause a painless scrotal mass?**
A hydrocele is a painless scrotal mass that is often larger in the evenings. It is caused by an abnormal collection of fluid between the visceral and parietal layers of the tunica vaginalis. Physical examination is significant for a fluctuant mass in the scrotum that may or may not be reducible. Since a hydrocele is fluid-filled, it can be transilluminated on examination, which helps to differentiate it from other scrotal masses. Many hydroceles resolve spontaneously, so surgical repair is often delayed until a patient is at least 24 months old.

Table 22.2 Features of Painless Scrotal Masses

FEATURE	HISTORY	PHYSICAL EXAMINATION	MANAGEMENT
Inguinal hernia	Increases with Valsalva maneuver; painful only when incarcerated or strangulated	Mass in groin or scrotum; palpable at internal inguinal ring; bowel feels "sausage-shaped"	Assess for obstruction; Trendelenburg position, ice packs, analgesia, muscle relaxation
Varicocele (dilated veins of pampiniform plexus due to incompetent valves located along spermatic cord)	15% prevalence in adolescence; left > right; if found on the right, consider tumor, situs inversus, or renal vein thrombosis	Decreases when supine; "wormy" vessels around the cord	Surgical ligation of internal spermatic vein only if causing testicular atrophy
Spermatocele (sperm-containing cysts of the epididymis or efferent duct system)	Postpubertal males; painless	Nontender, small, cystic nodule located posterior or superior to testicle	Surgical intervention only if painful or unusually large
Neoplasm	15-35 years old; incidence increased if undescended, worse if intra-abdominal; painless unless bleeding into the tumor	Hard mass, smooth or irregular, adherent to testicle; gynecomastia or other paraneoplastic phenomena from β-human chorionic gonadotropin or estrogen	Orchiectomy and investigation of preaortic lymph node involvement

A varicocele is a vascular lesion that is typically caused by increased pressure within the spermatic vein, which leads to dilation and tortuosity. Varicoceles are typically present in adolescent and young adult males. On physical examination, varicoceles are often described as a "bag of worms" within the scrotum. Varicoceles can lead to a decrease in testicular size and development. Management is typically conservative, with surgical repair reserved for patients who have associated pain and concerns for infertility (see Table 22.2).

16. **Every parent who feels a mass in their child's scrotum is worried about a tumor. Do children get testicular tumors?**
    While testicular tumors in pediatric males are rare, most of them are malignant. Testicular neoplasms account for only 1% to 2% of all pediatric solid tumors. They often present as a painless scrotal mass. Nonseminomatous germ cell tumors, such as yolk sac tumors, teratomas, embryonal carcinomas, and choriocarcinomas are the most common in children. Among these tumors, yolk cell tumors account for 80% of the cases and have a peak incidence at age 2 years. Yolk cell tumors can be diagnosed based on an elevated alpha-fetoprotein level and an ultrasound showing a heterogeneous solid mass.

KEY POINTS: FIVE IMPORTANT THINGS TO REMEMBER ABOUT THE SCROTAL EVALUATION

1. Testicular torsion should be diagnosed and repaired as soon as possible because delays in care lead to increased ischemia of the testicle.
2. A high TWIST score should prompt immediate surgical evaluation without waiting for any imaging.
3. A torsed appendix testis is the most common cause of acute scrotal pain.
4. Epididymitis can look a lot like testicular torsion but typically has a more gradual onset and has a normal testicular lie and cremasteric reflex.
5. Painless scrotal masses are mostly benign but given that a small number can be malignant tumors, an ultrasound should generally be obtained to determine their source.

KEY POINTS: DIFFERENTIATING TESTICULAR TORSION AND TORSION OF APPENDIX TESTIS

Testicular Torsion
1. It is most commonly seen in mid-to-late adolescence.
2. Pain is sudden in onset, located in the entire testicle.
3. Cremasteric reflex is absent.

Torsion of Appendix Testis
1. It is most commonly seen in children and early adolescents.
2. Pain can be more gradual, located in a specific area of the testicle.
3. Cremasteric reflex is brisk.

BIBLIOGRAPHY

1. Addas F, Yan S, Hadjipavlou M, Gonsalves M, Sabbagh S. Testicular rupture or testicular fracture? A case report and literature review. *Case Rep Urol.*. 2018;2018:1323780. PMID: 30538883; PMCID: PMC6261066. https://doi.org/10.1155/2018/1323780.
2. Bastianpillai C, Ryan K, Hamid S, Li CY, Green JSA. Testicular pain pathway in children: investigating where missed torsion occurs most often. *Pediatr Emerg Care.*. 2021;37(12):e1311–e1314. https://doi.org/10.1097/PEC.0000000000002026. PMID: 31977775.
3. Bowlin PR, Gatti JM, Murphy JP. Pediatric testicular torsion. *Surg Clin North Am.*. 2017;97(1):161–172. https://doi.org/10.1016/j.suc.2016.08.012. PMID: 27894425.
4. Cerulo M, Farina A, Caiazzo S, Cortese G, Servillo G, Settimi A. Current concepts in the management of inguinal hernia and hydrocele in pediatric patients in laparoscopic era. *Semin Pediatr Surg.*. 2016;25(4):232–240. https://doi.org/10.1053/j.sempedsurg.2016.05.006. PMID: 27521714.
5. Dagrosa LM, McMenaman KS, Pais Jr. VM. Tension hydrocele: an unusual cause of acute scrotal pain. *Pediatr Emerg Care*. 2015;31(8):584–585. https://doi.org/10.1097/PEC.0000000000000283. PMID: 26244726.
6. Dalton DM, Davis NF, O'Neill DC, Brady CM, Kiely EA, O'Brien MF. Aetiology, epidemiology and management strategies for blunt scrotal trauma. *Surgeon.*. 2016;14(1):18–21. PMID: 25151340https://doi.org/10.1016/j.surge.2014.06.006.
7. Frohlich LC, Paydar-Darian N, Cilento Jr BG, Lee LK. Prospective validation of clinical score for males presenting with an acute scrotum. *Acad Emerg Med.*. 2017;24(12):1474–1482. https://doi.org/10.1111/acem.13295. PMID: 28833896.
8. Graumann LA, Dietz HG, Stehr M. Urinalysis in children with epididymitis. *Eur J Pediatr Surg.*. 2010;20(4):247–249. PMID: 20440674https://doi.org/10.1055/s-0030-1253356.
9. McConaghy JR, Panchal B. Epididymitis: an overview. *Am Fam Physician.*. 2016;94(9):723–726. PMID: 27929243.
10. Mohammed A, Chinegwundoh F. Testicular varicocele: an overview. *Urol Int.*. 2009;82(4):373–379. PMID: 19506401https://doi.org/10.1159/000218523.
11. Nassiri N, Zhu T, Asanad K, Vasquez E. Testicular torsion from bell-clapper deformity. *Urology.*. 2021;147:275. PMID: 32650017https://doi.org/10.1016/j.urology.2020.06.045.
12. Osumah TS, Jimbo M, Granberg CF, Gargollo PC. Frontiers in pediatric testicular torsion: an integrated review of prevailing trends and management outcomes. *J Pediatr Urol.*. 2018;14(5):394–401. https://doi.org/10.1016/j.jpurol.2018.07.002. PMID: 30087037.
13. Taghavi K, Dumble C, Hutson JM, Mushtaq I, Mirjalili SA. The bell-clapper deformity of the testis: the definitive pathological anatomy. *J Pediatr Surg.*. 2021;56(8):1405–1410. PMID: 32762939https://doi.org/10.1016/j.jpedsurg.2020.06.023.

CHAPTER 23

SORE THROAT

Magdy W. Attia and Yamini Durani

1. **What are the common causes of sore throat in pediatric patients?**
   - Viral infection
   - Bacterial infection
   - *Candida* infection (infants)
   - Mucosal injury (due to physical, chemical, or thermal causes)
   - Foreign body
   - Systemic inflammation (i.e., Kawasaki disease)

2. **What is acute pharyngitis?**
   Acute pharyngitis is an infection of the tonsils or the pharynx. *Pharyngitis, tonsillitis*, and *tonsillopharyngitis* are interchangeable terms often used to describe the clinical diagnosis of sore throat, regardless of the etiology.

3. **What is the incidence of pharyngitis in children?**
   The exact incidence of pharyngitis is not known. It is, however, the second most common diagnosis in children 1 to 15 years of age in the ambulatory setting.

4. **What is the most common etiology for pharyngitis?**
   Viral agents account for most cases of pharyngitis (70%-80%). These include:
   - Rhinoviruses
   - Epstein-Barr virus
   - Parainfluenza viruses
   - Adenovirus
   - Influenza A and B
   - Herpes simplex virus types 1 and 2
   - Enteroviruses
   - Coronaviruses (including severe acute respiratory syndrome coronavirus 2 [SARS-CoV-2])
   - Cytomegalovirus
   - Human immunodeficiency virus (HIV)

5. **How can throat infection caused by these viruses be distinguished?**
   The signs and symptoms often overlap between different causes of throat infection. Some helpful diagnostic clues are as follows:
   - When pharyngitis is associated with conjunctivitis, the diagnosis of pharyngoconjunctival infection secondary to *adenovirus* is highly likely.
   - The presence of ulcerative lesions on an erythematous base on the posterior palate is associated with *coxsackie A virus*, a condition also known as herpangina. Hand, foot, and mouth disease is another variant of coxsackie pharyngitis, which is characterized by the presence of small vesiculopustular lesions or shallow ulcers on the soft palate, palms, and soles.
   - The association of significant cervical or generalized lymph adenopathy and hepatosplenomegaly is highly suspicious for infectious mononucleosis due to *Epstein-Barr virus* or, less commonly, *cytomegalovirus*.
   - SARS-CoV-2 should be suspected in the presence of symptoms such as fever, cough, congestion, fatigue, sore throat, myalgias, vomiting, and diarrhea and if there is a close contact exposure. Testing for SARS-CoV-2 should be performed in these circumstances.

6. **Which bacterial pharyngitis is the most common?**
   Streptococcus pyogenes, also known as group A β-hemolytic streptococcus (GABHS), is the most common bacterium causing pharyngitis in children and is often referred to simply as strep throat. It is implicated in as many as 20% to 30% of all cases of pharyngitis in children. Other bacterial causes of sore throat (group C β-hemolytic streptococci, group G β-hemolytic streptococci, *Mycoplasma pneumoniae, Neisseria gonorrhoeae*) are much less common. Neisseria gonorrhea should be considered in sexually active patients with symptoms of pharyngitis.

7. **What are the clinical features of GABHS pharyngitis?**
   - Sudden onset of fever and sore throat in a school-aged child. Fever is often low grade or absent.
   - Scarlatiniform rash—an erythematous, fine, sandpaper-like exanthem that generally appears in axillary and inguinal folds before it is generalized. It is pathognomonic for GABHS infection.

- Headache, vague abdominal pain, nausea, vomiting, and halitosis may be present.
- The pharynx is erythematous, and the tonsils are enlarged. Tonsillar exudate, palatine petechiae, and nasal excoriation may be present. Nasal excoriation is rare but more common in the younger child.
- Significant submandibular lymphadenopathy is usually present.
- Absence of cough or coryza is characteristic.

8. True or False: GABHS pharyngitis is usually obvious and easy to diagnose clinically.
   False. Initially, signs and symptoms are often absent because of the child's early presentation to clinicians. GABHS and viral pharyngitis have many overlapping clinical features and are often difficult to distinguish from one another.

9. Are some of the signs and symptoms more reliable than others in diagnosing strep throat?
   Yes. Scarlatiniform rash, large and tender submandibular lymph nodes, and the absence of coryza are more reliable than fever and tonsillar exudates in children. The latter two features are more common and reliable in adults.

10. Why is it important for clinicians to diagnose and treat GABHS pharyngitis?
    Early treatment of GABHS pharyngitis shortens the course of the disease and reduces transmission to contacts. Antibiotic treatment of GABHS pharyngitis prevents rheumatic fever and suppurative complications.

11. List the suppurative complications of GABHS.
    These include peritonsillar cellulitis or abscess (quinsy), retropharyngeal abscess, cervical adenitis, otitis media, and sinusitis.

12. What are the symptoms of a retropharyngeal abscess?
    A retropharyngeal abscess is an infection in the deep tissues of the neck, which may be a complication of a preceding pharyngitis or upper respiratory tract infection. It is generally more common in children under 5 years due to the more prominent lymph nodes in the retropharyngeal space in younger children. Typical symptoms include sore throat, fever, neck pain, neck stiffness or torticollis, dysphagia, odynophagia, and drooling.

13. What are the findings of a peritonsillar abscess?
    A peritonsillar abscess is another possible suppurative complication of pharyngitis that generally occurs in older children and adolescents. Patients often have a severe sore throat, which is worse or more inflamed on one side. Fever, dysphagia, a muffled-sounding voice, and drooling are other common symptoms. On physical exam, they have visible tonsillar inflammation, which is unilaterally more enlarged, often with a midline shift of the uvula to the contralateral side.

14. What are other important complications of GABHS infections? Does treatment of GABHS prevent these complications?
    Poststreptococcal glomerulonephritis (GN) is one of the complications of GABHS. Treating GABHS infection does not prevent poststreptococcal GN. Poststreptococcal GN can occur following non-GABHS, particularly groups C and D. Toxin-mediated diseases, such as scarlet fever and toxic shock syndrome, are also important complications of GABHS infection.

KEY POINTS: TREATMENT OF STREP THROAT

1. Shortens the course of the disease
2. Prevents suppurative complications
3. Prevents rheumatic fever
4. Reduces transmission to contacts
5. Does not prevent poststreptococcal GN

15. Can rheumatic fever occur after a skin GABHS infection or after non-GABHS pharyngitis?
    No. It is only known to occur after GABHS pharyngitis.

16. Is PANDAS (pediatric autoimmune neuropsychiatric disorder associated with streptococcal infections) a complication of strep pharyngitis?
    The existence of PANDAS is uncertain. It has been proposed that there is a possible association with group A strep infections and otherwise unexplained acute neurological changes in pediatric patients such as tics and obsessive-compulsive behavior. The data are limited, and these patients should be referred to specialists for management.

17. **What laboratory tests are available to diagnose GABHS infections? What are their advantages and disadvantages?**

    Throat culture is considered the gold standard for diagnosing GABHS pharyngitis, though it has limitations. Throat culture has a relatively high incidence of false-negative results (10%-20%). Also, a positive throat culture for GABHS without serologic evidence does not distinguish between carrier state and an acute infection. Finally, cultures may take 24 to 48 hours of incubation to detect GABHS, which may delay diagnosis and care.

    Alternative tests include serologic testing (Antistreptolysin O, anti-DNase) and rapid antigen tests. Serologic testing is impractical in the acute evaluation of suspected GABHS pharyngitis. Rapid antigen tests by a reference laboratory method are highly specific (few false-positive results), but the sensitivity varies (60%-90%) depending on the quality of sample. Hence, the clinical guidelines recommend the use of rapid antigen tests in conjunction with back-up throat cultures if the rapid test is negative. Positive rapid antigen tests do not require a throat culture since it is a highly specific test.

    Newer diagnostic tests such as polymerase chain reaction (strep A PCR) for amplification of nucleic acids are available, which are highly sensitive and can provide more timely results than a throat culture. Given these advantages, PCR can be used as a first-line diagnostic test whenever possible.

    Indiscriminate testing (i.e., in a patient with clear clinical diagnosis of viral upper respiratory tract infection) diminishes sensitivity and specificity of rapid antigen tests and throat culture.

18. **What is the carriage rate of GABHS in healthy children?**

    10% to 20% of healthy children have a positive throat culture for GABHS while they are asymptomatic (i.e., carriers).

19. **What is the antibiotic of choice for treating GABHS sore throat?**

    Penicillin is the mainstay of treatment for GABHS pharyngitis. Resistance to penicillin has not been documented. It is least expensive and has a proven efficacy. Oral penicillin V or a penicillin derivative such as amoxicillin is most often used (because liquid penicillin has an unpleasant taste). The recommended dose of amoxicillin is 50 mg/kg/day for 10 days. The maximum dose is 1000 mg/day and can be given once a day. While the symptoms improve rapidly, it is crucial to complete the entire 10-day period of therapy. If compliance is in question, intramuscular benzathine penicillin G (0.6-1.2 million units) is an effective, one-time alternative. Cephalosporins, clindamycin, clarithromycin, and azithromycin are alternate antibiotic choices for penicillin-allergic patients.

20. **Do GABHS carriers need to be treated with antibiotics?**

    Carriers do not need to be treated. Up to 20% of school-aged children may be carriers of GABHS. They are at low risk for disease transmission or development of suppurative and nonsuppurative complications.

21. **What should I do if symptoms of strep throat persist?**

    Determining the cause of symptoms' persistence is imperative and may include noncompliance, recurrent infection, infection with a different pathogen (commonly infectious mononucleosis and adenovirus) superimposed on a carrier state, or presence of suppurative complications such as peritonsillar abscess.

22. **Should sore throat secondary to non-GABHS be treated?**

    There is not enough evidence in the literature to answer this question, and there are currently no clear recommendations on the necessity of treating these infections. In one report, children with group G β-hemolytic streptococci seem to have improved more quickly with oral penicillin. Group C is usually seen in older adolescents and young adults and is generally a milder illness than GABHS pharyngitis.

KEY POINTS: GABHS PHARYNGITIS

1. Accounts for 20% to 30% of pharyngitis in children.
2. Sore throat, pharyngeal erythema, tender submandibular nodes, absence of cough, and coryza are characteristic. Scarlatiniform rash is almost always pathognomonic.
3. Indiscriminate testing is discouraged.
4. Penicillin or amoxicillin—still the drugs of choice for treatment.

23. **What is the current recommendation for tonsillectomy in patients with recurrent pharyngitis?**

    Tonsillectomy should be considered in patients with three or more episodes of pharyngitis per year for 3 consecutive years, or five episodes per year in 2 consecutive years, or seven episodes in 1 year despite adequate medical therapy.

24. **True or False: Tonsillectomy affects the incidence and the course of pharyngitis.**
    False. The presence or absence of the tonsils has no bearing on the overall incidence or the course of the disease. However, after tonsillectomy, the frequency of streptococcal pharyngitis diminishes for 1 to 2 years, after which the incidence returns to that of the general population.

25. **Should steroids be used routinely in patients with pharyngitis?**
    There are not sufficient data to support the routine use of steroids in patients with pharyngitis, but it may be helpful in some patients with severe symptoms of pain who are also on antibiotics. Steroids may decrease the time to onset of pain relief. There is not a defined dose, preparation, or duration for steroid use, but some clinicians use a single dose of dexamethasone. Other modalities of analgesia should be considered such as nonsteroidal antiinflammatory drugs and acetaminophen.

26. **How soon can children with GABHS pharyngitis return to school or childcare?**
    The American Academy of Pediatrics recommends that children receive at least 12 hours of an appropriate antibiotic before returning to school or childcare. Most schools require a period of afebrile state for 24 hours prior to return.

27. **How can recurrent episodes of rheumatic fever be prevented?**
    If GABHS pharyngitis develops in a patient who has already had rheumatic fever in the past, that person is at high risk for recurrent rheumatic fever. GABHS pharyngitis should therefore be prevented in any patient who has previously had rheumatic fever by administering continuous antibiotic prophylaxis. In most cases, intramuscular benzathine penicillin G every 4 weeks is preferred.

28. **Can GABHS pharyngitis occur in children <3 years?**
    Yes. Although it is a more prevalent disease in school-aged children, it is a common myth that GABHS pharyngitis does not occur in younger children. Studies have reported disease rates between 5% and 25% in this age group. Rheumatic fever is rare in these young children.

29. **Which diagnoses should you consider if a child has sore throat and respiratory distress?**
    It is rare for a child with sore throat to also have difficulty breathing. The combination of sore throat and respiratory distress suggests a serious condition of the pharynx (or near the pharynx) causing airway obstruction. Consider conditions such as epiglottitis, particularly with an unimmunized patient. In young children and infants, retropharyngeal abscess can lead to airway obstruction. Peritonsillar abscess is less likely to do so, since this is found in older children who have larger airways. Massive tonsillar hypertrophy may be seen with infectious mononucleosis, and this can cause airway obstruction. Patients with sore throat related to coronavirus disease 2019 (COVID-19) infection may also have pneumonia, leading to respiratory distress. A foreign body in the pharynx, such as a fish bone or toy, could lead to dysphagia and rarely airway obstruction.

BIBLIOGRAPHY

1. Attia MW, Zaoutis T, Klein JD, Meier FA. Performance of a predictive model for streptococcal pharyngitis in children. *Arch Pediatr Adolesc Med.* 2001;155:687–691.
2. Attia MW. Adding corticosteroids to antibiotics improves pain relief in patients with sore throat. *Ann Intern Med.* 2013;158(6):JC11.
3. Centers for Disease Control and Prevention. Group A Streptococcal Disease/Strep Pharyngitis. Information for Clinicians. Accessed 22.06.22.
4. Gerber MA. Diagnosis and treatment of pharyngitis in children. *Pediatr Clin North Am.* 2005;52:729–747.
5. Hayward G, Thompson MJ, Perera R, et al. Corticosteroids as standalone or add-on treatment for sore throat. *Cochrane Database Syst Rev.* 2012;10:CD008268.
6. Kimberline DWD, Barnett EDE, Lynfield RT, Sawyer MHK. *Group A streptococcal infections. Red Book (2021): Report of the Committee on Infectious Diseases.* 32nd ed. American Academy of Pediatrics (AAP); 2021:694–707. https://doi.org/10.1542/9781610025225-part03-ch130.
7. Morad A, Sathe N, Francis DO, et al. Tonsillectomy versus watchful waiting for recurrent throat infection: a systematic review. *Pediatrics.* 2017;139(2):e20163490.
8. Shapiro DJ, Lindgren CE, Neuman MI, Fine AM. Viral features and testing for Streptococcal pharyngitis. *Pediatrics.* 2017;139(5):e20163403.
9. Shulman ST, Bisno AL, Clegg HW, et al. Clinical practice guideline for the diagnosis and management of group A streptococcal pharyngitis: 2012 update by the Infectious Diseases Society of America. *Clin Infect Dis.* 2012;55:1279.
10. UptoDate. Treatment and prevention of streptococcal pharyngitis in adults and children. <https://www.uptodate.com/contents/treatment-and-prevention-of-streptococcal-pharyngitis-in-adults-and-children?search=treatment%20of%20pharyngitis%20in%20children&source=search_result&selectedTitle=1~150&usage_type=default&display_rank=1#H3972918375>; 2021 Accessed 22.06.22.

CHAPTER 24

STIFF NECK

Marla Friedman and Nicholas Tsarouhas

1. **What is meningismus?**

   This is a form of neck stiffness associated with meningeal irritation. The child with meningismus has difficulty flexing the neck. The patient often has fever. Meningitis is always a consideration in these children. Another infection, spinal epidural abscess, is a very rare cause of meningismus.

2. **What is the pathophysiology of meningismus?**

   Flexion of the neck stretches the inflamed nerve roots and meninges of the cervical region. Autoprotective muscle spasm manifests as neck stiffness or meningismus.

3. **Is meningismus usually seen in neonates with meningitis?**

   No. Neonates rarely manifest meningismus or nuchal rigidity. The most common symptoms of meningitis in neonates are lethargy, irritability, poor feeding, dyspnea, and apnea. Fever is uncommon in neonates; hypothermia is a more likely manifestation of sepsis/meningitis.

4. **At what age is meningismus or nuchal rigidity reliable in evaluation of children for meningitis?**

   Meningismus is usually seen after 18 to 24 months of age. Importantly, it is a late finding in meningitis in younger infants.

5. **What are the Kernig and Brudzinski signs?**

   These signs are physical examination maneuvers to evaluate for the presence of meningeal inflammation. The Kernig sign is positive when extension of the patient's hip and knee causes pain and flexion of the neck. The Brudzinski sign refers to involuntary flexion of the knees with flexion of the patient's neck.

6. **What are the most common causes of bacterial meningitis in children?**

   Bacterial meningitis is a serious infection, which must be recognized and treated in a timely manner. The most common organisms vary by age group and include *Streptococcus pneumoniae*, group B streptococcus, *Staphylococcus aureus*, *Neisseria meningitidis*, *Haemophilus influenzae*, and *Escherichia coli*. Empiric antibiotics are strongly recommended and also vary by age group. Sequelae of bacterial meningitis may include hearing loss, learning disabilities, and brain damage. Untreated bacterial meningitis can lead to organ failure and death.

7. **Can viruses and other organisms cause a stiff neck and meningitis?**

   Yes! The most common causes of viral meningitis are enteroviruses. Other common viral organisms include mumps, measles, herpesvirus, and influenza. Even the severe acute respiratory syndrome coronavirus disease 2019 (COVID-19) can cause meningitis in children. Most children recover from viral meningitis completely without permanent sequelae. While most cases of viral meningitis require only supportive care, there are some exceptions, including herpes simplex virus, which requires a treatment course of acyclovir.

   Lyme disease can also cause meningitis, resulting in neck stiffness and pain. A lumbar puncture (LP) will show pleocytosis of the cerebral spinal fluid, but bacterial culture will be negative. Often, serum Lyme titers support the diagnosis.

8. **What are the indications for LP in a child with a stiff neck?**

   Consider performing an LP to rule out meningitis in any febrile child with a stiff neck and no other obvious source of infection. This is especially important in children who are not well appearing. Lethargy and irritability should always raise concern for meningitis.

9. **What are the contraindications to doing an LP?**

   LP may be dangerous in an unstable, critically ill child. "Curling" the young patient into position for the LP may limit ventilation and lead to respiratory arrest in an already compromised infant. If the child is unstable, draw a blood culture and administer antibiotics. Defer the LP until the child is more stable. Other contraindications to LP include increased intracranial pressure, lumbosacral cutaneous infection, and coagulopathy.

10. **What other spinal infections may present with a stiff neck?**
Osteomyelitis, epidural abscess, and diskitis may occur in the cervical region. Focal spine tenderness in the presence of fever should raise suspicion for these infections. Conventional radiography is sometimes helpful, but magnetic resonance imaging is more diagnostic.

11. **Which serious deep neck infection can present with stiff neck?**
Retropharyngeal abscess. Retropharyngeal infections (cellulitis, adenitis, abscess) can develop in the potential space between the anterior border of the cervical vertebrae and the posterior wall of the esophagus. These infections generally occur in infants and toddlers and are rarely seen in children older than 5 years. They are usually caused by group A streptococcus, *S. aureus*, or anaerobes. These ill-appearing children may present with fever, respiratory distress, drooling, difficulty swallowing, stridor, and stiff neck. Although the neck is "stiff" with retropharyngeal abscess, the patient can often flex the neck (unlike a child with meningitis). These children have more difficulty with neck extension.
   Obtain a lateral neck radiograph to investigate for widening of the upper cervical prevertebral tissues. Computed tomography is confirmatory, though not always mandatory. Management includes intravenous (IV) antibiotics and, sometimes, surgical drainage.

12. **Define torticollis?**
Torticollis, which is derived from the Latin *tortus*, meaning "twisted," and *collum*, meaning "neck," is a characteristic tilting of the head to one side secondary to an underlying disorder. The child with torticollis may or may not have pain and usually holds the head tilted to one side with the chin rotated in the opposite direction. There is unilateral neck muscle contraction. This condition can be due to a variety of causes, including minor trauma and muscle strain.

13. **What are the most common causes of torticollis in well-appearing, *afebrile* children?**
Minor irritation, muscle spasm, and awkward sleep position are quite common in young children. The onset is usually sudden, often occurring after waking from sleep. These children have no history of fever or trauma and should have a completely normal neurologic examination. Supportive care and analgesics/anti-inflammatory agents are usually the only therapies indicated.

14. **What is a common cause of stiff neck in a well-appearing, *febrile* child?**
Cervical adenitis, which presents with an enlarged tender lymph node, may be associated with stiff neck. Group A streptococcus and *S. aureus* are the most likely organisms responsible, but *Bartonella henselae* (cat scratch disease) and mycobacterial disease should also be considered. Pharyngitis/tonsillitis and upper respiratory tract infections may also be associated with stiff neck. Finally, Kawasaki disease may present with a large tender lymph node and neck pain or stiffness, but these children should have other features of Kawasaki disease.

15. **What common pulmonary condition may be associated with torticollis?**
Upper lobe pneumonia, which causes referred pain to the neck. Tachypnea is the most reliable physical examination sign in patients with pneumonia. Of course, fever and cough are also usually seen.

16. **Which gastroenterologic condition may be associated with torticollis?**
Sandifer syndrome, which is characterized by intermittent torticollis, opisthotonus, and irritability, is caused by severe gastroesophageal reflux with esophagitis in infants. Many infants with this condition exhibit vomiting and failure to thrive.

17. **What is the most common oncologic cause of torticollis in children?**
Posterior fossa tumors. In addition to head tilt, torticollis, or stiff neck, children with these tumors may present with headache, early-morning vomiting, clumsiness, ataxia, strabismus, visual changes, or papilledema. Neck stiffness in these patients is thought to be due to irritation of the accessory nerve by the cerebellar tonsil, trapped in the occipital foramen. Every child with torticollis needs a careful neurologic exam to rule out a brain tumor.

18. **What is the most common form of torticollis in infancy?**
Congenital muscular torticollis (also called sternocleidomastoid [SCM] tumor of infancy or pseudotumor of infancy) usually presents in the first 2 weeks of life as a unilateral, hard, immobile, and fusiform swelling in the inferior aspect of the SCM muscle. The infant's head is tilted toward the affected side. The cause is controversial. The most common explanation implicates birth trauma with resultant hematoma formation followed by muscle contracture. Another theory postulates that intrauterine abnormal fetal position causes unilateral shortening of the SCM muscle. Ultrasonography may confirm that the palpable mass or swelling is muscular in origin. Passive stretching of the involved muscle is usually curative; recalcitrant cases may require surgical release (<5% of all cases). Intramuscular injections with botulinum toxin have also been employed.

19. **What is benign paroxysmal torticollis of infancy?**
This is a self-limited condition characterized by intermittent episodes of torticollis. It may last for minutes to hours and may recur for weeks to months. Onset is usually in the first few months of life and usually resolves by 2 to 3 years of age. These episodes are associated with pallor, ataxia, nystagmus, migraines, vomiting, agitation, and lethargy. The cause of the syndrome remains unknown and, at present, there is no effective therapy.

20. **Which congenital syndrome is identified by the triad of short neck (brevicollis), limited neck motion, and low occipital hairline?**
Klippel-Feil syndrome. This is a skeletal malformation characterized by the fusion of a variable number of cervical vertebrae. It may also be associated with other bony anomalies and significant scoliosis. These children may have anomalies of multiple organ systems (cardiovascular, genitourinary) as well. The cause is unknown.

21. **What is Sprengel deformity?**
This is a congenital failure of the scapula to descend to its correct position. In its most severe form, the scapula is connected by bone to the cervical spine and limits neck motion. The treatment of choice is surgery and physical therapy.

22. **What are the first priorities in managing a trauma victim with a stiff neck?**
While maintaining in-line stabilization of the cervical spine, ensure adequacy of the airway. Immobilize the cervical spine before further evaluation. The physical examination should then focus on the presence of neurologic deficits (weakness, paresthesias, bowel or bladder dysfunction). If neurologic deficits are present, obtain emergent neurosurgical consultation.

23. **Which initial radiographs should be obtained in the trauma victim with neck pain?**
The routine initial views include a lateral cervical spine (the most important view), an open-mouth odontoid view (difficult to obtain in younger children), and an anteroposterior cervical spine view.

24. **If the initial radiographs are inconclusive, which other images may be helpful?**
If plain radiographs are inconclusive, computed tomography of the cervical spine may be indicated. If focal neurologic findings are present, spinal magnetic resonance imaging should be considered.

25. **Are traumatic cervical spine injuries more common in the upper or lower cervical spine in young children?**
Traumatic cervical spine injuries are more common in the upper cervical spine in younger children, due to the higher fulcrum of the cervical spine, as well as the relative weakness of the neck muscles, compared with adolescents and adults.

26. **What is the most common anatomic abnormality identified in cases of traumatic torticollis?**
Atlantoaxial rotary subluxation. The ligamentous laxity of the pediatric cervical spine predisposes children to this condition, which may be seen after only a minor injury, such as a fall from a low height. These patients report stiff neck with pain but have no neurologic deficits. Plain films of the cervical spine may reveal asymmetry of the odontoid relative to the atlas. However, these films may not detect the subluxation. Computed tomography is usually confirmatory. In most cases, soft collar, rest, and anti-inflammatory agents or analgesics are curative. Severe cases, however, may require traction or surgery.

27. **Is atlantoaxial subluxation always a result of trauma?**
No, atlantoaxial subluxation may result from ligamentous laxity following an infection or inflammatory process. It may be associated with rheumatoid arthritis, systemic lupus erythematosus, or tonsillitis/pharyngitis.

28. **What is Grisel syndrome?**
Grisel syndrome is neck stiffness related to inflammatory atlantoaxial subluxation caused by ligamentous laxity, as noted above. Think of this condition if a child comes to the emergency department (ED) with a stiff neck following an otolaryngology procedure (e.g., tonsillectomy, adenoidectomy), in which the neck is maneuvered during surgery. These patients may also present with an upper respiratory infection. Fever and dysphagia are common. Usually, the condition is mild and there is no displacement of the axis. Children with Down and Marfan syndromes are particularly susceptible to this subluxation, secondary to the laxity of the transverse ligament of the atlas.

29. **Are there other injuries to consider in a child with a stiff neck after a minor fall?**
Some children with a clavicle fracture may hold their neck to one side and limit movement because of pain and SCM muscle spasm. Always remember to examine/palpate the clavicles of a child who has sustained a fall. Likewise, examine the spine of a child with a clavicle fracture to rule out a masked injury of the cervical spine or atlantoaxial rotary subluxation.

30. **What is the name given to drug-induced torticollis?**
Dystonic reaction. This is characterized by muscle spasm and abnormal postures, and it most commonly affects the eyes, face, neck, and throat. Patients with dystonic reactions may present with nuchal rigidity, opisthotonus, trismus, oculogyric crisis, or cogwheel rigidity. These patients are awake and often very distraught over their condition. The torticollis is caused by increased cholinergic activity and change in dopaminergic activity in the basal ganglia, which are responsible for muscle tone.

31. **Which drugs most commonly cause dystonic reactions in children?**
Metoclopramide (Reglan) and phenothiazines such as prochlorperazine (Compazine). These reactions are dose-related and usually begin within 2 to 5 days of initiating therapy.

32. **How are dystonic reactions treated?**
IV diphenhydramine (Benadryl) at a dose of 1 mg/kg usually terminates the reaction. Continue oral diphenhydramine for several days after the patient is discharged from the ED. Of course, discontinue the offending drug.

33. **What arachnid envenomation may be associated with torticollis?**
The bite of *Latrodectus mactans*, the dreaded black widow spider, is a neurotoxic envenomation that causes muscle pain and sometimes nuchal rigidity. There is little to no local reaction at the site of the bite. Black widow spider bites are the leading cause of death from spider bites in the United States.

34. **What is the differential diagnosis of stiff neck in children?**
The extensive differential diagnosis of stiff neck in children is summarized in Table 24.1.

Table 24.1 Causes of Stiff Neck in Children

Infectious
Meningitis,* brain/epidural abscess, encephalitis, septic arthritis/osteomyelitis, epiglottitis, diskitis, retropharyngeal abscess, viral myositis/myalgia,* tonsillitis/pharyngitis,* upper respiratory tract infection,* cervical adenitis,* pneumonia (upper lobe), otitis media, mastoiditis

Traumatic
Muscle contusion/spasm,* subarachnoid hemorrhage, atlantoaxial rotary subluxation, epidural hematoma, congenital muscular torticollis,* spinal cord injury, cervical spine fracture, clavicle fracture*

Congenital
Benign paroxysmal torticollis, skeletal malformation (Klippel-Feil syndrome, congenital muscular torticollis,* Sprengel deformity), atlantoaxial instability (Down syndrome), Arnold-Chiari malformation

Toxic
Dystonic reaction,* black widow spider bite

Oncologic
Posterior fossa tumors, lymphoma

Miscellaneous
Migraine, spasmus nutans, Sandifer syndrome, syringomyelia, collagen vascular disease (juvenile rheumatoid arthritis, pseudotumor cerebri, ankylosing spondylitis), psychogenic causes

*Denotes most common causes of stiff neck.

KEY POINTS: EVALUATING STIFF NECK IN CHILDREN AND INFANTS

1. Do not count on meningismus as a symptom of meningitis in neonates and young infants; instead, focus on the nonspecific signs and symptoms, which include lethargy, irritability, poor feeding, dyspnea, and apnea.
2. An LP may be dangerous in an unstable, critically ill child; if the child is very sick, draw a blood culture, administer antibiotics, and defer the LP until the child is more stable.
3. Consider the following common infectious causes of stiff neck:
   - **Meningitis:** This is characterized by ill appearance, irritability, lethargy; fever; pain with flexion.
   - **Tonsillitis/pharyngitis:** Tonsils are red and inflamed, but not always exudative; consider peritonsillar abscess if there is posterior, superior, soft palatal bulge, often with uvular deviation.

- **Retropharyngeal abscess**: The febrile, ill-appearing child may be drooling and will be unwilling to move the neck laterally or in extension.
- **Cervical adenitis**: Single enlarged, tender cervical node is seen; fever is common, but not universal.
- **Viral myositis/myalgia**: Cervical muscles are diffusely tender to palpation; other viral symptoms may be present.
- **Upper respiratory tract infection**: Appearance is similar to that for viral myositis, with prominent upper respiratory tract symptoms.

4. The most common cause of torticollis in an afebrile, well-appearing child with no history of trauma is minor irritation, muscle spasm, or awkward sleep malposition.

BIBLIOGRAPHY

1. Bedetti L, MarrozziniL Baraldi A, et al. Pitfalls in the diagnosis of meningitis in neonates and young infants: the role of lumbar puncture. *J Matern Fetal Neonatal Med.* 2019;32(23):4029–4035.
2. Ben Zvi I, Thompson DNP. Torticollis in childhood—a practical guide for initial assessment. *Eur J Pediatr.* 2022;181(3):865–873.
3. Bochner RE, Gangar M, Belamarich PF. A clinical approach to tonsillitis, tonsillar hypertrophy and pertonsillar and retropharyngeal abscess. *Pediatr Rev.* 2017;38(2):81–92.
4. Cronan K, Wiley J. Lumbar puncture. In: Henretig FM, King C, eds. *Textbook of Pediatric Emergency Procedures.* 2nd ed. Lippincott Williams & Wilkins; 2008:507.
5. Fafara-Les A, Kwiatkowski S, Marynczak L, et al. Torticollis as a first sign of posterior fossa and cervical spinal cord tumors in children. *Childs Nerv Syst.* 2014;30(3):425–430.
6. Greene KA, Lu V, Luciano MS, et al. Benign paroxysmal torticollis: phenotype, natural history and quality of life. *Pediatr Res.* 2021;90(5):1044–1051.
7. Litrenta J, Bi AS, Dryer JW. Klippel-Feil syndrome: pathogenesis, diagnosis and management. *J Am Acad Orthop Surg.* 2021;29(22):951–960.
8. Powell EC, Leonard JR, Olsen CS, et al. Atlantoaxial rotary subluxation in children. *Ped Emerg Care.* 2017;33(2):86–91.
9. Ta JH, Krishnan M. Management of congenital muscular torticollis in a child: a case report and review. *Int J Pediatr Otorhinolaryngol.* 2012;76(11):1543–1546.
10. Tzimenatos L, Vance C, Kuppermann N. *Neck stiffness. Fleisher & Ludwig's Textbook of Pediatric Emergency Medicine.* 8th ed. Wolters Kluwer; 2021:324–332.
11. Woodward GA, Keilman AE. *Neck trauma. Fleisher & Ludwig's Textbook of Pediatric Emergency Medicine.* 8th ed. Wolters Kluwer; 2021:1215–1253.
12. Yousefi K, Poorbarat S, Abasi Z, Rahimi S, Khakshour A. Viral meningitis associated with COVID-19 in a 9-year old child: a case report. *Pediatr Infect Dis Journ.* 2021;40(2):e87–e98.

CHAPTER 25

STRIDOR

Marisa Riverso

1. List the four primary diagnostic considerations in a febrile child with acute stridor.
   - Croup
   - Epiglottitis
   - Retropharyngeal abscess
   - Bacterial tracheitis

   Table 25.1 illustrates the clinical criteria helpful in distinguishing among the four.

2. What is the most common cause of acute stridor in young children?
   Laryngotracheobronchitis (croup) accounts for more than 90% of all emergency department (ED) visits for stridor in the pediatric population. The key features of croup include barky cough, stridor, and hoarseness, usually preceded by symptoms of a mild upper respiratory tract infection. Croup is most common in older infants and toddlers, though it also occurs in school-aged children.

3. How do you treat croup?
   Croup is caused by inflammation of the upper airway. Stridor results from airflow through the narrowed airway, almost like breathing through a pinched straw. The treatment goals are then aimed at reducing inflammation in the upper airway. The mainstay of treatment is oral dexamethasone 0.6 mg/kg given orally or intramuscularly. If the patient has stridor at rest (indicating a critical narrowing of the airway), treatment with nebulized epinephrine is indicated to reduce airway edema quickly as steroids take hours to reach full effect.

Table 25.1 Clinical Criteria Helpful in Distinguishing Among the Four Primary Diagnoses in a Febrile Child With Acute Stridor

CRITERIA	CROUP	EPIGLOTTITIS	RETROPHARYNGEAL ABSCESS	BACTERIAL TRACHEITIS
Anatomy	Subglottic	Supraglottic	Retropharyngeal nodes	Trachea
Cause	Viral: parainfluenza	Bacterial*	Bacterial: oral flora	Bacterial: *Staphylococcus aureus*
Age range	6 mo-3 years	Any, sporadic	6 mo-4 years	Any, sporadic
Onset	1-3 days	Hours (prodrome—days)	1-3 days	3-5 days
Toxicity	Mild to moderate	Marked	Marked	Marked
Drooling	No	Yes	Yes	No
Hoarseness	Yes	No	No	No
Cough	Barky	No	No	Yes, painful
White blood cell count	Normal	Elevated	Elevated	Elevated
Radiograph	"Steeple" sign (anteroposterior)	"Thumb" sign (lateral)	Widened prevertebral soft tissues†	"Shaggy" trachea

*Hib (*Haemophilus influenzae* type b) now accounts for less than 25% of cases; other causes include staphylococci, streptococci, and, in immunosuppressed patients, *Candida* species and herpes simplex virus.
†Expiratory film or poor positioning may also show significant widening; the best test is computed tomography of the neck.

4. **How long should you monitor a patient after administration of racemic epinephrine (RE) before discharge?**
   This is unclear. Many suggest observation in the ED for at least 2 to 3 hours. The peak onset of action for oral corticosteroids is between 1 and 2 hours. The effects of RE peak at 30 minutes and have been shown to last 2 hours. One study showed outpatient treatment failure (requiring a second dose of RE and subsequent admission) in patients monitored between 2.1 and 3 hours of 16.7% versus 7.1% in patients monitored for 3.1 to 4 hours (odds ratio = 2.44, $P < .01$).

5. **You decide to treat a child with croup and stridor at rest with nebulized epinephrine. Is it better to use RE rather than L-Epinephrine?**
   No, the two forms of epinephrine are equally effective, and the rate of side effects is not significantly different. The recommended dose of RE 2.25% is 0.05 mL/kg (maximal dose: 0.5 mL) or L-Epinephrine 1 mg/mL solution (1:1000) 0.5 mL/kg (maximal dose: 5 mL) via nebulizer. L-Epinephrine may be more readily available in clinical settings.

6. **Can COVID-19 cause croup?**
   Yes. While we are still learning about the many manifestations of acute severe acute respiratory syndrome coronavirus 2 (SARS-CoV-2) virus in children, there have been multiple case reports of patients presenting with classic symptoms of croup found to be positive for SARS-CoV-2 as well as a case report of a patient presenting early with stridor and subsequently developing multisystem inflammatory syndrome in children.

7. **Which infection should you consider when the young child with stridor is sitting in a tripod position with the neck extended (sniffing position)?**
   Epiglottitis. Children with this condition find a way to open their airways by sitting in this classic position. Epiglottitis is very rare since most children are vaccinated against *H. influenzae B*. However, the infection is still seen in unimmunized populations.

8. **An adolescent female cross-country runner presents to the ED for the third time in a month for "croup" worsened by running. What is the likely cause of her stridor? What is the treatment?**
   This teen athlete likely suffers from vocal cord dysfunction (also called Exercise-Induced Laryngeal Obstruction and Paradoxical Vocal Fold Movement). This is a condition in which the vocal cords adduct abnormally on inspiration, expiration, or both. It has been associated with exercise, gastroesophageal reflux, and irritant exposures. Stress or anxiety is found in many patients. The stridor often occurs during high-intensity exercise and resolves with cessation of exercise. It is not present during sleep. One case series found a mean age of 13 years and a female-to-male ratio of 3:1. It is often misdiagnosed as asthma or occurs concurrently with asthma. The gold standard for diagnosis is direct visualization of the abnormal vocal cord motion via fiberoptic laryngoscopy. Treatment with speech therapy and vocal cord relaxation exercises is often successful.

9. **What radiographic findings would you expect to find in croup versus epiglottitis?**
   The classic radiographic finding in croup is the "steeple sign," a narrowing of the laryngotracheal air column just below the vocal cords on an anteroposterior view (Fig. 25.1). Another finding includes "ballooning" (distention) of the hypopharynx during inspiration, seen on a lateral view. The steeple sign lacks sensitivity and specificity. Radiographs are not indicated for most children with suspected croup. Radiographs are reserved for the evaluation of children with stridor when other causes are considered or atypical cases. The classic radiographic finding in epiglottitis is the "thumb sign," referring to the lateral view of the swollen epiglottis resembling a lateral view of one's thumb (Fig. 25.2). The thumb sign is also subjective, and radiographs alone should not be used to diagnose epiglottitis. If clinical suspicion is high, imaging should be deferred in favor of direct visualization of the airway under controlled circumstances.

10. **Which bacterial infection of the upper airway most closely clinically mimics croup: epiglottitis, bacterial tracheitis, or retropharyngeal abscess?**
    The clinical presentation of bacterial tracheitis is nearly indistinguishable from that of severe croup. In fact, croup caused by parainfluenza and influenza type A may lead to bacterial superinfection in some cases. Bacterial tracheitis presents with symptoms of stridor, fever, and toxicity generally worsening over a 3- to 7-day period. RE and steroids are not effective, and many patients will require intubation and surgical débridement of the membranous tracheal exudates. The most common organism causing bacterial tracheitis is *Staphylococcus aureus*, though *Moraxella catarrhalis* infection is also prevalent and potentially more severe.

11. **Why are retropharyngeal abscesses uncommon in children over the age of 5 years?**
    The abscess is caused by seeding of the retropharyngeal nodes with bacteria, usually oral pathogens. After the age of 4 years, the retropharyngeal nodes atrophy. Older children are more likely to present with peritonsillar abscesses, and these very rarely lead to airway obstruction or stridor.

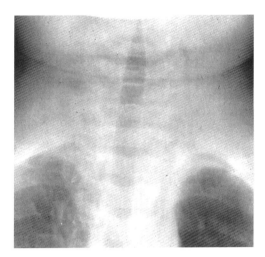

Fig. 25.1 Radiographic view of the steeple sign.

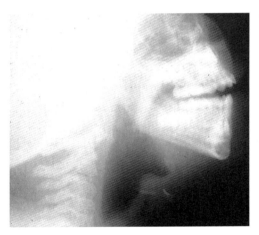

Fig. 25.2 Radiographic view of the thumb sign.

12. **What is stertor? How does it differ from stridor?**
    Stertor is the noise most aptly described as snoring. It refers to the low-pitched vibratory noise made when airflow is obstructed in the nose and soft tissues of the pharynx. Stridor is higher pitched and refers to the noise of turbulent airflow through the larynx and trachea. Thus a snoring patient is stertorous, and a "croupy" patient is stridulous (not stridorous!).

13. **Name four noninfectious causes of stridor in children.**
    - Foreign body
    - Laryngomalacia
    - Vascular ring or sling
    - Airway hemangioma

14. **When should you worry about a foreign body as a cause of stridor in a young child?**
    Always! When a toddler (usually age 2-3 years old) presents with sudden onset of stridor, a foreign body in the upper airway should always be considered. These children are afebrile, so infection is less likely. The foreign body ingestion/aspiration, such as a coin or button battery, may not be witnessed.

15. **A mother reports her infant has "always had noisy breathing." What is the most common cause of chronic stridor?**
    Laryngomalacia is the most common cause of chronic stridor in infants. Stridor is usually worse when the infant is feeding or sleeping. It is generally benign and resolves spontaneously as the child grows, usually by age 12 to 18 months. The exact cause is unknown, though it is usually related to one or more supraglottic abnormalities, including a long epiglottis that prolapses posteriorly, bulky arytenoids that prolapse anteriorly, or shortened aryepiglottic folds and is typically worse when crying.

16. **What is the best test for diagnosing laryngomalacia?**
    Clinical clues to the diagnosis of laryngomalacia include stridor that improves with prone positioning and worsens with crying. Airway fluoroscopy is suggestive of the diagnosis, but the gold standard for diagnosis is direct laryngoscopy in an awake, upright, spontaneously breathing infant. Direct laryngoscopy also rules out other, less common causes of congenital stridor, including vocal cord paralysis and laryngeal webs and cysts.

17. **A sedated patient develops acute stridor followed by sudden complete airway obstruction. What steps do you take to relieve suspected laryngospasm?**
    Stop the procedure and remove the offending stimulus. Make sure the upper airway is clear and in good position. Apply continuous positive airway pressure, and apply firm digital pressure to the laryngospasm notch (Fig. 25.3). If laryngospasm persists, deepen sedation with propofol or paralyze the patient with succinylcholine. Consider tracheal intubation if the patient remains heavily sedated or if bag-mask ventilation is difficult.

18. **What is the significance of stridor that is loudest in the expiratory phase?**
    Expiratory stridor suggests tracheal disease. The differential diagnosis includes complete tracheal rings, primary tracheomalacia (faulty tracheal development), and secondary tracheomalacia (associated with external compression). External compression may be caused by vascular abnormalities or mediastinal masses, such as thymic cysts, cystic hygroma, thyroid hyperplasia, or mediastinal tumors.

KEY POINTS: CLINICAL CLUES TO THE ETIOLOGY OF STRIDOR

1. Hoarseness in the presence of stridor indicates vocal cord inflammation and is reassuring for the lack of supraglottic diseases such as epiglottitis or retropharyngeal abscess.
2. Conversely, drooling with stridor is concerning for supraglottic obstruction.
3. Inspiratory stridor suggests an extrathoracic lesion (e.g., laryngeal, nasal, pharyngeal).
4. Expiratory stridor implies an intrathoracic lesion (e.g., tracheal, bronchial).
5. Biphasic stridor may represent subglottic or glottic disease.

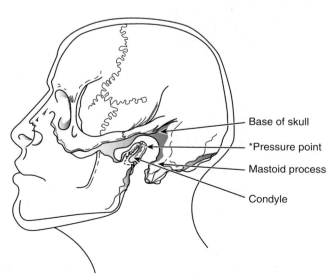

Base of skull
*Pressure point
Mastoid process
Condyle

Fig. 25.3 Laryngospasm notch. *Pressure point. (Adapted from Larson Jr PC. Laryngospasm—the best treatment [correspondence]. *Anesthesiology*. 1998;89(5):1293–1294.)

19. What are the three most common vascular anomalies associated with tracheal compression?
    - Double aortic arch (the most common anomaly, where two arches encircle the trachea and esophagus)
    - Pulmonary sling (aberrant left pulmonary artery arising from the right pulmonary artery, passing between the trachea and esophagus)
    - Aberrant innominate artery (arising from aortic arch or left carotid, causing pressure on the anterior tracheal wall)

20. A toddler born to a mother with a history of human papillomavirus (HPV) develops hoarseness over several months and presents with an acute exacerbation of stridor. What important pathologic condition must be considered?
    Recurrent respiratory papillomatosis, caused by certain strains of the HPV, may cause significant airway obstruction preceded by an indolent history of hoarseness, chronic or intermittent coughing spells, or poor feeding. HPV infection remains common, with a point prevalence of 10% in women with normal cytology worldwide. About 1% of infants born to mothers with vaginal condyloma will develop recurrent respiratory papillomatosis. Treatment includes both surgical (laser) and medical (antiviral) modalities.

21. Name five causes of stridor that are not directly related to the anatomy of the upper airway or infections.
    - **Allergic:** Anaphylaxis or hereditary angioedema
    - **Cardiac:** Vascular rings; surgical injury to recurrent laryngeal nerve
    - **Gastrointestinal:** Gastroesophageal reflux
    - **Neurologic:** Arnold-Chiari malformation with brainstem compression
    - **Psychiatric:** Paradoxical vocal cord adduction or vocal cord dysfunction

22. Name an injury that can result in acute stridor.
    Airway burns can cause significant respiratory distress. A child who ingests a caustic substance, intentionally or accidentally, will have immediate pain and distress. Stridor is possible. Likewise, a child who drinks (guzzles) very hot liquid, perhaps taken immediately from a microwave oven, will have a serious burn of the posterior pharynx and stridor may be noted. These are not usually mystery cases, as the etiology is immediately obvious.

23. What electrolyte abnormality has been associated with stridor?
    Hypocalcemia may be associated with laryngospasm and stridor, in addition to tetany and the characteristic Chvostek and Trousseau signs. This can be due to a poor diet resulting in vitamin D deficiency and rickets or hypoparathyroidism.

24. Why is it important to examine the skin of a baby who presents with stridor?
    Examine the skin and look for a hemangioma. A baby with a cutaneous hemangioma located in a cervicofacial, mandibular, or "beard" distribution (including the preauricular skin, mandible, lower lip, chin, or anterior neck) has an increased risk of an airway hemangioma (Fig. 25.4). A baby with an airway hemangioma may develop progressive hoarseness or stridor, most likely between the ages of 6 and 12 weeks when hemangioma proliferation is most rapid. Symptoms can progress from initial hoarseness or stridor to respiratory failure. Airway involvement can be confirmed using endoscopic visualization. Airway hemangiomas can also develop in children who do not have cutaneous hemangiomas.

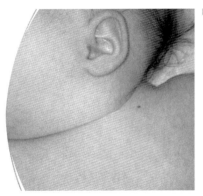

Fig. 25.4 Hemangioma of the neck. (Photograph courtesy J. Loiselle.)

KEY POINTS: METHODS TO DIAGNOSE LARYNGOMALACIA

1. Clinical diagnosis
2. Airway fluoroscopy
3. Direct laryngoscopy

BIBLIOGRAPHY

1. Adam DL, Eksteen E, Hicks EA. A 10-year-old girl with acute shortness of breath. *Paediatr Child Health*. 2021;26(5):264–265.
2. Al-alami A, Zestos M, Baraka A. Pediatric laryngospasm: prevention and treatment. *Curr Opin Anesthesiol*. 2009;22:388–395.
3. Brewster RC, Parsons C, Laird-Gion J, et al. COVID-19-associated croup in children. *Pediatrics*. 2022;149(6):e2022056492.
4. Casazza G, Graham ME, Nelson D, et al. Pediatric bacterial tracheitis-a variable entity: case series with literature review. *Otolaryngol Head Neck Surg*. 2019;160(3):546–549.
5. Gates A, Johnson DW, Klassen TP. Glucocorticoids for croup in children. *JAMA Pediatr*. 2019;173(6):595–596.
6. Lim C, Saniasiaya J, Kulasegarah J. Croup and COVID-19 in a child: a case report and literature review. *BMJ Case Reports*. 2021;14(9):e244769. https://doi.org/10.1136/bcr-2021-244769.
7. Mandal A, Kabra SK, Lodha R. Upper airway obstruction in children. *Indian J Pediatr*. 2015;82(8):737–744.
8. McCormick AA, Tarchichi T, Azbell C, et al. Subglottic hemangioma: understanding the association of facial segmental hemangioma in a beard distribution. *Int J Pediatr Otorhinolaryngol*. 2018;113:34–37.
9. Smith N, Giordano K, Thompson A, DePiero A. Failure of outpatient management with different observation times after racemic epinephrine for croup. *Clin Pediatr*. 2018;57(6):706–710. https://doi.org/10.1177/0009922817737075.
10. Worhunsky DJ, Levy BE, Spephens EH, Backer CL. Vascular rings. *Semin Pediatr Surg*. 2021;30(6):151128.
11. Yousefi Z, Aria H, Ghaedrahmati F, et al. An update on human papilloma virus vaccines: history, types, protection, and efficacy. *Front Immunol*. 2022;12:805695. https://doi.org/10.3389/fimmu.2021.805695.

CHAPTER 26

SYNCOPE

James M. Callahan

1. **What is syncope?**
   Syncope is a sudden, transient loss of consciousness and muscle tone due to a reversible impairment in cerebral perfusion or substrate delivery (oxygen or glucose). Unconsciousness usually lasts no longer than 1 to 2 minutes. Patients or their families may say they fainted, passed out, or blacked out.

2. **How common is syncope in the pediatric age group?**
   Syncope is common. It has been found to account for about 0.1% to 3% of visits to pediatric emergency departments (EDs). Syncope is more common in adolescents, with 15% to 50% of all adolescents experiencing at least one episode of syncope by adulthood. In younger children, there is no difference in incidence by gender. In adolescence, twice as many females as males have syncope.

3. **Is syncope in children serious?**
   Most syncope in children is due to benign causes. One-third to as many as 80% of cases are *simple neurocardiogenic or vasodepressor (vasovagal) episodes*. In the adult population, only 5% of episodes are vasodepressor events, and one-quarter are due to a cardiac cause. Even so, syncope may be due to a life-threatening condition in children and adolescents. Up to 25% of pediatric and adolescent patients with sudden deaths have had at least one prior episode of syncope.

4. **What are the common causes of syncope in children and adolescents?**
   More than one-half of patients have experienced a simple vasodepressor episode. Other disorders of autonomic control, including orthostatic hypotension (20% of cases in one series), breath-holding spells, situational syncope (e.g., tussive syncope, micturition syncope), and hyperventilation are also common. Hysterical faints (pseudosyncope) are common in adolescents.

5. **Name the potentially life-threatening causes of syncope in children and adolescents.**
   - Cardiac arrhythmias (including causes of long QT intervals and Brugada syndrome)
   - Structural heart disease (including hypertrophic cardiomyopathy)
   - Seizures
   - Subarachnoid hemorrhage
   - Carbon monoxide poisoning
   - Effects of medications and ingestions

6. **How is the cause of a syncopal event usually determined?**
   The history and physical examination are enough to suggest the most likely cause of syncope in the vast majority of patients. Even so, tachyarrhythmias often present in much the same way as vasodepressor syncope. Obtain an electrocardiogram (ECG) for all patients presenting with syncope.

7. **Are there historical factors that help identify serious causes of syncope?**
   Patients with vasodepressor syncope usually experience a prodrome or may faint after a precipitating event (e.g., pain, fright, startle). They can usually describe dizziness or lightheadedness, nausea, warmth, and a visual grey-out, often with tunnel vision, before fainting. They often have time to lower themselves slowly or brace themselves against something. Associated injuries such as lacerations or large hematomas are rare. Vasodepressor syncope usually occurs in a standing or sitting position. Syncope with associated injuries, that occurs with exertion, when the patient is supine, in infancy, and that is recurrent is more likely due to a serious etiology.

8. **Are there screening questions that may help identify children at risk of sudden cardiac arrest and sudden cardiac death?**
   An AAP Task Force has recommended four questions be asked of all children during preparticipation examinations (for athletics) and at a minimum of every 3 years or on entry to middle school, junior high school, and high school. These questions may be used to screen for a worrisome personal and family history in children with syncope.
   1. Have you ever fainted, passed out, or had an unexpected seizure suddenly and without warning, especially during exercise or in response to sudden loud noises?
   2. Have you ever had exercise-related chest pain or shortness of breath?

3. Has anyone in your immediate family or other relatives died of heart problems or an unexpected sudden death before age 50?
4. Are you related to anyone with hypertrophic cardiomyopathy, hypertrophic obstructive cardiomyopathy, Marfan syndrome, a history of arrhythmias or anyone younger than 50 years old with a pacemaker or implantable defibrillator?

9. **What is the goal of the evaluation of syncope in the ED?**
It has been said: "Syncope and death are the same—except that in one you wake up." The goal of the ED evaluation is to identify the rare pediatric patient with a serious underlying disorder, while realizing that most patients have probably suffered a vasodepressor episode (a diagnosis of exclusion). Extensive workups are rarely required, usually nondiagnostic, and often expensive.

10. **What should *every* patient with syncope have done in the ED?**
A thorough history (including family history and social history) and physical examination are the most important parts of the ED evaluation. Orthostatic vital signs and complete cardiac and neurological examinations should be performed. Screen all patients with an ECG, looking for signs of hypertrophy or abnormal conduction times (e.g., long QT syndrome) or ST changes (e.g., Brugada syndrome). Other diagnostic testing is guided by the results of the history, physical examination, and ECG. If there are still diagnostic questions or when syncope is recurrent, referrals for specialized testing (echocardiography, tilt table testing, Holter or event-recorder monitoring, or stress testing) may be made.

11. **How are episodes of vasodepressor syncope and seizures different?**
The description of the syncopal event and surrounding circumstances may distinguish between the two. With vasodepressor syncope, the patient is usually unconscious for only a matter of seconds, and incontinence is rare. Once awake, there may be some mild fatigue, but a true postictal period with decreased responsiveness and marked confusion is absent. Tonic-clonic movements usually occur near the end of a syncopal episode and last for only a few seconds. They are usually more persistent and last for at least a few minutes in patients with seizures. If the nature of the event is uncertain, an electroencephalogram may be helpful.

12. **What is the proposed pathophysiology of vasodepressor syncope?**
Typically, a prolonged upright position leads to venous pooling in the lower extremities, causing a decrease in left ventricular volume. In response to this and possibly a precipitating event, there is a catecholamine surge, causing increased contractility and a strong contraction against a relatively empty ventricle. Cardiac vagal fibers in the ventricular wall are activated and stimulate the medulla oblongata, causing a sympathetic withdrawal with or without vagal stimulation (Bezold-Jarisch reflex). These events produce bradycardia and a profound loss in systemic vascular resistance, decreased cerebral perfusion, and syncope. The term *vasodepressor* syncope is more accurate than *vasovagal* syncope, as it has been shown that vagal activity may contribute but is not necessary for these events.

13. **What are breath-holding spells?**
Breath-holding spells are common in infants and toddlers, probably related to developmental differences in autonomic control. There are two types. In *cyanotic* breath-holding spells, some provocation produces crying. The child develops a sustained expiration and becomes silent. There is deepening cyanosis, a loss of muscle tone, and, often, opisthotonos. There may be a brief period of tonic-clonic movements at the event's conclusion. The child then makes an inspiratory gasp, normal respirations resume, and the child slowly awakens.

With *pallid* breath-holding spells, there is usually an abrupt onset of pallor and loss of consciousness after one to two cries. Opisthotonos is followed by relaxation and gradual awakening. Pallid breath-holding spells have been associated with vasodepressor syncope in later life.

14. **How common are breath-holding spells, and at what ages are they seen?**
Breath-holding spells associated with unconsciousness are seen in up to 5% of all children. Onset is usually in the first year of life and almost always by age 2. These benign events resolve spontaneously. Spells cease occurring in 50% of children by age 4, 90% by age 6, and more than 99% by age 8.

15. **What types of syncope are associated with orthostasis?**
Orthostatic hypotension may be due to dehydration or anemia. *Micturition syncope, syncope with defecation*, and *syncope occurring during menses* are all related to orthostatic changes. A variety of medications (prescribed; accidentally or intentionally ingested) may cause orthostasis, including antihypertensives, antidepressants, phenothiazines, sedatives, and diuretics. Tussive syncope (seen in patients with pertussis and severe asthma) results when coughing, respiratory spasm, and Valsalva maneuver cause increased intrapleural pressure, decreased venous return, and decreased left ventricular filling.

16. **What do postural orthostatic tachycardia syndrome (POTS) (and pans?) have to do with syncope?**

    POTS is increasingly recognized in pediatric and adolescent patients. Orthostatic symptoms are common, including dizziness, lightheadedness, presyncope, weakness, nausea, visual changes, and occasionally syncope. POTS is diagnosed when there is orthostatic intolerance for >3 months and an increased heart rate when standing. In adults, an increase of 30 beats per minute or more, or a heart rate of 120 beats per minute or higher within 10 minutes of standing, is considered increased. In children and adolescents, an increase of 35 to 40 beats per minute or higher has been used. POTS may be associated with symptoms of chronic fatigue, fibromyalgia, and other somatic complaints. Iron deficiency, low iron stores, and vitamin B_{12} deficiency have been associated with POTS. A variety of therapies may be useful for various individuals, including improved hydration, medications, and improved physical conditioning.

    Pans are not related to syncope in children!

17. **What arrhythmias are associated with syncope in children and adolescents?**

    Ventricular tachycardia, although rare, is a potentially life-threatening cause of syncope. Supraventricular tachycardia may cause presyncopal symptoms, but rarely true syncope. Congenital complete heart block may not cause symptoms until later childhood or adolescence. Complete heart block may also be acquired (e.g., due to Lyme disease). Patients with structural heart disease and those who have had previous cardiac surgery are at increased risk of arrhythmias. Paroxysmal episodes of ventricular tachycardia may occur in the setting of a long QT interval.

18. **A very loud fire alarm went off at school. A group of schoolchildren were startled; one child had a syncopal episode and fell to the floor. Her classmates were amused. Should she be taken seriously in the ED?**

    Yes. Syncope related to a loud noise is no joke. This patient likely has long QT syndrome.

19. **How is the diagnosis of long QT syndrome made?**

    Long QT syndrome is diagnosed by finding a long QT interval on the patient's ECG. The QT interval must be corrected (QTc) for the patient's heart rate using Bazett's formula:

    $$QTc = (QT/\sqrt{RR'})$$

    The QT interval should be measured from the beginning of the QRS complex to the end of the T wave in lead II, V_5, or V_6. The measured RR' time should be the RR interval that immediately precedes the measured QT interval. The QTc should be less than 0.45 seconds in children younger than 16 years.

20. **What are the familial forms of long QT syndrome?**

    Long QT syndrome is associated with sensorineural hearing loss and autosomal recessive inheritance in the Jervell and Lange-Nielsen syndrome and with autosomal dominant inheritance and normal hearing in the Romano-Ward syndrome.

21. **If a diagnosis of long QT syndrome is made, what should be done?**

    Patients with long QT syndrome have a mortality rate of up to 70% if not treated. Immediate cardiology consultation is required. Beta-blockers are the usual initial treatment. Disposition may include admission for further monitoring. Family members should be told to have ECGs. A long QT interval may be acquired in the setting of electrolyte abnormalities (e.g., hypocalcemia) and may be due to certain medications.

22. **What medications and other drugs may be associated with tachyarrhythmias?**

    - Antiemetics (e.g., ondansetron)
    - Tricyclic antidepressants
    - Antipsychotics (e.g., haloperidol)
    - Cocaine (including crack)
    - Carbamazepine (usually in overdose only)
    - Amphetamines
    - Inhalants (especially Freon)

23. **Are there other cardiac causes of syncope?**

    Structural heart disease may cause syncope or sudden death. Hypertrophic cardiomyopathy (including hypertrophic obstructive cardiomyopathy [HOCM] or idiopathic hypertrophic subaortic stenosis) is associated with a thickened left ventricular wall, especially along the septum in the subaortic outflow tract. With exertion and increased contractility, outflow tract obstruction and syncope occur. *Hypertrophic cardiomyopathy* is the most common autopsy-proven cause of death in young athletes.

An aberrant coronary artery that courses between the aorta and pulmonary artery can also be associated with exertional syncope due to ischemia, resulting in arrhythmias. Other rare causes that result in ventricular outflow obstruction include valvar aortic stenosis and primary pulmonary hypertension. Also, consider atrial myxoma, a very rare cardiac tumor that may cause recurrent syncope in infants and toddlers. Finally, dilated cardiomyopathies and myocarditis due to a variety of infectious agents can be associated with arrhythmias or pump failure.

24. **Other than seizures, are there other central nervous system events that may precipitate syncope?**
Syncope may be a presenting symptom of *atypical migraines.* Often there is a history of aura and headaches. Nausea and vomiting are common. Pain is frequently unilateral and may be throbbing in nature. Basilar artery migraines may affect equilibrium and the patient's vision. A family history of migraines can help make the diagnosis.
Spontaneous subarachnoid hemorrhage is rare in children but may present with severe thunderclap headache (worst of the patient's life) and syncope.

25. **What metabolic derangements can cause syncope?**
Hypoglycemia can cause syncope. This is rare in children after infancy, except in children receiving insulin. A decreased level of consciousness due to hypoglycemia usually does not resolve spontaneously. Fasting, which leads to increased counterregulatory hormones including catecholamines, may play a role in vasodepressor syncope. Consider carbon monoxide poisoning, especially if several family members have symptoms. Consider anemia, especially in teenage girls with abnormal uterine bleeding. Dehydration and pregnancy may also cause syncope.

26. **How does a patient with pseudosyncope (hysterical faints) present?**
Hysterical faints are usually seen in adolescents. They typically occur in front of an audience in the absence of physical findings. There may be eye fluttering behind half-closed eyelids. Self-protective behaviors are preserved (e.g., patients will not allow their own hands to fall and hit their faces). Social history often reveals stress at home, in school, or in other social situations.

27. **What is the treatment for the most common causes of syncope (vasodepressor and orthostatic)?**
The most effective treatment for vasodepressor and orthostatic causes of syncope is to ensure adequate hydration. Older children and adolescents should drink at least 64 ounces of noncaffeinated fluids daily. The patient's urine should remain pale and clear. Small amounts of salty foods may help to maintain intravascular volume. Counsel patients to lie down when they have prodromal symptoms to prevent episodes of syncope. Refer patients who continue to have episodes of syncope for additional testing and possible pharmacological therapy.

28. **Which patients with syncope require referral to a cardiologist or neurologist?**
Refer patients to a cardiologist if they have syncope with exertion; syncope associated with chest pain, arrhythmias, or palpitations; or syncope that is recurrent or not responding to usual therapies. Also refer patients with syncope who have an abnormal cardiac history, physical examination, or ECG or those who have a family history of sudden death or who have atypical episodes of syncope. Patients with focal neurological findings, other neurological abnormalities, or a history that is consistent with the presentation of a seizure should be seen by a neurologist as soon as possible.

29. **Which patients with syncope require admission?**
Patients with cardiovascular disease or an abnormal cardiac examination, serious ECG abnormalities (e.g., long QTc interval or complete heart blocks), syncope with chest pain, or cyanotic spells, apnea, or focal neurological findings should be admitted. Also admit patients for observation, further diagnostic testing, and treatment if they have a toxic ingestion or orthostatic hypotension that does not respond to intravenous fluids.

KEY POINTS: SYNCOPE IS COMMON AND USUALLY BENIGN BUT MAY SIGNAL A LIFE-THREATENING CONDITION

1. Syncope is common in children. Although it usually has a benign etiology, it may be the first presentation of a serious condition.
2. Etiologies of syncope associated with fatal outcomes include cardiac arrhythmias, structural heart disease, seizures, subarachnoid hemorrhage, carbon monoxide poisoning, and syncope due to ingestion of medications.

KEY POINTS: WARNING SIGNS OF POTENTIALLY SERIOUS SYNCOPE

1. History of heart murmur or congenital heart disease, a new murmur on examination, or a murmur that is heard as a patient moves from squatting to standing; other abnormal findings on cardiac examination.
2. Family history of arrhythmias, sudden death, cardiomyopathy, sensorineural hearing loss.
3. Exertional syncope.
4. Syncope without a prodrome consistent with vasodepressor syncope.
5. Use of medications associated with arrhythmias.
6. Attacks associated with hyperpnea or cyanosis.
7. Syncope that leads to other injuries (lacerations, large hematomas).

KEY POINTS: INITIAL EVALUATION OF CHILDREN WITH SYNCOPE

1. All patients should have a complete history and physical examination.
2. Pay specific attention to the cardiac and neurologic examinations including orthostatic vital signs.
3. Order an ECG.

BIBLIOGRAPHY

1. Fischer JWJ, Cho CS. Pediatric syncope: cases from the emergency department. *Emerg Med Clin North Am.* 2010;28:501–516.
2. Erickson CC, Salerno JC, Berger S, et al. AAP Section on Cardiology and Cardiac Surgery, Pediatric and Congenital Electrophysiology Society (PACES) Task Force on Prevention of Sudden Death in the Young. Sudden death in the young: information for the primary care provider. *Pediatrics.* 2021;148(1):e2021052044.
3. Friedman KG, Alexander ME. Chest pain and syncope in children: a practical approach to the diagnosis of cardiac disease. *J Pediatr.* 2013;163:896–901.
4. Hurst D, Hirsh DA, Oster ME. Syncope in the pediatric emergency department: can we predict cardiac disease based on history alone? *J Emerg Med.* 2015;49(1):1–7.
5. Jarjour IT. Postural tachycardia syndromes in children. *Semin Pediatr Neurol.* 2013;20:18–26.
6. Steinberg LA, Knilans TK. Syncope in children: diagnostic tests have a high cost and low yield. *J Pediatr.* 2005;146:355–358.
7. Stewart JM. Common syndromes of orthostatic intolerance. *Pediatrics.* 2013;131:968–980.
8. Villafane J, Miller JR, Glickstein J, et al. Loss of consciousness in the young child. *Pediatr Cardiol.* 2021;42(2):234–254.
9. Zavala R, Metais B, Tuckfield L, et al. Pediatric syncope: a systematic review. *Pediatr Emerg Care.* 2020;36:442–445.

1. **What is the average age at menarche?**
   The average age of menarche is 12.43 years. Menarche occurs 2 to 3 years after the development of breast buds. Ninety-eight percent of females will have experienced menarche by 15 years.

2. **Describe the normal menstrual cycle**
   One menstrual cycle is the time between the onset of one menses to the onset of another. Normal cycle length varies (21-45 days in teens) in the first year following menarche, the mean cycle length is 34.5 days. Menses in adolescents typically last from 2 to 7 days and result in an average blood loss of 30 to 40 mL. The upper limit of normal blood loss is 80 mL. There are three phases of the menstrual cycle: follicular, ovulatory, and luteal. During the follicular phase (7-22 days), low levels of estradiol and progesterone result in elevated gonadotropin-releasing hormone levels and, thus, rises in both follicle-stimulating hormone (FSH) and luteinizing hormone (LH). FSH stimulates the maturation of one follicle, and LH stimulates the theca cells to produce androgens, which are converted to estrogens that stimulate proliferation of the endothelium. As estradiol levels rise, FSH levels begin to fall. During the ovulatory phase, a preovulatory estradiol surge causes an LH surge, resulting in release of the ovum. During the luteal phase, the corpus luteum produces large amounts of progesterone and estrogen, resulting in development of the secretory endometrium. If fertilization does not occur, the corpus luteum involutes, and there is a loss of estrogen and progesterone. Sloughing of the endometrium follows, and increased levels of FSH lead to a new cycle.

3. **What is abnormal uterine bleeding (AUB)?**
   AUB encompasses any menstrual bleeding that falls outside typical ranges and includes a lack of bleeding (amenorrhea), excessive menstrual flow or prolonged duration of bleeding (menorrhagia), and bleeding at irregular intervals (metrorrhagia). An orderly sequence of hormonal and endometrial events is responsible for the regular and limited bleeding that occurs in adult women. In adolescents, the most common cause of AUB results from anovulatory menstrual cycles due to "immaturity" of the hypothalamic-pituitary-ovary axis, with lack of normal negative feedback. During anovulatory cycles, estrogen levels are increased without increasing FSH responsible for the subsequent fall in the estrogen level. A lack of progesterone normally produced by the corpus luteum, which stabilizes the endometrium, results in sporadic growth and sloughing of the endometrium. In adolescents, it may be more useful to think of this as anovulatory uterine bleeding, because this term reflects the most common cause in adolescents.

4. **What is the most common cause of AUB in adolescents?**
   The most common cause of adolescent AUB is anovulation. After menarche, menstrual cycles are not always ovulatory. In fact, the older the age of the female at menarche, the longer it takes for cycles to become consistently ovulatory. Especially in the first 2 years after menarche, adolescent females are prone to having anovulatory cycles. This is important because an orderly sequence of hormonal and endometrial events is responsible for the regular and limited bleeding that occurs in adult women. In adolescents with anovulatory cycles, lack of ovulation causes no progesterone production by the corpus luteum, which in turn causes sporadic (and often excessive) growth and sloughing of the endometrium.

5. **List the causes of abnormal vaginal bleeding in the adolescent female**
   Although anovulation is the most common cause of abnormal vaginal bleeding in the adolescent, it remains a diagnosis of exclusion. The conditions listed in Table 27.1 must be considered when excessive vaginal bleeding is present.

6. **How should a clinician evaluate a patient to determine the source of vaginal bleeding?**
   In a hemodynamically unstable patient, begin initial evaluation with the ABDCEs (Airway, Breathing, Circulation, Disability, Exposure), obtaining intravenous access with two large bore IVs, administering crystalloids, and obtaining bloodwork including a complete blood count, coagulation studies, type and screen, and cross-matching of blood in preparation for transfusion. If a patient is hemodynamically unstable and no cross-matched blood is available, transfuse with type O negative blood. If needed, initiate a massive transfusion protocol. Pay special attention to the most common causes of life-threatening vaginal bleeding and subsequent management as appropriate.

Table 27.1 Causes of Abnormal Vaginal Bleeding in the Adolescent Female

Immediately Life-Threatening	
PREGNANT FEMALE	**NONPREGNANT FEMALE**
Ectopic pregnancy, septic abortion, complication of termination, placenta or vasa previa, placental abruption, uterine rupture, postpartum hemorrhage	Trauma (vaginal/cervical laceration), vascular malformation

Common Causes

Anovulation, sexually transmitted infections, pregnancy/complications of pregnancy, hormonal contraception

Complete Differential Diagnosis by Category		
Pregnancy-Related	**Systemic Disease**	**Genital Tract**
Pregnancy, ectopic pregnancy, threatened abortion, spontaneous abortion, hydatidiform mole	Coagulopathy, idiopathic thrombocytopenic purpura, renal failure, liver failure, systemic lupus erythematosus, malignancies, inflammatory bowel disease	Sexually transmitted infections, trauma, tumor, foreign body, malignancy, endometriosis, myoma, polyp, intrauterine device, vascular malformation

Endocrine	*Drugs*
Anovulation, pituitary disease, hypothalamic disease, thyroid disease, hyperprolactinemia, hypercortisolemia, Addison disease, polycystic ovary syndrome, premature ovarian failure, ovarian tumor	Hormonal contraceptives, anticonvulsants, anticoagulants, antipsychotics, corticosteroids, chemo-therapeutic agents, spironolactone

In a hemodynamically stable patient, obtain a careful history and perform a physical examination including a pelvic examination to evaluate the source of the bleeding and any evidence of abnormalities. Screens for sexually transmitted infections (STIs), a pregnancy test, and serum hemoglobin are useful. In the young teenager who is not sexually active and has mild symptoms, consider a pelvic examination but this may be deferred after discussion with the patient and family. As always, follow-up is an important part of patient care.

7. What are the recommended therapies for acute AUB?
Therapy is aimed at stopping the bleeding by converting the endometrium to the secretory state so that sloughing can occur under controlled conditions, correcting the anemia, restoring normal cyclic bleeding, and preventing recurrence and long-term sequelae of anovulation.
Hormonal treatment is recommended for patients with active bleeding, either a combination of estrogen and progesterone or progesterone only for those with contraindications to estrogen. For more information about whether it is appropriate for a specific patient to use estrogen-containing contraceptives, see The United States Medical Eligibility Criteria for Contraceptive Use at https://www.cdc.gov/reproductivehealth/contraception/ mmwr/mec/summary.html. A nonhormonal option for control of active bleeding is tranexamic acid orally, and while it does not regulate cycles, it has been shown to decrease the amount of bleeding. For patients with severe bleeding, who cannot tolerate oral hormonal therapy, consider IV estrogen. A potential side effect of this management is systemic thromboembolism. If hormonal treatment fails, other therapies include tranexamic acid orally, aminocaproic acid orally or intravenously, desmopressin intravenously, and surgical curettage. See Table 27.2 for more information.

8. What is primary dysmenorrhea, how common is it, and what is the cause?
Primary dysmenorrhea is painful menses without associated pelvic disease that typically appears 6 to 24 months following menarche. This is in contrast to secondary dysmenorrhea which is painful menses that can be ascribed to another condition such as endometriosis. Typical symptoms are crampy lower abdominal pain beginning a few days before, or at the start, of the menstrual cycle and lasting for 1 to 3 days. Additional symptoms include fatigue, back pain, headache, nausea, vomiting, and diarrhea. Half to three-quarters of teens experience dysmenorrhea that affects their daily activities. Fifteen percent of teens describe severe symptoms that incapacitate them for 1 to 3 days during each menstrual cycle. Dysmenorrhea typically occurs with ovulatory cycles, which become more frequent as the hypothalamic-pituitary-ovarian axis matures. It is unusual to have primary dysmenorrhea at the onset of menarche and the presence of painful periods at menarche should prompt evaluation for anatomical abnormalities. Occasionally, dysmenorrhea occurs with anovulatory cycles. Dysmenorrhea is caused by elevated prostaglandin F2 alpha (PGF2 alpha) or an elevated PGF2 alpha:prostaglandin E2 (PGE2) ratio.

	HEMOGLOBIN	
SEVERITY	**LEVEL (G/DL)**	**THERAPY**
Mild	>12	Menstrual calendar
		Iron therapy
		Follow-up 3-6 months
Moderate	8-12, not bleeding	*Hormonal therapy
		Iron therapy
		Follow-up in 2 weeks
	8-12, bleeding	*Hormonal therapy
		Admission versus discharge home with follow-up in 1-2 weeks
Severe	<8, hemodynamic symptoms	*Hormonal therapy
		IV conjugated estrogen (unstable patients)
		Hemostatic therapies: tranexamic acid, aminocaproic acid, or desmopressin
		Refractory bleeding nonresponsive to above therapies: surgical curettage
		Coagulation workup, blood transfusion prn
		Iron therapy
		Admission

Table 27.2 Therapies for Dysfunctional Uterine Bleeding

*Hormonal therapy typically consists of estrogens and progesterone, but types and doses may vary. Consult your institution's formulary.

9. **What is the approach and recommended treatment for a patient with primary dysmenorrhea?**

Teens who present 6 to 12 months after menarche, who are younger than 20 years, and who describe pain with menses can be treated and followed for resolution of symptoms. A pelvic examination is not necessary for young teens who are not sexually active. Pelvic examination, laboratory testing, and imaging are reserved for patients who have atypical symptoms; have signs, symptoms, or risk factors for other diseases; or do not respond to therapy.

Nonsteroidal anti-inflammatory drugs (NSAIDs) are the first-line therapy for dysmenorrhea; a majority (70%-80%) of patients experience relief with their use. Ibuprofen, naproxen, and naproxen sodium have all been used successfully. Begin the medication at the onset of the premenstrual symptoms or at the onset of menses and continue it for 1 to 3 days as needed to control symptoms. A second NSAID can be trialed if the first does not work. Mefenamic acid competes with prostaglandin-binding sites, antagonizes existing prostaglandin, and inhibits prostaglandin synthesis and thus may be more effective than other NSAIDs.

Arrange close follow-up. If patients do not respond to the described therapies, a reevaluation seeking secondary causes is indicated.

10. **What are the causes of secondary dysmenorrhea?**

The causes of secondary dysmenorrhea are listed in Table 27.3.

KEY POINTS: VAGINAL BLEEDING

1. Anovulation due to immaturity of the hypothalamic-pituitary-ovarian axis is the most common cause of AUB in the adolescent patient.
2. Dysmenorrhea is common in adolescents and begins 6 to 24 months after menarche when ovulatory cycles occur with more frequency. It is associated with significant morbidity.

Table 27.3 Causes of Secondary Dysmenorrhea	
GYNECOLOGIC DISORDERS	**NONGYNECOLOGIC DISORDERS**
Endometriosis, pelvic inflammatory disease, pelvic adhesions, ovarian cysts, mass, polyps, fibroids, congenital obstructive müllerian malformations (i.e., septate or bicornuate uterus), vaginal septum, intrauterine device	Inflammatory bowel disease, irritable bowel syndrome, ureteropelvic junction obstruction, renal stone, cystitis, psychogenic disorder

11. **When should a pregnancy test be included in a workup?**
    For any pubertal and peripubertal girl with vaginal bleeding, dysmenorrhea, abdominal pain, or genitourinary complaints, perform a pregnancy test.

12. **What are the symptoms and signs of ectopic pregnancy?**
    Consider this diagnosis in any postpubertal female with abdominal pain. Patients present with abdominal pain, with or without vaginal bleeding in the face of either missed menses or irregular vaginal bleeding. Other symptoms of pregnancy may also be present. A ruptured ectopic pregnancy will present with pain and hemodynamic instability. Importantly, remember that 50% of patients are asymptomatic. The differential diagnosis of lower abdominal pain includes PID, spontaneous/threatened abortion, ovarian torsion, ovarian or corpus luteal cyst, endometriosis, appendicitis, and urinary tract infection. Diagnosis is made by ultrasound (usually transvaginal) to determine the location of the gestational sac and a quantitative β-hCG test. A negative urine pregnancy test result rules out the presence of an ectopic pregnancy.

13. **What is the initial approach to a patient with suspected ectopic pregnancy?**
    Attention to the ABCDEs is important in these patients because they are at risk for severe hemorrhage. For the patient with unstable hemodynamics, see Question 6 in this chapter. Immediate obstetric-gynecologic consultation is mandatory.

KEY POINTS: PREGNANCY TESTING

1. Pregnancy is the differential diagnosis for many chief complaints in adolescents; have a low threshold for obtaining pregnancy testing.
2. Ectopic pregnancy is a consideration for any pubertal female with abdominal pain.
3. Ruptured ectopic pregnancy must be considered for a pubertal female with abdominal pain and unstable vital signs.

14. **What are the causes of vaginal discharge in children and adolescents?**
    Vaginal discharge is a common symptom among females of all ages and has many causes. Vaginitis is inflammation of the vagina, often characterized by vaginal discharge, pruritis, vulvar erythema, odor, and dysuria. Although the causes of vaginal discharge are the same across all age groups, the most common etiologies vary by pubertal status. Table 27.4 lists the most common causes of vaginal discharge by pubertal status.

15. **What are the physical exam findings in nonspecific vulvovaginitis?**
    Nonspecific vulvovaginitis is a common cause of vaginal discharge in the prepubertal female and accounts for the cause in up to 75%. Nonspecific vulvovaginitis presents with vaginal discharge, erythema, pruritis, and irritation. Physical exam usually reveals vulvar erythema, clear or white discharge, excoriations, and sometimes fecal matter.

16. **What is the recommended treatment for nonspecific vulvovaginitis in prepubertal females?**
    After other causes have been considered, therapy includes daily sitz baths in warm water, avoiding perfumed soaps and bubble baths, and good toilet hygiene. A hair dryer set at a cool temperature can be used to dry the genital area after the bath to help promote healing. Creams with zinc oxide, such as Triple Paste, may be used to protect areas of skin breakdown. Avoid tight-fitting clothes and pajamas.

17. **When should you consider STI testing in the prepubertal girl?**
    Consider STI testing for prepubertal patients with vaginal pain or itching, abnormal discharge, genital ulcers or warts, odor, or urinary tract symptoms. The rate of STIs in prepubertal children as a result of sexual abuse is only 1% to 3%. The decision for STI screening in victims of suspected assault/abuse is made based on the history

Table 27.4 Common Causes of Vaginal Discharge in Children and Adolescents

PUBERTAL STATUS	NONINFECTIOUS	INFECTIOUS
Prepubertal	Nonspecific vulvovaginitis, foreign body, trauma, urethral prolapse, atopic dermatitis, contact dermatitis, lichen sclerosis, scabies, polyps or tumors, systemic diseases, ectopic ureter	*Streptococcus pyogenes*, pinworms, respiratory organisms (*Haemophilus influenzae, Staphylococcus aureus, Moraxella catarrhalis, Streptococcus pneumoniae, Neisseria meningitidis*), enteric organisms (*Shigella, Yersinia*), candidiasis, sexually transmitted infections (*Neisseria gonorrhoeae, Chlamydia trachomatis, Trichomonas vaginalis*), Epstein-Barr, *Mycoplasma pneumoniae*
Pubertal	Physiologic leukorrhea, foreign body, allergies, chemical irritant, trauma, contact dermatitis, pregnancy, vulvar dermatosis, systemic diseases, polyps, tumors	Bacterial vaginosis, candidiasis, sexually transmitted infections (*N. gonorrhoeae, C. trachomatis, T. vaginalis*), *S. pyogenes*, pinworms, enteric organisms (*Shigella, Yersinia*), Epstein-Barr, *M. pneumoniae*

and physical examination findings. Testing is indicated if any of the following are present: (1) vaginal discharge, (2) genital/rectal lesions, (3) genital, oral, or anal trauma, (4) evidence of ejaculation, (5) history suggesting oral, genital, or anal penetration, (6) STI confirmed in another sibling or child in the same home, (7) confirmed STI in the perpetrator, or (8) assault by a stranger. Testing can also be obtained due to patient or parent request. Nucleic acid amplification tests (NAAT) for *N. gonorrhoeae, Chlamydia trachomatis*, and *Trichomonas vaginalis* are now Food and Drug Administration (FDA) approved and, if available, are the most sensitive and specific tests. Urine or vaginal testing for NAAT is appropriate. Do not obtain cervical specimens from prepubertal girls. Be aware of local regulations regarding forensic evidence as some jurisdictions will require culture confirmation of a positive result. Other methods of testing include culture for *N. gonorrhoeae* and *C. trachomatis*, and culture and wet mount for *T. vaginalis*. When obtaining testing for STIs, testing should include all common STIs such as HIV antigen and antibody testing, rapid plasma reagin (RPR) to screen for syphilis, and HBSAg hepatitis B if not fully immunized. If lesions concerning herpes simplex virus (HSV) are present, obtain an HSV polymerase chain reaction (PCR) from the vesicular fluid.

KEY POINTS: VAGINAL DISCHARGE

1. Nonspecific vulvovaginitis is a common cause of vaginal discharge in prepubertal females.
2. There are many infectious and noninfectious causes of vaginal discharge in prepubertal and pubertal females.
3. Decision to pursue STI testing in prepubertal females is made from the history and physical exam findings.

18. **What is pelvic inflammatory disease (PID)?**
    PID is a polymicrobial infection of the upper genital tract in postpubertal women frequently caused by STIs. This disease presents with a broad spectrum of clinical manifestations, making an accurate diagnosis challenging. Many teens have mild or subtle symptoms. Clinical diagnosis is imprecise; in symptomatic patients, salpingitis can be demonstrated by laparoscopy in 65% to 95% of cases. There is no single historical finding, physical examination finding, or laboratory test that is sensitive and specific to the diagnosis. Many cases of PID are missed. Common symptoms include crampy lower abdominal pain, abnormal vaginal discharge/bleeding, anorexia/vomiting, fever, diarrhea, dysuria, and dyspareunia. The differential diagnosis includes serious conditions, such as ectopic pregnancy, ovarian torsion, appendicitis, threatened abortion, and endometriosis. Teens are at high risk for this disease and, thus, include PID in the differential diagnosis of abdominal pain and have a low threshold for treatment due to significant morbidity associated with missed diagnosis.

19. **How is the diagnosis of PID made?**
    The diagnosis is considered in sexually active teens with abdominal or pelvic pain who have one or more of the following minimum criteria: (1) uterine tenderness, (2) cervical motion tenderness, or (3) adnexal tenderness.

If these signs are noted, treat the patient empirically unless another diagnosis is present. Additional criteria include oral temperature higher than 38.3°C, abnormal cervical or vaginal mucopurulent discharge, presence of white blood cells on saline microscopy of vaginal secretions, elevated erythrocyte sedimentation rate, and elevated C-reactive protein level. Laboratory evidence of *C. trachomatis* or *Neisseria gonorrhoeae* infection can be used along with the minimum criteria to increase specificity.

20. **What is the treatment for PID? When is hospitalization necessary?**
Regimens for the treatment of PID have been developed to cover the polymicrobial nature of the disease. Thus therapy must be effective against *N. gonorrhoeae* and *C. trachomatis* as well as anaerobes, *Streptococcus* spp., gram-negative enterics, and *Mycoplasma* spp. Outpatient treatment is effective and results in similar outcomes as compared to parenteral therapy. Consider hospitalization in the following instances: pregnancy, unclear diagnosis, vomiting, peritoneal signs, tubo-ovarian abscess present or suspected failed outpatient treatment, or patient's inability to follow the outpatient regimen. Instruct patients to take their medications, rest, and avoid intercourse. Testing and treatment of all sexual partners within the preceding 2 months is indicated.
The CDC 2021 STI Treatments Guidelines recommend several regimens for both outpatient and inpatient treatment for PID. The most common outpatient regimen in patients with no history of drug allergy includes intramuscular (IM) or IV ceftriaxone plus a 14-day course of doxycycline, with a 14-day course of metronidazole. Metronidazole enhances anaerobic coverage and also treats bacterial vaginosis (BV), which is often present. Arrange for reevaluation 2 to 3 days following initiation of therapy. Offer counseling about sexual health and STI screening.

KEY POINTS: PELVIC INFLAMMATORY DISEASE

1. The diagnosis is challenging and often missed.
2. Diagnosis of pelvic inflammatory disease is made from following minimum clinical criteria in a sexually active female with abdominal or pelvic pain: (1) uterine tenderness, (2) cervical motion tenderness, or (3) adnexal tenderness.
3. Outpatient and inpatient antibiotic regimens exist for pelvic inflammatory disease.

21. **What diagnostic tests should be considered when evaluating an adolescent with a suspected STI?**
The following laboratory tests may be helpful in the evaluation of postpubertal females with vaginal discharge/discomfort or suspected PID:
- *N. gonorrhoeae:* NAAT from urine, endocervical or vaginal; if concern for extragenital sites, can obtain NAAT from rectum and pharynx
- *C. trachomatis:* NAAT from urine, endocervical or vaginal; if concern for extragenital sites, can obtain NAAT from rectum and pharynx
- *T. vaginalis:* NAAT from urine, endocervical, or vaginal
- BV: Gram stain for clue cells, whiff test, vaginal pH
- HSV (based on clinical symptoms, examination): Viral culture or PCR taken from unroofed blister
- Candidiasis: clinical diagnosis, wet prep with budding yeasts, hyphae, or pseudohyphae, vaginal culture
- Urinalysis and urine culture
- Urine β-hCG (affects therapy choices)
- Hepatitis B serologic test (based on clinical symptoms, immunization history, and examination)
- Syphilis serologic test: nontreponemal test (Venereal Disease Research Laboratory or RPR), followed by treponemal test if positive
- Human immunodeficiency virus (HIV): HIV 1&2 Antibody/Antigen
- Suspected PID: Complete blood count, C-reactive protein, erythrocyte sedimentation rate

22. **What is BV?**
BV results from the replacement of the normal hydrogen peroxide-producing *Lactobacillus* spp. with overgrowth of facultative anaerobes, including *Gardnerella vaginalis, Prevotella* spp., *Mobiluncus* spp., and *Mycoplasma hominis.* The majority (50%-75%) of women with BV are asymptomatic. However, BV is also a leading cause of vaginal discharge. Symptomatic patients complain of thin, gray vaginal discharge or "fishy" odor. The presence of burning, itching, inflammation, dyspareunia, or dysuria suggests another cause. Epidemiologic studies strongly support sexual transmission of this infection, as the condition is more common in women who have had multiple partners

and rare in women who are not sexually active, although one specific sexually transmitted organism has not been implicated. BV is associated with an increased risk for premature labor, premature rupture of membranes, and postpartum or postprocedure endometritis or PID, as well as STI and HIV acquisition. It may also play a role in the development of precancerous cervical lesions. The clinical diagnosis is made when patients have three of the four following Amsel criteria: (1) presence of a homogeneous, gray-white discharge; (2) vaginal pH higher than 4.5; (3) clue cells present on Gram stain of vaginal fluid (epithelial cells studded with many small bacteria, producing a fuzzy border; offers a "clue" to the diagnosis); and (4) a malodorous, fishy smell before or after exposure to 10% potassium hydroxide (KOH). There are now commercially available point-of-care tests as well as NAAT tests.

23. **What is the treatment for BV?**
Treat all symptomatic women. Treatment options for nonpregnant patients include metronidazole orally, clindamycin cream 2% intravaginally, or metronidazole gel 0.75% intravaginally. There are also several alternative regimens available. The recurrence rate 1 month after therapy is 30%; accordingly, instruct patients to return if symptoms reappear. Patients with multiple recurrences can be treated with a greater than 3-month regimen using twice weekly either 0.75% metronidazole vaginal gel or 750 mg metronidazole vaginal suppository. Routine treatment of male partners is not recommended.

24. **What are genital ulcers? What causes them?**
Genital ulcers are lesions characterized by disruption of the epithelium/mucosa with associated inflammation. Infections associated with ulcers include HSV, syphilis, chancroid (*Haemophilus ducreyi*), and *Lymphogranuloma venereum* (*C. trachomatis* serovars L1-3). In the United States, HSV is by far the most common cause, followed by syphilis and then, rarely, chancroid. HSV causes multiple small vesicles on an erythematous base that are often very painful. Open vesicles appear as shallow ulcers. Syphilis usually causes a single, large, indurated ulcer with a smooth border that is usually painless. Chancroid causes multiple sharply circumscribed, deep ulcers with ragged undermined edges that are painful. Clinical diagnosis is challenging; laboratory testing is useful.

Causes of genital ulcers that are infectious but not sexually transmitted are mycoplasma and lipschutz ulcers with Epstein-Barr virus. Noninfectious causes of genital ulcers include inflammatory bowel disease, Behçet disease, fixed drug eruptions, trauma, and neoplasms.

25. **How are genital ulcers caused by HSV treated?**
In addition to analgesia and hygiene, antiviral therapy reduces the length of symptoms and recurrence rate. Treat all patients with their first episode of HSV. Options for initial episode treatment of genital herpes in adolescents include acyclovir 400 mg PO TID for 7 to 10 days, for adolescents weighing 45 kg or greater famciclovir 250 mg PO TID for 7 to 10 days, or valacyclovir 20 mg/kg (max 1000 mg) PO BID for 7 to 10 days. For patients with recurrent infection, antiviral treatment can be given either to suppress outbreaks or to shorten the duration and symptoms of a current outbreak. Regimens are available on the CDC's website, https://www.cdc.gov/std/treatment-guidelines/herpes.htm. The risk of drug-resistant HSV infection while on suppressive antiviral therapy is rare. Patients who are immunocompromised or who have severe or disseminated infection, such as hepatitis, pneumonia, encephalitis, or meningitis, require systemic acyclovir therapy.

KEY POINTS: STIS

1. NAAT has become the preferred test for diagnosis of *N. gonorrhoeae, C. trachomatis, and T. vaginalis.* Check with your health system to see if your available test is FDA approved.
2. BV is associated with an increased risk for premature labor, premature rupture of membranes, and postpartum or postprocedure endometritis or PID, as well as STI and HIV acquisition.
3. Treat all patients with their first episode of genital HSV with antivirals.

BIBLIOGRAPHY

1. COG Committee Opinion No. 651. American College of Obstetricians and Gynecologists Menstruation in girls and adolescents: using the menstrual cycle as a vital sign. Reaffirmed. *Obstet Gynecol.* 2015;126(6):e143–e146. Reaffirmed 2020.
2. Banikarim C. *Primary Dysmenorrhea in Adolescents.* UpToDate; 2021. Available at: www.uptodate.com. Accessed 13.05.22.
3. *Centers for Disease Control and Prevention.* Sexually transmitted infections treatment guidelines. <https://www.cdc.gov/std/treatment-guidelines/pid.htm>; 2021 Accessed 31.05.22.
4. Chuang JH, Dipasquale KJ, Verma A, Mascaro D. Vaginal discharge. In: Shaw KN, Bachur RG, eds. *Fleischer & Ludwig's Textbook of Pediatric Emergency Medicine.* 8th ed. Wolters Kluwer; 2020:543–547.
5. Gala PK, Akers AY, Wolff M. Gynecologic emergencies. In: Shaw KN, Bachur RG, eds. *Fleischer & Ludwig's Textbook of Pediatric Emergency Medicine.* 8th ed. Wolters Kluwer; 2020:747–768.
6. Kives SI, Hubner N. Normal menstrual physiology. In: Neinstein LS, Katzman DK, Callahan ST, Gordon CM, Joffe A, Rickert VI, eds. *Neinstein's Adolescent and Young Adult Health Care: A Practical Guide.* 6th ed. Wolters Kluwer; 2016:403–404.

7. Mirosh M, Jamieson MA. Ectopic pregnancy. In: Neinstein LS, Katzman DK, Callahan ST, Gordon CM, Joffe A, Rickert VI, eds. *Neinstein's Adolescent and Young Adult Health Care: A Practical Guide*. 6th ed. Wolters Kluwer; 2016:449–453.
8. Mitan LA, Schwartz BI. Abnormal uterine bleeding. In: Neinstein LS, Katzman DK, Callahan ST, Gordon CM, Joffe A, Rickert VI, eds. *Neinstein's Adolescent and Young Adult Health Care: A Practical Guide*. 6th ed. Wolters Kluwer; 2016:412–414.
9. Senthil MV, Rockey A, Zinns LE, Chuang JH, Posner JC. Vaginal bleeding. In: Shaw KN, Bachur RG, eds. *Fleischer & Ludwig's Textbook of Pediatric Emergency Medicine*. 8th ed. Wolters Kluwer; 2020:533–542.

CHAPTER 28

VOMITING

Elisabeth Rogers

1. **What is the pathophysiology of vomiting?**

   True vomiting is the forceful elimination of gastrointestinal contents through the mouth or nose. Vomiting is caused by coordinated diaphragmatic and abdominal contractions in conjunction with pyloric constriction and gastroesophageal relaxation. This motor activity occurs in response to stimulation of the medullary "vomiting center" by impulses from a variety of anatomic locations. Sources of these impulses include the pelvic and abdominal viscera, the heart, the peritoneum, the labyrinth, and the "chemoreceptor trigger zone," an area on the floor of the fourth ventricle that is sensitive to circulating drugs, toxins, and metabolic derangements.

2. **What is the clinical difference between vomiting and "spitting up"?**

   It is important to differentiate between vomiting and "spitting up" because the causes of spitting up are rarely serious, but vomiting may indicate a potentially life-threatening condition. Spitting up is characterized by effortless regurgitation of the stomach or esophageal contents, and in most infants and childrens it is due to gastroesophageal reflux or overfeeding. Vomiting, on the other hand, is forceful, may be accompanied by retching, and is frequently associated with autonomic symptoms, such as salivation, pallor, sweating, tachycardia, and mydriasis. Projectile vomiting suggests gastric outlet obstruction, such as in pyloric stenosis.

KEY POINTS: FORCEFUL VOMITING

1. Effortless regurgitation is usually caused by non–life-threatening conditions.
2. Forceful vomiting may be associated with more serious conditions, such as gastrointestinal obstruction, metabolic disease, or toxic ingestions.

3. **What is the differential diagnosis of vomiting in a pediatric patient?**

   Vomiting may be caused by abnormalities in a variety of organ systems. When preschool-aged patients report "vomicking," they help us to remember the wide-ranging differential diagnosis with the following mnemonic:
   - **V**: Vestibular: labyrinthine disorders, otitis media
   - **O**: Obstruction: malrotation, volvulus, adhesions, intussusception, obstipation, pyloric stenosis, incarcerated hernia, intestinal atresias, annular pancreas, duodenal hematoma
   - **M**: Metabolic: diabetic ketoacidosis, inborn errors of metabolism (e.g., urea cycle defects, carbohydrate or amino acid metabolic defects), congenital adrenal hyperplasia (CAH), Reye syndrome
   - **I**: Infection/inflammation: gastrointestinal (appendicitis, hepatitis, pancreatitis, cholecystitis, gastroenteritis, gastritis, necrotizing enterocolitis) or extragastrointestinal (upper respiratory tract infections, sinusitis, pharyngitis, pneumonia, sepsis, urinary tract infection, asthma)
   - **C**: Central nervous system disease: increased intracranial pressure (brain tumor, intracranial hematoma, cerebral edema), hydrocephalus, meningitis, idiopathic intracranial hypertension, concussion, migraine, ventriculoperitoneal shunt malfunction
   - **K**: Kidney disease: acute kidney injury, chronic kidney disease, pyelonephritis, renal calculi, renal tubular acidosis, obstructive uropathy
   - **I**: Intentional: eating disorders, rumination
   - **N**: Nasty drugs/poisons: chemotherapeutics, iron, salicylates, organophosphates, alcohols, lead and other heavy metals, poisonous mushrooms, cannabinoid hyperemesis syndrome (CHS)
   - **G**: Other GI/GU/GYN (gastrointestinal, genitourinary, gynecological) causes

     - Gastrointestinal: gastroesophageal reflux, formula intolerance, peptic ulcer disease, cyclic vomiting syndrome
     - Genitourinary: testicular torsion, epididymitis
     - Gynecological: dysmenorrhea, ovarian torsion, pregnancy, pelvic inflammatory disease

4. **How do I approach vomiting in a pediatric patient?**

   The first two considerations in any patient with vomiting are as follows: (1) What is the presumed etiology of the vomiting? and (2) How dehydrated is this patient?

   Vomiting due to self-limited viral gastroenteritis is one of the most common presentations to the pediatric emergency department (ED). However, because this is such a common complaint extra care must be given to look for a history or examination that does not fit with viral gastroenteritis. This should entail a more detailed history and examination looking for other red flag symptoms such as bilious or bloody emesis, bloody stool, "coke-colored" urine, abdominal pain or distention, testicular pain/swelling, urinary symptoms, pregnancy, polyuria/polydipsia, weight loss, possible ingestion, headaches, or neurological symptoms. The presence of any of those symptoms, or a failure to tolerate oral rehydration after ondansetron, should make you reconsider and expand your evaluation.

A general impression of activity level and alertness can be most helpful in determining the ability to orally rehydrate a patient. Other clinical findings that signify a higher degree of fluid loss are dry mucosal membranes, absent tears, decreased urine output, skin tenting, and prolonged capillary refill. Lethargy, irritability, or hemodynamic instability may necessitate intravenous (IV) fluid hydration with an isotonic crystalloid solution.

Most infants and children with a self-limited infectious course will benefit from a trial of oral ondansetron and oral rehydration alone. A trial of oral ondansetron has been shown to decrease episodes of vomiting, reduce the need for IV fluids, and decrease the rate of hospital admissions for viral gastroenteritis.

KEY POINTS: VOMITING

1. Carefully consider a noninfectious etiology for vomiting without fever or diarrhea.
2. Strongly consider ondansetron for use in the setting of vomiting as it helps with symptom relief, decreases the need for IV hydration and hospital admission, and does not mask underlying pathology.

5. The differential diagnosis for vomiting depends on the age of the pediatric patient. What are the life-threatening causes of vomiting in the different pediatric age groups?
The life-threatening causes of vomiting in the different pediatric age groups can be found in Table 28.1.

Table 28.1 Life-Threatening Causes of Vomiting by Age

AGE	CAUSE
Neonate	GI obstruction
	Congenital intestinal obstruction
	Atresias
	Malrotation with volvulus
	Renal
	Obstructive uropathy
	Uremia
	Trauma
	Abusive head trauma with subdural hematoma
	Abdominal trauma
	Metabolic
	Inborn metabolic errors
	Congenital adrenal hyperplasia
	Infectious
	Sepsis
	Meningitis
	Severe gastroenteritis
	Necrotizing enterocolitis
	Neurological
	Hydrocephalus
Older infant/toddler	GI obstruction
	Pyloric stenosis
	Intussusception
	Incarcerated hernia
	Malrotation with volvulus
	Renal
	Uremia
	Trauma
	Abusive head trauma with subdural hematoma
	Abdominal trauma

Continued

Table 28.1 Life-Threatening Causes of Vomiting by Age –cont'd	
AGE	**CAUSE**

Older infant/toddler	Infectious
	    Sepsis
	    Meningitis
	    Severe gastroenteritis
	Metabolic
	    Diabetic ketoacidosis
	Neurological
	    Hydrocephalus
	    Mass lesion
	Toxic ingestions

Older child/
  adolescent
	GI obstruction
	    Malrotation with volvulus
	    Small bowel obstruction
	Renal
	    Uremia
	Infectious
	    Meningitis
	Metabolic
	    Diabetic ketoacidosis
	Neurological
	    Intracranial mass lesions (e.g., tumor, hematoma)
	Toxic ingestions
	    Cannabinoid hyperemesis syndrome
	Inflammatory
	    Appendicitis

GI, gastrointestinal.

6. **What are the most common causes of vomiting in the different pediatric age groups?**
   The most common causes of vomiting in the different pediatric age groups are given in Table 28.2.

Table 28.2 Common Causes of Vomiting by Age	
AGE	**CAUSES**

Neonates	GI
	    GE reflux
	    Congenital GI obstruction (intestinal atresias, malrotation)
	    Milk-protein allergy
	Infectious
	    Sepsis/meningitis

Older infant/toddler	GI
	    GE reflux
	    Gastroenteritis
	    Foodborne allergy
	    Incarcerated hernia
	    Pyloric stenosis
	    Intussusception
	Infectious
	    Otitis media
	    Urinary tract infection
	Toxic ingestion

Table 28.2 Common Causes of Vomiting by Age

AGE	CAUSES

Older child/ adolescent	GI
	  Gastroenteritis
	  Appendicitis
	Infectious
	  Urinary tract infection
	  Pneumonia
	Metabolic
	  Diabetic ketoacidosis
	Toxic ingestion
	  Cannabinoid hyperemesis syndrome
	Other
	  Eating disorder

GE, gastroesophageal; GI, gastrointestinal.

Table 28.3 Clues From Appearance of Vomitus

APPEARANCE	SOURCE/CAUSE
Undigested food	Esophageal lesion or reflux
Digested food, milk curds	Stomach, proximal to pylorus
Yellow-green, bilious	Obstruction distal to ampulla of Vater or retrograde peristalsis during retching causing gastroduodenal reflux
Feculent	Distal obstruction, colonic stasis
Blood	Lesion proximal to the ligament of Treitz
Bright red blood	Esophagus or stomach above the cardia, minimal contact of blood with gastric secretions
Brown, "coffee grounds"	Gastric bleeding or swallowed blood mixed with gastric secretions
Mucous	Upper respiratory tract, gastric mucous hypersecretion

7. What information should be obtained in the history of a child who is vomiting?
   Useful historical information includes the following:
   • Appearance of the vomitus (e.g., bloody, bilious)
   • Duration, frequency, and forcefulness of vomiting.
   • Presence of other gastrointestinal symptoms (e.g., abdominal pain, diarrhea, constipation)
   • Presence of other nongastrointestinal symptoms (e.g., headache, neck stiffness, fever, polydipsia/polyphagia/polyuria, dysuria, respiratory symptoms, vaginal discharge, menstrual abnormality, and vertigo)

8. What clinical clues can be obtained from the appearance of the vomitus?
   When obtaining a history of a patient with vomiting, details about the appearance of the vomitus can help pinpoint the location of the problem (Table 28.3).

KEY POINTS: BILIOUS EMESIS

1. All infants and children with bilious emesis should be presumed to have a bowel obstruction until proven otherwise.

2. In a young infant with bilious vomiting, obtain abdominal x-rays and/or limited upper GI to look for congenital obstructive abnormalities such as intestinal atresia, web, or malrotation (see Fig. 28.1).

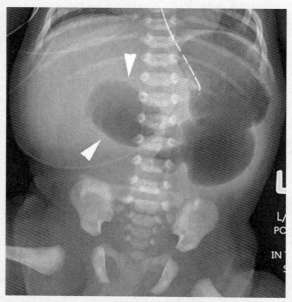

Fig. 28.1 Double bubble sign. (Reproduced with permission from Stanescu AL, Liszewski MC, Lee EY, Phillips GS. Neonatal gastrointestinal emergencies. *Radiol Clin N Am.* 2017;55(4):717–739.)

3. Only 10% to 38% of infants and children evaluated in the emergency department (ED) with yellow-green emesis are found to have a surgical emergency.

9. **What laboratory tests are indicated for a child with vomiting?**
In general, a basic metabolic profile and urinalysis are the most helpful. However, laboratory testing in a child with vomiting should be guided by the history and physical examination. Most children with viral gastroenteritis do not require any laboratory testing. In children with significant dehydration or those whose initial assessments suggest causes other than uncomplicated gastroenteritis, carefully selected laboratory tests can provide useful clues or confirm diagnoses (Table 28.4).

10. **When are radiographic tests indicated for a pediatric patient with vomiting?**
In the majority of patients with vomiting and a normal abdominal examination, radiographic studies are not useful or indicated. However, if another etiology is suspected, such as an obstruction, appendicitis, intussusception, or ovarian torsion, then a radiographic study may be crucial in the diagnosis. Plain radiographs of the abdomen are an appropriate initial study when an obstruction is suspected, especially in a patient with a history of abdominal surgery. Ultrasonography is the most useful and least harmful when looking at the pylorus, appendix, ovaries, or kidneys, and in the case of a possible volvulus or intussusception. The most useful radiographic tests for evaluating a child with vomiting in specified conditions are listed in Table 28.5.

11. **A 6-week-old infant presents with vomiting. What are the important historical findings that will help distinguish pyloric stenosis from gastroesophageal reflux?**
The typical history of an infant with pyloric stenosis is that of nonbilious vomiting that begins around 2 weeks of age and worsens in force and volume over the next several weeks. As the degree of obstruction increases, the vomiting becomes projectile and typically occurs during or soon after feeding. Most commonly seen in firstborn infants, pyloric stenosis affects males five times more often than females. By contrast, gastroesophageal reflux typically presents soon after birth and is characterized by effortless, nonprogressive spitting up, frequently occurring with burping or within 30 to 60 minutes after feeding. In most cases, the infant with gastroesophageal reflux will thrive despite the parent's impression that "he's been vomiting everything since birth."

Table 28.4 Laboratory Testing in Pediatric Patients With Vomiting

TEST	DIAGNOSTIC UTILITY

Serum electrolytes	Sodium
	  Elevated in hypernatremic dehydration
	  Decreased in hyponatremic dehydration, adrenal insufficiency
	Potassium
	  Elevated in renal failure, adrenal insufficiency
	  Decreased in pyloric stenosis
	Chloride
	  Decreased in pyloric stenosis, bulimia
	Bicarbonate
	  Elevated in significant or chronic vomiting (e.g., bulimia), pyloric stenosis
	  Decrease in inborn metabolic errors, renal tubular acidosis, and other causes of metabolic acidosis (sepsis, uremia, toxic ingestions, shock, diabetic ketoacidosis, acute gastroenteritis with dehydration)
	Glucose
	  Elevated in diabetic ketoacidosis
	  Decreased in inborn metabolic errors, starvation, toxic ingestion

Serum blood urea nitrogen/creatinine	Elevated in dehydration, renal failure
White blood cell count	Stress leukocytosis, a serious bacterial infection
Urinalysis	Glucose with or without ketones Specific gravity: elevated in dehydration Ketones: elevated in starvation, dehydration, inborn metabolic error Red blood cells: renal calculi, nephritis, UTI White blood cells: UTI
Urine pregnancy test	Pregnancy
Amylase, lipase	Elevated in pancreatitis
Aminotransferases	Elevated in hepatitis, Ebstein-Barr virus, acetaminophen ingestion

UTI, urinary tract infection.

Table 28.5 Radiographic Studies for Evaluating the Child With Vomiting

CLINICAL CONCERN	RADIOGRAPHIC STUDY OF CHOICE
Appendicitis	Abdominal ultrasonography, focused abdominal or noncontrast MRI, CT with IV contrast
Intussusception	Abdominal ultrasonography, air contrast enema for therapeutic reduction
Malrotation, intestinal atresias	KUB for signs of obstruction, abdominal ultrasonography can show a volvulus, and upper GI series is the definitive study if suspicion is still present.
Pyloric stenosis	Abdominal ultrasonography or upper GI series
Renal calculi	KUB, ultrasound may show stones or signs of obstruction, abdominal CT without contrast
Ovarian or uterine disease	Pelvic ultrasonography
Pancreatic disease	Abdominal CT with contrast
Duodenal hematoma/other intestinal disease	Abdominal CT with contrast
Abdominal mass	Abdominal CT with contrast

CT, computed tomography; GI, gastrointestinal; IV, intravenous; KUB, kidneys, ureters, and bladder; MRI, magnetic resonance imaging.

12. **What are the important physical examination and laboratory findings that will help distinguish pyloric stenosis from gastroesophageal reflux?**
If the vomiting has progressed significantly, the physical examination of an infant with pyloric stenosis may reveal a fussy, hungry infant who sucks vigorously unless weakened by dehydration. Peristaltic waves may be visible on inspection of the abdomen, and an olive-shaped mass (the hypertrophied pylorus) may be palpable in the subxiphoid region. The "olive" is rarely found on examination, especially when the infant presents early in the course of vomiting. The classic electrolyte abnormalities noted in pyloric stenosis are *hypochloremia, hypokalemia,* and *metabolic alkalosis.* Increasingly, however, infants are presenting for medical attention earlier in their course, so laboratory and physical findings are likely to be normal. This makes the differentiation of pyloric stenosis from other causes of infantile vomiting challenging and requires the physician to maintain a heightened index of suspicion for this condition. A focused abdominal ultrasound looking at the pylorus is a safe and effective way to screen for this disorder.

KEY POINTS: PYLORIC STENOSIS

1. A high index of suspicion for pyloric stenosis is necessary in young infants who present with vomiting because the characteristic physical examination and laboratory findings may not be present early in the course.
2. Infants with pyloric stenosis always have nonbilious vomiting.
3. Abdominal ultrasound is very useful to diagnose pyloric stenosis.

13. **A 12-month-old infant presents with vomiting and intermittent abdominal pain. How will you differentiate gastroenteritis from ileocolic intussusception in this patient?**
The classic patient with intussusception is between 3 months and 2 years of age and presents with the triad of episodic, paroxysms of cramping abdominal pain, vomiting, and bloody (currant jelly) stools. The pain typically lasts 5 to 10 minutes and is associated with crouching or drawing legs up, after which the infant may appear well or be lethargic. Many young infants with intussusception are lethargic without the other classic features.
Most often, the abdominal examination is soft and nontender. In 75% of patients with an intussusception the stool will be positive for occult blood or grossly bloody. However, currant jelly stools occur late in the course of illness. Gastroenteritis often starts with vomiting that progresses to diarrhea, fever, and nonspecific abdominal pain or cramping pain with defecation. An ultrasound will be diagnostic if intussusception is present.

KEY POINTS: INTUSSUSCEPTION

1. The classic triad of intermittent crampy pain, vomiting, and currant jelly stool is seen in fewer than 25% of children with intussusception.
2. Consider intussusception in any infant or toddler with unexplained lethargy.

14. **A 4-month-old infant presents with lethargy, vomiting, and pallor. This is her second such presentation, and after the first episode, she improved and went home following normal labs, IV hydration, and an ultrasound. They have recently started to supplement her diet with formula. What condition should be considered?**
Food protein–induced enterocolitis syndrome is a non-IgE mediated food allergy in which the acute form can cause a very impressive presentation and as such often presents to the ED. A recurrent history of such episodes should prompt this as a possibility in your differential. A detailed food history can help, as symptoms often occur at the introduction of new foods and rarely occur in breastfed-only infants.
Accurately identifying this as an allergy and identifying the food trigger can be crucial to the health of the patient. Close evaluation and follow-up by an allergist and/or pediatric gastroenterologist will help in their evaluation.

15. **A 2-week-old baby presents with significant vomiting and hypotension. Blood studies show hyponatremia, hyperkalemia, and severe metabolic acidosis. What condition is most likely?**
This infant likely has CAH due to a 21-hydroxylase deficiency. The electrolyte picture is classic and ambiguous genitalia may be another clue with such infants. This child should immediately be given stress dose steroids with IV hydrocortisone as well as other resuscitative measures.

16. An 8-year-old boy presents with headache and vomiting. How will you distinguish vomiting caused by an intracranial mass lesion from that associated with migraine headaches?

After headache, vomiting is the second most commonly noted symptom in children with intracranial mass lesions. However, vomiting is not likely to be the only abnormality. In more than 90% of children with vomiting from an intracranial mass, other neurological or ocular abnormalities will be present. Vomiting that accompanies brain tumors is commonly seen in the mornings, is usually effortless (although it may become projectile), and is not particularly associated with meals or abdominal pain. The vomiting may persist intermittently for weeks. Vomiting associated with migraine headaches is typically associated with infrequent, severe, diffuse headaches that resolve with sleep or when the cephalgia is treated. A careful neurological examination is essential.

17. A 15-year-old presents with forceful vomiting and nothing seems to help except for hot showers. When interviewed privately, she reports frequent use of marijuana. You suspect cannabinoid hyperemesis syndrome. What treatment should be provided, and what medications should you use to help her symptoms?

Treatment should be geared toward assessing for any electrolyte derangements, administering isotonic IV fluids, and evaluating for another obvious etiology. Ondansetron is often tried initially but is not as effective as benzodiazepines and haloperidol (0.05 mg/kg IV) for symptomatic relief. Cessation of marijuana use is the definitive treatment, and a subsequent resolution of symptoms confirms the diagnosis.

CHS was first documented in 2004 and has been on the rise in adolescent patients with the increased consumption and availability of highly potent tetrahydrocannabinol products. It is characterized by cyclical vomiting with profound nausea and abdominal pain. A history of illicit drug use may be hard to elicit from adolescent patients who are often resistant to acknowledging the use is contributing to their symptoms. A urine drug screen is very helpful when this condition is considered.

KEY POINTS: CHS

1. Persistent vomiting in adolescents should prompt you to consider cannabinoid hyperemesis as an etiology.
2. Effective treatments for CHS differ from those for other forms of vomiting.
3. A history of illicit drug use may be hard to elicit from adolescent patients who are often resistant to acknowledging that the use is contributing to their symptoms.

18. What is cyclic vomiting syndrome (CVS)?

CVS is a condition of recurrent episodes of frequent vomiting. This condition is usually found in older children or adolescents who do not have other significant medical problems. The vomiting episodes can last for days and the patients are usually well between cycles. There is usually associated abdominal pain, anorexia, and nausea. CVS is associated with migraine headaches and there is often a family history for this. Criteria for diagnosis include at least two episodes in the past 6 months. Episodes occur at least 1 week apart and last for less than a week. Treatment involves ondansetron, IV fluids, and attempts to avoid triggers (e.g., chocolate, caffeine, stress, sleep deprivation). Some may benefit from prophylactic treatment with cyproheptadine or amitriptyline.

BIBLIOGRAPHY

1. Benary D, Lozano JM, Higley R, Lowe D. Ondansetron prescription is associated with reduced return visits to the pediatric emergency department for children with gastroenteritis. *Ann Emerg Med*. 2020;76(5):625–634.
2. Lonsdale H, Wilsey MJ. Paediatric cannabinoid hyperemesis. *Curr Opin Pediatr*. 2022;34(5):510–515.
3. Merideth C, Doughty C. Vomiting. In: Shaw KN, Bachur RG, eds. *Fleisher & Ludwig's Textbook of Pediatric Emergency Medicine*. 8th ed. Wolters Kluwer; 2021:548–555.
4. Nowak-Węgrzyn A, Chehade M, Groetch ME, Spergel JM, et al. International consensus guidelines for the diagnosis and management of food protein–induced enterocolitis syndrome: executive summary—workgroup report of the Adverse Reactions to Foods Committee, American Academy of Allergy, Asthma & Immunology. *J Allerg Clin Immun*. 2017;139(4):1111–1126.
5. Nguyen HN, Kulkarni M, Jose J, Sisson A, et al. Ultrasound for the diagnosis of malrotation and volvulus in children and adolescents: a systematic review and meta-analysis. *Arch Dis Child*. 2021;106(12):1171–1178.
6. Rich BS, Dolgin SE. Hypertrophic pyloric stenosis. *Pediatr Rev*. 2021;42(10):539–545.
7. Rosen R, Vandenplas Y, Rudolph CD, Singendonk M, et al. Pediatric gastroesophageal reflux clinical practice guidelines: joint recommendations of the North American Society for Pediatric Gastroenterology, Hepatology, and Nutrition and the European Society for Pediatric Gastroenterology, Hepatology, and Nutrition. *J Pediatr Gastroenterol Nutr*. 2018;66:516–554.
8. Shields TM, Lightdale JR. Vomiting in children. *Pediatr Rev*. 2018;39(7):342–358.
9. Edwards EA, Pigg N, Courtier J, Zapala MA, et al. Intussusception: past, present and future. *Pediat Radiol*. 2017;47(9):1101–1108.

CHAPTER 29

ANAPHYLAXIS

Jillian Stevens Savage

1. **What is anaphylaxis?**
   Anaphylaxis is an acute, systemic hypersensitivity reaction that can be mild, life-threatening, or fatal. Signs and symptoms can be nonspecific, leading to underdiagnosis and undertreatment. Anaphylaxis develops rapidly as mast cells and basophils release potent biologically active mediators and clotting and complement cascades are recruited. Multiple organs may be affected, producing a constellation of signs and symptoms involving the skin, mucosa, respiratory, and gastrointestinal (GI) tracts, as well as the cardiovascular system.

2. **How is anaphylaxis diagnosed?**
   Diagnosis can be made if one of the following three criteria are present:
   - Acute illness with involvement of skin and/or mucous membranes AND one of the following:
     - Respiratory compromise
     - Reduced blood pressure (BP) and/or evidence of end-organ dysfunction
   - Two or more of the following criteria after LIKELY exposure to potential allergen
     - Involvement of the skin and/or mucosal tissue
     - Respiratory compromise
     - Reduced BP
     - Persistent GI symptoms
   - Reduced BP after a KNOWN exposure to an allergen

3. **How common is anaphylaxis?**
   The overall prevalence of anaphylaxis is rising. Newer data suggest that up to 2% of US citizens have experienced anaphylaxis.
   Allergic reactions occur frequently and represent 1% of emergency department (ED) visits. Of these encounters, anaphylaxis is diagnosed approximately 1% of the time. Incidence is on the rise, specifically in the 5 to 17-year-old age group.

4. **What makes anaphylaxis so dangerous?**
   Anaphylaxis usually occurs outside the hospital setting, it can evolve quite rapidly and fatality rates approach 1%. The majority of allergic reactions in children take place in school or daycare. Many schools lack full-time nurses, do not allow children to carry their own autoinjectable epinephrine, and are often noncompliant with written emergency management plans. In fatal reactions, the median time to respiratory or cardiac arrest is 5 minutes for reactions to medications or contrast material, 15 minutes for insect venom, and 30 minutes for food. These are sobering statistics, especially given the likelihood that patients with severe allergies seldom carry their epinephrine autoinjectors. To add to these worrisome anaphylaxis dangers, first-time exposure causes fatality up to 25% of the time due to the reaction being rapid and unrecognized.

5. **What are common causes of anaphylaxis?**
   Anaphylaxis in young children is mostly triggered by ingestion of cow milk, egg, or peanuts, though tree nuts, seafood, soy, wheat, and sesame can also cause severe reactions. The majority of reactions in teens and adults are due to peanuts, tree nuts, or seafood. In patients with known food allergies, anaphylaxis is often triggered by unknown ingredients or cross-contamination of foods believed to be safe. Peanuts and tree nuts are responsible for 90% of all food anaphylactic events, the majority of which occur in the setting of commercial catering. Among antibiotics, penicillin is the most common cause of anaphylaxis; contrary to common belief, cross-reactivity with cephalosporins is low. Aspirin and nonsteroidal anti-inflammatory drugs are the second most common cause of drug-induced anaphylaxis. Insect stings and allergen immunotherapy are also important but less common causes of anaphylaxis.

6. **Who is at the greatest risk for severe anaphylactic reactions?**
   Most deaths from anaphylaxis due to food occur in adolescents and young adults, who are more apt to take risks and less likely to carry their epinephrine autoinjectors. Patients with a history of previous anaphylaxis or poorly controlled asthma are at greater risk. Reactions to peanuts, tree nuts, fish, and shellfish are the most severe, with peanuts and tree nuts responsible for 94% of food-related deaths. Failure or delays in administration of epinephrine are associated with near-fatal and fatal reactions. Many severe reactions to foods and insect venom occur in children who have not required previous urgent medical intervention and thus lack access to epinephrine.

KEY POINTS: RISK FACTORS FOR SEVERE ANAPHYLAXIS

1. Adolescent or young adult
2. History of previous severe reaction
3. Peanuts, tree nuts, fish, or shellfish as inciting agent
4. Asthma, especially if poorly controlled
5. Failure to administer epinephrine promptly
6. Taking beta-blockers

Although large local reactions to insect venom are not predictive of anaphylaxis, 10% of children with generalized urticaria following a sting will develop severe reactions in the future.

7. **Which medications/interventions can trigger anaphylaxis in children?**
   - Neuromuscular blockers (succinylcholine, vecuronium, atracurium) account for 60% of episodes of anaphylaxis related to medical treatment. Airway obstruction and cardiovascular collapse may be mistaken for the effects of sedatives and anesthetic agents in this setting.
   - Latex, antibiotics, induction agents (etomidate, propofol, thiopental), and narcotics (fentanyl, meperidine, morphine)
   - Colloids, opioids, radiocontrast media, and blood products
   - All rabies vaccines, except Imovax, contain egg protein. Children with a history of systemic reaction to egg protein should undergo an allergy evaluation and vaccine testing prior to rabies vaccine administration.

8. **How does anaphylaxis typically present?**
   - Skin: generalized urticaria, pruritis, periorbital edema, angioedema
   - Oropharyngeal: tingling or pruritic sensation of the oropharynx, edema of the lips
   - Airway: swelling of the uvula, larynx, and epiglottis
   - GI: nausea, vomiting, and colicky pain.
   - Respiratory: nasal discharge, sneezing, cough, stridor, or wheezing
   - Cardiovascular: tachycardia, faintness, and hypotension
   - General: anxiety; sense of impending doom

9. **How can I recognize severe reactions requiring urgent intervention?**
   Onset of symptoms is generally rapid, with early signs of respiratory insufficiency and hemodynamic compromise. Cutaneous findings may be absent. Severe bronchospasm and upper airway swelling can both lead to asphyxia. Increased vascular permeability results in rapid shifts of intravascular fluid into the extravascular space. Concomitant vasodilation leads to a mixed distributive/hypovolemic shock, which may be refractory to aggressive fluid resuscitation and pressor support. Neurologic changes are ominous, signaling severe hypotension. Myocardial ischemia, conduction defects, T-wave abnormalities, and atrial and ventricular arrhythmias may result from direct mediator effects on the myocardium. Most deaths are caused by respiratory arrest or cardiovascular collapse.

10. **Which specific questions help confirm the diagnosis?**
    Confirm the diagnosis by a careful history that focuses on the nature and timing of known exposures, onset and description of symptoms, and response to medications. Ask about cutaneous, mucosal, and GI manifestations and signs of upper or lower airway obstruction. When the cause of anaphylaxis is unknown, ask about all foods and medications ingested in the hours preceding the reaction. Prepared or packaged foods safely consumed in the past may have undergone changes in ingredients or been subject to cross-contamination. Questions about preceding exercise (exercise-induced anaphylaxis) and sexual activity (latex or seminal plasma allergies; transfer of food or drug allergens by partner) may also yield important clues.

11. **What conditions can mimic anaphylaxis?**
    - **Vasovagal/neurocardiogenic syncope:** Bradycardia and pallor, but no hives or bronchospasm
    - **Scombroid poisoning:** Urticaria, nausea, headache, dizziness within 30 minutes of eating spoiled fish
    - **Physical urticaria:** Skin manifestations only (e.g., cold urticaria, cholinergic urticaria)
    - **Severe asthma exacerbations:** Bronchospasm and stridor, but no skin findings or GI symptoms
    - **Angioedema (hereditary form):** Difficult to distinguish from early anaphylaxis
    - **Panic disorder or vocal cord dysfunction**: Can present with functional stridor, but none of the other symptoms
    - **Oral allergy syndrome:** Reaction limited to lips and oropharynx after exposure to certain fruits/vegetables

12. Upon recognition of anaphylaxis, what is your first-line drug of choice?

Rapid administration of epinephrine should take priority. It can be repeated every 5 minutes as necessary for recurrent or persistent symptoms.

13. How is epinephrine best administered?

Epinephrine is best administered by the IM route, rather than IV or subcutaneous, as it is safer and more effective. Dosing recommendations are noted in Table 29.1.

14. How does epinephrine work in anaphylaxis?

Epinephrine is a direct-acting sympathomimetic with complex effects on many organs. Vasoconstriction, the primary α-adrenergic effect, reverses peripheral vasodilation and increases peripheral vascular resistance. Its β-adrenergic effects include downregulation of further release of inflammatory mediators, bronchodilation via smooth muscle relaxation, and increased heart rate and contractility via direct effects on the myocardium. Clinically, these effects decrease mucosal edema and cutaneous signs of angioedema and urticaria. More importantly, they lead to improvements in cardiovascular function by increasing BP and enhancing coronary blood flow.

15. What other adjuncts can be utilized in the management of anaphylaxis?

Epinephrine is the mainstay of therapy. In the setting of hypotension, IV crystalloids are indicated. For persistent wheezing after epinephrine, bronchodilators can be administered. Several additional adjuncts may be considered in the management of anaphylaxis including steroids and H1 and H2 blockers. See Table 29.2.

16. When should bronchodilators be used in anaphylaxis?

Most bronchospasm resolves after epinephrine administration, but if the patient is noted to have continuous wheezing after epinephrine, β-adrenergic agents (e.g., albuterol) will often alleviate the wheezing. Similarly, if the patient remains hypoxic after initial therapies, provide supplemental oxygen. Providers should have a low threshold to repeat epinephrine after 5 minutes if the patient continues to require respiratory support.

Table 29.1 Preferred and Alternative Dosing Recommendations for Epinephrine in the Treatment of Anaphylaxis

WEIGHT (KG)	PREFERRED	ALTERNATIVE
<10	Draw up 0.01 mg/kg (0.01 mL/kg of epinephrine 1 mg/mL)	0.1 mg autoinjector or 0.15 autoinjector if not available
10-25	0.15 mg autoinjector	Draw up 0.15 mg (0.15 mL of epinephrine 1 mg/mL)
>25	0.3 mg autoinjector	Draw up 0.3 mg (0.3 mL of epinephrine 1 mg/mL)

Adapted from Sicherer SH, Simons FER. Epinephrine for first-aid management of anaphylaxis. *Pediatrics*. 2017;139:e20164006.

Table 29.2 Acute Management of Anaphylaxis

Rapid and frequent assessment of ABCs
Patient placed in supine position, with legs elevated
Supplemental oxygen and airway management
Epinephrine IM
IV fluids for hypotension
Albuterol for bronchospasm persisting after IM epinephrine
H_1 and H_2 antagonists considered
Monitored for a minimum of 4-6 hr

ABCs, Airway, breathing, and circulation; IM, intramuscular; IV, intravenous.

17. Do steroids have a role in the management of anaphylaxis?

Steroids have no role in the acute management of anaphylaxis, though they were often administered for the theoretical benefit of minimizing the risk of biphasic response. Recently, however, a systematic review was unable to find the benefit of corticosteroid administration. Practice recommendations now recommend the avoidance of steroids in the management of anaphylaxis.

18. Do antihistamines have a role in the treatment of anaphylaxis?

Even when H1 antihistamines are given in combination with H2 blockers, such as ranitidine, they are considered to be second-line agents and should not be given in place of epinephrine. Though histamine is an important mediator in anaphylaxis, levels peak early and transiently. Antihistamines may provide symptomatic relief in limited cutaneous reactions, but they do not reduce the release of mediators, halt the progression of symptoms, or treat airway edema or hypotension.

19. What are the most common errors in the management of anaphylaxis?

Anaphylaxis continues to be underrecognized and undertreated in both prehospital and ED settings. Failure to administer epinephrine, delayed administration, and errors in dosing and route of administration are common among patients, caregivers, school health and EMS (emergency medical service) personnel, and ED providers. Hesitancy or failure to administer epinephrine by medical personnel, or delays until signs and symptoms are severe, not only sends the wrong message to patients and caregivers but is associated with increased morbidity and higher fatality rates.

20. How do you counsel caregivers on epinephrine administration for potential exposures after discharge?

When it comes to anaphylaxis, teach patients and practitioners to err on the side of injecting epinephrine. As the saying goes: "If you're thinking about it: Do it!" Serious adverse effects from epinephrine are rare in children receiving appropriate doses, and the transient pallor and palpitations that many experience "pale" in comparison to the symptoms of anaphylaxis itself and the potential consequences of delays in treatment.

Epinephrine is clearly indicated for allergic reactions with signs of respiratory distress or cardiovascular instability, or when hypotension develops following exposure to a known allergen. Epinephrine is also recommended for children exposed to allergens that previously caused anaphylaxis, even when initial symptoms are mild. Although generalized urticaria alone is not life-threatening, it should prompt epinephrine administration in children at risk for severe reactions, including those with a history of anaphylaxis, asthma, or severe atopy, or when the inciting agent is peanuts, tree nuts, shellfish, milk, or insect venom.

A good rule of thumb in all other situations is to give intramuscular (IM) epinephrine for acute systemic reactions involving two or more organ systems or any of the following severe symptoms: significant swelling of the lips, tongue, or uvula; throat tightness or trouble breathing or swallowing; persistent cough or respiratory compromise (dyspnea, bronchospasm, stridor, hypoxemia); persistent vomiting; cardiac effects (pallor, tachycardia, dizziness, syncope); or anxiety, confusion, or sense of impending doom.

KEY POINTS: EPINEPHRINE AND ANAPHYLAXIS

1. Most important medication in the treatment of anaphylaxis
2. Prevents further mediator release
3. Decreases upper airway edema
4. Reverses bronchospasm by relaxing bronchial smooth muscle
5. Increases BP via peripheral vasoconstriction
6. Increases heart rate and contractility
7. Delays in administration are associated with greater fatality

21. How common are biphasic anaphylactic reactions?

Biphasic reactions are rare but important. Recent literature suggests that these reactions occur approximately 5% of the time. These recurrent episodes occur up to 48 hours after initial reaction without recurrent exposure to the suspected causative agent. It is important to counsel the patient/caregivers about the potential risk of biphasic reactions and emphasize the importance of IM epinephrine accessibility, especially in the acute phase after treatment. Prompt administration of epinephrine during the initial episode is associated with decreased occurrence of biphasic reactions, but steroids have not been shown to have any effect.

22. How long should patients be monitored in the ED?

It is recommended to observe children presenting with systemic allergic reactions for at least 4 to 6 hours for progression or recurrence of symptoms. Those who have had a mild reaction, responded quickly to therapy and can be closely monitored at home, can then be discharged with detailed instructions about signs, symptoms, and treatment of a biphasic reaction. Admit to the hospital, or an extended-stay unit, those children with severe

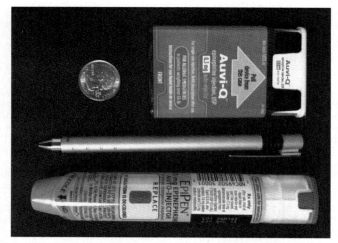

Fig. 29.1 Two frequently used autoinjectors and their relative size. *Directions for use of epinephrine autoinjectors:* EpiPen/EpiPen Jr. (1) Unscrew yellow or green cap and remove autoinjector from case. (2) Form a fist around the unit, with orange tip pointing downward. (3) Pull off the blue safety cap with other hand. (4) Firmly jab unit, at a 90-degree angle, into anterolateral thigh. (5) After a click is heard, hold firmly in place for 10 s. (6) Remove unit and massage area for 10 s. (7) Call 911 and seek immediate medical attention. The Auvi-Q autoinjector automatically activates step-by-step voice instructions for administration.

reactions or a history of severe reactions, those who live far from a medical facility or cannot return promptly if symptoms recur, and those who are unable to fill a prescription for autoinjectable epinephrine prior to discharge.

23. **Who should be discharged with epinephrine autoinjectors?**
    Prescribe autoinjectable epinephrine (Fig. 29.1) for all children meeting criteria for anaphylaxis, for those with generalized acute urticaria after an insect sting, and for systemic reactions in patients with a history of wheezing, a personal or family history of a severe reaction, or an allergy to peanuts, tree nuts, fish, shellfish, or milk. Teach caregivers when and how to administer IM epinephrine prior to discharge, using a trainer device. Epipen autoinjectors are most commonly prescribed, though the Auvi-Q autoinjectors are much smaller and provide step-by-step voice instructions for administration. The threshold for epinephrine administration should be lower if nonmedical caregivers are with the child; if the reaction is from peanuts, nuts, or seafood; or when the reaction occurs in a location that is more than 15 minutes from a medical facility. After epinephrine administration, emergency transport to a hospital is imperative.

24. **How is autoinjectable epinephrine dosed for home use?**
    The 0.15-mg dose is ideal for a 15-kg child and is generally prescribed for children weighing between 10 and 25 kg. The 0.3-mg units are intended for children who weigh 25 kg or more. For those above and below those weight parameters, assess the dosage based on the assessed risk of a severe reaction, taking history, specific inciting agents, and comorbid conditions into account. For children under 10 kg, there are two imperfect options. The 0.15 mg autoinjector will provide a fixed dose of epinephrine that exceeds 0.01 mg/kg. Parents may also be taught to draw up and administer a weight-based dose of epinephrine, though this method is highly prone to errors. Anticipatory guidance about allergen avoidance is particularly important in this group.

25. **What other discharge instructions should be given?**
    Discharge all patients with a caregiver who has been instructed to watch for signs and symptoms of a biphasic reaction. Include a written emergency action plan, to be accessible at all times, that details symptoms of anaphylaxis, medications prescribed, and indications for their use. Emphasize the importance of having autoinjectors available at all times, protecting them from direct sunlight or extreme temperatures, and promptly replacing expired medication. Provide education on allergen avoidance, particularly with respect to hidden ingredients in commercially prepared or catered foods and cross-contamination of food during factory processing and preparation in restaurants. Educational resources and allergy referrals are very helpful as well.

KEY POINTS: DISCHARGE PROCEDURE FOLLOWING ANAPHYLAXIS

1. Instruct a caregiver to watch for signs of a biphasic reaction.
2. Outline a straightforward management plan for future reactions, including names, doses, and indications for medications.
3. Provide education and links to resources on allergen avoidance.
4. Prescribe autoinjectable epinephrine for patients at risk of a severe reaction; demonstrate its usage with a trainer device; stress importance of carrying it at all times. Prescribe several devices for use at alternate locations (school/child care center).
5. Recommend timely follow-up with primary care provider; consider referral to an allergist.

Acknowledgment

The author would like to thank Dr. Linda Arnold for her excellent contributions in prior editions.

BIBLIOGRAPHY

1. Boyce JA, Assa'ad A, Burks AW, et al. Guidelines for the diagnosis and management of food allergy in the United States: report of the NIAID-sponsored expert panel. *J Allergy Clin Immunol.* 2010;126:S1–S58.
2. Campbell RL, Bashore CJ, Lee S, et al. Predictors of repeat epinephrine administration for emergency department patients with anaphylaxis. *J Allergy Clin Immunol Pract.* 2015;3:576.
3. Gupta RS, Springston EE, Warrier MR, et al. The prevalence, severity, and distribution of childhood food allergy in the United States. *Pediatrics.* 2011;128(1):e9–e17.
4. Michelson KA, Dribin TE, Vyles D, Neuman MI. Trends in emergency care for anaphylaxis. *J Allergy Clin Immunol Pract.* 2020;8:767.
5. Motosue MS, Bellolio MF, Van Houten HK, et al. Increasing emergency department visits for anaphylaxis, 2005-2014. *J Allergy Clin Immunol Pract.* 2017;5:171.
6. Sampson HA, Muñoz-Furlong A, Campbell RL, et al. Second symposium on the definition and management of anaphylaxis: summary report—Second National Institute of Allergy and Infectious Disease/Food Allergy and Anaphylaxis Network symposium. *J Allergy Clin Immunol.* 2006;117:391.
7. Sicherer SH, Simons ER. Section on allergy and immunology: self-injectable epinephrine for first-aid management of anaphylaxis. *Pediatrics.* 2007;119:638–646.
8. Shaker MS, Wallace DV, Golden DBK, et al. Anaphylaxis—a 2020 practice parameter update, systematic review, and Grading of Recommendations, Assessment, Development and Evaluation (GRADE) analysis. *J Allergy Clin Immunol.* 2020;145:1082.
9. Thomson H, Seith R, Craig S. Downstream consequences of diagnostic error in pediatric anaphylaxis. *BMC Pediatr.* 2018;18:40.
10. Turner PJ, Jerschow E, Umasunthar T, et al. Fatal anaphylaxis: mortality rate and risk factors. *J Allergy Clin Immunol Pract.* 2017;5:1169.
11. Worm M, Francuzik W, Renaudin JM, et al. Factors increasing the risk for a severe reaction in anaphylaxis: an analysis of data from the European Anaphylaxis Registry. *Allergy.* 2018;73:1322.
12. Wood RA, Camargo Jr CA, Lieberman P, et al. Anaphylaxis in America: the prevalence and characteristics of anaphylaxis in the United States. *J Allergy Clin Immunol.* 2014;133:461.

CHAPTER 30

CARDIAC EMERGENCIES

Alexandra A. Taylor and Susan M. Kelly

1. **What are the primary changes in the 2020 pediatric advanced life support (PALS) guidelines?**
   The 2020 PALS guidelines advise practitioners to:
   - Target a respiratory rate of 20 to 30 breaths per minute for patients receiving cardiopulmonary resuscitation (CPR) with an advanced airway and for infants/children with a pulse receiving rescue breaths.
   - Administer epinephrine early for all nonshockable rhythms to improve survival.
   - Intubate with cuffed endotracheal tubes to limit the need for tube replacement.
   - Avoid routine cricoid pressure during intubation.
   - Prioritize bag-valve-mask ventilation (BVM) over intubation in out-of-hospital arrests as both modes of ventilation have similar outcomes.
   - Recall that resuscitation does not end with the return of spontaneous circulation. Excellent postcardiac arrest care is essential to improve survival.

2. **What are the rates of compression: ventilation for infant and child CPR?**
   - 1-rescuer CPR 30 compressions: 2 ventilation
   - 2-rescuer CPR 15 compressions: 2 ventilation

3. **List the underlying causes of pulseless electrical activity (6 Hs and 4 Ts).**
   - Hypoxemia
   - Hypovolemia
   - Hydrogen ion (acidosis)
   - Hypoglycemia
   - Hypothermia
   - Hypokalemia/hyperkalemia
   - Tension pneumothorax
   - Tamponade (pericardial)
   - Thrombosis (pulmonary/coronary)
   - Toxins

KEY POINTS: PALS 2020 UPDATES

1. Postcardiac care is an essential part of the chain of survival.
2. Consider continued bag-valve-mask ventilation for out-of-hospital cardiac arrest, rather than intubation.

---

4. **How should bradycardia be evaluated?**
   PALS defines bradycardia as a heart rate of <60 beats per minute. Bradycardia in a pediatric patient requires immediate evaluation for cardiopulmonary compromise. Causes of bradycardia should be investigated (hypoxia, hypotension, hypoglycemia, hypothermia, acidosis, toxic ingestions).

5. **What are the steps in treating a patient with bradycardia associated with hemodynamic compromise?**
   - Ensure effective oxygenation and ventilation.
   - If bradycardia persists despite effective oxygenation and ventilation, start chest compressions immediately.
   - Administer 0.01 mg/kg (0.1 mL/kg of the 0.1 mg/mL concentration) epinephrine via intravenous/intraosseous (IV/IO) route. Repeat epinephrine every 3 to 5 minutes.
   - If IV/IO access unavailable, epinephrine may be administered via endotrachael (ET) tube 0.1 mg/kg (0.1 mL/kg of the 1 mg/mL concentration).
   - If increased vagal tone or primary atrioventricular (AV) block is suspected as the cause of bradycardia, administer atropine 0.02 mg/kg (minimum dose 0.1 mg; maximum single dose 0.5 mg). May repeat once after 5 minutes.
   - If complete heart block is discovered on electrocardiogram (ECG) or if there is a history of congenital or acquired heart disease, consider emergent pacing.

6. What is the most likely presentation for infants and children with SVT?
   - Signs: heart rate >220 beats per minute in an infant or heart rate >180 beats per minute in a child.
   - Symptoms: tachypnea, irritability, lethargy, poor perfusion, poor feeding, and other signs of congestive heart failure (infants); chest pain, palpitations, or dizziness (older children).

7. What is the treatment for SVT?
   - SVT with hemodynamic compromise:
     - Treat with synchronized cardioversion, 0.5 to 1 J/kg. If unsuccessful, treat with 2 J/kg.
   - SVT without hemodynamic compromise:
     - Establish IV access.
     - Administer supplemental oxygen.
     - Attempt vagal maneuvers
       - For infants and children, apply ice to the face.
       - Older children may be coached to perform a Valsalva maneuver such as bearing down, blowing into a straw.
     - If vagal maneuvers are ineffective, administer IV adenosine 0.1 mg/kg (maximum dose 6 mg). Use a three-way stopcock, immediately flushing with 5 to 10 mL normal saline (NS) after pushing adenosine rapidly. If the initial dose is ineffective, administer a second dose (0.2 mg/kg adenosine, maximum dose 12 mg).

8. What are the causes of sustained wide complex tachycardia?
   Consider ventricular tachycardia (VT) first in a patient with wide complex tachycardia (QRS >0.09 seconds). Other causes include SVT with bundle branch block or SVT with aberrant conduction.

9. According to the 2020 PALS guidelines, how should patients with wide complex tachycardia WITH a pulse be treated?
   - Patients with hemodynamic compromise, defined as acutely altered mental status, signs of shock, or hypotension, should be treated for possible ventricular tachycardia with synchronized cardioversion (0.5-3 J/kg). Notably, expert consultation is recommended prior to drug therapy.
   - In patients without hemodynamic compromise, if the rhythm is regular and the QRS is monomorphic, a trial of adenosine is recommended. Expert consultation is recommended prior to additional drug therapy.

10. How do patients with long QT syndrome present?
    - Abnormal ECG
      - Prolonged QT (using Bazett correction formula $QTc = QT/\sqrt{RR}$)
        - QTc >440 ms is the upper limit of normal for ages 1-15.
        - QTc >460 ms is prolonged.
      - Torsades de pointes
      - AV block
      - Premature ventricular contraction
      - Intermittent T-wave inversions (T-wave alternans)
    - Syncope
      - History of syncope precipitated by sudden stress or startle
      - History of syncope and family history of sudden unexplained death in an immediate family member under the age of 30 years
      - Syncope with a family history of long QT syndrome or familial deafness
      - Sudden death

11. What is the first-line treatment for patients with known congenital long QT syndrome?
    First-line treatment is a beta-blocker, such as propranolol (2-4 mg/kg/day). Treatment should be instituted regardless of the presence or absence of symptoms.

12. List several reasons for an abnormally long QTc interval that are not due to congenital long QT syndrome.
    - Electrolyte disturbances such as hypomagnesemia, hypocalcemia, or hypokalemia
    - Central nervous system insult (increased intracranial pressure, hypoxia)
    - Anorexia nervosa or liquid protein diets
    - Toxic ingestions

KEY POINTS: LONG QT SYNDROME

1. Normal QTc is less than 440 ms.
2. ECG changes include intermittent T-wave inversions, torsades de pointes, and bradycardia.
3. First-line treatment is the use of beta-blockers.

13. **Define heart failure for pediatric patients.**
    Heart failure occurs in children when excessive preload, excessive afterload, arrhythmias, or decreased contractility results in inadequate cardiac output to meet the metabolic demands of the body.

14. **What are the signs and symptoms of heart failure in children?**
    Infants may have poor feeding, easy fatigability, and failure to thrive. Older children may be sleepy and have poor exercise tolerance and anorexia. All children may have tachycardia, tachypnea, and dyspnea. On physical examination, grunting, S3/S4 gallop, hepatomegaly, crackles/rales, wheezing peripheral edema, and jugular venous distention may be present.

15. **What are the most likely causes of heart failure in neonates presenting to the emergency department (ED)?**
    Structural congenital heart disease is the most likely cause of heart failure in neonates. In the first week of life, transposition of the great vessels or total anomalous pulmonary venous return is the most likely cause. Between weeks 1 and 4, critical aortic stenosis, pulmonary stenosis and preductal coarctation of the aorta are the most likely causes.

KEY POINTS: HEART FAILURE

1. Heart failure is defined as a cardiac output that does not meet the metabolic demands of the body.
2. Infants may present with poor feeding, failure to thrive, and grunting.
3. Children may present with tachycardia, tachypnea, and dyspnea.
4. Structural heart disease is the most likely cause of heart failure in neonates.

16. **List the ECG findings of patients who have received overdoses of the following medications.**
    - Beta-blockers: bradycardia, increased PR interval
    - Calcium channel blockers: bradycardia, prolonged AV node conduction or block
    - Tricyclic antidepressants: tachycardia, prolonged QRS complex, decreased AV conduction time, VT, ventricular fibrillation, torsades de pointes
    - Phenothiazines: QTc prolongation, torsades de pointes
    - Type 1A antiarrhythmic medications (quinidine, procainamide, disopyramide): prolongation of QT interval, torsades de pointes, VT
    - Amiodarone: AV block, sinus node dysfunction (marked bradycardia), torsades de pointes

17. **Which chemotherapeutic agents cause cardiotoxicity?**
    - Anthracyclines (doxorubicin, daunorubicin) cause left ventricular dysfunction, which may lead to overt heart failure.
    - Bevacizumab causes hypertension and endothelial damage.
    - Imatinib causes QTc prolongation.

18. **What ECG changes are associated with hyperkalemia?**
    Peaked T waves, widened QRS, increased PR interval, flattened P waves, ventricular fibrillation, and asystole are associated with hyperkalemia.

19. **What are some cardiac causes of chest pain in children?**
    Fortunately, cardiac causes of childhood chest pain are rare. Consider hypertrophic cardiomyopathy, drugs of abuse (such as cocaine), myocarditis, pericarditis, mitral valve prolapse, supraventricular tachycardia, and ventricular tachycardia.

20. **Which ECG changes are associated with hypertrophic cardiomyopathy?**
    - Left ventricular hypertrophy (increased R-wave voltage in leads V5-V6)
    - Left atrial hypertrophy (widened, notched P waves)
    - Atrial fibrillation
    - Supraventricular tachycardia

21. **What risk factors are associated with sudden death in patients with hypertrophic cardiomyopathy?**
    Risk factors for sudden death in these patients include nonsustained VT on a Holter monitor, unexplained syncope, extreme left ventricular hypertrophy on echocardiogram, inadequate rise in blood pressure during exercise,

family history of sudden death in a first-degree relative, and left ventricular outflow tract obstruction seen on echocardiogram.

22. **How should chest pain from suspected cocaine ingestion be evaluated? What is the treatment?**
    - Clinical presentation: teen with chest pain and palpitations, anxiety, tachycardia, tachypnea, and hypertension.
    - Evaluation: urine drug screen (detects cocaine for 24-48 hours after use), ECG (may see findings consistent with acute coronary ischemia or arrhythmias). Consider a chest x-ray as pneumothorax can occur with snorting cocaine.
    - Treatment: nitroglycerin (may help decrease coronary artery vasospasm), aspirin (or clopidogrel), and benzodiazepines (to blunt the central stimulation effects of cocaine).

23. **How does a child with myocarditis present?**
    The classical presentation of myocarditis includes a viral prodrome (fever, upper respiratory infection symptoms), followed by chest pain or symptoms of heart failure. In the ED, they usually have tachypnea and tachycardia. They may have hypotension that is worse with standing and does not improve after fluid resuscitation. A chest radiograph usually shows cardiomegaly.

24. **What are the ECG changes in myocarditis?**
    ECG changes may include sinus tachycardia, low-voltage QRS complexes, abnormal T-wave inversion, heart block, arrhythmias, bundle branch blocks, infarct patterns, and ST-segment changes.

25. **What ECG changes are associated with pericarditis?**
    There is a progression of ECG abnormalities in pericarditis: diffuse ST-segment elevation (leads I, II, III, aVF, V2-V6), PR depression (with normalized ST segments), T-wave flattening/inversion, low-voltage QRS (due to evolving pericardial effusion).

KEY POINTS: PEDIATRIC CHEST PAIN

1. Most chest pain in pediatric patients is not cardiac in origin.
2. ECG changes associated with hypertrophic cardiomyopathy include left ventricular hypertrophy.
3. Maintain a high suspicion of ingestion (such as cocaine) as the cause of chest pain in adolescents.
4. Focus on possible viral prodrome symptoms in a child with suspected myocarditis.

26. **What is the differential diagnosis of congenital cyanotic heart disease?**
    - Ductal-dependent lesions: tetralogy of Fallot, tricuspid atresia, pulmonary stenosis, pulmonary atresia, VSD, hypoplastic left-sided heart syndrome
    - Ductal-independent lesions: truncus arteriosis, transposition of the great vessels, total anomalous pulmonary venous return

27. **What is the initial management of a distressed newborn presenting with suspected congenital cyanotic heart disease?**
    - Secure the airway and ventilate.
    - Maintain SpO_2 75% to 85%.
    - Obtain IV access and administer prostaglandin E1 at 0.05 to 0.1 µg/kg/minute.
    - Obtain a chest radiograph.
    - Consult cardiology.

28. **Describe the typical cardiac examination of a patient with tetralogy of Fallot.**
    Patients with unrepaired tetralogy of Fallot often have a single, loud S2. In addition, a harsh systolic ejection murmur will be heard, which is due to the obstructed pulmonary outflow tract. Though the constellation of abnormalities in the tetralogy of Fallot includes a ventricular septal defect (VSD), flow across the VSD is generally not turbulent and thus not audible.

29. **What is a hypercyanotic episode or "tet spell?"**
    Hypercyanotic spells occur in patients with an uncorrected tetralogy of Fallot. The rapid desaturation is related to acute and partial/complete obstruction of the subpulmonary outflow tract (thus rapidly decreasing pulmonary blood flow). After cyanosis develops, metabolic acidosis ensues, which results in increased pulmonary vascular

resistance and decreased systemic vascular resistance; this may lead rapidly to myocardial ischemia, lethargy, and death. Spells may be triggered by agitation or decreased hydration.

30. **How should a "tet spell" be managed?**
Manage "tet spells" at home by placing a child in a knee-chest position, which increases systemic vascular resistance and promotes systemic venous return to the heart.

    In the ED, obtain IV access and administer IV fluids to improve right ventricular preload. Give supplemental oxygen to decrease peripheral pulmonary vasoconstriction. Give intravenous morphine (0.1 mg/kg/dose) to decrease the release of catecholamines, which, in turn, results in decreased heart rate (increasing filling time) and relaxation of the infundibular spasm. If the "tet spell" persists despite IV fluids, oxygen, and morphine, give medications to paralyze the child and intubate the child's trachea. Then administer phenylephrine (to increase systemic vascular resistance).

31. **List some of the complications of repaired hypoplastic left-sided heart syndrome (Fontan operation) that may be encountered in the ED.**
    • Supraventricular arrhythmias: atrial flutter, AV reentry tachycardia, atrial ectopic tachycardia, pleural effusions
    • Thromboembolic complications: cerebrovascular accident, inferior or superior vena cava syndrome, pulmonary embolus
    • Protein-losing enteropathy
    • Pulmonary arteriovenous fistulas

KEY POINTS: CONGENITAL CYANOTIC HEART DISEASE

1. In an infant presenting with symptoms of heart failure, consider structural cardiac anomalies.
2. Have a low threshold for starting prostaglandin in a cyanotic neonate.
3. Treat "tet spells" in the ED with IV fluids, supplemental oxygen, and intravenous morphine (after placing the child in a "knee-chest position").

32. **When should echocardiography be performed in a patient with suspected Kawasaki disease?**
Obtain an echocardiogram as soon as Kawasaki disease is suspected; it may help to confirm the disease. If the disease is certain, an echocardiogram allows a baseline evaluation of cardiac function and determines the extent of coronary artery aneurysms. Notably, the echocardiogram may be normal in the first week of illness, as coronary artery dilation is not generally detected until after the first week of illness.

33. **What are the cardiac complications of Kawasaki disease?**
    • Coronary artery aneurysm (major complication)
    • Coronary artery stenosis
    • Myocarditis
    • Myocardial infarction
    • Valvular lesions

34. **What are the cardiac complications of multisystem inflammatory syndrome in children (MIS-C)? How frequently do they occur?**
    • Shock (cardiogenic or vasodilatory) (50%-80% of patients with MIS-C)
    • Left ventricular dysfunction, defined by BNP elevation or abnormal echocardiogram findings (51%-76% of patients with MIS-C)
    • Coronary artery dilation or aneurysm (14%-48% of patients with MIS-C)
    • Arrhythmia and conduction abnormalities (unknown prevalence)
    • Pericarditis (unknown prevalence)
    • Valvulitis (unknown prevalence)

35. **Which cardiac conditions cause sudden death in young athletes? How common are they?**
    • Hypertrophic cardiomyopathy (one-third of deaths)
    • Coronary artery anomalies (~15% of deaths)
    • Myocarditis (~7% of deaths)
    • Aortic rupture (Marfan syndrome)
    • Commotio cordis
    • Arrhythmogenic right ventricular hypertrophy ($\leq$6% of deaths)

36. **What is Brugada syndrome? What are the classic ECG abnormalities?**
Brugada syndrome is a genetic disorder associated with sudden cardiac death. Diagnosis depends on the combination of Brugada pattern on ECG plus clinical criteria. There are three types of Brugada syndrome: The ECG in Type I morphology has ST-segment elevation (≥ 2 mm) with a typical "coved" appearance in ≥ 1 leads in right precordial leads V1 and V2. There is an associated subsequent inverted T wave. Brugada types 2 and 3 are associated with ST-segment elevation (≥ 1 mm) in right precordial leads leading to a single or biphasic, upright T wave. Clinical signs of Brugada syndrome include a family history of sudden cardiac death, palpitations, syncope, a history of ventricular fibrillation, and self-terminating polymorphic VT.

BIBLIOGRAPHY

1. Ae R, Makino N, Kosami K, Kuwabara M, et al. Epidemiology, treatments, and cardiac complications in patients with Kawasaki disease: the nationwide survey in Japan, 2017-2018. *Journ Pediatr.* 2020:225.
2. Alsaied T, Tremoulet AH, Burns JC, et al. Review of cardiac involvement in multisystem inflammatory syndrome in children. *Circulation.* 2021;143:1.
3. Bailliard F, Anderson RH. Tetralogy of Fallot. *Orphanet J Rare Dis.* 2009;4:2.
4. Barbut G, Needleman JP. Pediatric chest pain. *Pediatr Rev.* 2020;41(9).
5. Behere S, Weindling S. Brugada syndrome in children: stepping into uncharted territory. *Ann Pediatr Cardiol.* 2017;10(3):248–258.
6. Clancy C. Cardiologic principles I: electrophysiologic & electrocardiographic principles. In: Nelson LS, Howland MA, Lewin NA, eds. *Goldfrank's Toxicologic Emergencies.* 11th ed. McGraw-Hill Education; 2019:244–259.
7. Colombo A, Meroni CA, Cipolla CM, Cardinale D. Managing cardiotoxicity of chemotherapy. *Curr Treat Options Cardiovasc Med.* 2013;15(4):410–424.
8. Green D, Green HD, New DI, Kalra PA. The clinical significance of hyperkalaemia-associated repolarization abnormalities in end-stage renal disease. *Nephrol Dial Transpl.* 2013;28(1):99–105.
9. Harris KM, Mackey-Bojack S, Bennett M, Nwaudo D, et al. Sudden, unexplained death due to myocarditis in young people, including athletes. *Am Journ Cardiol.* 2021;143.
10. Maron BJ, Doerer JJ, Haas TS, et al. Sudden death in young competitive athletes. Analysis of 1866 deaths in the US 1980-2006. *Circulation.* 2009;119:1085.
11. Madriago E, Silberbach M. Heart failure in infants and children. *Pediatr Rev.* 2010;13(1):4–12.
12. McCrindle BW, Rowley AH, Newburger JW, et al. Diagnosis, treatment, and long-term management of Kawasaki disease: a statement for health professionals from the American Heart Association. *Circulation.* 2017;135(17).
13. Reynisson B, Tanghöj G, Naumburg E. QTc interval-dependent body posture in pediatrics. *BMC Pediatr.* 2020;107.
14. Selbst S, Palermo R, Durani Y, Giordano K. Adolescent chest pain: is it the heart? *Clin Pediatr Emerg Med.* 2011;12(4):289–300.
15. Topjian AA, Raymond TT, Atkins D, et al. Part 4: pediatric basic and advanced life support: 2020 American Heart Association guidelines for cardiopulmonary resuscitation and emergency cardiovascular care. *Circulation.* 2020;142(16):S469–S523.

CHAPTER 31

CENTRAL NERVOUS SYSTEM EMERGENCIES

Nanette C. Dudley

1. Describe the physical findings in Bell palsy.

   Bell palsy refers to peripheral facial nerve weakness on one side of the face, including inability to wrinkle the forehead on the affected side, inability to close the affected eye, and flattening of the affected nasolabial fold. Bell palsy may also involve hyperacusis in the affected ear (noises sound excessively loud) because the site of injury is thought to be in the facial canal and may involve other branches of C7—including those to the stapedius muscle, which dampens sound waves.

2. Describe current recommendations for steroid treatment of Bell palsy in children.

   The literature on adult patients strongly supports the use of steroids for Bell palsy with improvement in facial nerve function and faster recovery. Overall, children have higher rates of recovery than adults, and the literature supporting steroid use is limited. Despite this, current guidelines recommend the treatment of children with steroids, involving caregivers in decision-making.

3. What is Todd paralysis?

   Todd paralysis refers to paresis or paralysis of one or more areas of the body after a seizure. This condition is transient, usually disappearing within 24 hours following a seizure.

4. List the drugs commonly used to stop seizures acutely in the emergency department (ED).

   Drugs commonly used to stop seizures in the ED are listed in Table 31.1.

5. In the absence of intravenous (IV) access, which pharmaceutical agents may be considered for abortive treatment for a seizure?

   - Rectal diazepam
   - Intranasal midazolam
   - Buccal midazolam
   - Intraosseous access (any medication listed in Table 31.1 can be given through an intraosseous line)

DRUG	DOSE ROUTE MAXIMUM DOSE (MG)	ROUTE	MAXIMUM DOSE (MG)
Table 31.1 Drugs Commonly Used to Stop Seizures in the Emergency Department			
First-Line Drugs			
Lorazepam	0.1 mg/kg	IV	4
Diazepam	0.2 mg/kg	IV	10
	0.5 mg/kg	PR	20
Midazolam	0.2 mg/kg	IN/IM	10
	0.3 mg/kg	Buccal	10
Second-Line Drugs			
Levetiracetam	60 mg/kg	IV	4500
Fosphenytoin	20 PE/kg	IV	1500 PE
Phenytoin	20 mg/kg	IV, IM	1000
Valproic acid	40 mg/kg	IV	3000
Phenobarbital	15–20 mg/kg	IV, IM	1000

IM, intramuscular; IN, intranasal; IV, intravenous; PE, phenytoin sodium equivalents; PR, per rectum.

6. Which is more effective at stopping a pediatric seizure within 10 minutes without recurrence by 30 minutes, IV lorazepam or IV diazepam?

   In a study comparing lorazepam and diazepam's effectiveness in pediatric status epilepticus, there was no difference.

7. Among the second-line drugs used to stop benzodiazepine refractory status epilepticus in a child, how does the provider decide which one to use?

   Recent studies demonstrated no difference in the primary safety and efficacy outcomes in the treatment of benzodiazepine refractory status epilepticus for three drugs: levetiracetam, fosphenytoin, and valproic acid. Each drug effectively stopped an episode of status epilepticus in 50% of patients. Endotracheal intubation occurred more frequently in children given fosphenytoin in one study. Selection of a second-line anticonvulsant may depend on provider experience, the patient's prior or ongoing use of one of the three anticonvulsants, or institutional guidelines.

8. Describe the characteristics of absence (petit mal) seizures.

   Absence seizures usually develop in school-age children before puberty. The seizures are characterized by abrupt onset of a brief loss of consciousness. Most are less than 30 seconds in duration. Children may appear to be staring or may have eye blinking or rhythmic nodding. The child does not fall, although he or she may drop things. These seizures are often easily precipitated by having the child hyperventilate.

9. What are infantile spasms?

   Infantile spasms usually present between 3 and 7 months of age. The seizures are usually of sudden onset and generalized, with bilateral and symmetric contraction of the muscles in the neck, trunk, and extremities. The initial contraction typically lasts less than 2 seconds and is then followed by a sustained contraction of 2 to 10 seconds. Typically, a 24-hour video-electroencephalogram (EEG) will confirm the diagnosis of infantile spasms; magnetic resonance imaging (MRI) is the preferred neuroimaging modality for these infants.

10. A 16-year-old boy presents after an early-morning generalized tonic-clonic seizure. The family describes occasional, brief jerking movements in the morning that make teeth brushing and hair combing difficult. These jerking movements resolve and do not recur later in the day. What does this symptom pattern suggest?

    Juvenile myoclonic epilepsy. This most commonly presents between 12 and 18 years of age with brief, bilateral flexor jerking movements of the arms. The seizures can be precipitated by sleep deprivation, alcohol ingestion, and awakening from sleep. Physical examinations and neuroimaging are typically normal. EEGs, and particularly sleep-deprived EEGs, are usually abnormal.

11. In what types of situations is phenytoin less effective and even contraindicated in the treatment of pediatric status epilepticus?

    In general, phenytoin or fosphenytoin should not be used for seizures caused by drug toxicity. Phenytoin is not typically effective at stopping seizures caused by drug effects and can worsen convulsions caused by drugs classified as class 1 antiarrhythmics such as quinidine, anesthetics (lidocaine, bupivacaine), cocaine, and tricyclic antidepressants.

12. What are the indications for urgent head imaging after a seizure?
    - Postictal focal neurologic deficits that do not resolve quickly
    - Signs of increased intracranial pressure
    - Persistent altered mental status
    - Posttraumatic seizures (not impact seizures)

      MRI is the preferred study in all cases but is usually not immediately available in the emergency setting. Patient stability may also be a factor, as computed tomography (CT) is typically faster and usually does not require sedation.

13. What are the indications for nonurgent MRI after a seizure?
    - Focal features of the seizure
    - Cognitive or motor impairment of unknown cause
    - Changes in seizure character, neurologic examination, or EEG
    - Age younger than 1 year

      Evaluation with MRI for the preceding indications avoids radiation exposure from CT.

14. What is the incidence of febrile seizures? When do they occur?

    About 2% to 5% of all children have a febrile seizure; most occur in children between the ages of 6 months and 6 years.

15. **What makes a febrile seizure "simple" or "complex"?**
    A simple febrile seizure has all of the following characteristics:
    - The seizure is brief (<15 minutes).
    - The seizure is generalized.
    - The child appears well shortly after the seizure stops.
        A complex febrile seizure has at least one of the following characteristics:
    - The seizure is prolonged (>15 minutes).
    - The seizure is focal.
    - The child has two or more seizures in 1 day.

16. **What is the recurrence risk for a febrile seizure?**
    Approximately 30%. This number varies by age at onset of the first febrile seizure.

17. **Is the risk of recurrence increased if the initial febrile seizure is complex?**
    No. Children may be at greater risk of recurrence if they have one or more of the following features:
    - Young age at onset
    - History of febrile seizures in a first-degree relative
    - Lack of hyperpyrexia in the ED
    - Brief duration between the onset of fever and the initial seizure

18. **Is the risk of epilepsy increased in a child with a simple febrile seizure?**
    No. The risk of developing epilepsy in a child after a simple febrile seizure is the same as that of a child without febrile seizures. However, children with multiple simple febrile seizures, those less than 12 months old at the time of the first simple febrile seizure, and those with a family history of epilepsy have a higher risk of developing epilepsy.

19. **What tests should be performed for children after a simple febrile seizure?**
    Perform laboratory testing or radiography only as appropriate for the diagnosis and management of the cause of the fever. There is usually no need for brain imaging studies or electroencephalography after a simple febrile seizure.

20. **When should you consider a lumbar puncture in a child with a febrile seizure?**
    - History or examination findings concerning meningitis
    - Cranky, irritable child who is difficult to console
    - Meningeal signs or bulging fontanel
    - Infants 6 to 12 months of age who are deficient in *Haemophilus influenzae* or *Streptococcus pneumoniae* immunizations or if immunization status is undetermined
    - Pretreatment with antibiotics

21. **In a child with suspected meningitis, what are some relative contraindications to performing an immediate lumbar puncture?**
    - Focal neurologic findings or concern for elevated intracranial pressure
    - Evidence of spinal cord trauma
    - Infection in the tissues near the puncture site
    - Coma
    - Papilledema
    - Severe coagulation defects (not corrected)
    - Cardiopulmonary instability
        In these cases, initiate antibiotic therapy presumptively and delay the lumbar puncture.

22. **A teenager with a headache needs a lumbar puncture (LP) with opening pressure measurement. How do you position the patient for the LP?**
    The patient should be lying on their side, with the head in line with the spine. The hips can be flexed or the body curled for needle insertion, but once cerebrospinal fluid (CSF) is obtained, straighten the legs and body. Leg flexion or the use of pillows can elevate the opening pressure. Anxiety or pain can also elevate the opening pressure, and sedation may be needed.

23. **How is a hyponatremic seizure managed?**
    Hyponatremic seizures are often managed with hypertonic saline to transiently raise plasma sodium levels by 5 to 10 mEq to stop the seizure. The dose is 2 to 4 mL/kg body weight of 3% sodium chloride (0.5 mEq/mL), given IV over 20 minutes.

Table 31.2 Guillain-Barré Syndrome Versus Transverse Myelopathy

SYMPTOM	GUILLAIN-BARRÉ SYNDROME	TRANSVERSE MYELOPATHY
Early pain/paresthesias	+	+
Progressive symmetrical weakness	Arms and legs	Legs
Bilateral facial weakness	+	−
Areflexia	+	+
Autonomic dysfunction	+	+
Sensory level*	−	+
Abnormal rectal tone	−	+

*A level below which the patient has the absence of sensation.

24. **What are some differentiating features of Guillain-Barré syndrome and transverse myelopathy?**
    The differentiating features of Guillain-Barré syndrome and transverse myelopathy are shown in Table 31.2.

25. **What does the term "transverse" in transverse myelitis refer to?**
    The term "transverse" refers to the band-like sensory level at which dysfunction occurs, leading to the common presenting symptoms.

26. **What is the Miller-Fisher variant of Guillain-Barré syndrome?**
    Patients with this form of Guillain-Barré syndrome also have ophthalmoplegia, areflexia, and ataxia.

27. **What simple grooming measure should be performed on any patient with acute onset of ascending paralysis?**
    Combing the hair. Tick paralysis can present very similarly to Guillain-Barré syndrome, although the rate of progression is faster and tick paralysis is accompanied by ataxia (not present in Guillain-Barré syndrome). Removal of the tick can bring about rapid improvement, and the tick is often found serendipitously.

28. **A 2-month-old baby with a history of hypotonia presents in acute respiratory distress. He has abdominal respirations and appears to be very tired. In preparing for intubation, what skeletal muscle relaxant is relatively contraindicated?**
    Succinylcholine. In children with undiagnosed skeletal myopathy, concern is raised about the use of succinylcholine and the potential for ventricular dysrhythmias and cardiac arrest from hyperkalemia.

29. **What is the initial symptom seen in infant botulism?**
    Constipation is often the first symptom in babies with infant botulism. Constipation may occur for days to weeks before the appearance of lethargy, feeding difficulties, diminished reflexes, weakness, hypotonia, and diminished gag reflex.

30. **What is the recommended treatment for infant botulism?**
    Human-derived botulism immune globulin (BabyBIG) decreases the duration of hospitalization, need for mechanical ventilation, and tube or parenteral feeding. Do not delay consultation with the Infant Botulism Treatment and Prevention Program while waiting for a definitive diagnosis.

31. **How would you differentiate a migraine headache from that due to idiopathic intracranial hypertension?**
    Headache due to idiopathic intracranial hypertension may be worse in the morning, and migraine symptoms are often relieved by sleep. Nausea, vomiting, and visual problems may also occur with both, and the neurologic examination may be normal. Papilledema is seen in most cases of idiopathic intracranial hypertension and is not present in migraine. Perform CT or MRI to rule out other causes of elevated intracranial pressure. If imaging does not demonstrate a mass lesion, perform a lumbar puncture to measure opening pressure, which will be elevated in idiopathic intracranial hypertension.

32. **Describe the worst complication of idiopathic intracranial hypertension.**
Elevated optic nerve pressure can lead to optic nerve ischemia and blindness.

33. **Describe the weakness in myasthenia gravis.**
Bilateral ptosis and eye muscle weakness are the most common manifestations of myasthenia gravis. Generalized myasthenia gravis can affect any skeletal muscle, including those involved with respiration, and can be life-threatening. The weakness is variable, and the specific muscles affected may vary with each examination. A history of worsening throughout the day or with continued activity may be reported. In the ED, easy fatigability of muscle strength may be demonstrated.

34. **Which electrolyte abnormality is responsible for periodic paralysis?**
Periodic paralysis can be due to hypokalemia or hyperkalemia. Paralytic episodes may occur after strenuous exercise. Persistent weakness is possible.

35. **Acute cerebellar ataxia is most commonly attributed to which viral illness?**
Varicella. Since varicella vaccination, other viruses have been associated with acute cerebellar ataxia, including Epstein Barr virus. Acute cerebellar ataxia typically occurs within 10 days of a viral illness and is most often post-infectious. The onset of ataxia is acute, and nystagmus and slurred speech can occur, but most children are otherwise normal. Recovery typically takes a few weeks, and residual neurologic deficits are possible.

36. **What is "milkmaid's hand"?**
Milkmaid's hand is found in patients with chorea. The child cannot maintain a continuous grasp when asked to squeeze the examiner's fingers but instead performs intermittent squeezing as if he or she were "milking" the finger. These low-amplitude jerking movements are characteristic of chorea.

37. **What is the most common cause of acquired chorea in children?**
Sydenham chorea, which is a manifestation of rheumatic fever.

38. **In uncal (unilateral transtentorial) herniation, is pupillary dilation present on the same side as the increased intracranial pressure or on the opposite side?**
The pupil dilates on the *same side* where the temporal lobe causes the uncus to bulge into the tentorial notch.

39. **Why does the pupil dilate in uncal herniation?**
Direct pressure on the oculomotor nerve (cranial nerve III) causes the ipsilateral pupil to dilate.

40. **How do brain abscesses occur?**
   - From the direct extension of chronic infection in the sinuses, ears, or dental structures
   - Following acute infections such as meningitis
   - Hematogenously from endocarditis or congenital heart disease (particularly with right-to-left shunting)
   - Following penetrating brain injury or neurosurgery

41. **What are the neurologic complications of sinusitis?**
   - Orbital cellulitis
   - Ophthalmoplegia
   - Cavernous sinus thrombosis
   - Intracranial empyema or abscess
   - Meningitis

42. **Why is the diagnosis of sphenoid sinusitis often difficult?**
The sphenoid sinuses are located posterior to the ethmoid sinuses, and the usual physical examination techniques, such as percussion and transillumination, are not useful. Headache is a common presenting symptom. The headache is usually severe but can mimic migraine and is often located on top of the head, behind the eyes, or at the back of the neck. Eighty percent of pediatric patients with intracranial complications of sinusitis have sphenoid involvement.

43. **Where are pediatric brain tumors most commonly located?**
Posterior fossa tumors account for 50% of brain tumors in children of all aged and are the most common location for brain tumors in children ages 1 to 8 years. This explains why gait disturbances are common in children with brain tumors.

44. A 7-year-old with a recent febrile illness developed new symptoms in the last 24 hours. She now has weakness and is unable to move her right arm. She is awake and alert, with low muscle tone in her right arm and absent reflexes. How would you diagnose this condition?
This patient has a classic presentation of acute flaccid myelitis. MRI imaging of the spinal cord demonstrates gray matter involvement spanning one or more vertebral segments. Specimen collection (CSF, blood, stool, respiratory) should be coordinated with your state Health Department on the day of presentation for this reportable disease. Biannual clusters of patients with acute flaccid myelitis did not occur in 2020, possibly due to precautions in place during the COVID-19 pandemic.

KEY POINTS: SEIZURES

1. Many common seizure types have characteristic presentations that can be identified with the initial history and physical examination.
2. Immediate testing or imaging is not always indicated after a seizure.
3. Workup after a febrile seizure should be directed to the cause of the fever.
4. When IV access is unavailable, absorption of benzodiazepines by the mucous membranes of the nose, buccal mucosa, or rectum may terminate the seizure.

KEY POINTS: INTRACRANIAL PRESSURE

1. A careful cranial nerve examination may be the clue to a mass lesion in the brain.
2. The presence of papilledema should prompt an imaging study of the brain.
3. A dilated unilateral pupil after head injury is concerning for herniation.
4. Headache from sinusitis may not be focused directly on the sinuses.

BIBLIOGRAPHY

1. *Centers for Disease Control and Prevention.* Acute Flaccid Myelitis (AFM). Available from: https://www.cdc.gov/acute-flaccid-myelitis/hcp/clinicians-health-departments.html
2. American Academy of Pediatrics, Steering Committee on Quality Improvement and Management, Subcommittee on Febrile Seizures, Febrile seizures: clinical practice guideline for the long-term management of the child with simple febrile seizures. *Pediatrics.* 2008;121(6):1281–1286.
3. American Academy of Pediatrics, Steering Committee on Quality Improvement and Management, Subcommittee on Febrile Seizures, Clinical practice guideline: febrile seizures: guideline for the neurodiagnostic evaluation of the child with a simple febrile seizure. *Pediatrics.* 2011;127(2):389–394.
4. Baugh RF, Basura GJ, Ishii LE, et al. Clinical practice guideline: Bell's palsy. *Otolaryngol Head Neck Surg.* 2013;149(3S):S1–S27.
5. Berg AT, Shinnar S, Darefsky AS, et al. Predictors of recurrent febrile seizures. A prospective cohort study. *Arch Pediatr Adolesc Med.* 1997;151:371–378.
6. Chamberlain JM, Kapur J, Shinnar S, et al. Efficacy of levetiracetam, fosphenytoin, and valproate for established status epilepticus by age group (ESETT): a double-blind, responsive-adaptive, randomized controlled trial. *Lancet.* 2020;395:1217–1224.
7. Chamberlain JM, Okada P, Holsti M, et al. Lorazepam vs diazepam for pediatric status epilepticus a randomized clinical trial. *JAMA.* 2014;311(16):238–240.
8. Cronan K, Wiley J. Lumbar puncture. In: King C, Henretig F, ed. *The Textbook of Pediatric Emergency Medicine Procedures.* Lippincott Williams & Wilkins; 2008:505–514.
9. Infant botulism treatment and prevention program. Available from: infantbotulism.org. Accessed 16.11.23.
10. Hirtz D, Ashwal S, Berg A, et al. Practice parameter: evaluating a first nonfebrile seizure in children. Report of the quality standards subcommittee of the American Academy of Neurology, The Child Neurology Society, and The American Epilepsy Society. *Neurology.* 2000;55:616–623. (reaffirmed 17.10.21).
11. Kapur J, Elm J, Chamberlain JM, et al. Randomized trial of three anticonvulsant medications for status epilepticus. *N Engl J Med.* 2019;381(22):2103–2113.
12. Pecina CA. Tick paralysis. *Semin Neurol.* 2012;32(5):531–532.
13. Peragallo JH. Pediatric myasthenia gravis. *Semin Pediatr Neurol.* 2017;24(2):116–121.
14. Takacs DS, Katyayan A. Clinical Features and Diagnosis of Infantile Spasms. *UpToDate;* 2022. Available from: http://www.uptodate.com. Accessed 29.03.22.
15. Wolf VL, Lupo PJ, Lotze TE. Pediatric acute transverse myelitis overview and differential diagnosis. *J Child Neurol.* 2012;27(11):1426–1436.

CHAPTER 32

ENDOCRINE DISORDERS

Danielle N. Mascarenas and Robert E. Sapien

1. **What are the severe outcomes of delayed recognition and treatment of endocrine emergencies?**
   The greatest consequence of an endocrine emergency such as hypoglycemia, adrenal insufficiency, hyperglycemia, and metabolic ketoacidosis is cerebral dysfunction, leading to coma or death.

2. **What is hypoglycemia?**
   Hypoglycemia (low glucose) is due to decreased availability of glucose, increased use of glucose, and/or inadequate alternatives to glucose. Preventing hypoglycemia requires a balance among glucose input, glycogenolysis, and gluconeogenesis controlled by the secretion of counterregulatory hormones. Any enzyme deficiency or inability to generate substrate during these pathways results in hypoglycemia.

3. **Name several causes of hypoglycemia.**
   Ketotic hypoglycemia is most common, which includes decreased intake (fasting, illness, transient neonatal hypoglycemia), decreased absorption (vomiting/diarrhea), defects in glycogenolysis or gluconeogenesis pathways, and increased use (sepsis/shock). If there is hypoglycemia in the absence of ketones, think of hyperinsulinism or fatty acid oxidation. Other complex mechanisms include toxin ingestion (diabetes medications, salicylate, ethanol), adrenal insufficiency, hypothyroidism, and hypopituitarism.

4. **Why are children susceptible to hypoglycemia?**
   Children utilize glucose at higher metabolic rates and have decreased reserves compared with adults. Rates of glucose utilization are the following:
   - Preterm infants: 10 mg/kg/minute
   - Term infants: 8 mg/kg/minute
   - Toddlers: 6 to 8 mg/kg/minute
   - Older children and adolescents: 4 to 6 mg/kg/minute
   - Adults: 2 to 4 mg/kg/minute

5. **How is hypoglycemia treated?**
   Hypoglycemia is generally defined as plasma glucose <50 mg/dL. In children who are awake and tolerating oral fluids, administer oral carbohydrates. Otherwise, obtain immediate intravenous (IV) access and administer dextrose. The preferred treatment is 5 to 10 mL/kg of 10% dextrose (D10) or 2 to 4 mL/kg of 25% dextrose (D25). These doses are equal to a rapid infusion of 0.5 to 1 g/kg of dextrose. Higher concentrations of dextrose (greater than D25) cause sclerosis of the peripheral veins. Maintain euglycemia with a glucose infusion at 6-8 mg/kg/minute. The goal is to keep glucose levels >70 mg/dL on multiple measurements. If no IV access, intramuscular (IM) glucagon can beadministered at 0.03 mg/kg, maximum dose of 1 mg.

6. **What initial studies should be obtained when a child presents with an unknown cause of hypoglycemia?**
   If possible, obtain studies prior to treatment with dextrose.
   - Blood glucose at bedside (do not delay)
   - Comprehensive metabolic panel
   - Liver function tests
   - Urine ketones
   - Others: lactate, insulin, beta-hydroxybutyrate, growth hormone, cortisol, C-peptide (consider exogenous insulin), free fatty acids, carnitine profile, amino acid profile, toxins (ethanol, salicylates), and urine amino and organic acids

---

KEY POINTS: HYPOGLYCEMIA

1. Rapid identification is crucial.
2. Children are susceptible because of their small glycogen stores and high glucose utilization.
3. Treatment of hypoglycemia: 5 to 10 mL/kg of D10 or 2 to 4 mL/kg of D25.

7. **What is the incidence of type 1 diabetes?**
Incidence of type 1 diabetes has increased by 1.9% per year among US youth between 2002 and 2015. Higher rates are seen among non-Hispanic White children, but steeper rates of increase are seen in Black and Hispanic youths.

8. **What is the pathophysiology of type 1 diabetes?**
Type 1 diabetes develops from the autoimmune destruction of beta cells in the pancreas. These include autoantibodies include to glutamic acid decarboxylase, tyrosine phosphatase, insulin, and zinc transporter 8.

9. **Define diabetic ketoacidosis (DKA).**
Nearly 30% of children newly diagnosed with type 1 diabetes present with DKA. In DKA, there is a relative or absolute decrease in circulating insulin, stimulating an increase in counterregulatory hormones (catecholamines, cortisol, glucagon, and growth hormone). This hormone surge increases gluconeogenesis and glycogenolysis, which in combination with low or no insulin result in hyperglycemia, hyperosmolality, ketosis, and acidosis.

10. **How does a patient with DKA typically present?**
Classically, there is a history of weight loss, polyuria, and polydipsia days to weeks prior to presentation. Once ketoacidosis develops, vomiting, abdominal pain, dehydration, and a fruity odor from ketones are evident. In severe forms, hyperpneic (Kussmaul) respirations, lethargy, and/or altered mental status are additional features. One percent of children with severe DKA develop cerebral edema. While the mortality and morbidity from DKA are low, the majority of deaths are from cerebral edema.
   Laboratory evaluation reveals glucose level >200 mg/dL, ketosis, glucosuria, venous pH <7.3, and serum bicarbonate level <15 mEq/L.

11. **Describe the goals of DKA treatment.**
Overall goals of treatment: (1) rehydrate, (2) correct acidosis, and (3) reverse ketosis while slowly correcting hyperglycemia. Most institutions have a management protocol that providers should be familiar with; there might be slight variations among them.
   Fluids: Fluid resuscitation begins immediately. Infuse crystalloid fluid boluses (0.9% normal saline [NS] or Lactated Ringer solution) at 10 to 20 mL/kg rapidly within the first 1 to 2 hours. After dehydration and shock are addressed, continue fluid administration for the next 24 to 48 hours to replace long-standing fluid losses. Children are usually 5% to 10% dehydrated at the time of presentation. Per the PECARN DKA FLUID clinical trials, ongoing fluid management can include either 0.45% or 0.9% saline, with no difference in patient outcomes correcting over 24 hours versus 48 hours.
   Hyperglycemia: Start insulin therapy at an infusion rate of 0.1 unit/kg/hour. Never give insulin as an IV bolus. Decrease glucose levels at 50 to 100 mg/dL/hour, using a two-bag system where bag 1 consists of saline (0.45% or 0.9% NS) plus 40 mEq/L of potassium acetate or potassium phosphate. Bag 2 contains 5% or 10% dextrose and NS, which is started when glucose levels drop ≤300 mg/dL as insulin infuses. Increase dextrose to a maximum of 12.5% if glucose drops too quickly.
   Electrolytes: There is a total body deficit of potassium due to shifts extracellularly, causing intracellular depletion. Therefore initial levels can be normal or elevated. As hyperglycemia resolves, potassium shifts back intracellularly. To correct this, add potassium to the fluid infusions of both bag 1 and bag 2 at 40 mEq/L. If the patient has hyperkalemia initially, add potassium at a lower concentration (0-20 mEq/L) and ensure the patient is urinating. Monitor sodium and phosphate closely.
   Alkali: Avoid bicarbonate therapy. Only consider with arterial pH ≤6.9, impaired cardiac function, or severe hyperkalemia.
   Cerebral edema: If suspected, start treatment immediately. Risk factors for developing cerebral edema include age ≤3 years, new-onset diabetes, treatment with bicarbonate, severe acidosis, low $PaCO_2$, elevated blood urea nitrogen, and failure of sodium to correct. Treat with mannitol (0.5-1 g/kg via IV over 20 minutes) or hypertonic saline 3% (2.5-5 mL/kg over 30 minutes). Hypertonic saline has increasingly been used, but the superiority over mannitol remains controversial.

KEY POINTS: DKA

1. The electrolyte, metabolic, and glucose abnormalities associated with DKA require prompt treatment, close monitoring, and frequent reassessments of the patient.
2. Cerebral edema has a high mortality/morbidity; recognize and treat early!
3. Do not discontinue insulin when treating DKA. Add dextrose when the serum level is <300 mg/dL to avoid hypoglycemia.

12. **Is type 2 diabetes a problem in children?**
Yes. The incidence of type 2 diabetes among patients less than 20 years old has been steadily increasing along with child obesity and is higher among racial and ethnic minorities. The rate of increase in incidence is higher for type 2 diabetes versus type 1 diabetes.

13. **What is the underlying mechanism of type 2 diabetes?**
Type 2 diabetes is a progressive illness that results in insulin resistance and impaired secretion, ultimately resulting in loss of beta cell function in the pancreas, causing a constant state of hyperglycemia. Persistent hyperglycemia leads to obesity, acanthosis nigricans, and anovulatory cycles.

14. **Describe hyperglycemic hyperosmolar syndrome.**
This is a medical emergency. Patients' glucose levels are ≥ 600 mg/dL with serum osmolality >330 mOsm/kg in the absence of ketosis and acidosis. Severe dehydration and cerebral edema contribute to high morbidity and mortality.

15. **What is diabetes insipidus (DI)?**
DI is a result of the renal system's inability to concentrate urine, characterized by polyuria and polydipsia. Patients present with dehydration, irritability, poor weight gain, and hypernatremia with dilute urine (specific gravity <1.010).

   There are two forms: central and nephrogenic. Nephrogenic DI results from an absent or decreased renal response to antidiuretic hormone (ADH), resulting in excessive free water excretion. Central DI is caused by ADH deficiency. Causes of DI include infections such as meningitis, genetic disorders, sickle cell disease, renal disease, drug-induced, structural problems (midline cleft palate), neoplasms (craniopharyngioma, optic nerve glioma), significant electrolyte abnormalities (hypercalcemia, hypokalemia), and head trauma.

16. **What studies should be obtained if DI is suspected?**
Obtain serum electrolytes plus serum and urine osmoles. Consider anterior pituitary disorders; obtain levels of adrenocorticotropic hormone (ACTH), thyroid, and growth hormone and check for hypogonadotropic hypogonadism.

17. **What is SIADH (syndrome of inappropriate antidiuretic hormone)?**
SIADH is a result of the inability to excrete free water, resulting in hyposmolality, hyponatremia, and concentrated urine. Significant hyponatremia results in confusion, weakness, or seizures.

   In SIADH, there is an increase in the release and activity of ADH without clear osmotic or hemodynamic triggers. Causes of SIADH include pulmonary disease, head trauma or neurological disease, medications, malignancy, gene mutations, and acute stress/pain.

   If SIADH is suspected, obtain electrolytes and serum and urine osmoles. First-line treatment is fluid restriction.

18. **What are the causes of adrenal insufficiency?**
This is a life-threatening emergency. The adrenal cortex cannot produce corticosteroids in response to stress (infection, trauma, surgery). Causes include the following:
- Primary destruction (congenital adrenal hyperplasia [CAH])
- Dysfunction (autoimmune: Addison disease, adrenoleukodystrophy)
- Impaired hypothalamic-pituitary-adrenal axis (septo-optic dysplasia, empty sella syndrome, tumor, surgery, radiotherapy)
- Acquired adrenal suppression (prolonged steroid therapy)

19. **What are the clinical features of adrenal insufficiency?**
- General malaise
- Fatigue
- Anorexia
- Weight loss
- Salt-craving
- Hyperpigmentation
- Altered mental status
- Severe cardiovascular or hemodynamic instability

20. **How is adrenal crisis treated?**
Provide hemodynamic resuscitation with boluses of 20 mL/kg of 0.9% NS. Subsequent IV fluid should contain D10 and sodium for both hypoglycemia and hyponatremia, but hold on potassium (severe hyperkalemia may be

present). Vasopressors may also be needed. Give hydrocortisone at 50 to 100 mg/m^2 intravenously. If body surface area cannot be calculated, give 1 to 2 mg/kg.

Obtain initial studies: random cortisol levels, electrolytes, glucose, ACTH levels, plasma renin activity, aldosterone level, and an electrocardiogram.

21. What is the most common cause of adrenal insufficiency in infancy?

CAH occurs in 1:10,000 to 1:18,000 live births, resulting from an inborn error of adrenal steroid biogenesis. Deficiency of 21-hydroxylase enzyme is the most common form, accounting for the majority of cases. Seventy-five percent of patients are deficient in aldosterone, causing salt-wasting. Twenty-five percent of patients present with virilization without salt-wasting. Newborn screening has significantly decreased morbidity and mortality.

22. How does a child with salt-wasting CAH present? What studies should be obtained?

Infants generally present at 2 to 5 weeks in a salt-wasting crisis with poor feeding, poor weight gain, lethargy, vomiting, and irritability. Genitalia often appear ambiguous.

Studies:
- Electrolytes (evaluating for hyperkalemia, hyponatremia)
- Glucose (typically found in hypoglycemia)
- Bicarbonate (usually low)
- Steroid profile (cortisol, 17-hydroxyprogesterone, dehydroepiandrosterone, androstenedione, testosterone, ACTH)

23. How is CAH treated acutely?
- Steroid: Give hydrocortisone at 50 to 100 mg/m^2 IV. If body surface area cannot be calculated, give 1 to 2 mg/kg.
- Fluids: Give 20 mL/kg of 0.9% NS for dehydration.
- Hyperkalemia: Generally tolerated better by infants. For arrhythmias secondary to hyperkalemia, give 10% calcium gluconate IV, 0.6 mL/kg.
- Hypoglycemia: Give 5 to 10 mL/kg of D10 or 2 to 4 mL/kg of D25.)
- Acidosis: Consider bicarbonate therapy for pH <6.9 with hemodynamic instability.

KEY POINTS: ADRENAL CRISIS

1. Do not delay steroid therapy.
2. Patients can present with severe electrolyte abnormalities (hyperkalemia, hyponatremia).
3. Fluid resuscitation and correction of hypoglycemia are imperative.

24. What is pheochromocytoma, and how do children present?

Pheochromocytomas are norepinephrine-, epinephrine-, and dopamine-secreting tumors. Eighty-five percent are located in the adrenal glands; 15% are in the extra-adrenal parasympathetic and sympathetic paraganglia. Children present with headaches, palpitations, flushing, excessive sweating, tremor, fatigue, and chest or abdominal pain.

Notable causes include von Hippel-Lindau syndrome, multiple endocrine neoplasia syndrome, and neurofibromatosis type 1.

Besides surgical resection, initial treatment includes the use of alpha-adrenergic blockade.

25. Describe normal menstruation and name common causes of amenorrhea in adolescents.

A normal cycle is 21 to 35 days, with periods lasting 3 to 7 days. Bleeding >7 days is considered prolonged. Primary amenorrhea is a lack of menses by age 15 years or >3 years after the onset of secondary sexual development. Secondary amenorrhea is the sudden absence of menstruation in someone who has previously menstruated.

Common causes of amenorrhea include pregnancy, polycystic ovarian syndrome, contraceptive use, genital outflow tract abnormalities (imperforate hymen, vaginal or uterine agenesis), hypoestrogenic states (anorexia, athletic activity), hypogonadotropic hypogonadism (hypothalamus/pituitary dysfunction, low follicle-stimulating hormone [FSH]), and hypergonadotropic hypogonadism (ovarian insufficiency, high FSH).

26. What workup should be completed for an adolescent with abnormal uterine bleeding?

First, check a pregnancy test! Generally, initial laboratory evaluation includes complete blood count to evaluate for anemia, hemoglobin A1C especially if obese, total and free testosterone, dehydroepiandrosterone sulfate, FSH, luteinizing hormone, thyroid-stimulating hormone (TSH), and prolactin levels. Consider pelvic ultrasound in the setting of pelvic/abdominal pain.

27. How do infants with congenital hypothyroidism present?

Congenital hypothyroidism, the most common cause of preventable intellectual disability in the world, results from iodine deficiency and embryological defects. Newborns are generally asymptomatic due to maternal protection but are diagnosed early through newborn screens, detecting hypothyroidism in 1 of 4000 newborns in the United

States annually. If undiagnosed, infants usually present between 6 and 12 weeks of age with hypothermia, hypoactivity, or hypotonia; poor feeding; constipation; prolonged jaundice; and large posterior fontanel. Laboratory studies show decreased T_4 and increased TSH.

28. **How is neonatal thyrotoxicosis different from congenital hypothyroidism?**
Neonates with thyrotoxicosis often present within 2 weeks of life *in extremis* with tachycardia, irritability, congestive heart failure, and poor weight gain. Goiter and exophthalmos may be present. Neonatal thyrotoxicosis is caused by maternal hyperthyroidism, where maternal thyroid-stimulating antibodies spur increased thyroid production by the neonatal thyroid. Laboratory studies show increased T_4 and decreased TSH.

29. **What is the leading cause of pediatric hyperthyroidism? How does thyroid storm differ from hyperthyroidism?**
Graves disease. This is more common in females than males (3:1) and is commonly associated with autoimmune disorders such as type 1 diabetes. Children present with tachycardia and weight loss in the setting of increased appetite, fatigue, diarrhea, hair loss, and behavioral issues.
Nearly all cases of thyroid storm occur in patients with known hyperthyroidism. It is a life-threatening emergency that has many features of hyperthyroidism, with distinguishing characteristics including high fever, hyperpyrexia, cardiovascular dysfunction with elevated heart rate and pressures, and altered mental status.

30. **How is thyroid storm treated?**
Initial treatment includes supportive care with IV fluids, cooling, and acetaminophen. IV beta-blockers (propranolol or esmolol) are also used, along with iodide and methimazole (iodine oxidation inhibitor). Propylthiouracil is contraindicated in children due to an association with liver failure.

BIBLIOGRAPHY

1. Alarcon G, Figueredo V, Tarkoff J. Thyroid disorders. *Pediatr Rev.* 2021;42(11):604–618. https://doi.org/10.1542/pir.2020-001420.
2. Auron M, Raissouni N. Adrenal insufficiency. *Pediatr Rev.* 2015;36(3):92–102.
3. Cashen K, Petersen T. Diabetic ketoacidosis. *Pediatr Rev.* 2019;40(8):412–420. https://doi.org/10.1542/pir.2018-0231.
4. Copeland KC, Silverstein J, Moore KR, et al. Management of newly diagnosed type 2 diabetes mellitus (T2DM) in children and adolescents. *Pediatrics.* 2013;131(2):364–382. https://doi.org/10.1542/peds.2012-3494.
5. Divers J, Mayer-Davis EJ, Lawrence JM, et al. Trends in incidence of type 1 and type 2 diabetes among youths - selected counties and Indian reservations, United States, 2002-2015. *MMWR Morb Mortal Wkly Rep.* 2020;69(6):161–165. https://doi.org/10.15585/mmwr.mm6906a3.
6. Dorney K, Agus MSD. Endocrine emergencies. In: Shaw KN, Bachur RG, eds. *Fleisher & Ludwig's Textbook of Pediatric Emergency Medicine.* 8th ed. Wolters Kluwer; 2021:653–679.
7. Edmonds S, Fein DM, Gurtman A. Pheochromocytoma. *Pediatr Rev.* 2011;32(7):308–310. https://doi.org/10.1542/pir.32-7-308.
8. Gan MJ, Albanese-O'Neill A, Haller MJ. Type 1 diabetes: current concepts in epidemiology, pathophysiology, clinical care, and research. *Curr Probl Pediatr Adolesc Health Care.* 2012;42(10):269–291. https://doi.org/10.1016/j.cppeds.2012.07.002.
9. Gray SH. Menstrual disorders. *Pediatr Rev.* 2013;34(1):6–18. https://doi.org/10.1542/pir.34-1-6.
10. Jackson S, Creo A, Al Nofal A. Management of type 1 diabetes in children in the outpatient setting. *Pediatr Rev.* 2022;43(3):160–170. https://doi.org/10.1542/pir.2020-001388.
11. Jones DP. Syndrome of inappropriate secretion of antidiuretic hormone and hyponatremia. *Pediatr Rev.* 2018;39(1):27–35. https://doi.org/10.1542/pir.2016-0165.
12. Kim SY. Endocrine and metabolic emergencies in children: hypocalcemia, hypoglycemia, adrenal insufficiency, and metabolic acidosis including diabetic ketoacidosis. *Ann Pediatr Endocrinol Metab.* 2016;21(2):111. https://doi.org/10.6065/apem.2016.21.2.111.
13. Kuppermann N, Ghetti S, Schunk JE, et al. Clinical trial of fluid infusion rates for pediatric diabetic ketoacidosis. *N Engl J Med.* 2018;378(24):2275–2287. https://doi.org/10.1056/NEJMoa1716816.
14. Lawrence JM, Reynolds K, Saydah SH, et al. Demographic correlates of short-term mortality among youth and young adults with youth-onset diabetes diagnosed from 2002 to 2015: the SEARCH for Diabetes in Youth Study. *Diabetes Care.* 2021;44(12):2691–2698. https://doi.org/10.2337/dc21-0728.
15. Nallasamy K, Jayashree M, Singhi S, Bansal A. Low-dose vs standard-dose insulin in pediatric diabetic ketoacidosis: a randomized clinical trial. *JAMA Pediatr.* 2014;168(11):999–1005. https://doi.org/10.1001/jamapediatrics.2014.1211.
16. Rewers A, Klingensmith G, Davis C, et al. Presence of diabetic ketoacidosis at diagnosis of diabetes mellitus in youth: the Search for Diabetes in Youth Study. *Pediatrics.* 2008;121(5). https://doi.org/10.1542/peds.2007-1105.
17. Ross DS, Burch HB, Cooper DS, et al. 2016 American Thyroid Association Guidelines for diagnosis and management of hyperthyroidism and other causes of thyrotoxicosis. [published correction appears in *Thyroid.* 2017;27(11):1462]. *Thyroid.* 2016;26(10):1343–1421. https://doi.org/10.1089/thy.2016.0229.
18. Weiner A, Vuguin P, Adam HM. Diabetes insipidus. *Pediatr Rev.* 2020;41(2):96–99. https://doi.org/10.1542/pir.2018-0337.
19. Zeitler P, Haqq A, Rosenbloom A, Glaser N. Hyperglycemic hyperosmolar syndrome in children: pathophysiological considerations and suggested guidelines for treatment. *J Pediatr.* 2011;158(1):9–14.e2. https://doi.org/10.1016/j.jpeds.2010.09.048.
20. Topjian AA, Raymond TT., Atkins D, et al. Part 4: Pediatric Basic and Advanced Life Support: 2020 American Heart Association guidelines for cardiopulmonary resuscitation and emergency cardiovascular care. *Circulation.* 2020;142(16 suppl 2):S469–S523. https://doi.org/10.1161/CIR.0000000000000901.

CHAPTER 33

FLUIDS AND ELECTROLYTES

Priyanka Joshi and Ronald F. Marchese

1. **Why are infants and young children sensitive to dehydration?**
   Infants and young children have higher fluid requirements secondary to higher metabolic rates, particularly in illness. They also have more insensible losses due to increased surface area. Furthermore, they may be less able to communicate their thirst to caregivers. Typical sites for fluid loss are the gastrointestinal tract, skin, and urine.

2. **How do you estimate the extent of dehydration in children?**
   Serial weights on the same scale are best but are rarely available in the emergency department (ED) setting. Although not as accurate, a physical examination is used to estimate the degree of fluid loss (Table 33.1).

3. **How do you determine degree of dehydration?**
   Infants and children with mild dehydration (less than 3% total body weight loss) may have minimal or no clinical change apart from decreased urine output.
   Children with mild-to-moderate dehydration (3%-10% total body weight loss) typically have prolonged capillary refill time (>2 seconds) and abnormal skin turgor, and may have abnormal respiratory patterns.
   Children with severe dehydration (>10% total body weight loss) typically present in a shock-like state with "ill" appearance, mottled skin, tachycardia, hypotension, and cool extremities. In children, hypotension is a very late sign of dehydration due to higher cardiac reserve to compensate for significant volume loss.

4. **What examination findings are most consistent with clinically significant dehydration?**
   Ill appearance, lack of tears, capillary refill time >2 seconds, and dry mucous membranes.

5. **How does the extent of dehydration translate into fluid loss?**
   The amount of fluid deficit should be calculated based on changes in weight or clinical signs. For each kilogram of weight loss, 1 L of fluid was lost. Using the weight obtained in the ED and your estimate of the percentage of

Table 33.1 Clinical Findings of Dehydration

SIGNS AND SYMPTOMS	DEGREE OF IMPAIRMENT		
	NONE OR MILD	MODERATE	SEVERE
General condition, infants	Thirsty; alert; restless	Lethargic or drowsy	Limp; cold, cyanotic extremities; may be comatose
General condition, older children	Thirsty; alert; restless	Alert; postural dizziness	Apprehensive; cold, cyanotic extremities; muscle cramps
Quality of radial pulse	Normal	Thready or weak	Feeble or impalpable
Quality of respiration	Normal	Deep	Deep and rapid
Skin elasticity	Pinch retracts immediately	Pinch retracts slowly	Pinch retracts very slowly (>2 sec)
Eyes	Normal	Sunken	Very sunken
Tears	Present	Absent	Absent
Mucous membranes	Moist	Dry	Very dry
Urine output (by report of the parent)	Normal to slightly reduced	Reduced	None passed in many hours

Adapted with permission from World Health Organization. *The Treatment of Diarrhea: A Manual for Physicians and Other Senior Health Workers.* 3rd ed. Division of Diarrheal and Acute Respiratory Disease Control, World Health Organization; 1995.

dehydration, you can calculate the "well" or rehydrated weight. The difference between the estimated well weight and current weight is converted into liters or kilograms. For example, a 9-kg ill-appearing baby presents with dry mucous membranes, crying with no tears, and a capillary refill time of longer than 2 seconds. She is estimated to have lost 10% of her body weight (severe dehydration).

To calculate the well weight, divide the current weight by 1 minus the dehydration percentage:

$$\text{Calculated well weight} = \text{current weight} / (1 - \text{dehydration percentage})$$
$$= 9 \text{ kg} / (1\% - 10\%)$$
$$= 9 \text{ kg} / 0.9$$
$$= 10 \text{ kg}$$
$$\text{Weight lost} = 10 \text{ kg} - 9 \text{ kg} = 1 \text{ kg} = 1 \text{ L}$$

6. **How much and what type of fluid do you use for a "bolus" to begin intravenous (IV) hydration?**
   If IV hydration is required, administer an initial 20 mL/kg of normal saline (NS) bolus and reassess the patient to determine the need for further 20 mL/kg aliquots. The goal is to restore blood pressure, reduce heart rate, restore perfusion to the tissues (return of capillary refill < 2 seconds), improve mental status or general appearance, and produce urine. If initial fluid boluses greater than a total of 60 mL/kg are needed, reconsider the diagnosis and management plan.

7. **Are there any children who should not receive a rapid fluid bolus?**
   Children with diabetic ketoacidosis or hypernatremic dehydration (serum sodium level > 150 mEq/dL) who are in a hyperosmolar state require more cautious fluid resuscitation. Additionally, children at risk for heart failure should receive fluid resuscitation in smaller aliquots of 10 mL/kg with reevaluation after each bolus.

8. **What stock should be used after the initial IV bolus or if the child is not dehydrated?**
   For patients greater than 28 days of age, administer dextrose-containing isotonic fluids (typically 5% dextrose with normal saline [D5NS]) with appropriate potassium supplementation (10-mEq/L KCl if <10 kg; 20 mEq/L if >10 kg) to decrease the risk of developing hyponatremia. Alternate approaches to fluid management may be warranted in different clinical situations such as children with burns, pyloric stenosis with hypochloremia, and diabetic ketoacidosis.

9. **At what rate should fluids run on a child who has orders to receive nothing by mouth? How is this maintenance rate adjusted for the dehydrated child?**
   All children who are unable to drink should receive maintenance fluids, and if they are dehydrated, the rate is higher to replace some of the remaining fluid deficit. Calculate all rates *by using the child's well or rehydrated weight*. Increase rates above maintenance if the child is febrile or has increased insensible or gastrointestinal losses.

   Maintenance IV Fluid Rate: 4-2-1 Rule.
   4 mL/kg/hour for the first 10 kg **PLUS**
   2 mL/kg/hour for the second 10 kg **PLUS**
   1 mL/kg/hour for each kg over 20 kg
   (Maximum rate of 120 mL/hour.)
   Example: Maintenance rate for a 16-kg child: 40 mL/hour (first 10 kg × 4 mL/hour) + 12 mL/hour (next 6 kg × 2 mL/hour) = 52 mL/hour (if the child is febrile, add 10% more, or 55-60 mL/hour). To determine the rate for the dehydrated child, half of the total fluid deficit (minus the fluid boluses already given) is added to the maintenance rate for the first 8 hours. The other half of the deficit is added to the maintenance rate over the next 16 hours (hopefully outside the ED). For children with hypertonic dehydration, the remaining fluid deficit after initial boluses is replaced evenly over the next 48 hours.
   Example: A 9-kg dehydrated baby was given 400 mL of NS (40 mL/kg) as an initial fluid bolus. The fluid deficit was 1000 mL. Half of the deficit is 500 mL. Because 400 mL was already given, 100 mL of the deficit should be added to the maintenance rate over the next 8 hours. Thus 100 mL/8 hours (=12.5 mL/hour) should be added to the maintenance rate of 40 mL/hour (based on 10-kg "well" weight) totaling 52 mL/hour of D5NS solution.

10. **What about children with syndrome of inappropriate antidiuretic hormone secretion (SIADH)?**
    Some children are at risk for secretion of antidiuretic hormone (ADH), which may cause retention of free water and hyponatremia. Conditions that have been associated with this state include bronchiolitis, meningitis, and pneumonia, as well as perioperative and postoperative states. These children may require fluid restriction.

In children with electrolyte abnormalities or prolonged IV fluid administration, serial electrolytes and urine output are monitored and fluid rates are adjusted on the basis of the child's hydration status, urine output, and presence or absence of increased ADH. Keeping children on isotonic parenteral maintenance solution may cause hypernatremia and may not replace insensible water loss, whereas hypotonic fluids may cause acute hyponatremia and encephalopathy. Therefore individualize the IV fluid rate and composition on a case-by-case basis.

11. **Which children may be treated with oral rehydration?**
Strongly consider oral rehydration in all children with mild or moderate dehydration who do not have uncompensated shock, severe vomiting, high stool output of more than 20 mL/kg/hour, or poor adherence. This is very effective in treating dehydration and has a low failure rate.

12. **Why are not more children treated with oral rehydration therapy (ORT)?**
ORT takes time, one-to-one care, and patience. Many parents bring their children to the ED because they want a "quick fix." Nevertheless, several studies have shown that ORT is as effective as IV rehydration and may require less time, and have a lower complication rate. In an effort to improve efficiency, many hospitals have adopted protocols for nurse-driven care to initiate ORT from triage, utilizing checklists and timers for caregivers.

KEY POINTS: DEHYDRATION

1. The first objective in treating a child with severe dehydration is to restore intravascular volume and treat shock, regardless of cause.
2. In children with electrolyte abnormalities or prolonged IV fluid administration, serial electrolytes and urine output are monitored and fluid rates are adjusted on the basis of the child's hydration status, urine output, and presence or absence of increased ADH.
3. Compared with IV therapy, ORT is equally effective in treating dehydration in most children with mild-to-moderate dehydration, has fewer complications, and may be faster.

13. **How do you calculate the amount of fluid to give for oral rehydration?**
Calculate the fluid deficit based on the estimate of the degree of dehydration, and give *the entire deficit by mouth over 4 hoursthe entire deficit by mouth over 4 hours*. Mildly dehydrated patients can receive 1 mL/kg every 5 to 10 minutes to start. Similarly, moderately dehydrated patients can receive 2 mL/kg every 5 to 10 minutes. This volume and frequency can be increased as tolerated. Nasogastric (NG) tubes can also be used to administer continuous volume replacement. This treatment should be initiated in the ED but can be completed at home as long as the child tolerates the initial doses and remains well appearing with stable vital signs.

14. **What type of fluid should be used for oral rehydration?**
We should use an oral rehydration solution (ORS). These solutions have the correct proportion of dextrose and salt to allow for maximal absorption of electrolytes. Although solutions with higher concentrations of sodium (75-90 mEq/dL) are recommended initially (Rehydralyte [manufactured by Ross], ORS packets [Jaianas]), solutions with a lower sodium content (40-60 mEq/dL) may be used and are more readily available (Pedialyte [Ross], Enfalyte [Mead Johnson]). Commonly used beverages such as apple juice, sports drink, and ginger ale are less effective for adequate ORT as they do not contain the correct sodium and glucose ratio to promote salt and water reabsorption across the gastrointestinal lumen.

15. **Why can I not use soda, juice, popsicles, or soups for ORT?**
These products have high sugar content and, thus, do not allow for maximum sodium/glucose transport across the cell membrane in the gastrointestinal tract. It is recommended to use flavored solutions from the manufacturer to ensure accurate electrolyte concentrations. Of note, however, one study showed that patients treated for mild gastroenteritis with a 50:50 mixture of apple juice and water were effectively treated with decreased treatment failures.

16. **When should oral rehydration not be used?**
   - Severe dehydration
   - Inability to tolerate oral fluids because of vomiting
   - Altered mental status with risk of aspiration
   - Ileus
   - Short gut or other conditions with carbohydrate malabsorption

17. Are there alternatives to ORT and IV therapy?

There is some evidence to suggest that recombinant human hyaluronidase-facilitated subcutaneous rehydration may be a reasonable alternative therapy in mild to moderately dehydrated children, especially with failed ORT or with difficult IV access. Additionally, fluid resuscitation can be completed via an NG tube.

18. When should ondansetron be used?

An antiemetic such as ondansetron, a serotonin 5-HT$_3$ selective receptor antagonist, may be useful for children with moderate or severe dehydration with nausea and persistent vomiting. Ondansetron can be administered orally, as an oral disintegrating tablet, or intravenously to reduce vomiting and improve a child's ability to maintain oral hydration. Oral ondansetron has been shown to improve the success rate of ORT in children with gastroenteritis.

19. What concerns should I have about a child with hypertonic dehydration?

The deficit in children with hypertonic dehydration may be underestimated. They appear less dry because their intravascular space is maintained longer. Their serum sodium will typically be greater than 150 mEq/L as their water loss exceeds the sodium loss. These children may present later for care due to their initial well appearance. Their examination is notable for "doughy" or "velvety" skin. Additionally, rapid rehydration can cause cerebral edema, hemorrhage, or thrombosis. These children should be monitored closely with slow correction of their sodium and fluid deficit over 48 hours. Hyperglycemia or hypocalcemia may also occur.

20. How do I treat hyponatremia?

Treat the patient, not the laboratory value. Treat children with seizures, severe lethargy, hypoventilation, coma, or shock immediately. For water-intoxicated children or those with SIADH—in whom sodium, not fluid, is needed—give 2 to 4 mL/kg of 3% saline to stop seizures, followed by 6 to 12 mL/kg of 3% saline over the next 2 to 4 hours. For children with more mild forms of hyponatremic dehydration, fluid boluses of 20 to 40 mL/kg NS quickly correct symptomatic hyponatremia.

21. How do I treat hypoglycemia?

For patients with hypoglycemia who are awake and tolerating oral fluids, administer oral carbohydrates. For patients with altered consciousness, ill appearance, or inability to tolerate oral fluids, place an IV and rapidly administer 2 to 5 mL/kg of D$_{10}$ (10% dextrose in water) and monitor glucose levels closely.

22. How and when do I treat metabolic acidosis?

Most children with dehydration correct their metabolic acidosis with fluid resuscitation and do not require bicarbonate. Bicarbonate should be given only for severe metabolic acidosis with pH < 7.1 and not for patients with respiratory acidosis. It is NOT indicated in patients with diabetic ketoacidosis due to the associated development of cerebral edema. Children with respiratory insufficiency should not receive bicarbonate. Bicarbonate does not cross the blood-brain barrier; however, its byproduct, carbon dioxide, does cross this barrier. Increases in carbon dioxide may cause cerebral acidosis, and therefore bicarbonate should be given slowly. Usually 0.5 to 1 mEq/kg is given over a minimum of 30 to 60 minutes.

23. How do I treat hyperkalemia?

The type and speed of treatment depend on the potassium levels and electrocardiogram changes. Potassium may be forced out of the cell by acidosis. Treatment of the acidosis causes potassium to return to the cell and out of the serum (Table 33.2).

KEY POINTS: ACIDOSIS/HYPERKALEMIA

1. Avoid bicarbonate—especially in the treatment of diabetic ketoacidosis—because it has been associated with cerebral edema
2. Treat hyperkalemia on the basis of the electrocardiogram, clinical picture, and cause, not just on the basis of serum value

24. How do I treat hypercalcemia?

Search for the causative etiology. For mild hypercalcemia (calcium < 12 mg/dL), no immediate treatment is needed. Chronic moderate hypercalcemia (12-14 mg/dL) is often well tolerated and may not need treatment. For severe hypercalcemia (>14 mg/dL), restore intravascular volume with IV isotonic saline. Consider giving calcitonin or bisphosphonates in consultation with a pediatric nephrologist or endocrinologist. Loop diuretics such as furosemide are no longer recommended due to the risk of electrolyte imbalance and hypovolemia. (Furosemide may be helpful if there is fluid overload from renal failure or congestive heart failure.)

Table 33.2 Treatment of Hyperkalemia

POTASSIUM LEVEL (MEQ/DL)	ECG FINDING	TREATMENT
<7.0	Peaked T waves only, or normal	Remove potassium source, treat acidosis with Kayexalate (1 g/kg orally or rectally) every 4-6 hr
7.0	Widespread ECG changes without arrhythmia	Glucose (0.5 g/kg or 5 mL/kg of D_{10} over 30-60 min) *and* insulin (0.1 U/kg over 30-60 min) *plus* bicarbonate (2 mEq/kg over 30-60 min)
8.0	Arrhythmia	10% calcium gluconate (0.5 mL/kg over 2-5 min with ECG monitoring; discontinue if heart rate < 100 beats/min) *plus* glucose *and* insulin, bicarbonate as earlier

ECG, electrocardiogram.

25. How do I treat hypocalcemia?
     First, check the ionized calcium and confirm the diagnosis. Oral supplementation is reasonable if symptoms are mild, chronic, or absent. IV formulation is reserved for patients with significant symptoms. For patients with cardiac disturbance, treat with calcium gluconate 50 to 100 mg/kg infused over 3 to 5 minutes. For patients with tetany, treat with 100 to 200 mg/kg infused over 5 to 10 minutes. Calcium carbonate is another option; however, this should only be infused via central access. Take caution to deliver calcium carbonate slowly to avoid bradycardia and arrest.

BIBLIOGRAPHY

1. Byerley JS. Is this child dehydrated? *JAMA*. 2004;291:2746–2754.
2. Feld LG, Neuspiel DR, Foster BA, et al. Clinical practice guideline: maintenance intravenous fluids in children. *Pediatrics*. 2018;142(6): e20183083.
3. Freedman SB, Adler M, Seshadri R, et al. Oral ondansetron for gastroenteritis in a pediatric emergency department. *N Engl J Med*. 2006;354(16):1698–1705.
4. Freedman SB, Willan AR, Boutis K, et al. Effect of dilute apple juice and preferred fluids vs electrolyte maintenance solution on treatment failure among children with mild gastroenteritis: a randomized clinical trial. *JAMA*. 2016;315(18):1966–1974.
5. Hartling L, Bellemare S, Wiebe N, et al. Oral versus intravenous rehydration for treating dehydration due to gastroenteritis in children. *Cochrane Database Syst Rev*. 2006;(3):CD004390.
6. Kaplan R, Burns R. Renal and electrolyte emergencies. In: Shaw KN, Bachur RG, eds. *Fleisher & Ludwig's Textbook of Pediatric Emergency Medicine*. 8th ed. Wolters Kluwer; 2021:965–989.
7. Powers KS. Dehydration: isonatremic, hyponatremic, and hypernatremic recognition and management. *Pediatr Rev*. 2015;36(7):274–283.
8. Meskill S, Morrow A. Dehydration. In: Shaw KN, Bachur RG, eds. *Fleisher & Ludwig's Textbook of Pediatric Emergency Medicine*. 8th ed. Wolters Kluwer; 2021:146–151.
9. Spandorfer PR, Alessandrini EA, Joffe MD, et al. Oral versus intravenous rehydration of moderately dehydrated children: a randomized, controlled trial. *Pediatrics*. 2005;115:295–301.

CHAPTER 34

GASTROINTESTINAL EMERGENCIES

Susan Fuchs

1. **What is the most common cause of vomiting in older children?**

   Acute gastroenteritis. Although usually associated with diarrhea, vomiting can occur alone in the early stages of gastroenteritis. The most common infectious viral causes are rotavirus, norovirus, and enterovirus. Bacterial causes include *Salmonella, Shigella, Yersinia, Campylobacter* sp., and *Escherichia coli.*

2. **What are other medical causes of vomiting in children?**

   Vomiting can be the leading symptom in a variety of diagnoses. Metabolic disorders, such as galactosemia, fructose intolerance, congenital adrenal hyperplasia, and amino acid or organic acid defects (phenylketonuria, urea cycle defects), usually present in infancy. Along with vomiting, symptoms such as lethargy, seizures, or coma may occur. Diabetes mellitus can cause vomiting because of ketoacidosis or slowed gastric motility. Other causes include milk/soy protein intolerance, strep pharyngitis, pancreatitis, urinary tract infection, neurologic disorders associated with increased intracranial pressure (tumor, hydrocephalus), migraines, pregnancy, toxic ingestions (lead, iron), and psychological causes (rumination, bulimia).

3. **Where are you most likely to find an ingested coin that has not passed?**

   In the esophagus. The cricopharyngeus/thoracic inlet (proximal third) is the most common place, with 60% to 70% lodged here. The level of the aortic arch (middle third) accounts for 10% to 20%, and the gastroesophageal junction/sphincter (lower third) accounts for the other 20%. Coins >23.5 mm such as an American and Canadian quarter are more likely to be impacted, especially in children <5 years. Other areas of the gastrointestinal (GI) tract where the coin may be found are the stomach, pylorus, ligament of Treitz, and ileocecal valve. Objects larger than 25 mm in diameter or longer than 6 cm are more likely to get "caught" at the pylorus.

4. **What is the best way to remove an esophageal coin?**

   When the foreign body has been lodged for less than 24 hours, no respiratory symptoms are present, and the child has no prior esophageal disease or surgery, 20% to 30% will pass spontaneously. If the child is asymptomatic, and the coin does not pass in 24 hours, it should be removed. However, if the child is symptomatic (unable to handle secretions, dysphagia, or respiratory symptoms such as wheezing or stridor), urgent removal by endoscopy is indicated. There are several methods of coin removal in infants and children with no respiratory symptoms and no history of esophageal disease. Some use Foley catheter extraction under fluoroscopic guidance for coins that have been lodged for less than 24 hours. Others use esophageal bougienage for coins lodged in the distal esophagus for less than 24 hours, which involves pushing the coin through the esophagus into the stomach. Another method is the penny pincher technique, which involves insertion of a grasping forceps through an NG tube under fluoroscopic guidance. Laryngoscopy with Magill forceps removal, esophagoscopy, or flexible or rigid endoscopy under general anesthesia are other options. The choice of method is often based on the expertise and availability of the specialists (radiology, otolaryngology, surgery, or gastroenterology) at a particular hospital.

   Fun fact: A dime is 18 mm, a nickel 21 mm, and a quarter 24 mm in diameter.

5. **What is the "big deal" about button batteries?**

   Although they are small (watch or hearing aid batteries), there is a risk of leakage of battery contents, electrical discharge, and pressure necrosis. If the battery remains in the esophagus, tissue damage may occur, with resultant erosions, tracheoesophageal fistulas, strictures, vocal cord paralysis, and aortoenteric fistula. Batteries larger than 12 mm are most likely to become lodged in the esophagus.

6. **How should an ingestion of a button battery be managed?**

   Button batteries range in diameter from 6 to 25 mm, notably similar to coins. X-rays can be helpful to decipher FB ingestion. On the lateral radiograph, batteries have a step-off (coins do not, but two coins could look like a battery). On anteroposterior (AP) radiographs, batteries have a double-ring or halo effect (coins do not). Button batteries in the esophagus should be immediately removed under direct visualization to assess for any damage to the esophageal mucosa. Pressure necrosis can result when the battery places pressure on surrounding tissue, leading to inflammation and irritation, which can lead to tissue necrosis. Lithium batteries tend to be larger (≥20 mm) and have the most complications.

   A recent recommendation from the National Capital Poison Center is to give honey, 10 mL every 10 minutes if the child is >12 months and a lithium button battery was ingested. This treatment can start at home but should not delay going to the Emergency Department (ED). When in the ED, give honey or sucralfate if less than 12 hours after ingestion. Honey is used to coat the battery and prevent the local generation of hydroxide, delaying alkali burns to adjacent tissue. If the battery is in the stomach, which is acidic, the seal of the battery may erode and potentially release alkali solutions that can cause liquefaction necrosis of the stomach mucosa. If there are no symptoms of GI injury (pain, hematemesis, hematochezia, and obstruction), and the patient is <5 years and the button battery is ≥20 mm, admit and consider endoscopic removal within 24 to 48 hours, if it does not pass spontaneously. If the patient is ≥5 years and/or the button battery is <20 mm, outpatient management can be considered. Repeat the radiograph in 48 hours for a button battery ≥20 mm, and repeat the radiograph in 10 to 14 days for a button battery <20 mm if it fails to pass in the stool.

Fun fact: Many batteries are made of mercuric oxide. There is little risk of mercury poisoning because mercuric oxide is poorly absorbed from the GI tract.

Fun fact: Battery identification can provide the chemical content, diameter, and height of the battery. The battery code uses letters followed by three or four numbers. The letters identify the chemical content (e.g., S, silver oxide; G, copper oxide; LR or AG, alkaline; CR, lithium/manganese oxide; BR, lithium carbon monofluoride). The three-number codes give the diameter (mm) in the first number and the height in tenths of millimeters in the last two. If there are four numbers, the first two are the diameter, then the last two are the height. For example, S712 is a silver oxide battery that is 7 mm in diameter and 1.2 mm high. CR2032 is a lithium/manganese battery that is 20 mm in diameter.

7. **If a child swallowed a magnet, should I be worried?**
   Yes. There is a high rate of complications from magnet ingestions. Although the Consumer Product Safety Commission (CPSC) raised the recommended age for magnetic children's toys to 6 years in 2006, the emergence of high-powered "rare earth" magnets in adult toys, cordless tools, and other household products has led to more cases of magnet ingestion. These magnets are made of neodymium, iron, and boron and are 5 to 10 times stronger than traditional magnets. The CPSC issued a ban on the sale of these magnets for children's use in 2009, and marketing of small high-powered magnets was initially restricted by recalls and a federal safety standard, but this was overturned in 2016. That has resulted in an increase in ED visits for magnet ingestions.

   The main concern is that loops of the bowel can be trapped between two magnets leading to intestinal obstruction, perforation, fistula formation, peritonitis, and even death. Even if a magnet is removed promptly (within 8 hours), ulcerations can occur. Obtain abdominal and chest radiographs in two views (AP [chest]/flat plate[abdomen] and lateral) to determine the number and position of the magnets. A concern is that radiographs do not reliably distinguish between one and two magnets.

8. **Do all magnets need to be removed?**
   If there are multiple magnets or a single magnet and another metallic object, and all are within the esophagus or stomach, it should be removed by GI or surgery, especially if <12 hours. If >12 hours, consult pediatric surgery for endoscopic removal, as there is concern that after this time, the risk of complications is increased. If there are multiple magnets beyond the stomach, asymptomatic patients should be admitted and followed by radiographs and physical examination every 4 to 6 hours. Magnets can also be removed by colonoscopy or enteroscopy. Symptomatic patients should undergo surgery for removal.

   If there is a single magnet within the esophagus or stomach, consult GI or surgery and consider removal if the child is at risk for further ingestions or follow-up with serial radiographs. If beyond the stomach, consider removal if possible or confirm passage with serial radiographs. If there is still a delay in passage, consider using a laxative.

9. **Distinguish among hematemesis, hematochezia, and melena.**
   - Hematemesis is the vomiting of bright red or denatured blood ("coffee-ground" appearance) and signifies an upper GI bleed. The source of the blood is proximal to the ligament of Treitz.
   - Hematochezia is bright red blood or maroon-colored blood or stools per rectum and implies a lower GI source (distal to the ligament of Treitz).
   - Melena is the rectal passage of black tarry stools (black from the bacterial breakdown of blood); the source is proximal to the ileocecal valve or from swallowed blood.

10. **What are some of the common tests used to determine the presence of blood? What causes them to be falsely positive or falsely negative?**
    The Hematest is a qualitative stool test that uses orthotolidine (a leukodye). False-positive results occur when the patient has ingested red meats, iron preparations, or plant peroxidases (found in horseradish, turnips, tomatoes, and fresh red cherries). False-negative results occur in the presence of ascorbic acid (vitamin C).

    The Hemoccult test is a qualitative stool test that uses guaiac (also a leukodye). False-positive results occur with red meats, broccoli, grapes, cauliflower, cantaloupe, turnips, iron preparations, plant peroxidases, and cimetidine. False-negative results occur with hard stool, penicillamine, antacids, and ascorbic acid.

    The HemoQuant test is the only quantitative test (2 mg hemoglobin per gram of stool) and uses a fluorescent antibody to porphyrin. It is falsely positive with red meat. Gastroccult tests check gastric fluids for blood.

11. **A child presents with bright red blood stools, but the qualitative study is negative and the child is well appearing. What did the child likely ingest?**
This is a relatively common ED presentation. Often, a careful history will reveal recent ingestion of fruit punch, Kool-Aid beverages (especially cherry or strawberry), red beets, red licorice, tomatoes, gelatin, rifampin, cefdinir, and red-dyed snack food ("red hot" snacks). Note that commercial dyes can also be found in breakfast cereals. Of note, *Serratia marcescens* in stool can cause red coloring in diapers.

12. **Similarly, what foods or items can cause black stools?**
Bismuth (Pepto-Bismol), iron preparations, charcoal, black licorice, beets, spinach, blueberries, grape juice, dark chocolate, and swallowed blood.

13. **What is the APT-Downey test? How is it used?**
This test is for fetal red blood cells and is used when an infant spits up blood. If the infant is breastfeeding, it is often unclear if the blood is from the baby's GI tract or maternal milk. Adult hemoglobin is denatured to alkaline globin hematin in an alkaline solution (sodium hydroxide), resulting in a yellow-brown color. Fetal hemoglobin resists the effect of alkali and stays pink. However, if the blood you use for the test is coffee-ground color (not red), it will be read falsely as adult blood.

14. **What are some common causes of <u>upper</u> GI bleeding in infants and children?**
- **Neonates:** Swallowed maternal blood, esophagitis, coagulopathy, vitamin K deficiency, hemophilia, sepsis, gastritis (stress ulcer), congenital anomalies (intestinal duplication or vascular anomalies), milk protein intolerance
- **Infants (age 1 to 12 months):** Gastritis, esophagitis, stress ulcer, Mallory-Weiss tear, duplication cyst, button battery ingestion, vascular malformation
- **Children (age 1 to 12 years):** Epistaxis, esophagitis, gastritis, peptic ulcers, Mallory-Weiss tear, esophageal varices, toxic ingestion, esophageal and GI foreign bodies
- **Adolescents:** Ulcers, esophagitis, varices, gastritis, Mallory-Weiss tear, nonsteroidal anti-inflammatory use, toxic ingestion

15. **What are some common causes of <u>lower</u> GI bleeding in infants and children?**
- **Neonates:** Swallowed maternal blood, anorectal lesions, milk- or soy-induced colitis, necrotizing enterocolitis, malrotation with midgut volvulus, Hirschsprung disease
- **Infants (age 1 to 12 months):** Anal fissure, malrotation with midgut volvulus, intussusception, Meckel diverticulum, infectious diarrhea, milk- or soy-induced colitis, intestinal duplication
- **Children (age 1 to 12 years):** Anal fissures, polyps, Meckel diverticulum, intussusception, infectious diarrhea, inflammatory bowel disease, duplications, hemangiomas, Henoch-Schönlein purpura, hemolytic uremic syndrome (HUS)
- **Adolescents:** Inflammatory bowel disease (ulcerative colitis, Crohn's disease), polyps, hemorrhoids, anal fissure, infectious diarrhea

16. **Distinguish between malrotation and volvulus.**
Malrotation is the incomplete or reverse rotation of the embryonic midgut about the superior mesenteric artery. The small bowel then hangs on a mesenteric stalk. Volvulus occurs when the midgut twists around the stalk, resulting in small bowel obstruction and vascular compromise due to compression of the mesenteric vessels. About 90% of intestinal rotation anomalies are found in children <1 year. One-third of children with malrotation present before 1 month with volvulus.

17. **What are the clinical features of malrotation with volvulus?**
An infant with malrotation and volvulus is typically less than 1 month. Symptoms include bilious vomiting, irritability, and abdominal pain. When volvulus is present, there are bloody or heme-positive stools. The infant can rapidly progress to a shock-like state. The physical examination reveals abdominal distention (from dilated loops of bowel), lethargy, pallor, and possibly hypotension. Therapy includes fluid resuscitation, nasogastric tube, broad-spectrum antibiotics, and emergent surgery (Ladd procedure).

18. **What is the radiographic finding in an infant with malrotation and volvulus?**
Abdominal radiographs may be normal (50%-60% of patients with malrotation and volvulus) or show duodenal obstruction ("double bubble"). In patients with high suspicion of malrotation with volvulus, an upper GI study should be promptly obtained. It is 96% specific and shows a displaced duodenal-jejunal junction (both to the right of the spine). There may be a corkscrew appearance of contrast material. A barium enema may show a displaced cecum, usually in the right upper quadrant, or an abnormally oriented superior mesenteric artery, but should not be used for the diagnosis of malrotation.

An ultrasound may be useful to diagnose malrotation, but a normal ultrasound does not exclude malrotation. It is more specific and sensitive for volvulus. Findings may include an abnormal position of the superior mesenteric vein, a dilated duodenum, the third part of the duodenum not in the normal position, or the "whirlpool sign" of volvulus (due to vessels twisting).

19. **A child who has had surgical correction for Hirschsprung disease presents with fever, vomiting, abdominal distention, and explosive diarrhea. What is your concern?**
    This child probably has Hirschsprung's enterocolitis. Enterocolitis is the most common cause of death in children with Hirschsprung disease. Other complications include persistent bowel obstructive symptoms, constipation, and fecal incontinence. This patient requires intravenous (IV) fluids, nasogastric drainage, broad-spectrum antibiotics, and decompression of the rectum or colon by rectal stimulation or irrigation.

20. **True or false: Pain is worse after meals in younger children with ulcers.**
    False. In most young children with ulcers, pain is not related to meals. In some older children and adolescents, pain may be exacerbated by acidic foods or spicy meals, as in adults. Symptoms in neonates include vomiting; infants may feed poorly or vomit; toddlers may have poorly localized abdominal pain or vomiting; adolescents may have epigastric pain. All age groups can have melena or upper GI bleeding.

21. **What is the relationship between *Helicobacter pylori* and gastritis/peptic ulcers in children?**
    H. pylori is a gram-negative, spiral-shaped bacterium that is the most common cause of peptic ulcers (both duodenal and gastric ulcers) and is associated with chronic gastritis in children. There is no relationship between gastroesophageal reflux and *H. pylori*.

22. **What is the best way to determine the presence of *H. pylori*?**
    Diagnosis can be made by invasive testing as well as noninvasive testing. Invasive testing by biopsy is the gold standard. The tissue can be tested for urease activity, can undergo histologic evaluation, and can be sent for bacterial culture. Noninvasive tests have been gaining in popularity as their sensitivity and specificity have improved but are not recommended for the initial diagnosis of *H. pylori*. The ^{13}C-urea breath test is based upon the hydrolysis of urea to CO_2 and ammonia by *H. pylori* and can be used for diagnosis in children ≥ 6 years. *H. pylori* stool antigen assay can be used in all ages but is preferred for younger children. Serologic testing to detect IgG or IgA antibodies is not recommended, due to wide sensitivity and specificity.

23. **What is the therapy for *H. pylori* infection in children?**
    Eradication therapy is recommended for children with a definitive peptic ulcer and *H. pylori* on histologic examination. Triple or quadruple therapy is recommended and is based on antibiotic sensitivity testing. This includes the following first-line therapies in a twice-daily fashion for 14 days:
    - Amoxicillin, 50 mg/kg/day (up to 1 g twice daily) (if allergic use metronidazole)
    - Clarithromycin, 15 mg/kg/day (up to 500 mg twice daily) (if resistant, use metronidazole)
      - Metronidazole 20 mg/kg/day (up to 500 mg twice daily). If there is resistance to both metronidazole and clarithromycin use high-dose amoxicillin or bismuth.
    - Proton-pump inhibitor (PPI; e.g., omeprazole), 1 mg/kg/day (up to 40 mg twice daily)
    - Quadruple therapy for children <8 years old is PPI, Amoxicillin, and Metronidazole with the addition of bismuth

24. Describe some of the anatomic and histologic differences between ulcerative colitis and Crohn's disease.
    - **Ulcerative colitis:** Inflammation of the mucosa and submucosa is limited to the colon and rectum, with continuous involvement in these regions. There are various degrees of ulceration, hemorrhage, and pseudopolyps.
    - **Crohn's disease:** The disease can involve any portion of the alimentary tract, including the upper GI tract (30%-40% of cases), small bowel (90%), and terminal ileum (50%-70%). There is transmural inflammation, with discrete lesions ("skip lesions"). Because of the full-thickness involvement, there can be focal linear ulcerations, granulomas, strictures, and a cobblestone appearance. There can also be perianal fistulas, abscesses, or large (>5 mm) skin tags.

25. What are some of the extraintestinal features of ulcerative colitis and Crohn's disease?
    Because both can present with bloody diarrhea, abdominal pain, weight loss, and fever, extraintestinal manifestations may help determine which is more likely prior to endoscopy.
    - **Ulcerative colitis:** Growth failure, arthropathy/arthritis, pyoderma gangrenosum
    - **Crohn's disease:** Growth failure, delayed puberty, perianal disease, stomatitis, erythema nodosum, arthritis, clubbing, uveitis, nephrolithiasis

26. What are some of the food allergy disorders of infancy and their treatment?
    Food protein-induced proctitis/proctocolitis is found in infants between 2 and 8 weeks who are breastfed or fed cow's milk or soy-based formulas. The infant presents with blood-tinged mucus or stool, may be fussy or irritable, and may have increased stool frequency, but not diarrhea. The problem resolves when the mother stops eating the presumed food antigen or the formula is changed.

    Food protein–induced enteropathy presents in infancy with diarrhea and poor weight gain. Vomiting and malabsorption also occur. Milk sensitivity is the usual culprit, but soy, egg, wheat, and other food can cause this. A biopsy of the small intestine shows villous atrophy with cellular infiltration. These symptoms also improve when the agent is removed, but these reactions often resolve on their own by 1 year of age.

    Food protein–induced enterocolitis syndrome is a non-IgE mediated gut reaction that occurs in the first few months of life and involves allergy mainly to milk protein and soy. The child has protracted vomiting and diarrhea (which can be bloody) and has poor weight gain/failure to thrive. These infants often present with lethargy, pallor and may present in shock due to dehydration. Lab abnormalities include hypoalbuminemia, leukocytosis, and anemia. In these cases, substitute whole cow's milk with casein hydrolysate formulas (Nutramigen, Pregestimil, Alimentum) or amino acid–based formulas (Elecare, Neocate, Puramino). Even whey hydrolysate or soy protein formulas are not appropriate, as some children have allergies to these as well.

27. What is eosinophilic esophagitis?
    Eosinophilic esophagitis is a chronic immune/antigen-mediated disease of the esophagus characterized by eosinophil-predominant inflammation that results in esophageal dysfunction. There may be a link between environmental (food allergies) and genetic factors. The clinical symptoms in children include vomiting, abdominal pain, feeding dysfunction, dysphagia, and food impaction. There is a family history of atopy in 35% to 45% of patients.

28. How do you diagnose eosinophilic esophagitis?
    Diagnosis requires symptoms related to chronic esophageal dysfunction, dysphagia, or gastrointestinal reflux. Upper endoscopy with biopsies should be performed after a course of acid suppression with a PPI and shows eosinophil predominate inflammation and a peak value of $\geq>15$ eosinophils per high power field (or 60 eosinophils per mm²). There is a scoring system that looks at findings such as basal zone hyperplasia, the presence of eosinophilic abscesses, and superficial layering of eosinophils.

    Fun fact. The main allergens for eosinophilic esophagitis are milk, egg, wheat, soy, peanuts/tree nuts, and seafood (fish/shellfish).

29. What is celiac disease?
    Celiac disease is an immune-mediated inflammatory disease of the small intestine due to gluten, a protein found in grains. The specific proteins are gliadin in wheat, secalines in rye, and hordeins in barley. Some patients may also have problems with oats. It is a human leukocyte antigen (HLA)–associated condition (HLA DQ2/DQ8). Presenting symptoms include weight loss/failure to thrive, chronic diarrhea, steatorrhea, and abdominal pain and distention. Some extraintestinal symptoms include arthritis or arthralgia, chronic fatigue, short stature or poor height gain, pubertal delay, dermatitis herpetiformis skin rash, dental enamel hypoplasia, recurrent aphthous stomatitis, and behavioral abnormalities. Lab findings include elevated liver enzymes (alanine transaminase, aspartate aminotransferase 2-3 times normal), and iron deficiency anemia.

30. **What is the treatment for celiac disease?**
A gluten-free diet is the treatment. This means avoiding barley, bran, couscous, durum, faro, matzo flour, orzo, panko, rye, seitan, semolina, spelt, udon, and wheat for the duration of the patient's life. Lots of other foods such as croutons, candy, energy bars, processed meats, pasta, stuffing, soy sauce, marinades, some prescription and over-the-counter medications, nutritional supplements, vitamins, and mineral supplements contain gluten, so families must read ingredient labels carefully. On the other hand, the following are gluten-free grains and starches and can be safely tolerated: amaranth, arrowroot, buckwheat, corn, flax, seeds, millet, potato starch, potato flour, quinoa, rice, sorghum, tapioca, and teff.

31. **What are some of the malignant neoplasms of the GI tract and liver in children?**
Lymphoma, colorectal carcinoma, neuroendocrine (carcinoid) tumors, soft tissue sarcoma, adenocarcinoma, hepatoblastoma, hepatocarcinoma, and biliary rhabdomyosarcoma.

32. **What is the classic triad of findings associated with HUS?**
Acute hemolytic anemia, thrombocytopenia, and renal injury (manifested by oliguria, abnormal urinalysis, and increasing blood urea nitrogen and creatinine levels). Although it is usually associated with bloody diarrhea, there are actually two phenotypes of HUS. One is Shiga toxin–associated HUS, which is associated with diarrhea (D-HUS, or typical HUS); the other is non–Shiga toxin–associated HUS, which does not present with diarrhea (D-HUS, or atypical HUS). The Shiga toxin is elaborated by *E. coli* O157:H7 or *Shigella dysenteriae* type 1. *Streptococcus pneumoniae* has also been associated with HUS and is usually accompanied by pneumonia with empyema or effusion.

33. **A child has diarrhea as a result of *E. coli* O157:H7. Should he receive antibiotics?**
No. The child has an increased risk of developing HUS if antibiotics are given during the diarrheal phase of the illness. In addition, the use of antimotility agents also increases the risk of HUS.

34. **Which laboratory tests should you order for a child you think has pancreatitis?**
Serum lipase is the test of choice for acute pancreatitis as it is more specific than amylase. A positive test is lipase activity >3 times the upper limit of normal. Serum lipase rises by 4 to 8 hours, peaks at 24 to 48 hours, and remains elevated for 8 to 14 days. Serum amylase usually rises within 6 hours after the onset of symptoms and returns to normal within 3 to 5 days. Because amylase is produced in the salivary glands and ovaries, an isolated serum amylase level does not necessarily reflect pancreatic origin.

35. **What causes pancreatitis in children?**
Acute pancreatitis in children is due to one of several causes:
- Anatomic/structural abnormalities (choledochal cysts, cholelithiasis, pancreatic duct abnormalities, tumors)
- Drugs and toxins (acetaminophen, antibiotics (tetracycline, metronidazole, sulfonamides), anticonvulsants (valproic acid), antihypertensives (enalapril, lisinopril), corticosteroids, antineoplastic agents (L-asparaginase, 6-mercaptopurine), ethanol)
- Infections (hepatitis A, *Ascaris lumbricoides*, Ebstein-Barr virus, mumps, coxsackievirus, influenza B virus)
- Trauma (disruption of pancreatic ducts, compression injury)
- Genetic disease (cystic fibrosis, gene mutations)
- Metabolic disorder (hyperlipidemia, hyperparathyroidism, malnutrition)
- Autoimmune and collagen vascular disease
- Solid organ transplant
- Idiopathic
  Fun fact: the pneumonic TIGAR-O can help remember etiologies of pancreatitis: toxic-metabolic, idiopathic, genetic, autoimmune, recurrent/severe, and obstructive.

36. **What is cyclic vomiting syndrome and its diagnostic criteria?**
This syndrome of vomiting in a cyclic pattern is severe, recurring, and stereotypical.
   Pediatric criteria include:
- At least five attacks in any interval or a minimum of three episodes of vomiting within a 6-month period
- Acute attacks of intense nausea and vomiting lasting 1 hour to 10 days, occurring at least 1 week apart
- Vomiting that occurs during attacks at least four times an hour for at least 1 hour
- Stereotypical pattern and symptoms for each patient
- No symptoms between episodes of vomiting
- No identifiable organic cause of the vomiting
   Vomiting is often precipitated by psychological stress, infection, exhaustion, a menstrual period, or certain foods (cheese, chocolate, caffeine, monosodium glutamate), and there is usually a strong family history of migraine headaches.

37. **What is ED treatment for cyclic vomiting?**
Treatment starts with IV fluids. Correct hypovolemia with 20 mL/kg normal saline boluses, then give 5% or 10% dextrose in 0.45 normal saline (D_{5-10}0.45-5NS) at 1.5 times maintenance, an antiemetic such as ondansetron, and a sedative such as lorazepam (or chlorpromazine or diphenhydramine). Keeping the room dark and quiet often helps. If headache or abdominal pain occurs, a nonsteroidal antiinflammatory agent such as ketorolac can be given.

38. **What is cannabinoid hyperemesis syndrome (CES)?**
CES is characterized by cyclic episodes of nausea and vomiting and abdominal pain, often relieved by hot showers. It occurs in those who have used cannabis regularly for at least 1 year. Vomiting can occur six to eight times an hour, with an episode lasting up to 48 hours. This cycle repeats every few weeks or months. Although often confused with cyclic vomiting, the chronic use of marijuana is the distinguishing feature. Those with CES do not usually have a migraine headache (like those with cyclic vomiting), and gastric emptying rates are delayed in CES but increased in cyclic vomiting. ED treatment includes IV fluids, antiemetics, and a PPI. Typical treatment with ondansetron may not be effective. Recent studies have shown that capsaicin cream (0.75%) applied to the abdomen and periumbilical region resulted in the resolution of the episode. The only cure is the cessation of the use of cannabis. Consider this condition in a teenager who has persistent vomiting despite usual treatment. A urine drug screen is helpful to make the diagnosis.

39. **What is the typical history of the GI symptoms associated with IgA vasculitis (Henoch-Schönlein purpura)?**
GI symptoms normally include nausea, vomiting, abdominal pain, and lower GI bleeding and can occasionally result in intussusception, bowel ischemia/infarction, and intestinal perforation. The GI symptoms usually develop within 8 days of the rash. Although palpable purpura is the presenting sign in 75% of cases, GI symptoms, including abdominal pain, precede the rash in about 15% to 35% of cases, making the diagnosis of this condition more challenging. Other symptoms include arthritis/arthralgia and hematuria without red cell casts and mild proteinuria, scrotal pain, and tenderness.

40. **What is the suggested imaging study in suspected intussusception associated with IgA vasculitis (Henoch-Schönlein purpura)?**
Abdominal ultrasonography is recommended as opposed to air or barium contrast enema, as ileoileal intussusception is seen in 75% of cases and contrast enemas cannot make the diagnosis of ileoileal intussusception.

41. **What is a Meckel diverticulum?**
Meckel diverticulum is a remnant of the vitellointestinal or omphalomesenteric duct that may result in painless rectal bleeding. It is present in 2% of the population, is 2 inches long (or less), and is found within 2 feet of the ileocecal valve. It contains ectopic gastric mucosa in 60% to 90% of patients and in almost all of those who have painless rectal bleeding. (The gastric mucosa can result in an ulcer, which bleeds.) Diagnosis is by a Meckel scan (technetium-99 m pertechnetate scan). Gastric mucosa concentrates the technetium-99. An intestinal duplication may also contain gastric mucosa and can cause GI bleeding or symptoms of obstruction or intussusception. A duplication occurs most commonly in the ileocecal region but also is found in the distal esophagus, stomach, and duodenum.

BIBLIOGRAPHY

1. Bonis PA, Gupta SK. In: Post TW, ed. *Clinical Manifestations, and Diagnosis of Eosinophilic Esophagitis.* UpToDate; 2021.
2. Brandt M.I. In: Post TW, ed. *Intestinal Malrotation in Children.* UpToDate; 2021.
3. Buccigrossi V, Spagnuolo MI. Bacterial infections of the small and large intestine. In: Guandalini S, Dhawan A, Branski D, eds.*Textbook of Pediatric Gastroenterology, Hepatology and Nutrition.* Springer; 2016:171–184.
4. Burke W. In: Post TW, ed. *Clinical Manifestations of Food Allergy: An Overview.* UpToDate; 2021.
5. Cucchiara Aloi M. Crohn's Disease. In: Guandalini S, Dhawan A, Branski D (ed): *Textbook of Pediatric Gastroenterology, Hepatology and Nutrition.* Springer, 2016, pp 323-334.
6. Crowley J, Hussey S. Helicobacter pylori in childhood. In: Wyllie R, Hyams JS, Kay M, eds.*Pediatric Gastrointestinal and Liver Disease.* 6th ed. Elsevier; 2021:275–292.
7. Cucchiara Aloi M. Crohn's disease. In: Guandalini S, Dhawan A, Branski D, eds.*Textbook of Pediatric Gastroenterology, Hepatology and Nutrition.* Springer; 2016:323–334.
8. Dedeoglu F, Kim S. In: Post TW, ed. *IgA Vasculitis (Henoch-Schönlein Purpura): Clinical Manifestations and Diagnosis.* UpToDate; 2021.
9. Eosinophilic Esophagitis Home. Eosinophilic esophagitis diet overview. https://eosinophilicesophagitishome.org, Accessed 18.04.22.
10. Di Lorenzo C. In: Post TW, ed. *Approach to the Infant or Child With Nausea and Vomiting.* UpToDate; 2021.
11. Galli J, Sawaya RA, Friedenberg FK. Cannabinoid hyperemesis syndrome. *Curr Drug Abuse Rev.* 2011;4(4):241–249.
12. Galloway D, Cohen MB. Infectious diarrhea. In: Wyllie R, Hyams JS, Kay M, eds.*Pediatric Gastrointestinal and Liver Disease.* 6th ed. Elsevier; 2021:398–415.
13. Gold B, Jones NL. In: Post TW, ed. *Helicobacter pylori: Diagnosis and Management in the Pediatric Patients.* UpToDate; 2021.

14. *GIKids.org*. Gluten-free diet guide for families. <https://toolbox.naspghan.org/nutitio/diets-for-diseases>. Accessed 15.04.22.
15. Gilger MA, Jain AK. *Foreign Bodies of the Esophagus and Gastrointestinal Tract in Children*. UpToDate; 2021.
16. Higuchi L, Bousvaros A. In: Post TW, ed. *Clinical Presentation and Diagnosis of Inflammatory Bowel Disease in Children*. UpToDate; 2021.
17. Higuchi LM, Regan B. Bousvaros. Ulcerative colitis. In: Guandalini S, Dhawan A, Branski D, eds. *Textbook of Pediatric Gastroenterology, Hepatology and Nutrition*. Springer; 2016:341–368.
18. Hill ID. In: Post TW, ed. *Diagnosis of Celiac Disease in Children*. UpToDate; 2021.
19. Hill ID, Fasano A, Guandalini S, Hoffenberg E, et al. NASPGHAN clinical report on the diagnosis and treatment of gluten-related disorders. *JPGN*. 2016;63(1):156–165.
20. *Poison Center Button: National Capital Poison*. National Capital Poison Center Button Battery Ingestion Triage and Treatment Guideline. <https://www.poison.org/battery/guideline>, 2021 Accessed 25.04.22.
21. Hyer W, Tavares M, Thomson M. Polyps and other tumors of the gastrointestinal tract. In: Guandalini S, Dhawan A, Branski D, eds. *Textbook of Pediatric Gastroenterology, Hepatology and Nutrition*. Springer; 2016:587–608.
22. Jarvis JR. Gastrointestinal bleeding. In: Shaw KN, Bachur RG, eds. *Fleisher & Ludwig's Textbook of Pediatric Emergency Medicine*. 8th ed. Wolters Kluwer; 2021:213–221.
23. Jones NL, Koletzko S, Goodman K, Bontems P, et al. Joint ESPGHAN/NASPGHAN guidelines for the management of Helicobacter pylori in children and adolescents (update 2016). *JPGN*. 2017;64(6):991–1003.
24. Kramer RE, Lerner DG, Lin T, Manfredi M, et al. Management of ingested foreign bodies in children: a clinical report of the NASPGHAN Endoscopy Committee. *JPGN*. 2015;60(4):562–574.
25. Kurkowski JA, Selvakumar PKC. Neoplasms of the gastrointestinal tract. In: Wyllie R, Hyams JS, Kay M, eds. *Pediatric Gastrointestinal and Liver Disease*. 6th ed. Elsevier; 2021:517–526.
26. Li BUK. In: Post TW, ed. *Cyclic Vomiting Syndrome*. UpToDate; 2021.
27. Lindley KJ, Koglmeier J. Vasculitides including Henoch-Schönlein purpura. In: Guandalini S, Dhawan A, Branski D, eds. *Textbook of Pediatric Gastroenterology, Hepatology and Nutrition*. Springer; 2016:369–376.
28. Markowitz JE, Venkatesh RD, Moye L, Liacouras CA. Allergic and eosinophilic gastrointestinal disease. In: Wyllie R, Hyams JS, Kay M, eds. *Pediatric Gastrointestinal and Liver Disease*. 6th ed. Elsevier; 2021:388–397.
29. Martinelli M, Staiano A. Hirschsprung's disease and intestinal neuronal dysplasia. In: Guandalini S, Dhawan A, Branski D, eds. *Textbook of Pediatric Gastroenterology, Hepatology and Nutrition*. Springer; 2016:261–268.
30. Mavis A, Goday PS, Werlin SL. Acute pancreatitis. In: Guandalini S, Dhawan A, Branski D, eds. *Textbook of Pediatric Gastroenterology, Hepatology and Nutrition*. Springer; 2016:385–394.
31. McConachie SM, Caputo RA, Wilhelm SM, Kale-Pradhan PB. Efficacy of capsaicin for the treatment of cannabinoid hyperemesis syndrome: a systematic review. *Ann Pharmacother*. 2019;53(1):1145–1152.
32. Mokha J. Vomiting and nausea. In: Wyllie R, Hyams JS, Kay M, eds. *Pediatric Gastrointestinal and Liver Disease*. 6th ed. Elsevier; 2021:70–87.
33. Mokha J. Vomiting and Nausea. In: Wyllie R, Hyams JS, Kay M, eds. *Pediatric Gastrointestinal and Liver Disease*. 6th ed. Elsevier; 2021:70–87.
34. Niaudet P. In: Post TW, ed. *Clinical Manifestations and Diagnosis of Shiga Toxin Associated (Typical) Hemolytic Uremic Syndrome*. UpToDate; 2021.
35. Patel N, Kay M. In: Post TW, ed. *Lower Gastrointestinal Bleeding in Children: Causes and Diagnostic Approach*. UpToDate,2022. Accessed October 26, 2023.
36. Piester T, Liu QY. Gastritis, gastropathy, and ulcer disease. In: Wyllie R, Hyams JS, Kay M, eds. *Pediatric Gastrointestinal and Liver Disease*. 6th ed. Elsevier; 2021:262–274.
37. Rela M, Reddy MS. Liver tumors in children. In: Guandalini S, Dhawan A, Branski D, eds. *Textbook of Pediatric Gastroenterology, Hepatology and Nutrition*. Springer; 2016:819–830.
38. Rus MC, Doughty C. Vomiting. In: Shaw KN, Bachur RG, eds. *Fleisher & Ludwig's Textbook of Pediatric Emergency Medicine*. 8th ed. Wolters Kluwer; 2021:548–555.
39. Sahn B, Mamula P, Friedlander JA. Gastrointestinal hemorrhage. In: Wyllie R, Hyams JS, Kay M, eds. *Pediatric Gastrointestinal and Liver Disease*. 6th ed. Elsevier; 2021:125–134.
40. Sato TT, Sato EH. Abnormal rotation and fixation of the intestine. In: Wyllie R, Hyams JS, Kay M, eds. *Pediatric Gastrointestinal and Liver Disease*. 6th ed. Elsevier; 2021:581–587.
41. Sinclair K, Hill ID. In: Post TW, ed. *Button and Cylindrical Battery Ingestion: Clinical Features, Diagnosis, and Initial Management*. UpToDate, 2022. Accessed October 26, 2023.
42. Sunku B, Li BUK. Cyclic vomiting syndrome. In: Guandalini S, Dhawan A, Branski D, eds. *Textbook of Pediatric Gastroenterology, Hepatology and Nutrition*. Springer; 2016:285–294.
43. Vege SS. In: Post TW, ed. *Clinical Manifestations and Diagnosis of Acute Pancreatitis*. UpToDate; 2021.
44. Villa X. In: Post TW, ed. *Approach to Upper Gastrointestinal Bleeding in Children*. UpToDate; 2021.

CHAPTER 35

GYNECOLOGIC EMERGENCIES

Kate M. Cronan

1. **A mother brought her 3-year-old daughter to the emergency department (ED) because she has noticed that her "vagina seems to be closing up." What could this be caused by?**
The description fits a diagnosis of labial adhesions. This is a benign condition occurring in 3% to 7% of girls between the ages of 3 months and 5 years (Fig. 35.1). The exact cause is not known, but it could be related to repeated bouts of vulvovaginitis. The majority heal on their own. The medial epithelial surfaces of the labia minora gradually adhere to one another, and the fusion proceeds anteriorly. Physical examination using labial traction reveals a flat area of adherent tissue, with a characteristic vertical raphe obscuring the introitus. A small opening remains through which urine may pass.

2. **What is the treatment for labial adhesions?**
Treatment for labial adhesions consists of twice-daily applications of estrogen cream at the point of the midline fusion. It is important to continue treatment until the lesions resolve. Once the adhesions have separated, instruct the caregiver to apply zinc oxide or petroleum jelly for an additional 2 weeks to prevent readherence. Medical therapy may rarely fail when the adhesions are thick (3-4 mm in width) with no evidence of a thin raphe.

3. **A healthy 14-year-old girl presents with urgency, frequency, and dysuria and complains of intermittent lower abdominal pain. The urinalysis is normal. She has not yet menstruated. What could be causing these symptoms?**
The somewhat late menarche is a clue to the diagnosis. To diagnose the problem, physical and genital examinations are necessary. Consider a congenital obstruction of the vagina, either an imperforate hymen or vaginal atresia. If this condition is not noticed during infancy, a young adolescent girl can present with large quantities of menstrual blood accumulated behind the hymen. The collection of blood is termed *hematocolpos*. Examination of the abdomen may reveal a mass that could initially be confused with a tumor or even pregnancy.

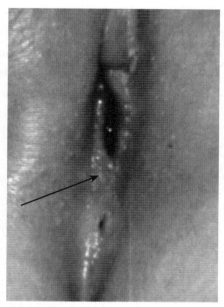

Fig. 35.1 Labial adhesions. (Modified from Stukus KS, Zuckerbraun NS. Review of the prepubertal gynecologic examination: techniques and anatomic variation. *Clin Pediatr Emerg Med*. 2009;10(9):3–9. Photograph courtesy Dr. Janet Squires, Children's Hospital of Pittsburgh.)

Examination of the genitalia shows a bulging, membranous covering over the introitus, often appearing bluish from the collection of blood. Treatment is surgical.

4. **How does hydrocolpos differ from hydrometrocolpos?**
Vaginal obstruction allows for vaginal secretions and occasionally urine to accumulate and cause vaginal dilation (hydrocolpos) and, in rare cases, dilatation of the uterus (hydrometrocolpos). This diagnosis is often made in utero or in an infant who may present with a palpable lower abdominal mass.

5. **How do hematocolpos and hematometrocolpos differ?**
If vaginal obstruction is not recognized until menarche, menstrual blood accumulates and distends the vagina, producing *hematocolpos*. In late puberty, the child may present with amenorrhea and cyclic episodes of lower abdominal pain occurring at monthly intervals. Eventually, urinary symptoms may develop as the collection of blood increases. A lower abdominal mass is often palpable (see Question 3). An ultrasound reveals a dilated vagina filled with blood products (hematocolpos). In severe cases, the uterus may also be dilated with blood products (hematometrocolpos).

6. **How does perineal trauma in young girls typically occur?**
Most perineal trauma in young girls results from a "straddle injury." This occurs when the girl falls on a narrow object (e.g., bicycle crossbar, jungle gym, chair arm, fence). The most common injuries are vulvar hematomas and superficial lacerations. Often, these may be treated conservatively with pain control and sitz baths several times a day. It is crucial to ensure that the patient can void prior to leaving the ED.

7. **What are the best ways to perform a genital examination on a prepubertal girl?**
First, examine the external genitalia with the child lying supine in a "frog-leg" position, either on the examining table or on the parent's lap. Use gentle lateral traction on the labia majora to obtain an adequate view of the introitus. To visualize the vaginal vault, examine the child in the "knee-chest" position. Have the child get up on her hands and knees ("like she is going to crawl") and rest her head on her folded arms. While the child relaxes her abdominal muscles, the labia and buttocks can be separated. An otoscope *without* a speculum or a small flashlight can be used as a light source. If discharge or bleeding is noted, return the child to the supine position to take samples/cultures. If you find that there is vaginal bleeding from an injury, it may be necessary to perform a speculum examination under sedation.

8. **How should urinary retention after a straddle injury be managed?**
In most cases, urinary retention is mild and brief, and it occurs because of the discomfort of the urine passing over the injured perineum. It is important to provide pain control. Girls may be more comfortable urinating while sitting in a tub of warm water.

9. **Describe possible injuries that can occur with more serious perineal trauma.**
With a very forceful straddle injury, deep lacerations may occur in the vagina and may extend into the rectum or urethra. Some hematomas may expand rapidly and become quite large, requiring evacuation. In these cases, the injuries must be explored thoroughly, either with effective sedation or under general anesthesia in the operating room. Consult colleagues from pediatric gynecology or pediatric urology as appropriate for surgical repair. Concerns are similar for penetrating trauma to the perineum by a foreign object.

10. **A 3-year-old African-American girl presents to the ED with vaginal bleeding and a donut-shaped mass of purplish tissue protruding from her vagina. Her mother is concerned that she might have been abused. What is your diagnosis?**
Although sexual assault must always be considered in the differential diagnosis of genital trauma, the soft donut-shaped mass in this child is most likely *not* protruding from the vagina. Consider a urethral prolapse (Fig. 35.2). This is the most common cause of *apparent* vaginal bleeding in childhood, with the bleeding resulting from ischemia of the protruding urethral mucosa. This happens mostly in African-American and Hispanic girls. If the segment of prolapsed urethra is not necrotic, warm compresses or sitz baths in combination with 2 weeks of topical estrogen may be effective. Dark red necrotic mucosa requires surgical reduction of the prolapse within several days.

11. **A 6-year-old girl has been urinating more frequently than usual and says that it hurts when she urinates. The symptoms seem like a urinary tract infection (UTI) but the urinalysis is normal. What could be causing her symptoms?**
Vulvovaginitis can include symptoms of urinary frequency and dysuria. It is often caused by irritation from poor hygiene or cleansing products such as bubble bath, soaps, and powders.
Infectious causes include *Shigella* spp., group A streptococci, *Neisseria gonorrhoeae*, and *Candida* spp. Pinworm infections may lead to intense itching and scratching resulting in perineal excoriations and bleeding.

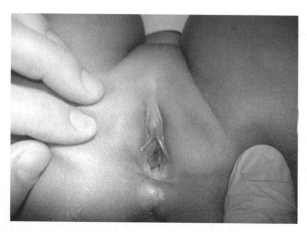

Fig. 35.2 Urethral prolapse. (Photograph by Steven M. Selbst, MD; used with permission.)

Vulvovaginitis can be treated with frequent sitz baths. If the vulva is irritated, the patient may be more comfortable voiding while sitting in a tub of warm water.

12. **What is the most common cause of foul-smelling vaginal discharge in young girls?**
Foul-smelling vaginal discharge usually signals a retained foreign body in the vagina. Toilet paper that may be contaminated with feces is the most common foreign body in this scenario. Other foreign bodies include crayons, toy parts, hair accessories, coins, and paper clips. To check for a foreign body, first place the patient in the knee-chest position to examine the vaginal area. Attach a 60-mL syringe filled with warmed saline to an 8-F feeding tube. Place the patient in the supine position and separate the labia majora. Viscous lidocaine may be applied prior to the insertion of the catheter. Then place the tube past the hymenal orifice and irrigate with saline.

13. **What is the first test to do on *any* adolescent patient with abnormal vaginal bleeding?**
A qualitative urine pregnancy test. An ectopic pregnancy can rapidly progress into a life-threatening emergency. In many instances, the urine sample can be obtained even before the physical examination is begun.

14. **What are the most common organisms causing sexually transmitted infection (STI) in the adolescent population?**
Chlamydia trachomatis and *N. gonorrhoeae* infections are the most commonly reported STIs among adolescent patients. The reported rates of chlamydial and gonorrheal infections are highest among females ages 15 to 19 years. Human papillomavirus and herpes simplex virus type 2 are also common. Neither are reportable diseases, so exact prevalence rates are not known. Human immunodeficiency virus (HIV) infection is increasing among adolescents, but rates of both primary and secondary syphilis have steadily declined in all age groups since peaking in 1990.

15. **True or false? Bacterial vaginosis (BV) occurs only in women who are sexually active.**
False. Women who have not been sexually active can also have BV. BV is the most prevalent reason for vaginal discharge in sexually active females and the most common vaginal condition in females ages 15 to 44 years. It is associated with having a new sexual partner, an increasing number of sexual partners, and a lack of condom use. Douching can upset the balance of vaginal bacteria and increase the risk of getting BV.

16. **Describe BV.**
BV is a clinical syndrome with changes in vaginal flora, usually due to a reduction in *Lactobacillus* species. Studies have shown that up to 50% of females with microbiologic criteria for a diagnosis of BV are not symptomatic. Classic signs are thin white or gray vaginal discharge with a fishy odor. Pruritus, abdominal pain, and vagina discharge are not usually seen with BV.

17. **What are the changes in microorganisms that cause pelvic inflammatory disease (PID)?**
C. trachomatis and *N. gonorrhoeae* are the pathogens most associated with PID. However, currently, less than half of PID cases have evidence of these bacterial pathogens. Evidence demonstrates that upper tract infection can be polymicrobial, involving both aerobic and anaerobic organisms. Isolates have included genital mycoplasmas, such

as *Mycoplasma hominis* and *Ureaplasma urealyticum*, aerobic and anaerobic streptococci, *Gardnerella vaginalis*, *Haemophilus influenzae*, cytomegalovirus, and enteric organisms such as *Escherichia coli* and *Bacteroides* spp.

18. **What is the differential diagnosis of pelvic inflammation disease?**
Appendicitis
Ectopic pregnancy
Endometriosis
Inflammatory bowel disease
Intrauterine pregnancy
Irritable bowel syndrome
Ovarian cyst or torsion
Nephrolithiasis
UTI

19. **What are the steps in diagnosing PID?**
Acute PID is often difficult to diagnose because of the nonspecific nature of symptoms and the broad differential diagnosis of abdominal pain in an adolescent female. Diagnosis is made based on the history of clinical clues. Laboratory and radiologic studies may be helpful.
    In evaluating an adolescent female with abdominal pain, it is imperative to interview her alone. Take a thorough gynecologic and sexual history, including menstrual history, number of sexual partners, contraceptive practices, and history of previous STIs. Clinicians should be attentive to signs of sexual abuse and/or sex trafficking during this interview. You may examine the patient with her preferred support person or with a staff chaperone. Focus the physical examination on the many possible causes of abdominal pain, including pregnancy, complications of prior abdominal surgery, appendicitis, pelvic inflammatory disease, and pneumonia. Perform a careful examination of the abdomen and a thorough pelvic examination (both speculum and bimanual examination, checking for cervical motion tenderness, adnexal masses, and/or tenderness). Take a culture or DNA probe samples for *Chlamydia* and *Neisseria*.

20. **What tests are very sensitive and specific in diagnosing genital gonorrhea and chlamydia?**
Nucleic acid amplification tests (NAATs) are very sensitive and specific if used on a female vaginal or endocervical swab or male urethral swab and male/female urine specimens. Using NAAT on urine specimens increases the likelihood of clinicians testing for STI and allows easier follow-up in young patients. Both gonorrhea and chlamydial infection can be detected through this method.

21. **When should you treat a teenager for PID?**
In the ED, have a low threshold for initiating empiric antibiotic treatment for any adolescent female patient with a history or physical examination suggestive of PID. Testing for gonorrhea and *C. trachomatis* should be performed. This minimizes the chance of missing PID in a patient presenting with only mild symptoms. If the patient presents with a severe clinical picture or is pregnant, undertake more extensive evaluation (laboratory and ultrasonography) to rule out other diagnoses. If no other definitive diagnosis is reached (e.g., appendicitis, UTI, pneumonia), start treatment.

22. **What is the recommended treatment for uncomplicated gonorrhea of the cervix, urethra, or rectum in adolescents?**
For treatment of uncomplicated gonorrhea, the Centers for Disease Control and Prevention (CDC) recommends one intramuscular (IM) dose of ceftriaxone: 500 mg for persons weighing up to 150 kg.
    If chlamydial infection has not been excluded, treat for chlamydia with doxycycline 100 mg orally two times/day for 7 days.

23. **What are the indicators for treating sexual partners?**
Identification and treatment of sexual partners are key in limiting the spread of STIs. Evaluate any sexual partners within the past 3 months and test for gonorrhea and chlamydial infection, whether or not they are symptomatic. In general, empiric treatment is appropriate for all sexual contacts of a patient with PID.

24. **What is expedited partner therapy (EPT)?**
EPT means that the clinician provides the patient's partner(s) with a prescription for treatment of infection without doing an evaluation or examination. This practice is not permitted in all states, and therefore, clinicians need to check the legal status of EPT. It is recommended that patients abstain from sexual contact until the therapy is completed and symptoms have resolved.

25. **After the CDC's recent changes to gonorrhea treatment recommendations, can EPT be used for gonorrhea?**
Due to new guidelines, make efforts to be sure that a patient's sex partners are evaluated and treated. This includes the recommended regimen (a single dose of ceftriaxone 500 mg IM). This may not always be feasible. Therefore, providers should still consider EPT for partners of patients diagnosed with gonorrhea who are unlikely to receive timely evaluation and treatment.

26. **Do all adolescents with PID need to be hospitalized for treatment?**
No. The CDC recommends hospitalization when "surgical emergencies" such as appendicitis cannot be excluded. Other reasons for hospitalization are the following: immunodeficiency, pregnancy, lack of clinical response to oral antimicrobial therapy; unable to follow or tolerate an outpatient oral regimen; severe illness, nausea and vomiting, or high fever; or the presence of tubo-ovarian abscess. There is no definite evidence that adolescents benefit from hospitalization for the treatment of PID.

KEY POINTS: INDICATIONS FOR ADMISSION OF PATIENTS WITH PID

1. Pregnancy
2. Surgical emergency that cannot be ruled out
3. No response to oral antimicrobial agents
4. Nonadherent patient
5. Evidence of severe illness
6. Tubo-ovarian abscess
7. Immunodeficiency

27. **What are the long-term complications of PID?**
Long-term complications may occur in as many as 25% of females who have had PID. These include chronic pelvic pain, tubo-ovarian abscesses, Fitz-Hugh-Curtis syndrome, ectopic pregnancy (6- to 10-fold increased risk), infertility as a result of scarring (with the risk of infertility increasing with the number of episodes of PID), dyspareunia, and chronic and recurrent pelvic pain.

28. **What are the most typical presenting features of ovarian torsion, and which patients are most likely to have this condition?**
- Sudden and severe pain in the lower abdomen
- Nonradiating pain
- Pain may be intermittent
- Colicky pain
- Nausea with and without vomiting
   A history of recent vigorous activity may be the precipitating event. Ovarian torsion is most frequently seen in postmenarchal females because it occurs more often when an ovarian cyst is present. However, ovarian torsion can occur in premenarchal females with normal ovaries.

29. **How is the clinical diagnosis of ovarian torsion made?**
In a female patient with symptoms of severe lower abdominal pain and vomiting, the differential diagnosis includes appendicitis, ovarian torsion, ectopic pregnancy, PID, tubo-ovarian abscess, endometriosis, and hemorrhagic cyst. Two-dimensional ultrasonography with Doppler and three-dimensional ultrasonography are the most effective modalities used to diagnose ovarian torsion. These studies demonstrate limited or absent blood flow in the ovary, which is suggestive of torsion; however, the diagnosis is made surgically. Open laparotomy provides definitive diagnosis.

30. **What are the risk factors for ectopic pregnancy?**
Risk factors include tubal abnormalities, history of assisted reproduction, use of an intrauterine device, prior upper gynecologic tract infection, certain STIs, PID, use of progestin-only contraceptives, previous ectopic pregnancy, and endometriosis.

31. **What is the most common presenting sign of early pregnancy in adolescents?**
A missed or abnormal period is the most common sign of pregnancy in teens. However, the menstrual history is often unreliable in adolescents because of anovulatory cycles. Therefore, other symptoms that should raise a red flag include fatigue, weight gain, nausea, morning sickness, cramping, and nonspecific gastrointestinal or genitourinary symptoms. Less common symptoms consist of vaginal bleeding or discharge, hyperemesis, and headache and moodiness.

32. **What is Plan B emergency contraception (EC)?**

Plan B provides a method to prevent pregnancy after unprotected sex. Specifically packaged products that contain a total dose of 1.5 mg of levonorgestrel (progestin only) for EC are available as Plan B. The two pills can be taken together with no risk of increased side effects. Plan B needs to be taken within 120 hours of unprotected sex. But it is more effective the sooner it is taken. It may prevent or delay ovulation, or it may interfere with the fertilization of an egg. It is not an abortion pill and will not interfere with implantation. Levonorgestrel for EC is available over the counter in pharmacies without a prescription or restriction of age.

33. **Why is Plan B called "Plan B"?**

It is a backup method of contraception and should not be considered a routine form of birth control.

34. **Are there side effects of the EC pills?**

There are no known serious complications after taking EC pills. The next period may not occur when expected. There may be irregular bleeding or spotting within the month after taking EC pills. Other short-term side effects may include headache, nausea and vomiting, abdominal pain, and dizziness.

35. **A patient comes to the ED and is concerned about having had sex with a person who has HIV. What would you advise?**

Postexposure prophylaxis (PEP) needs to be taken as soon as possible after a person has been exposed, ideally within 2 hours and not later than 72 hours (3 days). The sooner PEP is taken, the more likely it is to prevent HIV infection.

KEY POINTS: PLAN B EMERGENCY CONTRACEPTION

1. Progestin-only levonorgestrel
2. Can be taken up to 120 hours after unprotected sex (most effective closer to the time of unprotected sex)
3. Not a routine form of birth control
4. Will not affect a pregnancy
5. Levonorgestrel has no restriction of age

BIBLIOGRAPHY

1. Committee Opinion. Adnexal torsion in adolescents: ACOG Committee Opinion No, 783. 2019;134(2):e56–e63.
2. Chuang J, DiPasquale K, Archanan V, Mascaro D. Vaginal discharge. In: Shaw KN, Bachur RG, eds. *Fleisher & Ludwig's Textbook of Pediatric Emergency Medicine.* 8th ed. Wolters Kluwer; 2021:543–547.
3. Laufer MR. Congenital anomalies of the hymen and vagina. UpToDate. June 22, 2022. Chakrabarti A, Ed. UpToDate. https://www.uptodate.com/contents/congenital-anomalies-of-the-hymen-and-vagina
4. Mendez DR. Straddle injuries in children: evaluation and management. Wiley J, Deputy Ed. UpToDate. https://www.uptodate.com/contents/straddle-injuries-in-children-evaluation-and-management?search=undefined&source=search%20result&selectedTitle=1~40&usage%20type=default&display%20rank=1. Accessed 24.05.21.
5. Jenkins LK, Krywko D. *PID Pelvic Inflammatory Disease.* StatPearls; 2022. https://www.ncbi.nlm.NIH.gov., updated.
6. Red Book 2021-2024 Report of the Committee on Infectious Disease. 32nd ed. 221–223, 574–578
7. Senthil M, Rockey A, Zinns L, Chuang J, Posner J. Vaginal bleeding. In: Shaw KN, Bachur RG, eds. *Fleisher & Ludwig's Textbook of Pediatric Emergency Medicine.* 8th ed. Wolters Kluwer; 2021:533–542.
8. Turok D. Emergency contraception. In *UpToDate,* Eckler K, Ed. Accessed 05.10.21.
9. US Preventive Services Task Force: screening for Chlamydia and GC; 2021. https://www.uspreventiveservicestaskforce.org/uspstf/recommendation/chlamydia-and-gonorrhea-screening
10. https://www.cdc.gov/std/treatment-guidelines/gonorrhea.html; 2021.

CHAPTER 36

HEMATOLOGIC AND ONCOLOGIC EMERGENCIES

Paul Ishimine and Jenny Kim

HEMATOLOGIC EMERGENCIES

1. **What is anemia, and how is anemia categorized?**

   Anemia is defined as a reduction in red blood cells (RBC) or hemoglobin and is caused by increased RBC destruction or blood loss, decreased RBC or hemoglobin production, or a combination of these factors. Anemia can be divided into microcytic, normocytic, and macrocytic anemia. Common causes of anemia include:
   - Microcytic: Iron deficiency (most common childhood anemia), thalassemia, and anemia of chronic disease
   - Normocytic (with low or normal reticulocyte count): Infection, medication, lead poisoning, acute blood loss, renal disease, transient erythroblastopenia of childhood (TEC), and Diamond-Blackfan anemia (RBC bone marrow aplasia)
   - Normocytic (with high reticulocyte count): Hemorrhage, hemolytic anemias (e.g., sickle cell disease [SCD], hereditary spherocytosis, glucose-6-phosphatase deficiency, autoimmune hemolytic anemia, hemolytic-uremic syndrome)
   - Macrocytic: Medications, vitamin deficiencies (e.g., vitamin B_{12}, folate), liver disease, and aplastic anemia

2. **What history, physical examination findings, and laboratory tests are important considerations in evaluating a child with anemia?**

   How quickly the anemia develops will determine the degree of the patient's symptoms. The rapid development of anemia typically causes a patient to become more symptomatic, as the patient will not have to develop compensatory responses and acclimate to the anemia. After patient stabilization, the following features can help determine the underlying cause:
   - Historical features: Rapidity of onset, hemorrhage, diet, intercurrent illness, history of easy bruising or bleeding, previous episode of anemia, menstrual history, family history of blood disorders, pica
   - Physical examination findings: Pallor, icterus, jaundice, hepatosplenomegaly, enlarged lymph nodes, petechiae/purpura, blood on rectal examination
   - Laboratory studies: Complete blood count (CBC) with manual differential, mean corpuscular volume (MCV), peripheral smear, reticulocyte count, direct antiglobulin test (aka direct Coombs test), haptoglobin, direct/indirect bilirubin, lactate dehydrogenase, serum ferritin, serum iron, iron saturation, total iron-binding capacity

3. **An ill-appearing 6-year-old girl presents with weakness for 2 days. On examination, she has jaundice and pale conjunctivae but no bruising or petechiae. Her hemoglobin level is 4 g/dL, but her white blood cell and platelet counts are normal. Her reticulocyte count is elevated at 20%. She has unconjugated hyperbilirubinemia, and she has dark-brown urine, which is dipstick-positive for blood but has no RBCs on microscopic examination. This presentation suggests what broad cause of anemia?**

   Hemolytic anemia is suggested by her unconjugated hyperbilirubinemia and her hemoglobinuria, which result from RBC destruction. The elevated reticulocyte count is an appropriate compensatory response by this patient's bone marrow. Hemolytic disease may be seen in children with RBC membrane defects (e.g., hereditary spherocytosis) or enzyme defects (e.g., glucose-6-phosphate dehydrogenase deficiency). Autoimmune hemolysis occurs when antibodies directed against RBCs cause hemolysis. Nonimmune-acquired hemolysis may be caused by drugs, infections, or chemicals that cause direct RBC injury. Patients with hemoglobinopathies, such as SCD and thalassemias, can have periods of increased hemolysis and worsening anemia. Finally, mechanical causes of RBC fragmentation, such as hemolytic-uremic syndrome, may also cause hemolysis.

4. **What are the typical laboratory findings in iron deficiency anemia?**
   - Low hemoglobin and hematocrit
   - Low MCV and RBC count
   - High RBC distribution width
   - Low iron saturation and ferritin
   - Increased transferrin
   - Microcytosis, hypochromia, poikilocytosis, and anisocytosis on peripheral smear
   - Elevated platelet count

5. **Why is excessive cow milk consumption associated with iron deficiency anemia in young children?**
Overconsumption of cow milk decreases the toddler's appetite for other iron-containing foods, and cow milk does not contain adequate iron for nutrition. Calcium and casein in cow milk can also inhibit iron absorption. Additionally, there may be a concomitant cow milk enteropathy causing microscopic intestinal blood loss.

6. **Describe appetite abnormalities associated with iron deficiency anemia.**
Pica is associated with iron deficiency anemia and refers to an appetite for unusual substances not regarded as food, such as clay, paper, or dirt. Pagophagia, or pica for ice, is thought to be a specific finding in iron deficiency anemia.

7. **What is TEC? How does it present?**
TEC (transient erythroblastopenia of childhood) is an idiopathic disorder of acquired RBC aplasia characterized by a gradual onset of pallor. The median age at the time of diagnosis is 23 months, and there is often a history of an antecedent viral illness (e.g., parvovirus B19, human herpesvirus-6 [HHV6], echovirus 11). Except for pallor, the patient's physical examination is otherwise normal, with the absence of bruising, fever, lymphadenopathy, and hepatosplenomegaly. The CBC in a patient with TEC shows an isolated normochromic normocytic anemia with reticulocytopenia. TEC can be confused with leukemia, and bone marrow biopsy may be needed to exclude leukemia in a patient suspected of having TEC.

8. **What are some causes of methemoglobinemia?**
Methemoglobin is created when the heme iron is converted from a ferrous to a ferric state, resulting in hemoglobin with impaired oxygen binding. This manifests as cyanosis and results in tissue hypoxia. Methemoglobinemia may occur after exposure to oxidizing agents, such as certain drugs (e.g., benzocaine, sulfonamide antibiotics), well water that contains nitrites, mothballs, and aniline dyes. Acute gastroenteritis, usually with severe diarrhea, can lead to methemoglobinemia in infants. The heme iron is converted from a ferrous to a ferric state, resulting in hemoglobin with impaired oxygen binding, and manifests as cyanosis in these infants. Congenital methemoglobinemia is a rare cause of cyanosis in the newborn.

9. **How do patients with immune (or idiopathic) thrombocytopenic purpura (ITP) typically present?**
ITP most commonly presents in children ages 1 to 4 years with the acute onset of bruising and petechiae. There is often a history of a preceding viral illness. Children with ITP generally do not appear ill, and frank bleeding is surprisingly less common than would be expected in patients with severe thrombocytopenia.

10. **What is the most serious complication of ITP?**
The most serious concern in young children with ITP is intracranial hemorrhage. This is very rare. The risk of intracranial hemorrhage is highest in the first week after diagnosis and when the platelet count is less than 20,000 cells/mm^3. Intracranial hemorrhage is seen more frequently in patients who present with mucosal bleeding.

11. **How is ITP treated?**
The treatment of ITP is controversial, but guidelines from the American Society of Hematology recommend observation alone as the first intervention in patients with newly diagnosed ITP with no or minor bleeding (e.g., petechiae alone), given the generally benign bleeding associated with ITP and significant cost and side effects of treatment. ITP usually spontaneously remits within 6 months. Most patients with newly diagnosed ITP with no or mild bleeding can be managed as outpatients with close follow-up with a hematologist within 1 to 3 days. For patients with mucosal bleeding, corticosteroids, intravenous (IV) γ-globulin, anti-D immunoglobulin, or thrombopoietin receptor agonists can be considered. Rituximab, high-dose steroids, or splenectomy are reserved for patients who are unresponsive to initial treatments.

12. **Name the three most common bleeding disorders and the deficient factors associated with each.**
The most common inherited bleeding disorders are the following:
- Hemophilia A (factor VIII deficiency)
- Hemophilia B (factor IX deficiency)
- Von Willebrand disease (von Willebrand factor deficiency)

13. **What therapies can be used to treat patients with hemophilia?**
The mainstay of treatment for patients with hemophilia is factor replacement therapy. Monoclonal antibody-purified or recombinant factor VIII and factor IX are used most commonly to treat hemophilia A and hemophilia B, respectively. Patients with von Willebrand disease can be treated with desmopressin. Plasma-derived concentrates containing von Willebrand factor are used to treat more severe bleeding in patients with von Willebrand disease. For minor bleeding (e.g., epistaxis, gingival bleeding, menorrhagia), antifibrinolytic therapy with aminocaproic acid may be adequate treatment.

14. **What is the underlying pathophysiology of sickle cell disease?**
    SCD is caused by an inherited hemoglobinopathy in which a single mutation causes an amino acid substitution in the β-globin chain of hemoglobin. This results in distorted, elongated, sickle-shaped RBCs that are prone to aggregation. Combined with other cellular and plasma factors and endothelial interactions, this sickling results in vaso-occlusion, hemolysis, and resultant complications, such as stroke, acute chest syndrome, splenic sequestration, and pain from ischemia. There are many genotypes of SCD, all of which have enough abnormal hemoglobin to cause sickling.

15. **What causes vaso-occlusive crises in patients with SCD?**
    Vaso-occlusive crises are due to localized sickling and vascular occlusion and can occur in any organ, but most frequently affect bone and viscera, causing painful ischemia. Most older children report long bone, back, and abdominal pain. Adolescent boys can have vaso-occlusive crises causing priapism. Precipitating events may include infection, dehydration, fever, hypoxia, and exposure to cold.

16. **How should vaso-occlusive crises be treated?**
    Analgesia should be started as soon as possible upon ED arrival. Both nonsteroidal anti-inflammatory drugs and narcotic administration are often required. Alternative to IV routes of medication administration (e.g., intranasal, intramuscular) can be considered if there is a delay in obtaining IV access. Response to analgesic treatment should be reassessed frequently. If dehydration is present, IV fluids or oral rehydration is needed. IV fluid boluses should be reserved for patients who are severely dehydrated or hypotensive.

17. **What are some worrisome causes of headaches in patients with SCD?**
    Headaches are common in children with SCD. Although most headaches in children with SCD are idiopathic, children with SCD are at higher risk than the general pediatric population for ischemic stroke, intracranial hemorrhage, and cerebral venous thrombosis. Patients with SCD who develop severe headaches, altered levels of consciousness, speech disturbances, or other neurologic deficits require urgent head imaging and hematologic consultation. Patients with SCD who develop strokes need emergent exchange transfusion.

18. **Define acute chest syndrome and its causes and treatment.**
    Acute chest syndrome is a serious complication of SCD and can be life-threatening. This syndrome is defined as a new pulmonary infiltrate and chest pain, hypoxia, fever, tachypnea, wheezing, or cough, and often cannot be distinguished from pneumonia. The cause is uncertain but is likely multifactorial. Both infectious (e.g., chlamydia, mycoplasma, viruses, bacteria) and noninfectious (e.g., vascular occlusion due to sickle cells, fat embolism, pulmonary infarction) causes have been described. Admit all patients with suspected acute chest syndrome to the hospital. Treatment involves supportive care measures including analgesia, cautious hydration, oxygen, antibiotics, bronchodilators, and blood transfusions.

19. **What is splenic sequestration crisis?**
    Splenic sequestration crisis is a life-threatening complication of SCD that occurs when a large portion of a patient's blood volume becomes acutely trapped in the spleen. This crisis leads to massive splenomegaly, acute anemia, and hypovolemic shock. Treatment is supportive and includes fluid resuscitation and blood transfusion. Splenic sequestration is seen in young children, typically between 3 months and 5 years. It is important to quickly recognize severe splenomegaly in an ill-appearing young patient with SCD, as a hypovolemic shock due to massive splenic sequestration can be mistaken for septic shock, and delays in blood transfusion can result in cardiovascular collapse in these patients.

20. **How should patients with SCD and fever be treated in the ED?**
    Because these children are at high risk for serious bacterial infections, febrile children with SCD need rapid treatment with parenteral antibiotics after appropriate cultures are obtained. The greatest risk of serious bacterial infection is between the ages of 6 months and 3 years, when protective antibodies are not adequate and splenic function is greatly diminished. These patients require a dose of parenteral antibiotics (typically ceftriaxone because of its longer duration of action and good coverage of *Streptococcus pneumoniae*). Cautious outpatient management of selected low-risk febrile patients can be considered. A low-risk febrile patient is one with well-appearance, no focal physical examination abnormalities, temperature <40°C, white blood cell count >5000 cells/mm^3 but <30,000 cells/mm^3, no infiltrates on chest x-ray, and baseline hemoglobin, white blood cell, and platelet counts.

21. **Which virus frequently leads to aplastic crisis in children with chronic hemolytic diseases such as SCD?**
    Parvovirus B19 causes brief suppression of erythropoiesis, which is not tolerated in patients with SCD or other chronic hemolytic conditions because these patients have shortened RBC survival and rely on brisk erythropoiesis to maintain their baseline hemoglobin levels. Patients may present with fatigue, shortness of breath, and severe anemia with reticulocytopenia. Treatment is supportive, and RBC transfusions are often necessary.

22. **What is dactylitis?**
Dactylitis, or "hand-foot syndrome," results from vaso-occlusion of the nutrient arteries that supply the metacarpal and metatarsal bones, causing bone marrow infarction in patients with SCD. This form of vaso-occlusive crisis is most common in young infants (mostly under the age of 2 years) and results in pain and swelling of the hands and feet, irritability, and refusal to walk. It is usually bilateral, distinguishing it from cellulitis.

ONCOLOGIC EMERGENCIES

23. **What are the most common childhood malignancies?**
    - Leukemia is the most common childhood malignancy, and acute lymphoblastic leukemia (ALL) is the most common type of childhood leukemia.
    - The most common solid organ tumors are brain tumors, and most of these tumors are infratentorial. Medulloblastomas and cerebellar astrocytomas are the most common central nervous system tumors in children.

24. **Why are children with malignancies at risk for sepsis?**
Several factors contribute to the risk of severe infections and sepsis in pediatric oncology patients:
    - Malignant cells can replace the bone marrow, and chemotherapeutic agents can directly suppress granulocyte production, resulting in neutropenia.
    - Other mechanisms of defense against infection, including mechanical barriers (e.g., intact mucous membranes and skin), cell-mediated and humoral immunity, and splenic function, are frequently impaired in patients with cancer.
    - Indwelling central venous catheters, ventriculoperitoneal shunts, and other implanted devices may become sites of infection.

25. **How should febrile children with cancer be managed?**
Approach febrile children with cancer carefully! Any ill-appearing child needs broad-spectrum antibiotic coverage and admission to the hospital. If a febrile child is severely neutropenic (absolute neutrophil count < 500 cells/mm^3) or if the child's absolute neutrophil count is lower than 1000 cells/mm^3 and expected to drop further, administer broad-spectrum antibiotic therapy after blood and other appropriate cultures are obtained. These patients should be admitted to the hospital. Well-appearing febrile patients who are not neutropenic may be treated more selectively and can potentially be discharged from the ED, typically after receiving a dose of parenteral antibiotics. Discuss the treatment and disposition of all febrile children with cancer with the child's oncologist.

26. **An ill-appearing 6-year-old boy with acute myelogenous leukemia presents with fever and right-lower-quadrant abdominal pain. In addition to the usual causes of fever and right-lower-quadrant pain, what other entity needs to be considered in a neutropenic patient?**
Typhlitis, a necrotizing enterocolitis, can be seen in neutropenic patients. The cause is multifactorial and includes infection and mucosal injury from chemotherapy or radiation therapy, and most commonly involves the cecum. Typhlitis usually presents with fever, abdominal pain, and bloody diarrhea. The diagnosis is usually made by computed tomography, and treatment includes antibiotic therapy, and, rarely, surgery. The mortality rate with typhlitis is very high.

27. **What is the differential diagnosis of an anterior mediastinal mass in a child?**
The causes of anterior mediastinal masses are listed in Table 36.1.

28. **What are some of the risks associated with an anterior mediastinal mass?**
Anterior mediastinal masses are associated with superior mediastinal syndrome in 12% of patients at the time of presentation. This syndrome is defined as the compression of the structures of the superior mediastinum, including the superior vena cava (SVC) and trachea. Anterior mediastinal masses can also cause SVC syndrome, which refers to upper body venous congestion from either extrinsic compression of the SVC or a thrombus within the SVC. These conditions can lead to signs of airway compromise (e.g., stridor, cough, dyspnea, hemoptysis, orthopnea), facial edema, cardiovascular instability due to impaired venous return, and central nervous system findings (e.g., headache, mental status changes). Endotracheal intubation may be difficult because of tracheal or bronchial compression. Cardiac output may be compromised by positive-pressure ventilation. Avoid sedating these patients and avoid positioning them supine because doing so may result in cardiorespiratory arrest.

29. **A 4-year-old girl with lymphoma presents with shortness of breath. What are some possible causes of her symptoms?**
Causes of shortness of breath in patients with cancer are listed in Table 36.2.

Table 36.1 Causes of Anterior Mediastinal Mass

1. The "Terrible Ts":
   T-cell lymphoma/leukemia
   Thymoma
   Thyroid carcinoma
   Teratoma/germ cell tumors
2. Hodgkin disease
3. Non-Hodgkin lymphoma
4. Neuroblastoma
5. Cystic hygroma
6. Congenital diaphragmatic hernia

Table 36.2 Causes of Shortness of Breath in Patients With Cancer

Superior vena cava (SVC) syndrome: Compression or thrombosis of the SVC can cause dyspnea and may result in facial plethora, jugular venous distention, and headache

Superior mediastinal syndrome: Compression of the trachea by tumor; often used interchangeably with SVC syndrome

Pleural effusions

Pericardial effusion

Cardiomyopathy: Commonly associated with anthracycline chemotherapeutics

Arrhythmias: electrolyte disturbances

Pneumonia

Pulmonary embolism

Anemia

30. **What are neuroblastomas, and what are the most common presenting signs and symptoms?**
    Neuroblastomas are tumors that are derived from primitive neural cells. This is the third most common type of malignancy after leukemia and brain tumors. These tumors most commonly arise in the adrenal glands and along the sympathetic chain. Common presenting signs and symptoms of neuroblastoma include the following:
    Symptoms:
    - Abdominal pain
    - Bone pain
    - Back pain
    - Constipation
    - Fever
    - Weight loss
    Signs:
    - Abdominal mass
    - Horner syndrome
    - Hypertension
    - Periorbital ecchymoses
    - Proptosis

31. **An 8-year-old girl who has reported back pain intermittently for several months presents to the ED with a sudden inability to move her right leg. What does this presentation suggest, and what is the treatment?**
    Spinal cord compression from a mass can present with back pain (typically worse when lying down), leg paresis or paralysis, and bowel and bladder incontinence or retention. Examination may reveal back tenderness, leg

weakness, decreased rectal tone, and hyperreflexia or hyporeflexia. Plain radiography may reveal vertebral abnormalities, but the diagnostic study of choice is magnetic resonance imaging. Initiate treatment immediately to minimize permanent neurologic sequelae. Interventions may include a combination of steroids, chemotherapy, radiation therapy, and/or neurosurgical decompression.

32. **What is CAR T-cell therapy, and what are the most significant complications?**
Chimeric antigen receptor (CAR) T-cell therapy is a new treatment modality for refractory malignancies. In children, CAR T-cell therapy is most commonly used in the treatment of ALL and lymphoma. T-cells are extracted from the patient (or a donor), genetically modified to target malignant cells, and reintroduced back to the patient. The most important complications associated with CAR T-cell therapy are cytokine release syndrome (CRS) and immune effector cell-associated neurotoxicity syndrome (ICANS), also known as CAR T-cell-related encephalopathy. Patients with CRS present with fever and multiorgan dysfunction 1 to 14 days after CAR T-cell therapy, and patients with ICANS present with headaches, altered mental status, seizures, or other neurologic findings. These patients require stabilizing interventions, frequently requiring fluid resuscitation, vasopressors, and empiric antibiotics (as CRS may be indistinguishable from sepsis). Treat seizures in patients with ICANS. Avoid using steroids in patients with CAR T-cell if possible. However, treatment of life-threatening complications may require the use of steroids and/or tocilizumab. Early consultation with the patient's oncologist is necessary.

33. **What is tumor lysis syndrome (TLS)?**
TLS is a metabolic syndrome of hyperkalemia, hyperphosphatemia, hyperuricemia, hypocalcemia, and acute kidney injury resulting from the release of intracellular contents from dying cells. TLS is seen most commonly in cancers with large tumor burdens and rapid cellular turnover, such as lymphomas and leukemias. Although TLS usually occurs soon after the initiation of chemotherapy, patients can present at the time of initial diagnosis with TLS, especially those who present with Burkitt lymphoma or leukemia. TLS can cause numerous complications, such as arrhythmias and renal failure.

34. **How is TLS treated?**
The mainstay of treatment is IV hydration. Administer allopurinol or rasburicase to reduce uric acid levels, and start aluminum hydroxide or calcium carbonate for treatment of hyperphosphatemia. Hyperkalemia can be treated with a potassium-binding resin, calcium gluconate, sodium bicarbonate, or insulin with glucose, depending on the patient's clinical status. Urinary alkalinization is no longer recommended. Hemodialysis may be used for uncontrolled TLS and severe kidney injury.

35. **A teenager with a diffuse headache is found to have a white blood cell count of 200,000 cells/mm^3. What treatment should be initiated in the ED?**
This child has hyperleukocytosis, which is highly suggestive of leukemia. This degree of white blood cell elevation increases blood viscosity, which, in turn, predisposes a patient to thrombosis, leading to neurologic, pulmonary, and hemorrhagic symptoms. These patients are also at high risk for TLS. Treatment includes hydration and management of TLS; more refractory cases are treated with cytoreduction (either via chemotherapy or by leukapheresis). Give platelet transfusions if the platelet count is lower than 20,000 cells/mm^3 to reduce the risk of central nervous system hemorrhage. Give RBC transfusions judiciously because they can increase blood viscosity.

36. **A 5-year-old girl with ALL presents with fever and hypotension. Antibiotics and IV fluid resuscitation are started immediately, but she has persistent hypotension. In addition to fluids and vasopressors, what other therapies should be considered?**
Consider adrenal suppression in patients with persistent hypotension who recently (in the past year) have been treated with steroids. Treatment protocols for ALL usually include frequent and sometimes prolonged courses of corticosteroids. These patients may need stress-dose hydrocortisone. If worsening hypotension is associated with flushing of the central line or infusion of IV antibiotics through the central line, be suspicious of a central line infection.

KEY POINTS: PEDIATRIC HEMATOLOGY AND ONCOLOGY

- Iron deficiency anemia is the most common childhood anemia, and excessive cow's milk intake is a common cause of this condition.
- SCD is associated with several life-threatening complications, including sepsis, stroke, splenic sequestration crisis, hemolytic crisis, and acute chest syndrome.
- Children with cancer are at high risk for sepsis, and febrile children with cancer generally require antibiotics.
- Tumor lysis syndrome can lead to numerous complications, including dysrhythmias and kidney injury.

BIBLIOGRAPHY

1. American College of Emergency Physicians. Managing sickle cell disease in the ED. <https://www.acep.org/sickle-cell/>. Accessed 15.06.22.
2. Brandow AM, Carroll CP, Creary S, et al. American Society of Hematology 2020 guidelines for sickle cell disease: management of acute and chronic pain. *Blood Adv.* 2020;4(12):2656–2701.
3. Burns RA, Woodward GA. Transient erythroblastopenia of childhood. *Pediatr Emerg Care.* 2019;35(3):237–240.
4. Jones GL, Will A, Jackson GH, et al. British Committee for Standards in Haematology. Guidelines for the management of tumour lysis syndrome in adults and children with haematological malignancies on behalf of the British Committee for Standards in Haematology. *Br J Haematol.* 2015;169(5):661–671.
5. Long B, Yoo MJ, Brady WJ, et al. Chimeric antigen receptor T-cell therapy: an emergency medicine focused review. *Am J Emerg Med.* 2021;50:369–375.
6. National Institutes of Health/National Heart, Lung, and Blood Institute. *Evidence-Based Management of Sickle Cell Disease.* Expert Panel Report, 2014. National Institutes of Health; 2014.
7. Neunert C, Terrell DR, Arnold DM, et al. American Society of Hematology 2019 guidelines for immune thrombocytopenia. *Blood Adv.* 2019;3(23):3829–3866. Erratum in: *Blood Adv.* 2020;4(2):252.
8. Rensen N, Gemke RJ, van Dalen EC,, et al. Hypothalamic-pituitary-adrenal (HPA) axis suppression after treatment with glucocorticoid therapy for childhood acute lymphoblastic leukemia. *Cochrane Database Syst Rev.* 2017(11):Article No.: CD008727.
9. Ware RE, de Montalembert M, Tshilolo L, Abboud MR. Sickle cell disease. *Lancet.* 2017;390:311–323.

CHAPTER 37

INFECTIOUS DISEASE EMERGENCIES

Robert P. Olympia, Kaynan Doctor, Lauren McNickle and Nevena Rose

FEVER

1. **What is the risk for serious bacterial illness (SBI) in a febrile infant?**
   In a prospective observational study of infants <60 days old presenting with fever, 9.2% of infants had at least one positive culture for serious bacterial infection. Febrile infants <30 days had a 23.9% rate of serious bacterial infection versus infants 30 days old or greater had a rate of serious bacterial infection of 12.2%.

2. **Which bacterial agents are of most concern in an infant <28 days old presenting to the emergency department (ED) with a fever?**
   These agents are group B streptococci, gram-negative enteric organisms (*Escherichia coli, Enterococcus* spp.), *Listeria monocytogenes*, and, less commonly, *Streptococcus pneumoniae, Haemophilus influenzae, Staphylococcus aureus, Neisseria meningitidis*, and *Salmonella* spp. Currently, the most common bacteria to cause bacteremia are *E. coli*, group B streptococci, and *S. aureus*.

3. **A 14-day-old well-appearing infant presents to the ED with a 1-day history of fever, temperature up to 39°C rectally. What should your initial management include?**
   The American Academy of Pediatrics (AAP) released clinical practice guidelines on the evaluation and management of infants 8 to 60 days old. Per these guidelines, the initial workup for a febrile infant 8 to 21 days old should include the following:
   - A complete history (including prenatal history) and physical examination of the newborn.
   - Obtain laboratory studies:
     - Complete blood count (CBC) with differential.
     - Blood culture.
     - Urinalysis (UA).
     - Cerebrospinal fluid (CSF) for protein/glucose, cell count, polymerase chain reaction (PCR), Gram stain, and bacterial/viral cultures.
     - Consider herpes simplex virus (HSV) studies if increased risk (surface cultures of mouth, nasopharynx, conjunctivae, and anus along with serum HSV PCR).
     - Chest radiograph if signs of respiratory distress (tachypnea, cyanosis, wheezing, retractions, grunting, nasal flaring, rales, rhonchi, or decreased breath sounds).
     - Stool for heme testing and culture if bloody or watery stool is noted.
   - Admit the patient to the hospital and administer parenteral antibiotics (ampicillin plus cefotaxime or gentamicin).
   - Consider intravenous (IV) acyclovir if neonatal herpes is suggested by history, physical examination, or laboratory findings.

4. **Name the risk factors for neonatal HSV infection that should prompt evaluation.**
   Maternal risk factors include maternal history of HSV and fever within 48 hours pre- and postdelivery. Neonate risk factors include vesicular rash, seizures, hypothermia, mucous membrane ulcers, and CSF pleocytosis in the absence of positive Gram stain, leukopenia, thrombocytopenia, or elevated alanine transaminase (ALT).

KEY POINTS: HSV INFECTION IN NEONATES

1. Maternal risk factors: history of HSV or vesicular rash and fever 48 hours pre- or postdelivery
2. Neonatal risk factors: vesicular rash, seizures, hypothermia, CSF pleocytosis (without + Gram stain), thrombocytopenia
3. If there is increased risk, obtain surface cultures of the mouth, nasopharynx, conjunctivae, and anus
4. Obtain serum HSV PCR
5. Consider prompt treatment with acyclovir

5. **A 26-day-old well-appearing infant presents to the ED with fever and temperature up to 39.6°C. How does your management differ from the management of the 8- to 21-day-old group?**
   Per the AAP guidelines, clinicians should obtain UA, blood culture, and inflammatory markers (IMs) as initial workup. If UA is positive, urine should be sent for culture. Chest x-ray and stool studies are not routinely obtained;

only if clinically appropriate.
- If IMs (procalcitonin [PCT] or C-reactive protein [CRP] if PCT is unavailable) are elevated, lumbar puncture (LP) is recommended.
  - If LP reveals pleocytosis or is uninterpretable, administer parenteral antimicrobials and observe in the hospital.
  - If the LP is negative and the patient will be observed at home, administer parenteral antibiotics and ensure follow-up with PCP in 24 hours. If the LP is negative and the patient will be observed in the hospital, the clinician may admit on parenteral antibiotics or admit OFF antibiotics for observation.
- If IMs are normal, clinicians MAY complete the LP.
  - If the LP is NOT performed, admit the patient to the hospital.
    - May administer antibiotics or admit OFF antibiotics for observation.
  - If LP is completed and
    - CSF reveals pleocytosis or uninterpretable, MAY administer parenteral antimicrobials, and observe in the hospital.
    - CSF negative and the patient will be observed at home, administer parenteral antibiotics, and ensure follow-up with PCP in 24 hours. If the LP is negative and the patient will be observed in the hospital, the clinician may admit on parenteral antibiotics or admit OFF antibiotics for observation.

6. **A 6-week-old male infant presents to the ED with a temperature of 38.4°C. The infant appears nontoxic and is without an obvious source for the fever. What is your workup?**
Per the AAP guidelines, your initial workup for an infant 29 to 60 days old should consist of:
- CBC with differential.
- UA.
- Blood culture.
- IMs (PCT or CRP if PCT is unavailable).
- Chest radiograph only if signs of respiratory distress (tachypnea, cyanosis, wheezing, retractions, grunting, nasal flaring, rales, rhonchi, or decreased breath sounds).
- Stool for heme testing and culture if bloody or watery stool is noted.
If the IMs are NOT elevated (CRP <20 mg/L, PCT <0.5 ng/mL, absolute neutrophil count [ANC] <4000 mm^3):
- If UA is positive, send for urine culture, no need for LP; send home with oral antimicrobials, and close follow-up in 12 to 24 hours.
- If UA is negative, no need to perform LP or administer antibiotics. May observe closely at home with close follow-up in 24 to 36 hours.
If IMs are elevated (CRP >20 mg/L, PCT >0.5 ng/mL, ANC >4000 mm^3):
- If UA is positive, send for a urine culture.
- May perform LP:
  - If the LP result is positive:
    - Start parenteral antimicrobials and admit to the hospital.
  - If LP is negative, uninterpretable, or UA is negative or positive:
    - May start parenteral antimicrobials (or oral).
    - May admit or send home.

7. **What is the likelihood of a neonate having bacteremia and a viral illness?**
A retrospective cross-sectional study examined 0- to 60-day-old infants presenting with fever and the results of blood cultures and viral studies. Infants with documented respiratory viral pathogens were less likely to have an SBI or bacteremia than infants with negative viral testing (17.5% had SBI with negative viral testing vs. 4.7% with positive viral testing).

8. **Do infants with hyperpyrexia have a higher risk of having an SBI?**
Yes, according to a prospective observational study of infants <60 days old presenting with fever. This study demonstrated that as temperatures went up, the rate of SBI increased. For example, febrile infants with a temperature of 38.0°C had about a 5% rate of SBI versus infants with a temperature of 39.9°C who had about a 30% rate of SBI.

9. **Discern early from late-onset group B streptococcal (GBS) infection.**
Early-onset (birth to 7 days) GBS infection, which may be secondary to maternal obstetric complications, prematurity, or lack of prophylactic antibiotics prior to delivery commonly causes septicemia and respiratory illness. Late-onset GBS infection (7 days to 3 months) commonly causes meningitis and bacteremia without focus.

10. **A 54-day old infant presents to the ED with a temperature of 38.6°C after receiving his 2-month immunizations. He otherwise appears well. What should his workup be?**
A published study investigated the prevalence of SBI in febrile infants aged 6 to 12 weeks without a source of infection who received immunizations within the preceding 72 hours. Among febrile infants, the prevalence of

SBI is less in the initial 24 hours following immunizations (0.6% vs. 8.9%). The authors recommended only urine testing (no blood or CSF testing) in febrile infants who present within 24 hours of immunization. Infants who present greater than 24 hours after immunization with fever should be managed similarly to infants without recent immunization.

11. **How helpful are IMs (CRP and PCT) in detecting serious bacterial infection in febrile neonates?**
IMs (CRP and PCT) have gained popularity in the workup of febrile neonates as more data becomes available regarding their accuracy in predicting SBI. Studies have found CRP levels rise within 6 to 8 hours of infection and peak at 24 hours. Viral infections are usually not associated with a CRP level >5 mg/L.
   PCT can also be useful as the normal level for neonates >72 hours is usually <0.1 ng/mL. PCT has been found to be even more sensitive for the early detection of sepsis than CRP and is more likely to be elevated during bacterial infections than viral infections.

12. **A 4-week-old infant presents to the ED in January with a temperature of 38.6°C, cough, and is noted to have wheezing bilaterally. Respiratory syncytial virus (RSV) PCR is positive. Should this affect your fever workup?**
A retrospective study examining infants 4 weeks and younger with fever determined that the incidence of serious bacterial infection was less in infants with (+) RSV compared to the overall incidence (7% vs. 11.4%). In infants with RSV, 5.4% also had a urinary tract infection (UTI), 1.1% also had bacteremia, and 0% also had meningitis. Therefore in infants less than 60 days with fever and (+) RSV, an LP may not be necessary but the clinician should still obtain blood and urine cultures.

13. **Are febrile infants with influenza infection at lower risk for a serious bacterial infection?**
A prospective observational study of infants aged 0 to 60 days presenting to the ED with fever demonstrated that febrile infants with influenza infection had lower prevalence of a serious bacterial infection (3.1%) compared with infants who were negative for influenza A (13.3%).

SEPSIS

14. **Distinguish among bacteremia, systemic inflammatory response syndrome (SIRS), sepsis, severe sepsis, and septic shock.**
   - Bacteremia: The presence of bacteria in the blood
   - SIRS: Presence of at least two of the following four criteria, one of which must be abnormal temperature or leukocyte count
     - Core temperature >38.5°C or <36°C
     - Tachycardia (heart rate [HR] >2 SD above normal range or age) or, for children <1 year old bradycardia (HR <10th percentile for age)
     - Tachypnea (respiratory rate [RR] >2 SD above normal for age)
     - Leukocyte count elevated or depressed for age or >10% bands
   - Sepsis: SIRS in the presence of a suspected or known invasive infection
   - Severe sepsis: Sepsis plus one of the following criteria:
     - Cardiovascular organ dysfunction
     - Acute respiratory distress syndrome
     - Two or more other organ dysfunctions
   - Septic shock: Sepsis plus cardiovascular organ dysfunction

15. **What are the criteria for organ dysfunction in sepsis?**
Refer to Table 37.1 for the criteria.

16. **What are the antibiotic choices for empiric therapy in infants and children presenting with septic shock?**
Table 37.2 shows the antibiotic choices for empiric therapy in infants and children.

FEVER AND RASH

17. **What is the differential diagnosis of fever and petechiae?**
Children and infants who present to the ED with fever and petechiae require immediate attention because there are life-threatening causes that may progress rapidly to death. Fever and petechiae are associated with the following infections:
Bacterial:
   - *Neisseria meningitidis* (meningococcemia)
   - *Neisseria gonorrhoeae* (gonococcemia)

- *Pseudomonas aeruginosa*
- *Streptococcus pyogenes*
- *Rickettsia prowazekii* (epidemic typhus)
- *Rickettsia rickettsii* (Rocky Mountain spotted fever [RMSF])
- *Staphylococcus aureus* (endocarditis)

Viral:
- Adenovirus
- Rubeola (atypical measles)
- Enterovirus
- Epstein-Barr virus (EBV)

18. **When is fever associated with a petechial rash less concerning?**
A child with fever and petechiae is less likely to have SBI if he or she appears well and has one isolated petechial lesion, petechiae only above the nipple line, a mechanical cause of the petechiae (coughing, emesis, screaming or crying, blood pressure cuff, or tourniquet), and normal white blood cell (WBC) count. Most can be safely discharged from the ED.

19. **What factors predict poor prognosis in infants and children with meningococcemia?**
- Clinical findings:
  - Rapidly evolving hemorrhagic skin lesions

Table 37.1 Criteria for Organ Dysfunction in Sepsis

SYSTEM	CRITERIA
Cardiovascular	• Hypotension <5th percentile for age despite 40 mg/kg fluid bolus in 1 hr • Vasoactive requirement to maintain BP despite 40 mg/kg fluid bolus in 1 hr • Two or more signs of abnormal perfusion
Respiratory	• PaO_2/FiO_2 <300 • Hypercarbia • Required FiO_2 >50% to maintain SpO_2 >92% • Need for nonelective invasive or noninvasive mechanical ventilation
Neurologic	Altered mental status, GCS <11, or >3 point change in patient's baseline
Hematologic	Platelet count <80,000, INR >2.0
Renal	Serum creatinine >2 times upper limit of normal for age or twofold increase in patient's normal creatinine
Hepatic	• Total bilirubin >4 mg/dL • ALT more than two times the upper limit of normal for age

ALT, alanine transaminase; BP, blood pressure; FiO_2, fraction of inspired oxygen; GCS, Glasgow Coma Scale; INR, international normalized ratio.

Table 37.2 Antibiotic Choices for EmpiricTherapy in Pediatric Septic Shock

AGE	BACTERIAL ETIOLOGY	EMPIRIC ANTIBIOTIC THERAPY
Neonate	GBS	Ampicillin plus aminoglycoside or cefotaxime; if nosocomial add vancomycin
	Gram-negative bacilli	Cefotaxime plus vancomycin (if suspect gram-positive infection)
Child	*Streptococcus pneumoniae, Neisseria meningitidis, Staphylococcus aureus,* GAS	If nosocomial, vancomycin plus antibiotic against gram-negative bacteria (ceftazidime, cefepime)
	Invasive GAS (e.g., post varicella)	Aminoglycoside, carbapenem, or extended-spectrum penicillin with β-lactamase-inhibitor penicillin and clindamycin

GAS, group A streptococci; GBS, group B streptococci.

- Shock
- Hyperpyrexia
- Laboratory findings:
  - Leukopenia
  - Absence of CSF pleocytosis
  - Thrombocytopenia
  - Low plasma levels of fibrinogen
  - Disseminated intravascular coagulation
  - Metabolic acidosis
  - Low serum CRP level
  - Low ANC
  - Low serum potassium level

20. What is acute arthritis and dermatitis syndrome?

Also known as disseminated gonococcal infection, acute arthritis and dermatitis syndrome occurs in approximately 0.5% to 3% of persons with untreated mucosal gonorrhea. Clinical findings occur in two stages. A bacteremic stage and a joint-localized stage with suppurative arthritis. Often a clear delineation of these stages is difficult to make. The bacteremic stage consists of high fever and rigors as well as dermatitis (tender necrotic pustule with an erythematous base located distally on an upper extremity). The joint-localized stage consists of migratory polyarthralgias or tenosynovitis affecting smaller joints and arthritis (pyogenic monoarticular or polyarticular with effusion, especially of knee, ankle, or wrist).

21. List clinical criteria that define toxic shock syndrome.

Table 37.3 shows criteria for staphylococcal toxic shock syndrome and Table 37.4 shows criteria for streptococcal toxic shock syndrome.

Organ system involvement:
- Gastrointestinal (vomiting or diarrhea)
- Mucus membrane involvement
- Muscular (elevated CPK two times the upper limit of normal)
- Renal (blood urea nitrogen [BUN] or creatinine (Cr) two times the upper limit of normal or urinary sediment with sterile pyuria)
- Hepatic (total bilirubin, aspartate aminotransferase [AST], or ALT two times the upper limit of normal)
- Hematologic (platelets <100,000/mm^3)
- Neurologic (altered mental status)

Classification:
- Probable: More than four clinical criteria and laboratory criteria met.
- Confirmed: Five clinical criteria and laboratory criteria met, including desquamation.

Table 37.3 Criteria for Staphylococcal Toxic Shock Syndrome

STAPHYLOCOCCAL	CLINICAL CRITERIA	LABORATORY CRITERIA (MUST BE NEGATIVE IF OBTAINED)
	Fever: >38.9°C or 102°F	Blood or cerebrospinal fluid cultures (blood may be positive for *Staphylococcus aureus*)
	Rash with diffuse macular erythroderma	Serologies for Rocky Mountain spotted fever, leptospirosis, or measles
	Hypotension as defined by age	
	Three or more organ system involvement	

Table 37.4 Criteria for Streptococcal Toxic Shock Syndrome

STREPTOCOCCAL	CLINICAL CRITERIA	LABORATORY CRITERIA
	Hypotension as defined by age	Group A streptococcal isolation from culture
	Two or more organ system involvement	

Organ system involvement:
- Gastrointestinal (vomiting or diarrhea)
- Mucus membrane involvement
- Muscular (elevated creatine phosphokinase two times the upper limit of normal)
- Renal (BUN or Cr two times the upper limit of normal or urinary sediment with sterile pyuria)
- Hepatic (total bilirubin, AST, or ALT two times the upper limit of normal)
- Hematologic (platelets $<100,000/mm^3$, disseminated intravascular coagulation)
- Neurologic (altered mental status)
- Acute respiratory syndrome
- Skin (generalized erythematous macular rash that can desquamate)
- Soft tissue necrosis (gangrene, myositis, necrotizing fasciitis)

Classification:
- Probable: All clinical criteria met and absence of other etiology for illness with isolation of Group A Streptococcus from nonsterile sites
- Confirmed: All clinical criteria met and isolation of Group A streptococcus from sterile sites (blood, CSF, synovial fluid, pleural/pericardial fluid)

22. **Distinguish between staphylococcal and streptococcal toxic shock syndrome.**
    Table 37.5 shows the distinction between staphylococcal and streptococcal toxic shock syndrome.

CENTRAL NERVOUS SYSTEM INFECTIONS

23. **What are the most common etiologic agents of bacterial meningitis?**
    - 0 to 4 Weeks: Group B streptococci, *E. coli*, *Klebsiella pneumoniae*, *Salmonella* spp., other gram-negative bacilli, *L. monocytogenes*, enterococci
    - 4 Weeks to 3 months: Group B streptococci, *S. pneumoniae*, *N. meningitides*, *E. coli*, *H. influenzae*, *L. monocytogenes*
    - 3 Months to 18 years: *S. pneumoniae*, *N. meningitides*, *H. influenzae*

24. **A 2-week-old newborn presents with fever and focal seizures. What therapy should be instituted immediately?**
    In addition to parenteral antibiotics for bacterial infections, administer acyclovir as soon as possible. This child's presentation, especially seizures, is consistent with HSV encephalitis. Typically, fever, lethargy, and seizures occur at 2 to 3 weeks of age. Skin lesions are present in about 50% of patients, and in most will appear late in the illness if at all. CSF examination usually reveals fewer than 100 WBCs but may have an increased number of red blood cells. CSF cultures are usually negative for HSV. HSV DNA in the CSF can best be detected using a PCR study. Neonatal infections are serious, with high mortality and morbidity rates even with prompt treatment. About one-third of neonatal HSV infections involve the central nervous system (CNS), and while most patients survive, there is a high incidence of neurologic impairment.

25. **Why is ampicillin used to treat meningitis in 0- to 3-month-old infant?**
    It is used to provide adequate antimicrobial coverage for *L. monocytogenes*, a rare infection. Frequently, an aminoglycoside, such as gentamicin, is added to improve the effectiveness of the ampicillin. Penicillin-allergic patients may be treated with trimethoprim-sulfamethoxazole (TMP-SMZ).

Table 37.5 Staphylococcal Versus Streptococcal Toxic Shock Syndrome

FEATURE	STAPHYLOCOCCAL	STREPTOCOCCAL
General presentation	Acute onset of severe symptoms	Gradual onset of mild symptoms
Fever	High; abrupt onset	Gradual onset (if even present)
Rash	Erythroderma	Scarlatina
Shock	Responds to aggressive intravascular volume expansion	Unpredictable response to intravascular volume expansion
Source of infection	Menses, sinusitis, surgical wound	Cellulitis, necrotizing myositis, fasciitis, pneumonitis
Response to antibiotics	Treatment of acute infection; β-lactamase-resistant penicillins or cephalosporins	More difficult to treat acute infection; clindamycin is superior to β-lactam agents
Complications	Infrequent: coagulopathies, complicated hospitalizations, gangrene	Common: coagulopathies, complicated hospitalizations, gangrene
Mortality rate	10%	30%-50%

26. A 6-month-old infant presents with a 1-day history of fever, lethargy, vomiting, and poor feeding. You are concerned about bacterial meningitis following your physical examination. After performing an LP, what antibiotics should be administered?
Ceftriaxone and vancomycin. For all infants and children with bacterial meningitis presumed to be caused by *S. pneumoniae*, add vancomycin because of the possibility of resistance. Specific choice and duration of antibiotic therapy should be guided by culture and susceptibility results: 10 to 14 days for *S. pneumoniae*, 7 to 10 days for *H. influenzae*, and 5 to 7 days for *N. meningitidis*. For a child with hypersensitivity to β-lactam antibiotics, consider the combination of rifampin plus vancomycin. Vancomycin should not be given alone.

27. A 12-month-old infant presents with bacterial meningitis. In addition to antibiotics, should corticosteroids be administered as adjunctive therapy?
Corticosteroids have been shown to reduce hearing loss and neurologic sequelae in children with *H. influenzae* B (Hib) meningitis. The effectiveness of corticosteroids in diseases caused by *S. pneumoniae* and *N. meningitidis* is less clear, although retrospective studies have shown significant reductions in hearing loss among those treated with dexamethasone with antibiotics versus antibiotics alone. Benefits also include a reduction in the mean number of days before the resolution of fever. There is evidence that dexamethasone reduces the incidence of neurologic complications in adults with *S. pneumoniae* meningitis. Current recommendations suggest that dexamethasone be considered for children with pneumococcal meningitis. If used, dexamethasone should ideally be given before or at the time of antibiotic administration.

28. A 6-year-old child presents with fever, severe headache, and neck stiffness. What is the significance of the Kernig and Brudzinski signs?
Kernig sign is resistance to extension of the lower leg while the hip is flexed at 90 degrees and the child is supine. Brudzinski sign is flexion of the hips and knees in response to neck flexion while the child is supine. Often seen with bacterial meningitis, a positive Kernig or Brudzinski sign may be absent with aseptic meningitis or Lyme meningitis.

29. What is aseptic meningitis?
This term has become synonymous with viral meningitis but in fact describes meningitis caused by viruses, fungi, or certain bacteria that cannot be seen on Gram stain. It also applies to meningitis caused by drugs (nonsteroidal anti-inflammatory drugs), systemic illness, neoplasms, or parameningeal conditions. This term does not imply an aseptic course of illness or an aseptic-appearing child. A more accurate term would be *Gram stain–negative meningitis*.

30. How can viral meningitis be distinguished from bacterial meningitis?
It is often difficult to distinguish these two clinical entities. Both can present with fever, headache, stiff neck, vomiting, and photophobia. Young infants may show nonspecific signs such as irritability, poor oral intake, and somnolence. The typical CSF findings can sometimes be used to distinguish viral from bacterial meningitis, although considerable overlap can exist (Table 37.6). Gram stain is highly specific, but it is falsely negative in up to 40% of cases of bacterial meningitis.
More recent studies have demonstrated the utility of the Bacterial Meningitis Score (predictors of bacterial meningitis being a positive CSF Gram stain, CSF protein 80 mg/dL or greater, CSF neutrophils 1000 cells/μL or greater, peripheral ANC 10,000 cells/μL or greater, seizure before or at the time of presentation).

31. On a summer day, a 9-year-old female presents with fever, headache, and photophobia. You suspect meningitis and perform an LP. The CSF evaluation reveals a WBC count of 400 cells/mL with a polymorphonuclear cell predominance, normal glucose, normal protein, and negative Gram stain. What is the most likely diagnosis?
Enteroviral meningitis is the most likely diagnosis. Nonpolio enteroviruses are the leading cause of viral meningitis, accounting for 80% to 90% of all cases from which an etiologic agent is identified. This group includes group A and B coxsackie viruses, echoviruses, and enteroviruses (types 68-71 and 73). They are called *summer viruses*

Table 37.6 Typical CSF Findings in Viral and Bacterial Meningitis		
CSF VARIABLE	**BACTERIAL**	**VIRAL**
WBC count (cell/mm³)	>1000	<500
Neutrophils (%)	>50	<50
Glucose level (mg/dL)	<20	>30
Protein level (mg/dL)	>100	50-100

CSF, cerebrospinal fluid; WBC, white blood cell.

because resulting infections occur during the warmer months. The CSF examination in this patient is typical of enterovirus infection. The predominance of neutrophils is often seen *early* in the course of the disease. The presence of other identifiable enteroviral syndromes in the community, such as herpangina and hand-foot-mouth disease, can be useful in diagnosis because outbreaks tend to be epidemic and seasonal. Reliable enteroviral PCR tests for CSF are helpful.

32. **A 12-year-old male presents with fever and acute onset of "acting strangely," with combative behavior and garbled speech. What is the differential diagnosis for this presentation?**
Fever in combination with a change in mental status suggests a diagnosis of encephalitis. Encephalitis is defined as altered mental status for more than 24 hours accompanied by two or more findings concerning inflammation of the brain parenchyma: fever, seizures or other focal neurologic disorders, CSF pleocytosis, and abnormal neuroimaging and electroencephalographic findings. Increased intracranial pressure without signs of meningitis can also be seen. Infectious causes of encephalitis are predominately viral in origin. Epidemic acute encephalomyelitis is usually due to arboviruses (arthropod-borne viruses) such as West Nile and LaCrosse viruses. Sporadic acute encephalitis can be due to many viruses such as enteroviruses, HSV, varicella, cytomegalovirus (CMV), and EBV. Bacterial causes are less common, but in a child with exposure to cats (especially kittens), consider infection with *Bartonella henselae* (cat-scratch disease). Other infectious diseases that cause encephalitis include RMSF, Lyme disease, and *Mycoplasma pneumoniae* infection. Autoimmune causes of encephalitis, concurrent with an infectious etiology, should prompt the clinician to order a broad testing panel to detect the etiologic agent and consider immunomodulatory therapy.

33. **What is acute disseminated encephalomyelitis (ADEM)?**
ADEM, also known as postinfectious encephalomyelitis, is a rare monophasic inflammatory disorder of the CNS that can present with altered mental status including coma. Patients can have vision changes, unsteady gait, and severe weakness. ADEM has a propensity to occur after minor upper respiratory tract infections. CSF, by definition, reveals no bacterial or viral etiology. The existence of bilateral optic neuritis and transverse myelitis is consistent with the diagnosis of ADEM. Diagnostic evaluation for ADEM involves neuroimaging and laboratory studies to exclude potential infectious, inflammatory, neoplastic, and genetic mimics of ADEM. Acute treatment modalities include high-dose IV corticosteroids, therapeutic plasma exchange, and IV immunoglobulin. Most patients begin to recover after a few days of treatment and many recover completely within 6 months.

KEY POINTS: ACUTE DISSEMINATED ENCEPHALOMYELITIS

1. Postinfectious encephalomyelitis occurs after minor illness such as upper respiratory infection (URI).
2. Presents with altered mental status, weakness, ataxia, and coma.
3. Neuroimaging is useful for diagnosis.
4. Treatment includes high-dose IV steroids, and IV immunoglobulin.
5. Many patients have good recovery.

34. **A 14-year-old male with a 2-week history of sinusitis presents with persistent fever, headache, and altered mental status. What serious complication of sinusitis should be considered?**
Brain abscess is an uncommon but serious complication of frontal sinusitis. It is seen in older children and teenagers because of the late development of the frontal sinuses. Maintain a high index of suspicion when patients with sinusitis present with persistent symptoms, such as fever, frontal headache, altered mental status, and signs of increased intracranial pressure. Other potential complications include epidural abscess, meningitis, or Pott puffy tumor.

35. **An 8-year-old female has fever and back pain. What is your approach to diagnosis and management?**
Back pain is an unusual complaint for children in the ED. Fever and back pain may indicate significant disease. The differential diagnosis includes infectious, autoimmune, vascular, neoplastic, and rheumatologic disorders. The major infections producing back pain in children include discitis, vertebral osteomyelitis, spinal epidural abscess, and sacroiliac joint infection (Table 37.7).

OPHTHALMIC INFECTIONS

36. **This 9-year-old male presents with right eye swelling (Fig. 37.1). How do you differentiate between preseptal and orbital cellulitis in children?**
The differentiation between preseptal and orbital cellulitis in children is shown in Table 37.8.

Table 37.7 Description of Infections Causing Back Pain in Children

VARIABLE	DISCITIS	VERTEBRAL OSTEOMYELITIS	SPINAL EPIDURAL ABSCESS	SACROILIAC JOINT INFECTION
Age (years)	<5	<8	>8	Any
Symptoms	Gradual onset Increased with activity	Gradual onset Constant and dull	Acute onset Constant Radiation to the legs	Gradual onset Buttock pain Sciatica
Fever	Low grade	High	High	High
Physical examination	Local tenderness Decreased lumbar lordosis Decreased spinal mobility Refusal to walk	Local tenderness Decreased spinal mobility	Local tenderness Decreased spinal mobility Decreased deep tendon reflexes Decreased strength	Local tenderness Decreased spinal mobility

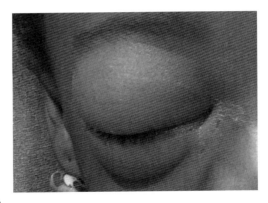

Fig. 37.1 Periorbital swelling.

Table 37.8 Preseptal Versus Orbital Cellulitis in Children

FEATURE	PRESEPTAL CELLULITIS	ORBITAL CELLULITIS
Location	Infection of the eyelids and periorbital soft tissues anterior to the orbital septum	Infectious process posterior to the orbital septum involving the tissues within the orbit (eye, fat, muscles, and optic nerve)
Etiology	Direct inoculation following trauma or insect bite Direct spread from adjacent structures (skin)	Extension of bacterial infection from sinuses (90%) Direct inoculation from penetrating trauma or surgery Spread from adjacent structure (skin)
Clinical presentation		
• Fever/malaise	+/−	Usually, +
• Conjunctival hyperemia or swelling	+	+
• Upper-/lower-eyelid edema, tightness, or erythema	+	+

Continued

Table 37.8 Preseptal Versus Orbital Cellulitis in Children–cont'd

FEATURE	PRESEPTAL CELLULITIS	ORBITAL CELLULITIS
• Signs of external trauma (insect bite, etc.)	+	+
• Fluctuance	+/−	+/−
• Photophobia	−	+/−
• Proptosis*	−	+
• Orbital pain	−	+
• Pain in eye movement	−	+
• Normal movement of eye*	+	−
• Visual loss or abnormal pupillary reactivity*	−	+ (if severe)
• Signs of cavernous sinus thrombosis, meningitis, or intracranial abscess formation	−	+ (if severe)

+ indicates present, − indicates absent.
*The three most important features.

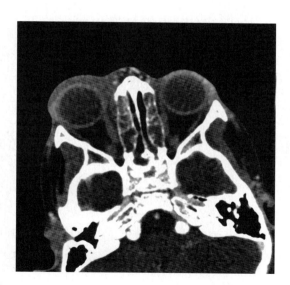

Fig. 37.2 Orbital cellulitis.

In this patient, it may be very difficult to perform an eye examination as his eye is swollen shut. In addition to laboratory work, a computed tomography (CT) scan of the orbits may be indicated to confirm if the infection has extended posterior to the orbital septum.

37. **Following his evaluation, the contrast-enhanced CT scan of the orbits (Fig. 37.2) shows findings concerning orbital cellulitis. How would you further manage this patient?**
Orbital cellulitis commonly arises as an extension of a sinus infection (most often an ethmoiditis). The usual infectious agents are similar bacteria as those seen in bacterial sinusitis and include *S. pneumoniae* and *H. influenzae* (especially in undervaccinated patients). Gram-negative rods may arise from trauma, while anaerobes may be seen with dental infection extension.

History: Assess for ear, nose, throat, or sinus infections, tooth pain, recent dental disease, history of periorbital infection (e.g., infected hordeolum/dacryocystitis), prior orbital trauma, penetrating foreign body or prior surgery to local structures (orbital or paranasal sinus surgeries), and immunocompromised state.

Examination: Be vigilant for an afferent pupillary defect on the swinging light test, pain with extraocular movements, and proptosis. Also check for other cranial neuropathies, mental status change, or neck stiffness. Additional investigations/management besides contrast-enhanced CT scan of the orbits:

- WBC count (often reveals leukocytosis with predominance of bands).
- Blood cultures obtained before antibiotic administration.
- COVID-19 testing. Although conjunctival congestion is the most common ophthalmological finding associated with severe acute respiratory syndrome coronavirus 2 (SARS-CoV-2) infection, there have been case reports of associated periorbital inflammation.
- LP if meningeal signs are present (only after negative findings on CT of the head for signs of increased intracranial pressure).
- Admission to the hospital for parenteral antibiotics. Protocols may be institution-dependent. In many cases, IV vancomycin should be considered if there is a high community rate of methicillin-resistant *S. aureus* (MRSA). This should be combined with one of the following: ceftriaxone or cefotaxime. Ampicillin/sulbactam or piperacillin-tazobactam with metronidazole may also be appropriate combinations.
- Consultation with ophthalmology and otolaryngology is essential. Consider infectious disease or neurosurgery consultation.

38. What are the considerations for hospital admission of infants and children who present with preseptal cellulitis?
- Age <1 year
- Moderate-to-severe illness
- Inability to rule out extension of infection (orbital cellulitis)
- Incomplete vaccination (in this case against *H. influenzae*)
- Toxic appearance and/or signs of meningitis/sepsis
- Anorexia and/or inability to tolerate oral medications/antibiotics
- Presence of subcutaneous abscess or radiological concern for worsening infection
- Failure of outpatient management/concerning or unreliable social situation

39. For children discharged from the ED with the diagnosis of preseptal cellulitis, which antibiotics are best?
Treatment is geared toward combatting common infecting organisms, such as *S. aureus*, *S. pneumoniae*, *H. influenzae*, and anaerobes. High-dose amoxicillin/clavulanate, cefpodoxime, or cefdinir are mainstay therapies. In penicillin-allergic patients, consider TMP-SMZ. If MRSA is suspected, TMP-SMZ or clindamycin are appropriate choices.

40. A 10-year-old autistic male presents with right eye pain, erythema, discharge, and periorbital rash as shown in Fig. 37.3. The patient has been constantly rubbing at the right eye for days despite oral antibiotics and erythromycin eye ointment prescribed by a telehealth provider. She is reluctant to undergo an examination.
The photo of this patient's eye shows a vesicular rash that can be seen with HSV infection. Compared to adults, children with HSV eye involvement can present with a more severe illness that can affect both the eyelid, conjunctiva, and cornea. This can be sight-threatening with significant morbidity. The patient will need a thorough eye examination (which may be facilitated in this case with sedation) to assess for corneal involvement. Look for

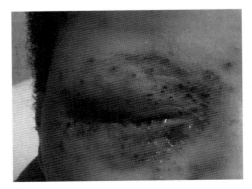

Fig. 37.3 Periorbital vesicular lesions.

dendrites on fluorescein staining or corneal clouding. With HSV eye infection, emergent aggressive topical antiviral therapy such as acyclovir is warranted. Urgent evaluation by ophthalmology is also indicated to further assess and treat for complications such as corneal ulcers and keratitis.

41. A 17-year-old female patient fell asleep wearing contacts and reports that she removed them the next morning. She presents 2 days later with left eye pain, conjunctival injection, and photophobia. How would you assess and manage her complaints?

This is a presentation of Contact Lens-induced Associated Red Eye (CLARE). As with any acute red eye presentation, a history to assess for visual disturbance/diplopia, inciting events, and exposures is paramount. At minimum your examination should consist of visual acuity assessment, swinging light test, visual field testing, assessment of extraocular movements, and fundoscopy as tolerated. In this case, everting the eyelids to assess for retained foreign body, looking for corneal clouding, and fluorescein staining (with/without topical anesthesia) are also very important before making the call to ophthalmology. With contact lens wearers, complications following CLARE can be sight-threatening and include microbial keratitis and contact lens-induced peripheral ulceration. A consult with ophthalmology is essential to coordinate prompt follow-up and further management.

42. What is ophthalmia neonatorum?

Ophthalmia neonatorum, also known as **neonatal conjunctivitis**, is defined as conjunctival inflammation during the first 4 weeks of life. Infants typically present with eyelid edema, chemosis, conjunctival hyperemia, and purulent or mucopurulent ocular discharge. Maternal history may reveal exposure to sexually transmitted diseases or previous genital infections. Birth history may reveal prematurity or premature rupture of membranes in infants born via cesarean section, or vaginal discharge with a vaginal delivery. Bacterial infectious causes include *Chlamydia trachomatis, N. gonorrhoeae,* and *P. aeruginosa.* However, 30% to 50% of bacterial causes are due to other microbes such as *S. aureus, S. pneumoniae, H. influenzae, Corynebacterium, Moraxella catarrhalis, E. coli,* and *K. pneumoniae.* Viral agents such as HSV, adenovirus, Coxsackie virus, CMV, echovirus, and even SARS-CoV-2 can also cause this condition.

The time of onset and type of eye discharge may help with the diagnosis, but this is confirmed using a Gram stain, culture on chocolate or Thayer-Martin agar (*N. gonorrhoeae*), chlamydial culture, direct immunofluorescent monoclonal antibody testing for chlamydia, and HSV immunochemical testing/PCR. Ideally, this should be ordered on every infant with these symptoms. Dacryostenosis or periorbital cellulitis may also have a similar presentation on examination.

43. Distinguish between the most concerning causes of ophthalmia neonatorum.

Such differentiation is shown in Table 37.9.

Table 37.9 Causes and Features of Ophthalmia Neonatorum

FEATURES	CHLAMYDIA TRACHOMATIS	NEISSERIA GONORRHOEAE	HERPES SIMPLEX VIRUS	PSEUDOMONAS AERUGINOSA
Proportion of cases (%)	2-40	<1	<1	<1
Presentation/ incubation period	First 1-2 wk of life	72-96 hr after birth	6-14 days	5-28 days
Distinctive clinical features	Initially mild swelling, hyperemia, tearing, mucopurulent discharge with pseudomembrane formation with possible bloody discharge Unilateral or bilateral	Initially mild conjunctival hyperemia but can progress to severe chemosis with purulent conjunctival discharge with marked eyelid edema	Cloudy cornea, conjunctival injection, and tearing. Classic herpetic vesicles may not be seen in the newborn A corneal dendrite may be seen on fluorescein staining	Seen in preterm infants. Eyelid edema, erythema, purulent drainage, and pannus formation

Table 37.9 Causes and Features of Ophthalmia Neonatorum –cont'd

FEATURES	CHLAMYDIA TRACHOMATIS	NEISSERIA GONORRHOEAE	HERPES SIMPLEX VIRUS	PSEUDOMONAS AERUGINOSA
Severity of conjunctivitis	Mild	Severe	Mild	Severe
Potential complications	Self-limited Rarely conjunctival or corneal scarring Potential development of upper and lower respiratory tract infections	Corneal ulceration and perforation Septicemia, meningitis, or arthritis	Ulceration, keratitis Disseminated infection, Meningoencephalitis	Corneal perforation, endophthalmitis, sepsis Meningitis
Diagnosis	ELISA, EIA, direct antibody tests, PCR, DNA-hybridization probe	Gram-negative diplococci seen on Gram stain	Viral culture/PCR Multinucleated giant cells seen on Giemsa stain	Gram stain and culture of exudate to identify gram-negative bacilli
Treatment	Oral erythromycin for 2 weeks with erythromycin ointment	Assess for systemic complications (e.g., blood and CSF studies as needed). Parenteral ceftriaxone or cefotaxime. Also treat for concurrent suspected chlamydial infection.	Assess for systemic complications (e.g., blood and CSF studies as needed). Parenteral acyclovir coupled with vidarabine, ganciclovir, or trifluridine ophthalmic preparations	Topical and systemic (parenteral) antipseudomonal antibiotic therapy

Adapted from Kimberlin D, Barnett E, Lynfield R, Sawyer M. Neonatal ophthalmia. In: *Red Book: 2021-2024 Report of the Committee on Infectious Diseases.* Committee on Infectious Diseases, American Academy of Pediatrics; 2021; Gervasio KA, Friedberg MA, Rapuano CJ. Pediatrics; 8.9 Ophthalmia neonatorum (newborn conjunctivitis). In: Gervasio KA, Peck TJ, Fathy CA, Sivalingam MD, eds. *The Wills Eye Manual Office and Emergency Room Diagnosis and Treatment of Eye Disease.* 8th ed. Wolters Kluwer; 2022:407–410.
CSF, cerebrospinal fluid; EIA, enzyme immunoassay; ELISA, enzyme-linked immunosorbent assay; PCR, polymerase chain reaction.

44. A 5-year-old girl presents to the ED with "burning and itchy" eyes. She describes a sensation of "chalk in her eyes," with some blurry vision. On physical examination, she has bilateral conjunctival hyperemia, chemosis, ocular discharge, and preauricular lymph nodes bilaterally. What is the differential diagnosis?
    The presence of preauricular lymph nodes and conjunctivitis is associated with conjunctivitis caused by *N. gonorrhoeae* (rare) and adenoviral keratoconjunctivitis (common). Adenoviral keratoconjunctivitis is often associated with fever, other upper respiratory symptoms, vomiting, and diarrhea. This could also be a presentation of COVID-19 infection.

45. What is the treatment for adenoviral keratoconjunctivitis?
    Treatment includes cold compresses and acetaminophen to help with ocular discomfort, gentle removal of conjunctival membranes with a cotton swab, and possibly topical corticosteroids for marked follicular conjunctivitis and pseudomembrane formation (Fig. 37.4). Ophthalmologic consultation is strongly recommended before using ophthalmic steroids. Prevention of transmission includes frequent hand washing and the recommendation to keep the child out of daycare or school until complete resolution of the conjunctival hyperemia.

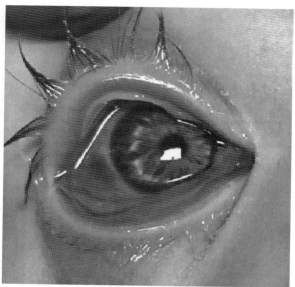

Fig. 37.4 Keratoconjunctivitis.

EAR, NOSE, AND THROAT INFECTIONS

46. A 3-year-old boy with a history of eczema presents with left ear pain and drainage. On physical examination, his tympanic membrane is neither erythematous nor bulging; however, his external auditory canal is swollen. He winces with pain when you manipulate the tragus and pinna. There is no lateral displacement of the ear and no mastoid tenderness. What is the likely diagnosis?

These clinical findings are consistent with acute otitis externa, which most commonly arises due to *Pseudomonas* infection of the outer ear. *Escherichia, Proteus, Enterobacter*, and *Klebsiella* spp. *Staphylococcus* and *Streptococcus* have been causative factors when otitis externa occurs as an extension of a focal infection. Fungal pathogens such as *Aspergillus* and *Candida* account for 5% of the cases. HSV and varicella may also cause otitis externa. Otitis externa is more commonly diagnosed in the summer months. It is associated with eczema, seborrhea, psoriasis, contact dermatitis, external auditory canal foreign bodies, earbuds, and hearing aids as well as cotton swab cleaning/washing/excoriations and swimming.*Escherichia, Proteus, EnterobacterKlebsiellaStaphylococcusStreptococcusAspergillusCandida*

47. How should otitis externa be managed?

For the intact tympanic membrane, a 7-day course of topical antibiotic drops such as neomycin, polymyxin B, or trimethoprim sulfate with hydrocortisone helps to reduce pain and inflammation.

For the perforated tympanic membrane or tympanostomy-tube-associated otorrhea, otic ofloxacin and ciprofloxacin, combined with either hydrocortisone or dexamethasone, are recommended. Immunocompromised individuals or those with treatment failure may be treated with a course of oral antibiotics as well.

If there is severe canal edema, administration using a wick may also be helpful. Avoidance of submersion until canal edema has resolved is also recommended. Culturing of the exudate is not indicated except for severe, refractory cases or when a fungal organism is suspected.

48. What is the best treatment for a young child with coryza, cough, sore throat, and fever?

The "common cold" or rhinosinusitis is caused by viruses (most commonly rhinoviruses). Antibiotics should not be used to treat the common cold because of their lack of efficacy, risk of side effects, and, more importantly, to curb increasing drug resistance among some bacterial pathogens. Over-the-counter cold remedies, such as antihistamines and decongestants, have not been proven to be safe, nor have they been shown to be effective in young children. They should not be given to children 4 years and under. Nasal saline drops can be safely used for nasal congestion (although aggressive suctioning should be avoided). A cool mist vaporizer can also help alleviate congestion symptoms. Antipyretics such as ibuprofen (for children older than 6 months) and acetaminophen could be used for fever and malaise. Avoid aspirin as it has been associated with Reye syndrome. Additionally, vaporub has been clinically shown to help with symptomatic relief and sleep disturbance associated with nocturnal cough and congestion caused by URIs in patients 3 months or older. *Echinacea purpura* extract, a commonly used alternative supplement for the treatment of common cold has not shown significant benefit in treating children aged 2 to 11 years. Similarly, vitamin C supplementation does not shorten or ameliorate the symptoms of the common cold. For children 12 months and older, honey has been found to be better than placebo and over-the-counter cough medications in reducing the frequency of cough.

49. **List the three major causes of exudative pharyngitis in children.**
    - Group A β-hemolytic streptococcus (GAS)
    - Adenoviruses
    - EBV
      In developing countries, add *Corynebacterium diphtheriae* to the differential. In sexually active adolescents or abused children, consider *N. gonorrhoeae*. More recently, *Arcanobacterium haemolyticum* has been shown to cause exudative pharyngitis, especially in adolescents, and is associated with a maculopapular rash. Although rare, oropharyngeal tularemia should be considered in children with exudative pharyngitis resistant to common antibiotic treatment and/or organisms that cannot be isolated via standard diagnostic testing.

50. **What are the CENTOR criteria?**
    The CENTOR (**C**ough, **E**xudate, **N**ode, **T**emperature, young **OR** old modifier) criteria is a useful risk stratifying tool to help decide if a patient needs to be tested for Group A streptococcal pharyngitis. One point is provided for each of the following: age 3 to 14 years, exudate or swelling on tonsils, tender swollen anterior lymph nodes, temperature >100.4°F, and absence of cough. A score of 2 or higher warrants testing.

51. **What is the recommended treatment for streptococcal pharyngitis?**
    Amoxicillin (50 mg/kg/day) or penicillin for a full 10-day course to prevent rheumatic fever is the oral drug of choice. In penicillin-allergic patients without anaphylactic reaction to penicillin, first-generation cephalosporin such as cephalexin can be used. Alternatively, 10-day courses of clindamycin or clarithromycin are appropriate. A single dose of intramuscular penicillin G benzathine (600,000 U if <27 kg or 1,200,000 U if >27 kg) may be considered if there is concern about compliance or medication availability.

52. **How is otitis media diagnosed clinically?**
    Per current AAP guidelines, acute otitis media is diagnosed by visualizing a moderate-to-severe bulging tympanic membrane AND a middle ear effusion. Otorrhea that is not due to acute otitis externa is also considered diagnostic. Acute otitis media can also be diagnosed in a child with a mild bulging of the tympanic membrane who has associated recent (less than 48 hours) onset of otalgia (holding, tugging, or rubbing of the ear in a nonverbal child) or if there is intense erythema of the tympanic membrane. Otitis media should not be diagnosed in children who do not have a middle ear effusion.

53. **Which pathogens are implicated in acute otitis media?**
    - *S. pneumoniae* (35%)
    - *H. influenzae*, nontypeable (25%)
    - *M. catarrhalis*
    - Viruses: Adenoviruses, coxsackie virus, measles virus, parainfluenza virus, rhinoviruses, RSV
    - Others: Anaerobes; *Chlamydia*, *Mycoplasma*, and *Staphylococcus* spp., *M. tuberculosis* agent

54. **What are the risk factors for developing acute otitis media?**
    - Tobacco smoke exposure
    - URI
    - Previous acute otitis media
    - Persistent middle ear effusion or otitis media with effusion
    - Family history of acute otitis media and atopy
    - Daycare attendance
    - Pacifier use
    - Daycare attendance

55. **When is watchful waiting appropriate in the case of acute otitis media?**
    Young children who have mild otitis media symptoms can be watched to see if there is a spontaneous resolution. This applies to children aged 6 to 24 months with unilateral or bilateral otitis media and children older than 24 months with bilateral otitis media. This approach requires patients to be reevaluated within 72 hours.
      In contrast, the following patients are at increased risk of severe infection and warrant antibiotic therapy instead of observation:
    - Age <6 months
    - Patients with severe signs and symptoms, for example, toxic appearance, temperature >39°C, and otalgia
    - Immunocompromised patients
    - Patients with known craniofacial abnormalities (e.g., cleft palate)

56. What is the first-line antibiotic treatment of acute otitis media?

High-dose amoxicillin (90 mg/kg/day) divided twice daily is the first-line antibiotic treatment for otitis media provided the patient does not meet the criteria for immediate second-line antibiotic treatment and is not penicillin-allergic. Duration of therapy varies according to age and severity:
- Children younger than 24 months: 10-day course
- Children between 2 and 5 years of age: 7-day course
- Children >5 years: 5- to 7-day course

57. Which antibiotics are considered second-line agents for the treatment of acute otitis media?

If there is purulent conjunctivitis (which can be a sign of *H. influenzae* infection), recent amoxicillin administration (within 30 days), or a history of otitis media refractory to penicillin, second-line treatment in the form of an antibiotic with additional β-lactamase coverage such as amoxicillin-clavulanate (90 mg/kg amoxicillin) is recommended.

Alternative therapies for otitis media (e.g., in the penicillin-allergic patient) include cefdinir, cefuroxime, or cefpodoxime. In cases where cephalosporins are not tolerated, clindamycin could be considered an alternative antimicrobial.

Intramuscular ceftriaxone should be reserved for children who are vomiting and cannot tolerate oral medication or for those with possible concomitant occult bacteremia.

58. What is the mechanism of pneumococcal antimicrobial resistance?

Pneumococcal drug resistance is mediated by alterations in the penicillin-binding proteins. In contrast, resistance of *H. influenzae* and *M. catarrhalis* is mediated by a β-lactamase enzyme which breaks open the beta-lactam ring, thus inactivating the antibiotic. The difference in the mechanism of antibiotic resistance has important therapeutic implications, since β-lactamase-stable agents, such as amoxicillin-clavulanate, are more effective against *H. influenzae* and *M. catarrhalis*. However, they do not provide an advantage over amoxicillin in treating penicillin-resistant pneumococci. Pneumococcal resistance is overcome via a high dosage of amoxicillin (90 mg/kg/day).

59. A toddler presents with fever, stridor, and increased work of breathing. He has nasal flaring, grunting, and retractions. His respiratory status acutely worsens in triage. The child was seen 2 days ago for fever and a barky cough. He was diagnosed with mild croup, treated with dexamethasone, and was subsequently discharged with no notable stridor at rest. At the bedside you note that the child is hypoxemic, somnolent, and in severe respiratory distress. You decide to intubate the trachea and find purulent tracheal secretions in the airway. What is the likely diagnosis?

This child has bacterial tracheitis, also called exudative tracheitis or acute laryngotracheobronchitis. This is a relatively rare, but potentially life-threatening, infection and requires emergency evaluation and treatment. Younger children are particularly vulnerable due to their small-caliber airways, as copious secretions can obstruct the trachea or a major bronchus, causing subsequent respiratory failure. Tracheitis in previously healthy children may be preceded by a viral URI such as influenza and parainfluenza with subsequent bacterial superinfection. The key distinguishing feature of bacterial tracheitis from viral croup is hypoxemia and biphasic (inspiratory and expiratory) stridor. Drooling and tripod posture are also characteristic, thus foreign-body aspiration and epiglottitis may be considered. The most common causative organisms include *S. aureus*, *H. influenzae*, *S. pyogenes*, *S. pneumoniae*, and *M. catarrhalis*. Treatment includes endotracheal intubation and IV antibiotics with MRSA coverage for endemic areas, such as vancomycin in combination with a third-generation cephalosporin.

60. What are the common causes of stomatitis? How can they be distinguished?

Inflammation of the oral mucous membrane (stomatitis) is a common finding in children, usually presenting with ulcers or vesicles (canker sores). The differential diagnosis is based on the location of the lesions and clinical picture:
- Buccal stomatitis may be due to infectious agents, Behçet syndrome, or trauma.
- Gingivitis may be due to HSV or enteroviruses (coxsackie virus: hand-foot-mouth disease).
- Gingivostomatitis may be due to an infectious agent: (HSV, *Candida albicans*) or Stevens-Johnson syndrome.
- Glossitis may be due to group A streptococci or HSV.

Recurrent lesions may be due to abnormalities in the immune system, such as in cyclic neutropenia or chemotherapy-induced neutropenia and chronic granulomatous disease. In association with recurrent fever, stomatitis may be due to **PFAPA** (**p**eriodic **f**ever, **a**denitis, **p**haryngitis, and **a**phthous stomatitis).

61. What are the clinical manifestations and management of a child with suspected acute mastoiditis?

Mastoiditis is a severe complication of otitis media and occurs when infection invades the mastoid portion of the temporal bone resulting in osteitis and subperiosteal abscess. Patients with mastoiditis present with fever, erythema, pain, and swelling behind the ear with posterior-inferior displacement of the auricle. The tympanic membrane is often erythematous and bulging; however, this finding may be absent if a patient has been taking antibiotics. Complications of mastoiditis can include intracranial extension with cranial nerve palsy, meningitis, labyrinthitis, petrositis, bacteremia, sigmoid sinus thrombosis, cranial osteomyelitis, as well as subdural empyema and brain abscess. Imaging is not required for all patients but can help confirm the diagnosis. A contrast-enhanced CT scan of the temporal bones is the gold standard and can be used as part of the assessment of the toxic patient in whom there is concern for intracranial or extracranial spread of infection or if there has been a poor response to antibiotics. Treatment involves hospital admission with parenteral antibiotics such as ampicillin/sulbactam, ceftriaxone, vancomycin, or piperacillin/tazobactam if there is a suspected *Pseudomonas* infection. If there is no improvement despite antibiotics, surgical management directed by otolaryngology may be indicated based on disease progression and site.

62. A healthy 9-year-old child is brought to the ED for persistent congestion, runny nose with thick secretions, and decreased appetite for 12 days. Parents report intermittent fever and cough that seems to be worse at night with no current or prior history of wheezing. There is no associated headache, vomiting, or rash. On physical examination, the child's vital signs are normal for age, and yellow purulent discharge is noted from the nares, along with malodorous breath. There are no signs of dental caries and no pharyngeal exudates, erythema, or abscess is present. There is mild tenderness over the maxillary sinus. What is the likely diagnosis?

The likely diagnosis in this child is acute bacterial sinusitis. According to the most recent AAP guidelines, a presumptive diagnosis of bacterial sinusitis should be made in a child/adolescent between the ages of 1 and 18 years presenting with a URI and any of the following additional features:

- Persistent illness, that is, nasal discharge (of any quality) or daytime cough or both lasting more than 10 days without improvement
  OR
- Biphasic illness with worsening or new onset of nasal discharge, daytime cough, or fever after initial improvement
  OR
- Severe onset, that is, concurrent fever (temperature $\geq 39°C/102.2°F$) and purulent nasal discharge for at least 3 consecutive days

63. What are the typical organisms causing sinusitis?
- *S. pneumoniae* (40%).
- Nontypable *H. influenzae* (20%).
- *M. catarrhalis* (20%).
- *S. aureus* is rarely isolated unless the sinusitis is associated with a dental infection. However, it is common when sinusitis is complicated by orbital or CNS involvement.

64. What is the role of role of diagnostic imaging for a child presenting with suspected sinusitis in the ED?

Sinusitis is a clinical diagnosis based on the established AAP criteria. Indications for imaging include suspected orbital or CNS involvement and should not routinely be utilized to differentiate between bacterial sinusitis and viral URI. However, CT or magnetic resonance imaging (MRI) could be helpful in children with drainable fluid collection within the cranium and orbit or those with persistent or recurrent infections that do not respond to medical management.

65. What is the recommended treatment for acute bacterial sinusitis?

Amoxicillin-clavulanate (80-90 mg/kg/day in two divided doses) is recommended as first-line therapy. In children who have a penicillin allergy, oral cephalosporins or levofloxacin are alternatives. Children who are unable to tolerate oral antibiotics can be treated with a single dose of IV/IM ceftriaxone. Admit those with severe infection and treat with a parenteral third-generation cephalosporin, coupled with vancomycin or metronidazole based on initial response to therapy.

66. What is Pott puffy tumor?

Pott puffy tumor (Fig. 37.5) was first described by Sir Percivall Pott in 1768. The patient presents with soft, fluctuant, painful forehead, or scalp swelling usually associated with frontal sinusitis. However, it can also develop as sequelae from head trauma, surgery in the frontal sinus region, dental infections, and cocaine use. Pott puffy tumor represents osteomyelitis of the frontal bone with subsequent subperiosteal elevation. Patients tend to be febrile and appear toxic. It is usually seen in older children who have developed frontal sinuses, with higher incidence noted in adolescence. Contrast-enhanced CT is the first-line radiology study for diagnosis in the ED, while MRI might aid in evaluating the degree of intracranial involvement. Treatment includes surgical drainage and an extended course of parenteral antibiotics.

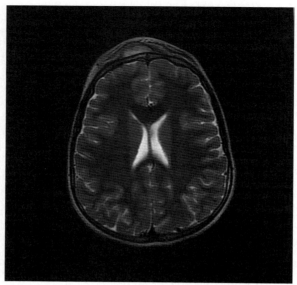

Fig. 37.5 Pott puffy tumor.

NECK INFECTIONS

67. What organisms are associated with deep neck infections (peritonsillar abscess, retropharyngeal abscess, and lateral pharyngeal abscess) in children?
Aerobic (*S. pyogenes, S. aureus,* and *H. influenzae*) and anaerobic (*Prevotella, Fusobacterium, and Peptostreptococcus* spp.) organisms are typically associated with deep neck infections in children. Almost 66% of deep neck abscesses contain β-lactamase-producing organisms.

68. Distinguish the features of deep neck infections in children.
For the features of deep neck infections in children, see Table 37.10.

69. What is Lemierre syndrome?
This is a relatively rare condition but has significant morbidity and mortality. It is a complication of a primary oropharyngeal infection. There is metastatic spread of the infection along with a suppurative thrombophlebitis of the internal jugular vein. Patients can initially present with pharyngitis and fever. Neck stiffness, pain, and mass can develop. When there is a clinical suspicion, a Doppler ultrasound or contrast-enhanced CT scan can point you to the diagnosis. *Fusobacterium* is a common isolate from cultures; however, Lemierre syndrome can arise secondary to *Streptococcus, Staphylococcus, Enterococcus, Proteus, Klebsiella, and Pseudomonas.* Hospital admission and treatment with broad-spectrum antibiotics are paramount.

70. Which IV antibiotics are appropriate for retropharyngeal abscess?
This is often institution-dependent. Ampicillin/sulbactam, clindamycin, third-generation cephalosporins, and metronidazole can be utilized for uncomplicated infection. With severe infection, one may need to consider vancomycin and linezolid as second-line parenteral antibiotics.

71. Do all children with retropharyngeal abscesses require surgical treatment?
Most patients with retropharyngeal abscesses (even those larger than 2 cm) can be treated successfully with IV antibiotics. Surgical incision and drainage have potential complications and should only be reserved for cases that do not respond to antibiotic therapy or in cases of persistent large abscess and/or airway compromise.

LYMPH NODES

72. What lymph node characteristics help distinguish infectious versus malignant causes?
Such characteristics are shown in Table 37.11.

Table 37.10 Features of Deep Neck Infections in Children

DEEP NECK INFECTION	AGE-ASSOCIATED	HISTORICAL/CLINICAL FEATURES	MANAGEMENT
Peritonsillar abscess	Adolescents and young adults	Difficulty swallowing or speaking, throat pain radiating to the ear, foul breath, swelling of one tonsil with lateral displacement of the uvula, trismus, drooling	Hospitalization, possible surgical drainage, IV antibiotics, tonsillectomy
Retropharyngeal abscess	<5 years (commonly 6 mo to 1 year)	High fever, preceding URI, or local infection, drooling, odynophagia dyspnea, hyperextension of the neck, unilateral posterior pharyngeal fullness Torticollis, trismus, difficulty breathing	Hospitalization, lateral neck x-ray (retropharyngeal space > half diameter of adjacent vertebral body), possible surgical drainage, stay in position of comfort, ENT consultation, IV antibiotics
Lateral pharyngeal/ parapharyngeal abscess	Older children, adolescents, and young adults	Ill-appearing, high fever, odynophagia, dysphagia, dyspnea; if anterior compartment (swelling of parotid region, trismus); if posterior compartment (minimal pain or trismus)	Hospitalization, possible surgical drainage, IV antibiotics

ENT, ear, nose, and throat; IV, intravenous; URI, upper respiratory infection.

Table 37.11 Characteristics of Lymph Nodes

VIRAL INFECTION	BACTERIAL INFECTION	MALIGNANCY
Soft	Soft to firm	Firm or rubbery
Tender or nontender	Tender	Nontender
Mobile	Fixed	Fixed or mobile
Nonerythematous	Erythematous	Nonerythematous
Small; usually <2 cm	Large; usually 2-3 cm	Increase in size over time
Discrete in a specific region or generalized/ bilateral Often cervical involvement	Unilateral Often submandibular followed by upper cervical, submental, occipital, and lower cervical nodes	Matted with adjacent nodes Left-sided supraclavicular lymphadenopathy is concerning
Duration 7-10 days	Medium duration (3-4 wk)	Duration >6 wk
Often associated with upper respiratory infections	Can be associated with dental, ear, throat, or scalp infections	Age >10 years Associated with fever, night sweats, and weight loss over the preceding 6 months

73. **How does a child with cat-scratch disease typically present?**

Chronic tender regional lymphadenopathy with overlying erythema is the hallmark of cat-scratch disease. Typically, there is a recent history of a scratch by a kitten followed by the appearance of a macule, papule, or vesicle (at around 12 days after the inoculation), which may last several days to weeks. Lymphadenopathy, proximal to the site develops 1 to 2 weeks after the scratch in approximately 50% of children and could be suppurative in nature. The axillary lymph nodes are most commonly involved, however, cervical, submandibular, submental, epitrochlear, or inguinal nodes can also be affected. Other clinical manifestations of cat-scratch disease include prolonged low-grade fever (30% of patients), malaise/fatigue, headaches, splenomegaly, anorexia/emesis/weight loss, sore throat, exanthems, conjunctivitis, and parotid swelling. The lymphadenopathy associated with cat-scratch disease is self-limited, lasting 2 to 4 months. CNS manifestations (encephalopathy, seizures, encephalitis, radiculitis, polyneuritis, myelitis, facial nerve palsy, acute hemiplegia) are rarely seen with this condition.

74. A healthy 5-year-old child presents with a rapidly growing, painless cervical mass for the past few days. On examination, the mass is unilateral and nontender. Induration and violaceous skin discoloration over the mass are noted. The overlying skin has a thin "paper-like appearance." The child has no fever. Which of the following is the most likely diagnosis?

The most likely organism is a nontuberculous mycobacterium (NTM). Classically, NTM lymph node infection is described as a unilateral, nontender cervical lymph node with a violaceous discoloration in an otherwise asymptomatic patient; usually without systemic signs or fever. There may have been a prior history of unsuccessful antistreptococcal/antistaphylococcal systemic antibiotic treatment. NTM affects both healthy and immunocompromised children and is found in contaminated soil and water (swimming pools, aquariums, and lakes). The recommended approach to the diagnosis of NTM adenitis is surgical excision of the affected node, as incision and drainage can be complicated by a sinus tract or a fistula formation.

RESPIRATORY INFECTIONS

75. A 3-month-old infant presents with a 2-day history of fever, nasal congestion, cough, and poor feeding. On physical examination, the infant has an RR of 60 breaths per minute and oxygen saturation of 90% in room air. You notice nasal flaring, intercostal retractions, and abdominal breathing. You hear faint expiratory wheezes throughout. What is the most likely diagnosis? Describe your initial management.

This infant likely has viral bronchiolitis, a disorder of the lower respiratory tract in infants characterized by acute inflammation, edema, and necrosis of the lining of the small airways as well as increased mucous production. Symptoms often start with nasal congestion and cough, progressing to signs of respiratory distress (tachypnea, nasal flaring, use of accessory muscles, wheezes, or rales). The most common etiology is RSV, but other causes are human rhinovirus, influenza, coronavirus, human metapneumovirus, and parainfluenza.

According to the AAP's Clinical Practice Guidelines, it is recommended to diagnose bronchiolitis and assess disease severity based on history and physical examination. Assess risk factors for severe disease (age <12 weeks, history of prematurity, underlying cardiopulmonary disease, immunodeficiency) and administer supplemental oxygen if the oxygen saturation is <90% on room air after performing nasal suctioning. Routine chest x-rays, albuterol, epinephrine, hypertonic saline, systemic corticosteroids, antibiotics, chest physiotherapy, and continuous pulse oximetry are not recommended.

76. Despite nasal suctioning, your 3-month-old infant with bronchiolitis demonstrates more tachypnea and increased work of breathing, with oxygen saturation of 86% on room air that does not improve with supplement oxygen via nasal cannula. What is your next step?

Noninvasive ventilation is often beneficial if initiated early in the management of pediatric acute respiratory failure associated with bronchiolitis. This will decrease the work of breathing, improve oxygenation and ventilation while avoiding complications associated with endotracheal intubation and invasive mechanical ventilation, and preserve spontaneous respiration and airway protective reflexes.

Although continuous positive airway pressure is a reasonable option, recent literature advocates for the use of high-flow nasal cannula therapy as a first-line modality for severe bronchiolitis. Recommended initial settings are 2 L/kg/minute for the first 10 kg of body weight and an additional 0.5 L/kg/minute for each kilogram greater than 10 kg with a maximum setting as indicated on the device equipment packaging. Set the fraction of inspired oxygen (FiO_2) at 0.40 and titrate to achieve a peripheral capillary oxygen saturation >92%.

77. A 10-year old otherwise healthy male presents to the ED with 3 days of high daily fever (temperature up to 104°F) associated with headache, nonproductive cough, chills, myalgias, and malaise. Today, his cough has become worse, associated with shortness of breath, and he complains of difficulty walking due to muscle pain. What infectious disease are you concerned about, and what are the potential complications?

This child likely has an influenza infection. Although most children recover fully after 3 to 7 days of illness, complications include the following:

- Neurologic complications—febrile seizures, severe encephalopathy, or encephalitis
- Reye syndrome—associated with the use of aspirin
- Myositis
- Myocarditis

- Complicated community-acquired pneumonia (parapneumonic effusion, empyema, necrotizing pneumonia, and lung abscess)
- Invasive secondary infections with *S. aureus* (including MRSA), *S. pneumoniae*, group A streptococcus, or other bacterial pathogens

78. What are the indications for the use of oseltamivir in influenza?

Oseltamivir is approved for the treatment of influenza A and B in children as young as 2 weeks and should be offered as early as possible to the following individuals, regardless of influenza vaccination status:

- Any hospitalized child.
- Any child, hospitalized or outpatient, with severe, complicated, or progressive illness.
- Children at high risk for complications (chronic pulmonary diseases, such as asthma, neurologic and neurodevelopmental disorders, hemodynamically significant cardiac disease, obesity, immunosuppression, metabolic diseases such as diabetes, and hemoglobinopathies such as sickle cell disease).
- Any previously healthy, symptomatic outpatient not at high risk for complications if treatment can be initiated within 48 hours of illness onset.
- Children whose sibling or household contact are either younger than 6 months or have a high-risk condition that predisposes them to complications of influenza.

79. A 2-month-old presents to the ED with nasal congestion, low-grade fever, and a paroxysmal cough for a few days. Prior to presentation, the infant had a coughing episode resulting in apnea and perioral cyanosis. What is the likely etiology?

Pertussis. This infection often starts with mild upper respiratory tract symptoms, with or without fever, similar to the common cold (catarrhal stage), and progresses to paroxysmal coughs, characterized by inspiratory "whoop" after repeated coughs on the same breath (paroxysmal stage), at times followed by vomiting. In young infants, you may not hear the characteristic whoop. Symptoms improve over weeks to months (convalescent stage). In infants <6 months, the paroxysmal stage may be associated with gagging, gasping, bradycardia, or apnea. Pertussis in infants has a high mortality and morbidity. Complications in infants with pertussis include pneumonia, seizures, encephalopathy, and death. Pertussis should be considered in any infant with a cough longer than 10 to 14 days. Adolescents and adults in the household are a major reservoir for the transmission of pertussis because of their waxing vaccine-induced immunity.

80. What is the antibiotic choice for a child with pertussis?

Antibiotic therapy administered during the catarrhal stage may ameliorate the infection, and therefore, therapy is indicated before test results have returned if the clinical history is suggestive or if the patient is at high risk of severe or complicated disease (such as infants <4 months). A 5-day course of azithromycin is the first-line choice for the treatment of all pediatric patients; erythromycin, clarithromycin, and TMP-SMZ are alternative choices.

81. A 12-year-old healthy female presents with a 1-week history of fever and cough and reports difficulty breathing. Her temperature is 38.4°C, her RR is 22 breaths per minute, and her oxygen saturation is 98% in room air. She is breathing comfortably and speaking in full sentences. She has crackles in the right lower posterior chest. Do you need a chest x-ray to diagnose pneumonia?

In an effort to decrease exposure to radiation and because of the difficulty distinguishing between consolidation and atelectasis on radiography, the Infectious Diseases Society of America and the Pediatric Infectious Diseases Society recommend against the use of routine chest radiographs for the confirmation of suspected community-acquired pneumonia in children not requiring hospitalization. Clinical diagnosis of pneumonia is often made in a child who presents with fever and cough, the presence of auscultatory findings (crackles, rales, rhonchi), and evidence of respiratory distress (tachypnea, grunting, retractions, hypoxia).

82. Are there other methods to aid in the diagnosis of pneumonia in children?

Chest ultrasound may be used for the evaluation of local complications of pneumonia, such as parapneumonic effusions and empyema. Recent studies have also demonstrated high sensitivity and specificity for detecting lung consolidation compared with chest radiography.

Blood cultures identify a pathogen in 2% to 7% of children with community-acquired pneumonia, and 10% to 15% of children with a parapneumonic effusion.

Pleural fluid cultures are positive in up to 35% of children with pneumonia and should be performed whenever pleural fluid is obtained.

In terms of acute-phase reactants, CRP (>40-60 mg/L) is elevated in 64% of children with bacterial pneumonia and a PCT cutoff value of 0.25 ng/mL demonstrated a sensitivity of 85% and specificity of 45% in children with bacterial pneumonia.

83. **What are the most common etiologies of pneumonia in children?**

Pneumonia is a disease caused by a variety of pathogens, including viruses and bacteria. Viruses were identified in greater than 70% of pneumonia in children. The most common viruses include RSV, human rhinovirus, human metapneumovirus, and adenovirus. The most common bacteria associated with pediatric pneumonia are *S. pneumoniae, H. influenzae, S. pyogenes,* and *S. aureus.* In older children, consider atypical pneumonia caused by *M. pneumoniae* and *Chlamydia pneumoniae.* Other pathogens less commonly seen are *Mycobacterium tuberculosis,* fungi, *Burkholderia cepacia, Aspergillus fumigatus,* and *P. aeruginosa.*

84. **A 9-year-old child presents with nonproductive cough, low-grade fever, and malaise. On physical examination, the patient appears well, has no evidence of respiratory distress, and has bilateral lower lung field crackles. What is the most likely cause of this child's symptoms?**

This is a classic presentation of a child with atypical pneumonia caused by *M. pneumoniae* or *C. pneumoniae.* Before modern diagnostic tests were available, researchers and clinicians noted that some pneumonias had different characteristics compared to "typical" pneumonias; children with "atypical" pneumonia had slightly different symptoms and appeared less sick, had chest radiographs with different findings, and had clinical courses that responded differently to antibiotics.

M. pneumoniae is a common cause of atypical pneumonia in older children and young adults. It accounts for about 40% of community-acquired pneumonias in certain populations. Bilateral diffuse infiltrates are the most common radiographic findings, which are frequently out of proportion to clinical findings. Extrapulmonary manifestations, including a maculopapular rash (10%), CNS disease, hemolytic anemia, arthritis, and hepatitis, are occasionally seen in atypical pneumonia syndromes caused by *M. pneumoniae.*

85. **You have made the diagnosis of bacterial pneumonia, and what are your strategies for antimicrobial therapy?**

Such strategies are shown in Table 37.12.

86. **What should you suspect in a child who was recently diagnosed with bacterial pneumonia with worsening symptoms over 48 to 72 hours despite oral antibiotics?**

Complicated community-acquired pneumonia should be suspected in any child with pneumonia not responding to appropriate antibiotic treatment within 48 to 72 hours. Complicated community-acquired pneumonia is characterized by a combination of local complications (parapneumonic effusion, empyema, necrotizing pneumonia, and lung abscess) and systemic complications (bacteremia, metastatic infection, multiorgan failure, acute respiratory distress syndrome, disseminated intravascular coagulation, and rarely death). Causative organisms include *S. pneumoniae* and *S. aureus,* and diagnosis is often made by chest radiography and ultrasound (CT scan is not usually indicated), and treatment includes prolonged IV antibiotics. There may be a role for systemic corticosteroids; more studies are needed.

87. **You are managing a 4-year-old refugee who has been having 6 weeks of cough, weight loss, fatigue, fever, and night sweats. You suspect tuberculosis (TB). What risk factors would make him prone to this illness, and how do you confirm your suspicion?**

M. tuberculosis infection can mimic several infective and noninfective etiologies. The patient described above has some of the classic symptoms of active pulmonary TB but many children who have TB or latent TB may be asymptomatic. Think of TB as a possibility in a patient with the following risk factors:

Table 37.12 Antibiotic Therapy for Pneumonia in Children Based on Ages

AGE	BACTERIAL PNEUMONIA	ATYPICAL PNEUMONIA
Neonates	Outpatient—N/A Inpatient—Ampicillin + gentamicin	N/A
1-3 mo	Outpatient—Amoxicillin Inpatient—Cefotaxime; azithromycin if suspect *Chlamydia trachomatis* or *B. pertussis*	N/A
3 mo to 5 years	Outpatient—Amoxicillin Inpatient—Ampicillin or ceftriaxone; clindamycin; or vancomycin in methicillin-resistant *Staphylococcus aureus*-prevalent regions	Outpatient—azithromycin Inpatient—azithromycin, doxycycline, or levofloxacin
5 years to 17 years	Outpatient—Amoxicillin Inpatient—Ampicillin or ceftriaxone; clindamycin or vancomycin in methicillin-resistant *S. aureus*-prevalent regions	Outpatient—azithromycin Inpatient—azithromycin, doxycycline, or levofloxacin

- Contact with people who have confirmed or suspected TB (e.g., in the case of a positive tuberculin skin test [TST]).
- Contact with people who are homeless, have been incarcerated or in other congregate settings, or those who inject or use drugs or excessive alcohol.
- Radiological or clinical findings suggestive of TB.
- Immigrated from countries with endemic infection, for example, Asia, the Middle East, Africa, and countries of the former Soviet Union. Also, consider international adoptees.
- A history of travel to a country with endemic infection where they had direct contact with the population.
- Chronic or complex medical history including diabetes mellitus, chronic renal failure, malnutrition, congenital or acquired immunodeficiencies (e.g., human immunodeficiency virus [HIV] infection), and neoplasms.
- Taking medications such as prolonged high-dose corticosteroid therapy, chemotherapy agents, or tumor necrosis factor-alpha antagonists.

A patient presenting with the above symptoms would likely need an extensive workup that starts with a CBC, looking for markers of bone marrow dysfunction, electrolytes, and a chest x-ray. For children younger than 2 years, the TST can be utilized. For those 2 years and older the TST or interferon gamma release assay (IGRA) testing can both be used. The IGRA may be more accurate in patients previously vaccinated with Bacillus Calmette-Guérin vaccine. Note that these tests cannot distinguish between TB infection and TB disease. TB is a public health sentinel event. Airborne precautions need to be taken.

KEY POINTS: COMMON ETIOLOGIC AGENTS OF PNEUMONIA IN CHILDREN

1. Neonate: Group B streptococcus, *E. coli*, *L. monocytogenes*
2. Infant (<3 months): RSV, human metapneumovirus, influenza virus, parainfluenza virus, adenovirus, *C. trachomatis*
3. Infant to toddler (<5 years): Respiratory viruses, *S. pneumoniae*, *M. pneumoniae*
4. School-age to adolescent: *M. pneumoniae*, *C. pneumoniae*, S. *pneumoniae*, respiratory viruses

CARDIAC INFECTIONS

88. How does myocarditis present in children?

Myocarditis is a life-threatening condition and is the leading cause of cardiogenic shock in the pediatric population. There are multiple etiologies including toxic, pharmacologic, autoimmune, and vasculitic processes. Viral infection is the most common etiology, and Coxsackie B, echovirus, and adenovirus are the most frequent viruses found. Initial presentation can be frustratingly nonspecific and can even be missed on the first encounter. A flu-like illness or viral prodrome is most commonly reported in history. Infants may present with feeding difficulties, lethargy, or respiratory distress. Chest pain and abdominal pain are common presenting symptoms in older children. A combination of fever, malaise, dyspnea, tachypnea, chest pain, pallor, cool extremities are often noted, and other signs of hypoperfusion can be seen in older children who present with shock.

The cardiac examination can reveal signs of cardiac dysfunction or heart failure such as tachycardia at rest, muffled or distant heart sounds, lateral displacement of the point of maximal impulse, and a gallop rhythm. Other clinical findings include jugular venous distention, weak pulses, cyanosis, poor perfusion, hepatosplenomegaly, edema, and altered mental status. In rare occurrences, sudden cardiac death may be the initial presentation of myocarditis. Think of myocarditis with an ill-appearing child presenting with tachycardia and other signs of cardiogenic shock.

89. What is the recommended diagnostic workup for suspected myocarditis?

- Chest radiography may demonstrate cardiomegaly, interstitial pulmonary edema, or pulmonary vascular congestion and pleural effusions.
- Electrocardiography is usually abnormal but is not specific. There may be sinus tachycardia, mild to moderate PR interval prolongation, generalized low-voltage QRS complexes, ST-segment elevation or depression, T-wave inversion, decreased precordial voltages, high-grade atrioventricular block, and complex ventricular or supra-ventricular arrhythmias as well as atrial and ventricular enlargement.
- Point-of-care, bedside ultrasound is helpful in the early diagnosis of cardiomyopathy. An experienced user may note global left ventricular or biventricular dysfunction and pericardial effusions.
- Echocardiography typically demonstrates left ventricular dysfunction, global cardiac chamber enlargement with poorly contracting ventricles, wall motion abnormalities, or atrioventricular valve regurgitation. Pericardial effusion may also be present.
- Cardiac biomarkers such as troponin reflect cardiac injury and strain. Elevated troponin is seen in most patients with myocarditis. The degree of elevation does not consistently correlate with the severity of disease, and unfortunately, a normal biomarker does not exclude myocarditis.
- Natriuretic peptides such as B-type natriuretic peptide and NT-proBNP may be elevated in myocarditis and suggest cardiac etiology of symptoms as compared to a respiratory etiology.

- WBC count, erythrocyte sedimentation rate, and creatine kinase-MB fraction may be abnormal but are nonspecific.
- Based on the possible etiologies of infective myocarditis a blood culture and viral studies including those testing for SARS-CoV-2, EBV, and CMV may also be helpful.
- Cardiac MRI is becoming a common tool in the diagnosis of myocarditis and is perhaps the gold standard for diagnosis. This modality may require sedation.
- Beyond the emergency department, endomyocardial biopsy is rarely performed and is reserved for cases refractory to standard treatment.

90. **What is the acute management of infective myocarditis in infants and children?**
    - Stabilization of airway, breathing, and circulation.
    - Aim to reduce ventricular filling pressure, decrease systemic vascular resistance, and maximize oxygen delivery.
    - Intubation and ventilatory support under the guidance of pediatric cardiology and pediatric cardiac anesthesiology are often required in fulminant cases. Deployment of extracorporeal membrane oxygenation for further stabilization is based on individual hospital/cardiac/cardiothoracic protocols.
    - Judicious fluid resuscitation (e.g., a 5-10 mL/kg bolus) was administered slowly in the hypovolemic patient with constant reevaluation of vital signs and clinical examination to assess for heart failure.
    - Diuretics, inotropic agents, angiotensin-converting enzyme inhibitors, β-blockers, and antiarrhythmics.
    - Admission to an intensive care setting/cardiac intensive care setting for serial echocardiography, electrocardiography, and monitoring.
    - Specific antibiotics if a bacterial etiology is considered.
    - Continue care in conjunction with a pediatric cardiology team.

91. **What are the common symptoms, signs, and laboratory findings in infants and children with infective endocarditis?**
    Such symptoms, signs, and laboratory findings are shown in Table 37.13.

92. **Differentiate among Osler nodes, Janeway lesions, and Roth spots.**
    - **Osler nodes** are painful, red, nodular lesions seen most frequently on the pulp areas of the distal digits. Think of "ouch"-lers nodes.
    - **Janeway lesions** are small, erythematous, nontender areas typically on the palms and soles.
    - **Roth spots** are retinal hemorrhages with central clearing.
      Although commonly seen in adults, these findings are rare in infants and children with infective endocarditis. Other embolic phenomena associated with endocarditis include splinter hemorrhages and conjunctival hemorrhages.

93. **How would you clinically diagnose bacterial endocarditis?**
    Two major criteria or one major plus three minor OR five minor criteria according to the modified Duke criteria are required for *definitive clinical diagnosis* of infective endocarditis.
    Major criteria: (1) Positive blood culture for typical bacterial endocarditis-causing organisms (ideally from two to three separate initial blood cultures); (2) Single positive blood culture for *Coxiella burnetii* or antiphase 1 IgG antibody titer >1:800; (3) Evidence of endocardial involvement by echocardiogram.

Table 37.13 Symptoms, Signs, and Laboratory Findings in Infective Endocarditis

SYMPTOMS	SIGNS	LABORATORY FINDINGS
• Unexplained, prolonged fever (especially in patients with congenital heart defects or prosthetic valves) • Night sweats • Chills • General malaise • Irritability • Anorexia/weight loss • Fatigue/weakness • GI symptoms • Headaches • Altered mental status • Chest pain	• New-onset diastolic murmur • Abnormal systolic murmur (regurgitant or holosystolic) • Hypoxemia • Petechiae • Splenomegaly • Circulating immune complex deposits/embolic phenomena (Osler nodes, Janeway lesions, and Roth spots splinter hemorrhages) • Heart failure	• Positive aerobic blood culture • Anemia, hemolytic anemia bandemia on CBC • Elevated ESR and CRP • Microscopic hematuria on UA • Rheumatoid factor • Hypocomplementemia

CBC, complete blood count; CRP, C-reactive protein; ESR, erythrocyte sedimentation rate; UA, urinalysis.

Minor criteria: (1) Predisposing cardiac condition or history of IV drug use; (2) Fever >38°C; (3) Vascular manifestations (septic pulmonary infarcts, mycotic aneurysm, intracranial and/or conjunctival hemorrhages, Janeway lesions, major arterial emboli); (4) Immunological manifestations: glomerulonephritis, positive rheumatoid factor, Osler nodes, Roth spots; and (5) Microbiological evidence that is not included in the major criteria.

94. What antibiotics are recommended for the presumptive diagnosis of infective endocarditis?
Although viridans group streptococci are the most common etiological agents, it is not essential and may even be harmful to immediately administer antibiotics without definitive knowledge of the causative organism. In emergency cases, consider an aminoglycoside such as gentamicin combined with a penicillinase-resistant penicillin, for example, ampicillin/sulbactam. Alternative therapy includes ampicillin/sulbactam with gentamicin with the addition of vancomycin.

95. What are the clinical manifestations associated with pericarditis?
    - Substernal chest pain is worse with inspiration and lying flat and relieved by sitting upright and forward. Pain may radiate to the scapular ridge.
    - Abdominal pain, vomiting.
    - Irritability.
    - Grunting expiratory sounds.
    - Fever.
    - Exercise intolerance.
    - Pericardial friction rub is best heard in the second to fourth intercostal spaces, midclavicular line, and left sternal border during deep inspiration with the patient kneeling or in the knee-chest position. This is a pathognomonic finding and has been described as "scratchy" or "creaking leather" on auscultation.
    - In the unstable patient be vigilant for signs of tamponade; look for Beck's triad (hypotension, muffled heart sounds, and jugular venous distension). In addition to tachycardia, peripheral vasoconstriction, decreased arterial pulse pressure, or pulsus paradoxus (a fall in systolic blood pressure by >10 mm Hg with inspiration).

96. What are the diagnostic findings associated with pericarditis?
    - WBC count, CRP, erythrocyte sedimentation rate (ESR), and troponin may be elevated
    - Blood culture and testing for TB in at-risk populations
    - Pericardial fluid analysis suggestive of infection
    - Increased size of cardiac shadow in the absence of pulmonary congestion on chest radiography (water bottle heart)
    - Electrocardiography (50% of patients may not follow the electrocardiac progression as outlined below):
      - Stage I: Diffuse ST elevation and PR depression
      - Stage II: Normalization of ST and PR segments
      - Stage III: Widespread T-wave inversions
      - Stage IV: Normalization of T waves
    - Echocardiography/point-of-care ultrasound: presence of pericardial fluid
    - Microbiological evaluation of the pericardial fluid by pericardiocentesis
    - Viral cultures, serologic tests, and molecular genetic techniques

GASTROINTESTINAL INFECTIONS

97. A 5-year-old child presents with a 2-day history of fever, bloody diarrhea, and severe abdominal pain. Which infectious agents are most likely responsible?
The most common agents are *Salmonella, Shigella*, and *Campylobacter* spp.; shiga toxin-producing *E. coli* (*E. coli* O157:H7); and *Yersinia* spp. Other infectious agents, including *Vibrio parahaemolyticus, Aeromonas* spp., and acute amebiasis, should be considered. Viral etiologies of diarrhea often cause low-grade fever and watery, non-bloody diarrhea.

98. Which bacterial stool pathogens require antimicrobial treatment?
    - ***Shigella:*** Most infections are self-limiting; however, antibiotics can reduce the length of symptoms. Antibiotics are therefore recommended for severe disease with dehydration, or in immunocompromised individuals.
    - ***Salmonella:*** Treatment does not shorten the duration of the symptoms and may actually prolong the carrier state. However, bacteremia is common in infants younger than 3 months, in patients with sickle cell disease, and in other immunocompromised individuals. Therefore treatment should be considered if bacteremia is suspected, as well as for children with chronic gastrointestinal disease, malignant neoplasms, hemoglobinopathies, HIV infection, or other immunosuppressive illnesses or therapies.
    - ***Campylobacter:*** Antibiotics may shorten the duration of illness and excretion of suspected organisms and may prevent relapse.
    - ***Yersenia:*** Antibiotics may decrease the duration of shedding.
    - ***E. coli* O157:H7:** No treatment because there is no proven benefit. A meta-analysis failed to confirm an increased risk of hemolytic uremic syndrome in patients treated with antibiotics.

99. A 2-year-old presents with vomiting, profuse diarrhea, and new-onset seizures. What could be the etiology of this clinical picture?

    Shigella infections are associated with CNS symptoms, including seizures and toxic encephalopathy. Severe diarrhea regardless of the etiology, however, may cause electrolyte abnormalities that result in seizures.

100. Should antimotility agents, probiotics, and prebiotics be used to manage gastroenteritis in children?

    Antimotility agents have limited benefits and have a high rate of side effects. Products with opiate derivatives are actually contraindicated. Non-narcotic antimotility agents may be used in afebrile patients with nonbloody diarrhea. Probiotics are live microorganisms that work by stimulating the host immune system, may be associated with reduced severity and duration of illness, and are most effective if started early in the disease course. Prebiotics, oligosaccharides that stimulate the growth of intestinal flora, have failed to show a decrease in diarrheal severity or length of illness in children, and thus are not recommended.

101. What are indications for hospitalization in children with gastroenteritis?

    - Infants <3 months who appear ill (fever, irritability, abdominal distension)
    - Children with underlying chronic illness (diabetes, renal disease, cardiopulmonary disease, immunodeficiency, gastrointestinal disease, etc.)
    - Evidence of shock (hypoperfusion) or significant dehydration
    - Persistent vomiting, especially if bloody or bilious
    - Severe abdominal pain or distension or concern for a surgical abdomen
    - Neurologic abnormalities (altered mental status, seizures)
    - Failure of oral rehydration

102. Which organisms cause foodborne illnesses?

    The list of onset, symptoms, and etiology of foodborne illnesses is shown in Table 37.14.

103. A 3-month-old infant presents with a 3-day history of constipation, progressively poor feeding, and lethargy. On physical examination, you notice a quiet, inactive infant who is otherwise alert with good perfusion. The neurologic examination reveals a weak cry, poor suck, and hypotonia. What is the likely diagnosis?

    Infant botulism. Infants with botulism may appear to be septic, but usually are afebrile and have stable vital signs. Botulism occurs after ingestion of airborne spores from soil or dust. The ingested spores produce toxins in

Table 37.14 Onset, Symptoms, and Etiology of Foodborne Illnesses

TIME OF ONSET	MAIN SYMPTOMS	ORGANISM OR TOXIN
1-6 hr	Nausea, vomiting, usually febrile	*Staphylococcus aureus*
1-6 hr	Nausea, vomiting, afebrile	*Bacillus cereus* (emetic form)
8-16 hr	Diarrhea, febrile	*B. cereus* (diarrheal form)
6-24 hr	Foul-smelling diarrhea, cramps, afebrile	*Clostridium perfringens*
16-48 hr	Abdominal cramping, diarrhea, fever	*Vibrio cholerae, Norwalk virus, Escherichia coli* O157:H7, *Cryptosporidium* spp.
16-72 hr	Bloody diarrhea, fever, abdominal cramping	*Salmonella, Shigella, Campylobacter* spp., and *E. coli*
16-72 r	Bloody diarrhea, fever, pseudoappendicitis, pharyngitis	*Yersenia enterocolitica*
1-6 wk	Mucoid diarrhea (fatty stools), abdominal pain, weight loss	*Giardia lamblia*
12-36 hr	Neurologic manifestations: vertigo, diplopia, areflexia, weakness, difficulty breathing and swallowing, constipation	*Clostridium botulinum*
14 days	All the above, plus vomiting, rose spots, constipation, abdominal pain, fever, chills, malaise, swollen lymph nodes	*Salmonella typhi*

the intestine of the infant. Peak incidence is in infants 6 weeks to 6 months. Breast-feeding is a significant risk factor. The ingestion of honey or corn syrup is often implicated, but not proven to be a risk factor. A history of soil disruption, which occurs near construction sites, has been a common epidemiologic finding in reported cases. Admit all infants with botulism and observe for progressive weakness and respiratory failure. Botulism immune globulin IV is an antitoxin that, when given early, decreases the duration of illness and hospital stay.

KEY POINTS: INFANT BOTULISM

1. Consider in septic appearing infant who is afebrile, with normal vital signs.
2. Peak ages 6 weeks to 6 months.
3. Etiology—spores in soil that are ingested produce toxins in the gut.
4. Nearby construction sites are often implicated.
5. Honey may also contain spores (honey is not recommended for young infants).
6. Constipation, weak cry, hypotonia, and poor suck are early features.
7. Progressive weakness may lead to respiratory failure.
8. Admit all patients, treat with antitoxin, botulism immune globulin.

104. **A 5-year-old child who resides in a group home is transported to your ED because he appears "yellow" in color. What are the diagnostic considerations?**
Hepatitis A virus (HAV) is highly contagious and spreads among children with poor hygiene or those in close quarters. Outbreaks at childcare facilities usually represent an extension of a community outbreak. HAV infection is abrupt in onset and self-limiting, consisting of fever, anorexia, nausea, and headache. Jaundice is uncommon in young children compared with older children and adults, in whom jaundice can occur in 70% of cases. Liver failure in HAV is not common. The differential diagnosis should include hepatitis B or C (obtain a good history for associated risk factors: maternal history, blood transfusions, sexual contact), EBV, adenoviruses, enteroviruses, varicella zoster, and HIV.

105. **A 17-year-old girl complains of fatigue, abdominal pain, nausea, and vomiting for a few days. She had a URI last week. On physical examination, she is afebrile and has tachycardia without tachypnea. Eyes are icteric. She has right upper quadrant tenderness to palpation without guarding or rebound. Skin is jaundiced. Capillary refill prolonged. What do you think is going on?**
Her presentation is consistent with hepatitis. Often the disease process starts with a 5- to 7-day prodrome of low-grade fever, anorexia, malaise, fatigue, nausea/vomiting, and epigastric/right upper quadrant abdominal pain, followed by an acute onset of scleral icterus, jaundice, dark urine. About 25% to 50% of patients will have splenomegaly. Laboratory findings consistent with hepatitis include hyperbilirubinemia, elevated liver transaminases, elevated WBC, elevated PT, hypoglycemia, and normal albumin and globulin. Treatment includes IV fluids for dehydration, vitamin K and/or clotting factors as needed, and lactulose/neomycin for hepatic encephalopathy. Indications for hospital admission include dehydration due to anorexia and vomiting, bilirubin >20 mg/dL, abnormal PT, WBC >25k, and transaminases >3000 U/L.

URINARY TRACT INFECTIONS

106. **How common are UTIs in infants and children?**
A UTI is the second most common bacterial infection seen in children following acute otitis media. In the first year of life, UTIs are more common in males (3.7%) compared to females (2%), partly due to a higher incidence of congenital urinary tract anomalies. After infancy, females have a higher incidence of childhood UTI at 8% compared to males at 1% to 2%. The risk of UTI recurrence following an initial infection is 12% to 30% in the first 6 to 12 months. In febrile infants less than 3 months who present without a source of infection, the incidence of a UTI is approximately 7% to 9% regardless of gender. This decreases to 2% for both males (after 3 months) and females (after 12 months). Circumcised infant males have a lower risk of developing a UTI in infancy.

107. **A father brings his 9-month-old daughter to the ED following a 3-day history of fever, temperature up to 102.5°F, and reported irritability. The examination reveals no signs of focal infection. You are concerned for a UTI and recommend obtaining a catheterized sample. The patient's father is reluctant to pursue this option but is willing to discuss the pros and cons. How do you proceed?**
The AAP has identified risk factors for UTIs in febrile infants. This includes a temperature >39°C (102.2°F), and a fever for more than 2 days in a female or uncircumcised male who is less than 12 months old without other sources of fever. A UTI probability score can be shown to families by keying in this data on an online UTI calculator

(https://uticalc.pitt.edu). In this at-risk patient, the only definitive, timely method to confirm a UTI is with a urine culture obtained by catheter. The risks of this procedure, which include minor trauma and a relatively minor risk of bladder infection, are far outweighed by the short- and long-term morbidity of missing a UTI which can include the following:

- Worsening dehydration, fever, and fussiness
- Ascending infection (perinephric abscess/ pyelonephritis)
- Hematogenous uropathogenic spread, bacteremia, urosepsis, and meningitis
- Renal injury and scarring leading to long-term renal dysfunction, hypertension, chronic kidney disease
- Missed identification of an anatomical anomaly making the child prone to UTI

108. **What other comorbidities make patients vulnerable to developing UTIs?**
- High-grade vesicoureteral reflux
- Congenital anomalies of the kidneys and the urinary tract
- Bowel and bladder dysfunction
- Instrumentation of the urinary tract (indwelling bladder catheterization)
- Kidney stones*
- Sexual activity*
- Diabetes*

*In older children and adolescents

109. **What are the signs and symptoms of a UTI?**
Signs and symptoms of a UTI are shown in Table 37.15.

The most common presentation of UTI in all age groups is fever. In infants, additional symptoms such as lethargy, irritability, hypothermia, or failure to thrive are nonspecific and often occur with other infectious and noninfectious conditions.

In the child who is 2 years and older, there may be reports of dysuria, urinary frequency, and suprapubic tenderness. However, these symptoms are also seen in the setting of non-UTI conditions such as constipation, vulvovaginitis, epididymal-orchitis, meatal stenosis, or *Candida* infection and it is also worth assessing for these by a thorough physical examination and/or additional testing. The history of foul-smelling urine is nonspecific. With urinary symptoms and concerning or inconsistent history in the patient who is unable or unwilling to communicate, sexual assault or nonaccidental trauma must also be on the differential.

Adolescents have a more reliable symptom correlation with UTIs, in part, due to their maturity and development. However, in this age group, UTI symptoms may also arise in the setting of a sexually transmitted illness or pregnancy.

110. **What is the definition of pyuria?**
Pyuria is defined as the presence of 5 WBCs per high-power field (centrifuged) or 10 WBCs/mm³ (uncentrifuged) specimens. On urine dipstick analysis, positive leukocyte esterase (≥trace) is used as proxy for pyuria. Without other findings, this is not adequate to diagnose a UTI and is not a substitute for a urine culture. A sterile pyuria (one without significant bacterial growth on urine culture) may also be seen with multiple conditions including recent antibiotic use, viral infections, appendicitis, group A *Streptococcal* infection, renal tubular acidosis, glomerulonephritis, Kawasaki disease, and TB.

Table 37.15 Signs and Symptoms of Urinary Tract Infections According to Age

NEWBORNS	INFANTS AND TODDLERS	SCHOOL-AGED CHILDREN
(Unexplained) fever	Fever	Fever
Failure to thrive	Failure to thrive	Dysuria
Vomiting	Vomiting	Frequency
Irritability	Irritability	Urgency
Lethargy	Diarrhea	Enuresis
Jaundice	Suprapubic tenderness	Abdominal pain
Sepsis	Flank pain	Flank pain
Hypothermia		

111. **You are lecturing medical students regarding specificity and sensitivity. What is the most specific component of the chemical UA in testing for UTI?**
Sensitivity refers to the ability of a test to correctly identify patients with a disease while specificity is defined as the ability of a test to correctly identify people without the disease. Most urinary pathogens can metabolize urinary nitrate to nitrite. Nitrite testing has a relatively low sensitivity for UTI; therefore a negative test cannot reliably rule out or screen out a UTI. However, a positive nitrite is highly specific at 98% to 99% (as there are very few other sources of urinary nitrite besides infection) and therefore it is used to rule in and preliminarily, yet accurately diagnose UTI in any age-pending cultures (the gold standard).

112. **What constitutes a contaminated versus accurate urine sample?**
Urine samples obtained via urine bags have high contamination rates. The most common urine sample contaminants are feces and skin flora. The presence of ≥10 per high-power field squamous epithelial cells on UA, along with insignificant bacterial colony count, or the identification of two or more pathogens on urine culture obtained via midstream urine specimen is suggestive of contamination. Additionally, the growth of nonuropathogenic organisms such as *Lactobacillus, Corynebacterium, Viridans streptococci,* or *Staphylococcus epidermidis* in urine culture suggests a contaminated sample. On the other hand, the presence of confirmed uropathogens such as *Enterococcus, Klebsiella,* and *Pseudomonas* species in the following numbers: 50,000 colony-forming units (CFU)/mL (catheterized sample), 100,000 CFU/mL (clean catch sample), or 1000 CFU/mL (suprapubic aspiration sample) are confirmatory of a UTI.

113. **What treatment options are available for infants and children with simple cystitis and pyelonephritis?**
Outpatient therapy may be considered for well-appearing, well-hydrated patients, without underlying urological conditions, who can tolerate oral medications and have reliable caregivers.
Empiric therapy should be based on patterns of local antimicrobial sensitivity, and treatment adjusted according to urine cultures. A 3- to 7-day course of oral antibiotics is recommended. As of 2022, most uropathogens causing UTIs in children were sensitive to third-generation cephalosporins. Antibiotics such as amoxicillin and SMZ/TMP should no longer be utilized due to increased resistance.

114. **When should you consider inpatient treatment of a UTI in young children?**
Criteria for admission and parenteral antibiotic treatment include dehydration, inability to tolerate oral medication (vomiting), ill appearance, hemodynamic instability, worsening progression despite oral antibiotics, and presence of chronic diseases such as sickle cell or diabetes mellitus. Furthermore, the AAP recommends admission and IV antibiotics for febrile infants younger than 2 months with findings of UTI.

KEY POINTS: HOSPITAL ADMISSION FOR UTI

1. Vomiting—cannot tolerate oral antibiotics
2. Ill child, hemodynamic instability
3. Worsening condition despite oral antibiotics
4. Comorbid conditions: for example, diabetes mellitus, sickle cell disease, renal disease
5. Febrile young infants <2 months old

GYNECOLOGIC INFECTIONS

115. **A 17-year-old sexually active female complains of unilateral groin swelling. On physical examination of her labia minora, she has a deep and painful ulcer with ragged edges and a friable base. The base is covered with a yellow exudate. She has left-sided inguinal adenopathy, which is mildly tender. What is your differential diagnosis of genital ulcers?**
Differential diagnosis for genital ulcers is shown in Table 37.16.

116. **A 17-year-old female presents with a chief complaint of vaginal discharge. She states that it is foul-smelling, white, and non-pruritic. She has had similar symptoms in the past. What is your differential diagnosis of infectious causes of vaginal discharge?**
Such differential diagnosis is shown in Table 37.17.

117. **A 14-year-old female presents with right lower quadrant (RLQ) abdominal pain. No vomiting or diarrhea. She admits to unprotected sexual activity with multiple partners. She reports scant vaginal discharge. Vital signs are normal. Abdominal examination reveals mild RLQ tenderness to palpation without rebound or guarding and you suspect pelvic inflammatory disease (PID). Describe this condition.**
PID is an ascending infection of the genital tract including endometritis, salpingitis, tubo-ovarian abscess, and pelvic peritonitis. The etiologic agents causing PID primarily include *N. gonorrhoeae* and *C. trachomatis.* The

Table 37.16 Differential Diagnosis for Genital Ulcers

DISEASE	CLINICAL PRESENTATION	DIAGNOSIS	TREATMENT

Herpes genitalis (herpes simplex 1, 2)	Single or multiple vesicles on the genitalia that rupture to form shallow ulcers; very painful and resolve without scarring; may be preceded by tingling or burning sensation	• Viral detection
		  • DNA PCR—high sensitivity and specificity
		  • Immunofluorescence
		  • Culture—low sensitivity (dependent on stage of lesion, primary vs. recurrent) and high specificity
		• Serologic testing (IgM, IgG)
			Primary
			• Acyclovir 400 mg PO TID for 7-10 days, OR
			• Acyclovir 200 mg PO 5x/day for 7-10 days, OR
			• Valacyclovir 1 g PO BID for 7-10 days OR
			• Famciclovir 250 mg PO TID for 7-10 days

Syphilis *(Treponema pallidum)*	Chancre at the site of the inoculation (painless, papule eroding to an indurated ulcer) with lymphadenopathy; heals in 4-6 wk	• Non-treponemal—Venereal Disease Research Lab or rapid plasma reagin • Treponemal fluorescent treponemal antibody absorption or *T. pallidum* passive particle agglutination assay	• Primary, secondary, and early latent (contracted in the last year) • Benzathine Penicillin G 2.4 million units IM × 1
Lymphogranuloma venereum (*Chlamydia trachomatis* L1, L2, L3)	Non-painful genital papule or ulcer associated with tender suppurative inguinal adenopathy (buboes) and fever, chills, and malaise	• Clinical + positive serology	• Doxycycline 100 mg PO BID × 21 days OR • Erythromycin base 500 mg PO QID × 21 days
Chancroid *(Haemophius ducreyi)*	Usually single, superficial, painful ulcer surrounded by an erythematous halo; bleeds easily with purulent exudate; unilateral adenopathy (buboes)	• Culture/PCR is often difficult, diagnosis of exclusion	• Azithromycin 1 g PO × 1 OR • Ceftriaxone 250 mg IM × 1 OR • Ciprofloxacin 500 mg PO BID × 3 days OR • Erythromycin base 500 mg PO TID × 7 days

BID, two times daily; Ig, immunoglobulin; IM, intramuscular; PCR, polymerase chain reaction; PO, orally; TID, three times daily; QID, four times daily.

diagnosis is made in a sexually active female at risk for sexually transmitted infections experiencing pelvic or lower abdominal pain if no other cause is identified, AND at least one of the following is present: cervical motion tenderness, uterine tenderness, or adnexal tenderness. Additional criteria not required but which may increase specificity include oral temperature >101°F, cervical mucopurulent discharge or friability, abundant WBCs on saline microscopy, elevated ESR, elevated CRP, and laboratory documentation of cervical infection for gonorrhea/chlamydia. Indications for hospitalization with PID include inability to exclude a surgical emergency, tubo-ovarian abscess, pregnancy, severe illness, nausea or vomiting, high fever, non-response to oral therapy, and inability to tolerate an outpatient oral regimen.

118. **What is the treatment of PID?**
   • Recommended parenteral
     • Cefotetan 2 g IV Q 12 hours PLUS
     • Doxycycline 100 mg PO or IV Q 12 hours
   OR
     • Cefoxitin 2 g IV Q 6 hours PLUS
     • Doxycycline 100 mg PO or IV Q 12 hours

Table 37.17 Differential Diagnosis of Vaginal Discharge in a Postpubertal Female

DISEASE	CLINICAL PRESENTATION	DIAGNOSIS	TREATMENT

Bacterial vaginosis (*G. vaginalis, Mycoplasma hominis*)	• Thin, homogeneous, gray-white vaginal discharge
	• Pruritis
	• "Fishy" odor
		• Amsel criteria
		• At least three of the following:
		  • Clue cells (on at least 20% of epithelial cells)
		  • pH >4.5
		  • +amine or whiff test—"fishy odor"
		  • Homogeneous thin, whitish vaginal discharge, adheres to vaginal walls
		• OSOM BVBLUE test
			• Metronidazole 500 mg PO BID × 7 days, OR
			• Metronidazole gel 0.75 % 1 applicator (5 g) intravaginal daily × 5 days, OR
			• Clindamycin cream 2% 1 applicator (5 g) intravaginal QHS × 7 days

Vulvovaginal candidiasis (*Candida albicans*)	• Pruritis, external dysuria, dyspareunia, thick white "cottage cheese" vaginal discharge	• Vulvar/vaginal erythema/edema with satellite lesions or fissures, whitish discharge • pH <4.5 • KOH prep: pseudohyphae or blastospores and WBC	• Clotrimazole 1% cream 5 g intravaginal daily × 7-14 days, OR • Clotrimazole 2% cream 5 g intravaginal daily × 3 days • Intravaginal prescription • Butoconazole 2% cream 5 g intravaginal × 1 • Terconazole 0.4% cream 5 g intravaginal daily 7 days • Terconazole 0.8% cream 5 g intravaginal daily × 3 days • Fluconazole 150 mg PO × 1

Trichomonas (*T. vaginalis*)	• Pruritis, dysuria, dyspareunia, lower abdominal pain, postcoital bleeding
	• Vaginal discharge—malodorous, greenish-yellow, frothy
	• Vulvar irritation
		• Wet prep
		  • motile trichomonads
		  • Sensitivity (60%-70%)
		• KOH—malodorous
		• pH >4.5
		• Culture
		• NAATs
		• Rapid Antigen Test—OSOM TV
		• DNA Probe—Affirm VP III
			• Metronidazole 2 g PO × 1 dose OR
			• Tinidazole 2 g PO × 1, OR
			• Metronidazole 500 mg PO BID × 7 days

Cervicitis (Chlamydia trachomatis, Neisseria gonorrhoeae)	• Symptoms
	  • Abnormal vaginal discharge
	  • Abnormal bleeding/postcoital bleeding
	  • Dysuria
	• Physical examination
	  • Friable cervix
	  • Erythema
	  • Discharge from os
	  • No CMT
	  • Cervical petechiae—"strawberry cervix"
		• – Nonamplified test
		• – NAAT (gen probe)
		• – Culture
			• Azithromycin 1 g PO× 1, OR
			• Doxycycline 100 mg PO BID × 7 days
			• PLUS
			• Ceftriaxone 250 mg IM × 1 dose, OR
			• Cefixime 400 mg PO × 1

BID, two times daily; IM, intramuscular; KOH, potassium hydroxide; NAAT, nucleic acid amplification test; os, left eye; PO, orally; QHS, every night at bedtime; WBC, white blood cell.

OR
- Clindamycin 900 mg IV Q 8 hours PLUS
- Gentamicin 2 mg/kg IV or IM followed by 1.5 mg/kg Q 8 hours
- Recommended IM/oral
  - Ceftriaxone 250 mg IM × 1 PLUS
  - Doxycycline 100 mg PO BID × 14 days
  - with or without metronidazole 500 mg BID PO × 14 days
  OR
  - Cefoxitin 2 g IM × 1 and probenecid 1 g PO × 1 PLUS doxycycline 100 mg PO BID × 14 days
  - with or without metronidazole 500 mg BID PO × 14 days

ORTHOPEDIC INFECTIONS

119. **What are the most common sites for septic arthritis?**
The lower-extremity joints, such as the hip, knee, and ankle are the common sites for septic arthritis. Always consider associated osteomyelitis when the joint "looks septic," that is, if there is warmth, stiffness, tenderness, and swelling over the joint (seen only in 10% of cases).

120. **A 2-year-old presents with fever and limp. He is favoring his left lower extremity. Radiographs of the left hip and femur show no osseous abnormality. Have you successfully ruled out osteomyelitis?**
No. In the first 2 weeks of osteomyelitis, plain radiographs are not sensitive for the detection of osteomyelitis (osteolytic changes or periosteal elevation may not be evident yet). Newborn infants are an exception to the rule as their radiographs often show findings concerning osteomyelitis at the time of presentation. MRI is the best option to confirm the diagnosis of osteomyelitis. Cultures of blood, bone, and soft tissue may increase the yield of pathogen identification.

121. **What is the classically described position that the leg is held in by a child with septic arthritis of the hip?**
The leg is externally rotated and abducted.

122. **Which bones are most commonly affected by osteomyelitis?**
The metaphysis of the long bones of the leg is most affected by osteomyelitis. This is partly due to the increased vascularity of long bones in children. In neonates and infants, osteomyelitis may affect any bone, including the humerus, pelvic bones, the calcaneus, or the mandible.

123. **A 2-year-old presents with fever and limp and undergoes a joint aspiration, which reveals a WBC count of 60,000 cells/mm³ with a neutrophil predominance. What is the most likely diagnosis?**
The most likely diagnosis is septic arthritis. Refer to Table 37.18 for diagnosis based on the WBC count and differential; however, note the considerable overlap. Epidemiology, presence of fever, and detailed history may help narrow the correct diagnosis.

124. **What are the most common infectious organisms in bone and joint infections, and what is the recommended mode of diagnosis and treatment?**
The most common infectious organisms are shown in Table 37.19.

Table 37.18 Differential Diagnosis of Septic Arthritis Based on White Blood Cell Count and Neutrophils

DIAGNOSIS	WHITE BLOOD CELLS (CELLS/MM³)	NEUTROPHILS (%)
Normal	<200	10-20
Traumatic effusion	<2000	10-30
Rheumatologic	10,000-50,000	50-80
Septic arthritis	>50,000	>80
Lyme arthritis	15-125,000	>50

Table 37.19 Organisms Most Commonly Found in Bone and Joint Infections

AGE	SEPTIC ARTHRITIS	OSTEOMYELITIS
Neonate	*Staphylococcus aureus* Group B streptococci Gram-negative bacilli	*S. aureus* Group B streptococci Gram-negative bacilli
Toddler	*S. aureus* Group A streptococcus *Kingella kingae*	*S. aureus* Group A streptococcus *K. kingae*

Diagnosis	• ↑ WBC (70%), CRP (95%), sedimentation rate (90%), (+) blood culture (40%)
	• Synovial fluid analysis
	• Kocher criteria (60%-98% sensitivity)
	   • Fever ≥38.5°C
	   • Inability to bear weight
	   • WBC ≥12k
	   • ESR ≥40
	   • CRP ≥20
		• Leukocytosis, ↑ CRP (95%), ↑ sedimentation rate (90%), (+) blood culture (35%-50%), bone aspirate (50%-80%)
		• Radionuclide bone scan (80%-100%)
		• MRI (92%-100%)

Treatment	• IV clindamycin or vancomycin (or oxacillin) for 3-4 wk	• IV clindamycin or vancomycin (or oxacillin or ceftriaxone) for 3-6 wk

CRP, C-reactive protein; ESR, erythrocyte sedimentation rate; IV, intravenous; MRI, magnetic resonance imaging; WBC, white blood cell.

125. What is pyomyositis and how does it present?
    Pyomyositis is a bacterial infection with microabscesses of the skeletal muscle that may be associated with prior trauma to the area or immunodeficiency. The most common organisms in pyomyositis are *S. aureus* or GAS in immunocompetent children, and gram-negative organisms in immunocompromised children. Clinical manifestations include fever, cramping muscle pain localized to a single muscle group, tenderness to palpation, and swelling of the involved muscle. Diagnosis is confirmed with contrast-enhanced MRI or CT scan. Treatment includes surgical drainage of abscesses and IV antibiotics.

126. What organism should you consider in daycare attending children aged between 6 months and 4 years as a cause for bone infection?
    Although *S. aureus* is overall the most common bacterial pathogen, *Kingella Kingae* is one of the most common pathogens in young children with osteomyelitis, spondylodiscitis, and septic arthritis. It is associated with microtrauma and has a milder course. However, it is difficult to culture. Identification is with PCR-based assays. Patients with underlying hemoglobinopathies can be prone to *Salmonella* species.

127. A child presents with significant knee swelling but is able to ambulate. He has had intermittent knee pain for a few months since visiting relatives in Pennsylvania. What is the likely cause, evaluation, and treatment of this condition?
    Lyme disease is commonly caused by the spirochete *Borrelia burgdorferi*, transferred through the bite of the Ixodes scapularis tick that is endemic to certain areas within the United States. Lyme arthritis is a late manifestation of the disease and can occur within 1 to 12 months following inoculation. There is usually a monoarticular manifestation involving the knee (80%-90% of cases), with the hip being the second most common affected joint. Joint swelling is described as out of proportion to the degree of pain. Fever can be absent or low grade. Lyme disease is diagnosed via two-tiered testing: A serum enzyme-linked immunosorbent assay with positive results is subsequently confirmed by a western immunoblot for IgG antibodies to *B. burgdorferi*. Treatment for Lyme arthritis is a 4-week course of either oral doxycycline, amoxicillin, or cefuroxime.

BITES

128. A 3-year-old girl was bitten by the family dog while she was playing with its food. Her mother reports that the dog was a rescue and they do not have access to the rabies vaccination status. The dog is acting normally and is being observed in the home. Does the child need a rabies vaccine?
    Most recorded rabies cases from 2000 to 2017 have been due to contact with bats. However, raccoons, skunks, foxes, coyotes, bobcats, and mongoose are other wild animals that can harbor this RNA virus. It is very rare to see rabies in small rodents or lagomorphs (rabbits and hares). Rabies transmission from domestic animals (cats and dogs) who have been healthy is also rare in the United States. Typically the animals should be

watched for 10 days. There is no need for rabies prophylaxis unless the animal starts to develop rabid symptoms during this time such as fearfulness, aggression, excessive drooling, difficulty swallowing, staggering, paralysis, or seizures.

129. Parents report that they found a bat flying in the room of their 11-month-old boy where he had been sleeping. The bat escaped prior to capture. No obvious bite wounds are found on the examination. What are your next steps?

This patient cannot reliably recall a bite or mucous membrane exposure with the bat. However, bat bites can be small. Therefore one cannot rule out exposure to a species that has a high risk of transferring rabies (depending on local prevalence). Unless the bat can be caught, euthanized, and tested, the patient requires rabies prophylaxis. Without this crucial protection, the patient is prone to a terminal and rapid progression of central neurological symptoms that include anxiety, radicular pain, dysesthesias, pruritus, hydrophobic, and dysautonomia, likely culminating in death.

KEY POINTS: RABIES PROPHYLAXIS FOR BAT BITES

1. Bats are the leading cause of rabies deaths in the United States.
2. If the bat cannot be caught and tested for rabies, give rabies postexposure prophylaxis:
   - When known bite or scratch from bat.
   - When patient was asleep and bat was found in room (may not know if bitten).

---

130. A 14-year-old was bitten by a stray dog. There is a moderate-sized bite wound to the right wrist. The patient's neurovascular examination is reassuring. X-rays are normal. The patient has an allergy to penicillin. What wound care and antimicrobial measures should you pursue?

Unless gaping, or occupying the face, bite wounds to the extremities should be left open or closed loosely due to the high risk of infection. There should be extensive irrigation with the assessment of tetanus coverage (especially if there have been more than 5 years since the last vaccination). With moderate-to-severe bite wounds, initiate antibiotic prophylaxis. In a well patient who can tolerate oral antibiotics, this would consist of amoxicillin-clavulanate. However, if there is a true penicillin allergy, an extended-spectrum cephalosporin or TMP-SMZ coupled with clindamycin is appropriate coverage.

131. How would you administer rabies immunoglobulin (RIG)?

RIG and human rabies vaccine (HRV) should be given as soon as possible. RIG should be infiltrated around the wound with the rest administered intramuscularly. Since this is often a viscous solution, there may be some benefit in locally anesthetizing the wound with 2% lidocaine. RIG and HRV should be administered in sites that are anatomically distant to avoid potential inactivation. The patient will need repeat doses of HRV on days 3, 7, and 14 after the first dose for a total of four doses.

132. A 12-year-old boy presents with pain and swelling of his right forearm 12 hours after getting bitten by his cat. He has a low-grade fever, temperature of 38.0°C (100.4°F) with erythema, edema, and purulent drainage from a puncture wound on his right arm. Based on the examination, which infectious organisms do you suspect?

The most likely organism is *Pasteurella multocida*, which is the most frequent isolate from dog and cat bites. Symptoms usually develop within 24 hours of initial injury and can be seen as early as 3 hours following a cat bite. Cat bites are also associated with the development of osteomyelitis and septic arthritis more often than dog bites, due to the cats' smaller and sharper teeth that can easily penetrate the periosteum. Deep wounds should not be sutured. *Staphylococcal* and *Streptococcal* species can also be found in animal bites.

TICK-BORNE DISEASE

133. What are the typical symptoms of Lyme disease, and how can they be further characterized?

Lyme disease symptoms can be characterized as early localized, early disseminated, and late disseminated (see Table 37.20).

134. What is the appropriate treatment for a child who presents with erythema migrans?

Erythema migrans is characterized as a red macule or papule that expands over days to weeks to form a large annular (>5 cm in diameter) erythematous lesion, often with a partial central clearing. The lesion itself is usually

Table 37.20 Clinical Stages Associated WithLyme Disease

CHARACTERIZATION	TIMING	SYMPTOMS
Early localized	3-32 days	Single erythema migrans lesion, myalgia, headache, arthralgia, fever
Early disseminated	3-10 wk	Single or multiple erythema migrans lesions, arthralgia, neck pain and/or stiffness, facial nerve palsy, meningitis, radiculoneuritis
Late disseminated	2-12 mo	Arthritis, carditis, encephalomyelitis

Table 37.21 Treatment for Lyme Disease

DISEASE CATEGORY	DRUG(S) AND DOSE
Early localized Erythema migrans (single or multiple)	Any age: Doxycycline, 4.4 mg/kg/day, BID, for 10 days OR Amoxicillin 50 mg/kg/day, TID, for 14 days OR Cefuroxime 30 mg/kg/day, BID, for 14 days OR Azithromycin 10 mg/kg/day, daily, for 7 days
Isolated facial palsy	Doxycycline 4.4 mg/kg/day, BID for 14 days
Arthritis	Oral agent from "early localized" for 28 days
Atrioventricular block or carditis	Oral agent from "early localized" for 28 days OR Ceftriaxone 50-75 mg/kg, IV, daily, for 14 days, may transition to oral to complete 14-21-day course
Meningitis	Doxycycline 4.4 mg/kg/day, BID, 14 days OR Ceftriaxone 50-75 mg/kg, IV, daily for 14 days

BID, two times daily; IV, intravenous; TID, three times daily.

not bothersome. If this cutaneous finding is present, then a clinical diagnosis of Lyme disease can be made. Any antibiotic chosen from the early localized category of treatment is appropriate (see Table 37.21).

135. **What is the recommended treatment for Lyme disease in children?**
To understand the recommended treatment, see Table 37.21.

136. **A child presents with bilateral facial palsy. What disease entities would you consider?**
In areas that are endemic for Lyme disease in the United States (Northeast, Upper Midwest, and Pacific Northwest), Lyme disease should always be suspected. It is one of the few diseases that can produce bilateral facial palsy. Other causes of facial palsy, usually unilateral, include mastoiditis, Guillain-Barré syndrome, HSV infection, and tumors.

KEY POINTS: POSSIBLE PRESENTATIONS OF LYME DISEASE IN CHILDREN

1. Rash
2. Arthritis
3. Heart block
4. Meningeal signs
5. Facial palsies

137. **List the common presenting symptoms of RMSF and its characteristic rash distribution.**
RMSF is a small vessel vasculitis caused by *R. rickettsii*. Typical symptoms include fever, myalgia, severe headache, photophobia, nausea, vomiting, anorexia, and a hallmark rash. The rash begins within the first 2 to 4 days of symptoms and initially presents as erythematous macules that become more confluent and purpuric. It characteristically begins on the wrists and ankles and spreads rapidly to the trunk and distally to the palms/soles. Although the rash is pathognomonic, its absence should not rule out RMSF.

138. **What laboratory abnormalities are commonly associated with RMSF?**
Hyponatremia (sodium level <130 mEq/L) is seen in about 20% to 50% of affected patients. Other laboratory abnormalities commonly include thrombocytopenia, anemia, leukopenia, and elevated transaminases.

139. **What is the treatment for RMSF?**
Doxycycline is the gold standard for RMSF in any age group. Begin treatment as soon as RMSF is suspected. Testing will often take weeks to return. Treatment started after the fifth day of symptoms is less likely to prevent morbidity or mortality.

KEY POINTS: RMSF

1. Rickettsial infection
2. Presents with severe headache, photophobia, nausea, fever, myalgia
3. Classic rash on wrists and ankles after 2 to 4 days of symptoms
4. Rash spreads to palms, soles, and trunk, and evolves from erythematous macules to purpura
5. Laboratory findings: hyponatremia, thrombocytopenia, anemia, leukopenia, elevated transaminases
6. Treat with doxycycline

SKIN AND SOFT TISSUE

140. **What are the most common organisms causing cellulitis based on location and type of exposure?**
Table 37.22 shows that the most common cause of cellulitis overall is group A streptococcus (GAS), or *S. pyogenes* followed by *S. aureus*. Exceptions are noted when oral flora is involved or if there is an immunocompromised state.

141. **Are blood or wound cultures helpful in diagnosing cellulitis?**
In a published study looking at uncomplicated skin and soft tissue infections (SSTIs), 94% of patients had a blood culture drawn, none were positive, however, three were positive for contaminants.
With regards to wound cultures, previous studies have examined their efficacy and have found 58% to 66% of cultures have been helpful in identifying the causative organism.

142. **What are the oral antibiotics of choice for simple cellulitis?**
Antimicrobial therapy should be aimed at treating *S. aureus* and group A-beta-hemolytic *streptococci*. For mild cases of cellulitis, treat with a β-lactam alone (first-generation cephalosporin such as Keflex). Consider MRSA coverage with TMP-SMZ or clindamycin can be considered if there is a high incidence rate or the patient is at high risk (i.e., family member with MRSA or family member that works in a health care setting).

143. **When is parenteral treatment recommended for cellulitis?**
Criteria for parenteral antibiotics include signs of systemic toxicity, a rapidly progressing lesion, involvement of the face or neck, and absence of improvement following 48 hours of outpatient management. Consider clindamycin for suspected MRSA infection. For critically ill patients use vancomycin or linezolid.

144. **What are some epidemiologic concerns regarding community-acquired MRSA?**
Community-acquired MRSA infections continue to be of higher incidence than hospital-acquired. While younger children still remain at higher risk for invasive MRSA infections, there has been an overall decrease in invasive MRSA infections in hospitalized infants, suggesting the success of strict infection prevention strategies. There are apparent differences between racial groups, with African-American children having a higher incidence of these infections.

145. **Necrotizing infection can complicate cellulitis. How does this present?**
When evaluating for cellulitis, if there is crepitus, a violaceous skin discoloration, and severe pain that is out of proportion with manipulation, it is important to consider a necrotizing infection. This is a dangerous skin,

Table 37.22 Most Common Causes of Cellulitis Based on Location

PRESENTATION	BACTERIAL ORGANISM
Facial cellulitis	*Staphylococcus aureus*, GAS, p*neumococcus*
Erysipelas	GAS
Odontogenic cellulitis	Viridans streptococcus, *Fusobacterium*, *Prevotella*
Perianal cellulitis	GAS
Water exposure cellulitis	*S. aureus*, GAS, *Vibrio vulnificus*, *Aeromonas*
Animal bite cellulitis	*Pasteurella multocida*, *S. aureus*, GAS, *Capnocytophaga canimorsus*
Cellulitis after clenched fist injury (fight bite)	Polymicrobial oral flora and anerobes; *Eikenella corrodens*
Plantar cellulitis from puncture wound	*S. aureus*, GAS, *Pseudomonas aeruginosa*
Neutropenic and other immunocompromised hosts	*P. aeruginosa*, GNR, anaerobes

GAS, group A streptococcus or *S. pyogenes*; GNR, gram-negative rods.
Adapted from Shaw KN, Bachur RG, Chamberlain JM, eds. *Fleisher & Ludwig's Textbook of Pediatric Emergency Medicine.* 7th ed. Wolters Kluwer Health; 2016.

limb, and life-threatening complication of cellulitis and warrants emergent IV antibiotic administration in addition to surgical consultation. Antimicrobial management includes broad-spectrum coverage with vancomycin for MRSA, and carbapenem or beta-lactam with beta-lactamase inhibitor, along with clindamycin for toxin suppression.

146. **What findings may be associated with an invasive skin or soft tissue infection?**
   - Necrosis of skin or soft tissue
   - Crepitance on physical examination
   - Nonadherence of skin and subcutaneous tissue to the underlying fascia on exploration
   - Abnormal skin color other than erythema (such as bronzed, cyanotic, violaceous)
   - Severe systemic toxicity, anxiety, or confusion
   - Pain on palpation out of proportion to physical findings
   - Tachycardia out of proportion to fever (suggestive of clostridial infection)
   - Hypocalcemia (calcium deposition in necrotic subcutaneous fat)
   - Gas present on radiograph
   - Failure to respond to medical management
   - Bullae with thin, brown discharge with "sweet but foul" odor (clostridial infection), or "dishwater" fluid (anaerobic fluid)

147. **When should oral antibiotics be considered for abscesses, if ever?**
   Small abscesses can resolve by themselves without any treatment through spontaneous drainage or an incision and drainage can be performed at the bedside. The need for systemic antibiotics following drainage is currently up for debate. Some studies, conducted mostly on adults, have not found any evidence to support the routine use of antibiotics while other studies, which have included both children and adults, showed a 7- to 10-day course of TMP-SMZ after incision and drainage can help to prevent treatment failure and recurrence of abscesses. Other studies suggest clindamycin may be a better choice of antibiotic to prevent treatment failure than TMP-SMZ. When considering the use of antibiotics, consider your institution's choice for MRSA coverage as well as the severity of the abscess and the patient's history (i.e., previous abscesses, age, location).

148. **What soft-tissue infections are seen predominantly in neonates?**
   Omphalitis and mastitis are soft-tissue infections seen in the neonatal period. Omphalitis is rare in developed countries and is an infection of the umbilical stump and surrounding tissues. It can arise due to poor cord hygiene and presents with purulent, malodorous drainage with surrounding erythema, tenderness, and induration. Fever may be a later finding, along with hypothermia and lethargy. If untreated, omphalitis is extremely dangerous, resulting in sepsis, septic umbilical arteritis, portal vein thrombosis, liver abscess, and necrotizing fasciitis. Common organisms include *S. aureus*, GBS, GAS, and gram-negative enterococci. Mastitis is an infection of the breast tissue within the first three weeks of life. It manifests with unilateral erythema, pain, and induration of the breast bud. Fever is often absent, even when there is bacteremia.

Cultures from the purulent drainage are often positive for *S. aureus*, and less commonly GBS, *E. coli*, and *Salmonella*.

149. **An 8-year-old patient presents after stepping on a nail while wearing sneakers. He did not bring this to attention of his parents until he was found to be limping 4 days later. On arrival he has erythema and warmth of the plantar surface of his foot with point tenderness at the proximal end of his fifth metatarsal. How would you manage him?**
This is the classic presentation of a nail puncture wound through a rubber-soled shoe. It can result in deep *S. aureus* and *P. aeruginosa* infectious complications including deep space abscesses, septic arthritis, necrotizing soft tissue infection, tenosynovitis, and osteomyelitis. Initial assessment includes wound care, assessing for tetanus status and a retained foreign body using x-rays, potentially coupled with bedside ultrasound. However, these patients may also need to be admitted to the hospital for broad spectrum parenteral antibiotic treatment (consider piperacillin-tazobactam or meropenem with vancomycin). Surgical or orthopedic consultation is warranted for possible debridement. In this scenario, remember "Shoe-da-monas" (*Pseudomonas*) deep infection in addition to other causes of SSTI.

150. **Match the superficial bacterial skin infection with its classic presentation and respective treatment.**
A. Impetigo
B. Ecthyma
C. Erysipelas
D. Paronychia
E. Folliculitis
F. Furuncles/carbuncles
1. May begin following minor trauma or an insect bite; initially vesiculopapular with surrounding erythema and later developing a thick, adherent crust that, when removed, reveals a punched-out, painful ulcerative lesion. Treatment includes cleansing, and topical and systemic antibiotics covering streptococci and S. aureus, typically seen in immunocompromised patients.
2. Results from local injury to the nail fold are seen in children who suck their fingers or bite their nails; lateral nail fold becomes warm, erythematous, edematous, and painful. Treatment includes warm compresses and, for deep infections, incision and drainage and antibiotics covering mixed oral flora.
3. Either isolated nodular subcutaneous abscesses or multiple abscesses separated by connective tissue septae clinically presenting as painful red papules or boils in a nontoxic-appearing child. Treatment includes local care, incision and drainage, and systemic antibiotics for larger lesions.
4. Superficial infection of the skin caused by either S. aureus or group A beta-hemolytic streptococci appearing as mildly painful lesions with an erythematous base and honey-crusted exudates in a nontoxic child; absence of constitutional symptoms; and presence of regional adenopathy. Treatment includes topical mupirocin or systemic antibiotics (widespread lesions, lesions near the mouth, evidence of deeper infection, constitutional symptoms).
5. Clearly demarcated, raised, and advancing red border extending from the site of inoculation with lymphangitic streaks extending from the involved area; shiny and warm to touch; and the presence of systemic signs and high fever. Treatment with IV antibiotics until the patient is afebrile and lesion begins to regress, then oral antibiotics.
6. Small, red pustules at the site of hair follicles. Treatment includes local care and topical antibiotics.
Answers: 1, B; 2, D; 3, F; 4, A; 5, C; 6, E.

151. **A 4-year-old boy presents with a boggy, purulent mass measuring 5 × 5 cm on his right temporal scalp area. He also has alopecia and right-sided posterior chain cervical adenopathy. What is the likely diagnosis?**
This presentation is consistent with a kerion, which is a local cell-mediated response to tinea capitis often confused with a bacterial skin infection as it can be boggy like an abscess and is often covered in pustules. Therapy includes a minimum of 4 weeks of oral antifungal therapy (griseofulvin or ketoconazole) plus or minus 1 week of systemic steroids. Systemic antibiotics or drainage of the area are not indicated.

152. **Which infectious agents are most commonly associated with erythema multiforme minor and major, respectively?**
Erythema multiforme minor is most commonly associated with HSV, and erythema multiforme major is most commonly associated with *M. pneumoniae*.

153. **What is staphylococcal scalded skin syndrome?**
Staphylococcal scalded skin syndrome is a superficial blistering skin disorder caused by the exfoliative toxins of certain strains of *S. aureus*. It generally affects children <5 years old. Symptoms are abrupt and usually begin

with widespread erythroderma and tissue paper-like wrinkling of the skin (spares mucosal membranes), often accentuated in the flexural and periorificial area. Fluid-filled blisters develop within 24 to 48 hours and enlarge, creating bullae that rupture easily. When the bullae rupture, skin may peel off in sheets (desquamation) leaving skin with a moist erythematous appearance, giving rise to the term scalded. The presence of the Nikolsky sign (wrinkling of the upper layer of the epidermis and removal of the layer by light stroking, like the peeling of wet tissue paper) may be present. The mortality rate is <5%. Hospitalization is often required for skin care, fluid management, and IV antibiotics.

154. **What are the typical cutaneous findings associated with scarlet fever?**
Patients with scarlet fever usually have abrupt onset of fever, headache, nausea, vomiting, malaise, myalgia, and sore throat. After a 2- to 4-day incubation period, they often develop:
- Erythematous oral mucous membranes with scattered palatal petechiae.
- White or red strawberry tongue.
- Circumoral pallor.
- Erythematous, punctate rash with sandpaper-like texture; first appears (12-48 hours) on abdomen and chest, and then becomes more generalized (more intense in skin folds of axillae, antecubital, popliteal, and inguinal regions, and sites of pressure such as buttocks and small of back). The rash is rapidly evolving which can be useful in distinguishing it from viral rashes.
- Pastia lines (transverse areas of hyperpigmentation with petechial character in antecubital fossa, axilla, and inguinal regions).
- Scaly exfoliation on the hands, palms, knees, feet, and perineum which occurs within 1 week of sandpaper rash. This can potentially last 3 to 6 weeks.

155. **What precautions and antibiotic prophylaxis are needed for the ED staff when managing/ resuscitating a patient with meningococcemia?**
Institute droplet precautions. This includes the use of a respiratory mask if within 3 feet of the child. Chemoprophylaxis for the staff is strongly recommended if mouth-to-mouth resuscitation is provided or there is unprotected contact during endotracheal intubation. Options for chemoprophylaxis include oral rifampin for 2 to 4 days, intramuscular ceftriaxone for one dose, or oral ciprofloxacin for one dose.

156. **An 18-year-old male is escorted to the ED from prison with a chief complaint of "coughing up blood." He has had a chronic cough for approximately 6 months and has lost 10 pounds over the last year. What should the ED staff do to protect themselves from exposure to this infection?**
This patient likely has TB. Institute airborne precautions. This includes a private room with negative air-pressure ventilation. Health care providers in contact with the patient must wear properly fitted or sealed respiratory masks.

157. **A 16-year-old boy with cerebral palsy and developmental delay, who lives in a long-term care facility has extensive infected purulent decubitus ulcers on his buttocks and lower extremities. What should the ED staff do to protect themselves from exposure to this infection?**
The patient likely has an infection related to MRSA. Institute contact precautions, including a private room for the patient. Staff must wear gloves and gowns at all times. Hand washing with an antimicrobial agent is essential, including after glove removal.

VIRAL ILLNESSES/EXANTHEMS

158. **What is the classic description of roseola infantum? (Primary human herpes virus-6 [HHV6] infection?)**
Patients will commonly develop a maculopapular rash following 3 to 4 days of high fevers (>36°C). The rash is characteristically widespread with discrete pink macules that do not coalesce, first appearing on the trunk and extending peripherally. The HHV6 or "Sixth disease" rash can last from hours to days. Appearance of the rash within 24 hours of fever defervescence is pathognomonic. Unlike measles (rubeola), the rash of roseola presents in the afebrile, well-appearing child and does not begin on the face, nor does it spread caudally. The course of roseola is usually benign, although in 10% to 15% of patients, febrile seizures can occur. Rarely HHV6 infection has been associated with aseptic meningitis, encephalitis, and thrombocytopenia purpura.

159. **A 7-year-old child presents with fever with an erythematous rash on the cheeks. What is the typical presentation and the potential complications associated with this infection?**
Erythema infectiosum is the most common manifestation of parvovirus B19 infection, also known as "Fifth disease." This infection is associated with a rash, characterized by intense erythema of the cheeks (the

"slapped-cheek" appearance) with circumoral pallor. In addition, a lacey rash may appear on the trunk and extremities with a symmetric distribution. Rarely patients may develop the atypical "gloves and socks" syndrome. This is described as pruritic, erythematous, papular lesions occupying the hands and feet with purpuric lesions on the palms and soles. Complications of parvovirus include hepatitis, small joint arthritis, and myocarditis. It can cause aplastic crisis in children with sickle cell disease. It is therefore prudent to isolate patients with parvovirus from those with hemoglobinopathies. It is also important to keep children with parvovirus away from pregnant women, as it can cause fetal hydrops, intrauterine growth retardation, and fetal demise.

160. A 15-year-old male just returned from spring break. He presents with 4 days of fever, fatigue, headache, and an exudative pharyngitis with tender posterior lymphadenopathy. His COVID-19 PCR was negative. He was treated at another center with amoxicillin despite a negative strep test. He subsequently developed a maculopapular rash. What testing will help isolate the cause of his symptoms?
A heterophile antibody or "Monospot" may be positive in adolescents after the first week of illness. There is poor sensitivity of this test in children less than 4 years old (who often have a less severe or asymptomatic course). However, the heterophile antibody may also return positive in cases of leukemia, lymphoma, CMV, lupus, HIV, rubella, and pancreatic cancer. Therefore a CBC ordered concurrently may be helpful; in the case of infectious mononucleosis a lymphocytosis or atypical lymphocytosis would be seen. EBV titers may help confirm diagnosis in a symptomatic patient with negative Monospot but can also be falsely positive for CMV infection. There can be an associated hypersensitivity rash with amoxicillin.

161. What should you recommend to a patient with infectious mononucleosis upon discharge from the ED?
Due to the associated splenomegaly with infectious mononucleosis, patients should avoid contact sports until the spleen is no longer palpable. Spontaneous and traumatic rupture of the spleen is a life-threatening complication in 1 to 2/1000 cases often between 2 and 21 days after onset of clinical symptoms. Treatment for infectious mononucleosis is supportive. There is a paucity of data to suggest that patients who develop rare, life-threatening complications such as severe tonsillitis with impending airway obstruction, hemophagocytic syndrome, fulminant liver failure, massive splenomegaly, hemolytic aplastic anemia, and carditis may benefit from corticosteroid therapy.

162. Match the disease with the clinical description.
   1. Varicella (chicken pox)
   2. Measles
   3. Rubella (postnatal)
   A. High fever, nonproductive cough, coryza, and conjunctivitis. Confluent maculopapular rash beginning at hairline and spreading caudally; can involve palms and soles. You may see a cluster of bluish-white papules with erythematous border on the buccal mucosa before this illness fully manifests.
   B. Fever with coalescent, pink, maculopapular rash that begins on the face and extends downwards; tender postauricular, suboccipital, and posterior cervical lymph nodes. Additionally, there can be associated arthralgias and arthritis.
   C. Prodrome of fever, malaise, pharyngitis, and loss of appetite with the development of a vesicular rash within 24 hours. Lesions may be seen in different stages of evolution; scabbed lesions at the same time with crop distribution. They may be described as "dew drops on a rose petal." Initial lesions typically start on the face and scalp and can involve oral mucosa.
   Answers: 1: C; 2: A; 3: B.

163. Compare the contagious period for a child with varicella versus measles.
The period of communicability for varicella begins 1 to 2 days prior to the outbreak of lesions and lasts until all lesions are crusted over. By contrast, the contagious period for measles is from 5 days before the appearance of rash to 4 days afterward regardless of the stage of the lesions.

164. If a child with a primary varicella infection presents with high fever and toxic appearance, what should you suspect?
Examine the child for evidence of a secondary bacterial infection with *S. aureus* and *S. pyogenes* (group A). Secondary bacterial infection is the most common cause of morbidity in children with varicella infection. Clinical features include high fever, toxic appearance, and a varicella lesion that has become erythematous, warm, and painful. Superinfection with group A streptococci can progress to soft tissue necrosis, necrotizing fasciitis, and toxic shock syndrome.

165. What are the neurologic complications of varicella?
Neurological sequalae include meningoencephalitis, acute cerebellar ataxia, and Reye syndrome (described as nausea, vomiting, headache, excitability, delirium, and agitation with progression to coma in the setting of salicylate use).

MISCELLANEOUS INFECTIONS

166. A 4-year-old boy presents with a chief complaint of body temperature of 40°C for 7 days. On physical examination, you notice bilateral conjunctivitis, a strawberry red tongue, anterior cervical lymphadenopathy, and diffuse erythema of the perineal area. How should you proceed?

Investigate about Kawasaki disease. This is a multisystem vasculitis with a peak incidence in childhood; 80% to 90% of cases occur in children less than 5 years old and is the most common cause of acquired childhood heart disease in developed countries.

167. What are the diagnostic criteria for Kawasaki disease?

Fever for at least 5 days is the said criteria.

   PLUS

It also involves the presence of four of the following:
- Swelling and erythema of hands and feet
- Cervical lymphadenopathy
- Bilateral, nonpurulent conjunctival injection (limbic sparing)
- Mucous membrane changes
- Diffuse polymorphous rash

168. What is the differential diagnosis of Kawasaki disease?
- Adenovirus
- Cervical adenitis
- SARS-CoV-2 infection
- Multisystem inflammatory syndrome in children (MIS-C), a complication of COVID-19
- Enterovirus
- Enterovirus
- EBV
- Leptospirosis
- Measles
- RMSF
- Streptococcal scarlet fever
- Toxic shock syndrome

169. What laboratory findings support the diagnosis of Kawasaki disease?
- Normal or increased WBC count with left shift
- Elevated CRP/erythrocyte sedimentation rate
- Platelets increased during the second week of illness
- Sterile pyuria
- Mild elevation of aminotransferase levels
- Hypoalbuminemia
- Hyponatremia

170. What is the management of a patient with suspected Kawasaki disease?

Management includes admission to the hospital for treatment with high-dose aspirin and IV immunoglobulin, given within 10 days of fever onset. Obtain echocardiography during the initial hospital evaluation and then arrange to repeat the test 6 to 8 weeks after onset. Treatment within the first 10 days of the illness has been shown to substantially decrease the risk of coronary artery disease (a known complication of Kawasaki disease).

171. What are the noncardiac complications of Kawasaki disease?

Urethritis, hepatitis, hydrops of the gall bladder, arthritis, aseptic meningitis, vasculitis and even Macrophage activation syndrome are potential noncardiac complications.

172. When should MIS-C be on your differential?

MIS-C is a new and evolving illness. It should be considered in any child (<21 years) who is positive for current or recent COVID-19 infection or COVID-19 exposure within 4 weeks prior to onset of symptoms AND with 3 or more days of fever who is moderate-to-severely ill with clinical signs of organ dysfunction.

   Symptoms can include the following:
- Persistent fever
- Kawasaki disease–like features
- Gastrointestinal symptoms
- Toxic shock–like features
- Cytokine storm/macrophage activation or hyperinflammatory features

- Thrombosis or acute kidney injury
- Shortness of breath suggestive of congestive heart failure of pulmonary embolism

173. **What are typical laboratory findings of MIS-C?**
- Elevated CRP, ESR, ferritin, LDH
- Lymphopenia <1000
- Thrombocytopenia <150,000
- Neutropenia
- Elevated BNP
- Elevated D-dimer
- Hyponatremia

174. **What is the current treatment for MIS-C?**
Current treatment includes IVIG. Refractory cases can be treated with steroids and anakinra.

BIOTERRORISM AND TROPICAL INFECTIONS

175. **What distinguishes agents of bioterrorism?**
- **Category A agents/diseases** provide the greatest risk as they are easily transmitted from person to person and tend to have the highest mortality rates: *Bacillus anthracis* (anthrax), *Variola major* (smallpox), *Yersinia pestis* (plague), *Francisella tularensis* (tularemia), filoviruses and arenaviruses (viral hemorrhagic fever), and *Clostridium botulinum* toxin (botulism). *Variola major Yersinia pestis Francisella tularensis Clostridium botulinum*
- **Category B agents/diseases** have lower mortality rates and are not as easily spread as Category A agents: *Coxiella burnetii* (Q fever), *Brucella* species (brucellosis), *Burkholderia mallei* (glanders), *Burkholderia pseudomallei* (melioidosis), *Chlamydia psittaci* (psittacosis), *Clostridium perfringens*, ricin toxin, viral encephalitis (alphaviruses), *Salmonella* species, *Shigella dysenteriae*, *E. coli* O157:H7 (hemolytic uremic syndrome), *Staphylococcus* enterotoxin B, *R. prowazekii* (typhus fever), *Vibrio cholerae* (cholera), and *Cryptosporidium parvum*.
- **Category C agents** can be engineered to be biological weapons of mass destruction with the potential for high morbidity and mortality rates: Hantavirus, Nipah virus.

176. **Match the bioterrorism disease with the agent and symptoms.**
1. Anthrax
2. Tularemia
3. Plague
4. Botulism
A. Gram-negative rods resulting in pneumonia-like illness with fever, cough, dyspnea, large lymph node swelling, and hemoptysis 2 to 4 days after exposure. Chest radiographs reveal bilateral infiltrates or lobar consolidation. Sepsis or acute respiratory distress syndrome can further complicate this condition.
B. Spore-forming gram-positive bacillus causing a flu-like illness with fever, chills, malaise, and nonproductive cough with the absence of rhinorrhea. Chest radiographs can reveal a "widened mediastinum."
C. Gram-negative coccobacillus resulting in biphasic high fevers, chills, tender lymphadenopathy, and maculopapular lesions that later ulcerate. There is associated pharyngitis as well as conjunctival injection. Chest radiographs reveal hilar adenopathy.
D. Anerobic, gram-positive, spore-forming bacillus. The spores release a neurotoxin that causes descending flaccid paralysis without fever or mental status changes within 6 hours of inhalation. Characteristic features include ptosis, diplopia, dysphagia, and progression to ventilatory failure requiring mechanical ventilation. Diagnosis is often clinical with emerging PCR assays. Botulism antitoxin is available through the CDC.
Answers: 1: B; 2: C; 3: A; 4: D.

177. **What are the three major criteria for diagnosing smallpox?**
1. Febrile prodrome: Fever of ≥101°F, 2 to 4 days prior to rash onset with associated prostration, headache, backache, chills, vomiting, or severe abdominal pain
2. Classic smallpox lesions: Deep-seated, firm/hard, round well-circumscribed vesicles or pustules; lesions may umbilicate or become confluent
3. Lesions are all in the same stage of development

178. **What are the five minor criteria for diagnosing smallpox?**
1. Centrifugal distribution of lesions
2. Initially lesions involve the oral mucosal palate, the face, or forearms
3. Malaise
4. Lesions that evolve from macule to papule to vesicle (with 1-2 days duration in each stage)
5. Lesions on the palms and soles

Table 37.23 Transmissible Illnesses

GEOGRAPHICAL LOCATION	INFECTIONS CAUSING FEVER
Caribbean	Chikungunya, acute histoplasmosis, dengue fever, Zika virus, cholera, leptospirosis, malaria (*P. falciparum*)
Central America	Chikungunya, acute histoplasmosis, dengue fever, Zika virus, malaria (*P. vivax*), coccidioidomycosis, tuberculosis
South America	Chikungunya, dengue fever, Zika virus, malaria (*P. vivax*)
South Central Asia	Dengue fever, Typhoid fever, malaria (non-falciparum)
Southeast Asia	Chikungunya, dengue fever, malaria (non-falciparum), yellow fever, Japanese encephalitis virus
Sub-Saharan Africa	Dengue, malaria (*P. falciparum*), rickettsioses, acute schistosomiasis, yellow fever, meningococcus

Illness is not in order of prevalence or severity.
Adapted from Abdel-Haq N, Asmar BI. Fever in the returned pediatric traveler. *Glob Pediatr Health*. 2021;8:2333794X211026188. doi: 10.1177/2333794X211026188. PMID: 34423077; PMCID: PMC8375340.

179. A 7-year-old presents with 5 days of fever after traveling back to the United States from India. In the room next door, another teenager is febrile upon return from Nigeria. What infectious conditions should you consider in each of these ill-returning travelers?
Table 37.23 shows some of the transmissible illnesses based on geographical (tropical) location that a provider must be aware of when encountering the returned febrile traveler. It is also important to consider COVID-19 as a probable cause of fever in the returned traveler.

180. What are the clinical features of malaria?
Malaria is characterized by paroxysms of fever, occurring at certain time intervals along with chills, malaise, headaches, and muscle or joint pain often accompanied by nausea, vomiting, or diarrhea. Symptoms typically start 7 to 30 days after exposure (usually following return to the patient's home country). Children may present to the ED without a measurable fever. With any tropical illness, a CBC, comprehensive metabolic panel, cultures, UA, peripheral blood smears, and radiographs are common initial investigations. While awaiting thick and thin smears, a CBC may show anemia and thrombocytopenia. Infection with *Plasmodium falciparum* carries high morbidity and mortality (due to the risk of cerebral malaria along with renal and respiratory failure). The *Plasmodium* parasite is transferred by the *Anopheles* mosquito.

181. What is the purpose of the thick and thin smear in the workup for malaria?
Smears are best obtained near the end of a fever episode. Thick peripheral smears are specifically looking for small numbers of parasites. The thin peripheral smear is to identify malarial species.

182. Describe dengue and chikingunya.
These are also mosquito-borne illnesses. Dengue and chikungunya are viral illnesses transferred by the *Aedes* mosquito. Dengue is the second most common cause of fever in travelers from tropical areas. It has a shorter incubation period compared to malaria and presents with fever, retro-orbital pain, rash, myalgias and can progress to hemorrhagic fever due to plasma leak. As with dengue, chikungunya can cause fever, rash, and painful arthralgias. However, in contrast, there is an even shorter incubation period and no associated hemorrhagic fever.

Acknowledgments
The authors would like to thank Dr. Julie-Ann Crewalk, Dr. Theoklis Zaoutis, Dr. Joel Klein (deceased), Dr. Robert Wilkinson, Dr. Sanjeev Swami, and Dr. Stephen Eppes for their contributions to this chapter in previous editions.

BIBLIOGRAPHY

1. Committee on Infectious Diseases, American Academy of Pediatrics, Kimberlin DW, Barnett ED, Lynfield R, Sawyer MH, eds. *Red Book: 2021-2024. Report of the Committee on Infectious Diseases.* 32nd ed. American Academy of Pediatrics; 2021.
2. American Academy of Pediatrics. Multisystem Inflammatory Syndrome in Children (MIS-C) interim guidance. COVID-19 interim guidance. <https://www.aap.org/en/pages/2019-novel-coronavirus-covid-19-infections/clinical-guidance/multisystem-inflammatory-syndrome-in-children-mis-c-interim-guidance/>; 2021.
3. Coulthard MG. Using urine nitrite sticks to test for urinary tract infection in children aged <2 years: a meta-analysis. *Pediatr Nephrol.* 2019;34(7):1283–1288.
4. Bendig DW. The differential diagnosis of sterile pyuria in pediatric patients: a review. *Glob Pediatr Health.* 2021;8: 2333794X21993712.
5. Bullimore MA. The safety of soft contact lenses in children. *Optom Vis Sci.* 2017;94(6):638–646.
6. CaJacob NJ, Cohen MB. Update on diarrhea. *Pediatr Rev.* 2016;37(8):313–322.
7. Cox DA, Tani LY. Pediatric infective endocarditis: a clinical update. *Pediatr Clin North Am.* 2020;67(5):875–888.
8. Daniels HL, Sabella C. Bordetella pertussis. *Pediatr Rev.* 2018;39(5):247–257.
9. Davis J, Lehman E. Fever characteristics and risk of serious bacterial infection in febrile infants. *J Emerg Med.* 2019;57(3):306–313.
10. DeBenedictis FM, Kerem E, Chang AB, et al. Complicated pneumonia in children. *Lancet.* 2020;396:786–798.
11. DeBlasio D, Real FJ. Tracheitis. *Pediatr Rev.* 2020;41(9):495–497. https://doi.org/10.1542/pir.2019-0181.
12. Bhattacharya J, Mohandas S, Goldman DL. Nontuberculous mycobacterial infections in children. *Pediatr Rev.* 2019;40(4):179–190.
13. Fraley CE, Pettersson DR, Nolt D. Encephalitis in previously healthy children. *Pediatr Rev.* 2021;42(2):68–77.
14. Gervasio KA, Peck TJ, et al. Chapter 6.10 Preseptal cellulitis. In: Gervasio KA, Peck TJ, Fathy CA, Sivalingam MD, eds. *The Wills Eye Manual Office and Emergency Room Diagnosis and Treatment of Eye Disease.* 8th ed. Wolters Kluwer; 2022.
15. Greenfield BW, Lowery BM, Starke HE, Mayorquin L, et al. Frequency of serious bacterial infections in young infants with and without viral respiratory infections. *Am J Emerg Med.* 2021;50:744–747.
16. Gottlieb M, Long B, Koyfman A. The evaluation and management of toxic shock syndrome in the emergency department: a review of the literature. *J Emerg Med.* 2018;54(6):807–814.
17. Greenhow TL, Hung Y, Herz AM. Changing bacteremia in infants aged 1 week to 3 months. *Pediatrics.* 2012;129(3):e590–596.
18. Gupta A, Eckenswiller T. Point-of-care ultrasound in early diagnosis of cardiomyopathy in a child with viral myocarditis: a case report. *Clin Pract Cases Emerg Med.* 2021;5(2):186–189.
19. Hamiel U, Bahat H, Kozer E, Hamiel Y, et al. Diagnostic markers of acute infections in infants aged 1 week to 3 months: a retrospective cohort study. *BMJ Open.* 2018;8(1):e018092. https://doi-org.umassmed.idm.oclc.org/10.1136/bmjopen-2017-018092.
20. Hasbun R, Rosenthal N, Balada-Llasat JM, et al. Epidemiology of meningitis and encephalitis in the United States, 2011-2014. *Clin Infect Dis.* 2017;65(3):359–363.
21. Iwamoto M, Mu Y, Lynfield R, Bulens S, et al. Trends in invasive methicillin-resistant *Staphylococcus aureus* infections. *Pediatrics.* 2013;132(4):817–824.
22. Jaramillo D, Dormans JP, Delgado J, Laor T, et al. Hematogenous osteomyelitis in infants and children: imaging of a changing disease. *Radiology.* 2017;283(3):629–643.
23. Katz SE, Williams DJ. Pediatric community-acquired pneumonia in the United States: changing epidemiology, diagnostic and therapeutic challenges, and areas for future research. *Infect Dis Clin N Am.* 2018;32:47–63.
24. Kaufman J, Temple-Smith M, Sanci L. Urinary tract infections in children: an overview of diagnosis and management. *BMJ Paediatr Open.* 2019;3(1):e000487. https://doi.org/10.1136/bmjpo-2019-000487.
25. Khudan A, Jugmohansingh G, Islam S, Medford S, et al. The effectiveness of conservative management for retropharyngeal abscesses greater than 2 cm. *Ann Med Surg.* 2016;11:62–65.
26. Koltsidopoulos P, Papageorgiou E, Skoulakis C. Pott's puffy tumor in children: a review of the literature. *Laryngoscope.* 2020;130(1):225–231.
27. Kulik DM, Uleryk EM, Maguire JL. Does this child have bacterial meningitis? A systematic review of clinical prediction rules for children with suspected bacterial meningitis. *J Emerg Med.* 2013;45(4):508–519.
28. Kynion R. Mastoiditis. *Pediatr Rev.* 2018;39(5):267–269. https://doi.org/10.1542/pir.2017-0128.
29. Malone JR, Durica SR, Thompson DM, Bogie A, et al. Blood cultures in the evaluation of uncomplicated skin and soft tissue infections. *Pediatrics.* 2013;132(3):454–459.
30. Law YM, Lal AK, Chen S, iháková D, et al. American Heart Association Pediatric Heart Failure and Transplantation Committee of the Council on Lifelong Congenital Heart Disease and Heart Health in the Young and Stroke Council Diagnosis and management of myocarditis in children: a scientific statement from the American Heart Association. *Circulation.* 2021;144(6):e123–e135.
31. Leung AK, Barankin B, Leong KF. Staphylococcal-scalded skin syndrome: evaluation, diagnosis, and management. *World J Pediatr.* 2018;14(2):116–120.
32. Levine DA, Platt SL, Dayan PS, Macias CG. Multicenter RSV-SBI Study Group of the Pediatric Emergency Medicine Collaborative Research Committee of the American Academy of Pediatrics Risk of serious bacterial infection in young febrile infants with respiratory syncytial virus infections. *Pediatrics.* 2004;113(6):1728–1734.
33. Li R, Hatcher JD. Gonococcal arthritis. *StatPearls.* StatPearls Publishing; 2021.
34. Mahajan P, Browne LR, Levine DA, Cohen DM, et al. Risk of bacterial coinfections in febrile infants 60 days old and younger with documented viral infections. *J Pediatr.* 2018;203:86–91.
35. Mameli C, Genoni T, Madia C, et al. Brain abscess in pediatric age: a review. *Childs Nerv Syst.* 2019;35(7):1117–1128.
36. Martin K, Weiss SL. Initial resuscitation and management of pediatric septic shock. *Minerva Pediatr.* 2015;67(2):141–158.
37. Mattoo TK, Shaikh N, Nelson CP. Contemporary management of urinary tract infection in children. *Pediatrics.* 2021;147(2): e2020012138.
38. McCrindle B, Rowley A, Newberger J, Burns J, et al. Correction to: Diagnosis, treatment, and long-term management of Kawasaki disease: a scientific statement for health professionals from the American Heart Association. *Circulation.* 2017;140(5):927–999.
39. McGrath A, Barrett MJ. Petechiae. *StatPearls.* StatPearls Publishing; 2021.
40. Mintegi S, Garcia S, Martin MJ, et al. Clinical prediction rule for distinguishing bacterial from aseptic meningitis. *Pediatrics.* 2020;146(3):e20201126.
41. Mogilner L, Katz C. Pasteurella multocida. *Pediatr Rev.* 2019;40(2):90–92.

42. Nolt D, Starke JR. Tuberculosis infection in children and adolescents: testing and treatment. *Pediatrics*. 2021;148(6): e2021054663. https://doi.org/10.1542/peds.2021-054663. PMID: 34851422.
43. Noor A, Krilov LR. Necrotizing fasciitis. *Pediatr Rev*. 2021;42(10):573–575.
44. Oduwole O, Udoh EE, Oyo-Ita A, Meremikwu MM. Honey for acute cough in children. *Cochrane Database Syst Rev*. 2018;4(4):CD007094 https://doi.org/10.1002/14651858.CD007094.pub5. PMID: 29633783; PMCID: PMC6513626.
45. Pantell RH, Roberts KB, Adams WG, Dreyer BP, et al. Clinical practice guideline: evaluation and management of well-appearing febrile infants 8 to 60 days old. *Pediatrics*. 2021;148(2): e2021052228.
46. Pecora F, Abate L, Scavone S, Petrucci I, et al. Management of infectious lymphadenitis in children. *Children (Basel)*. 2021;8(10):860.
47. Pereda MA, Chavez MA, Hooper-Miele CC. Lung ultrasound for the diagnosis of pneumonia in children: a meta-analysis. *Pediatrics*. 2015;135(4):714–722.
48. Pinninti SG, Kimberlin DW. Neonatal herpes simplex virus infections. *Semin Perinatol*. 2018;42(3):168–175.
49. Ralston SL, Lieberthal AS, Meissner HC, et al. Clinical practice guideline: the diagnosis, management, and prevention of bronchiolitis. *Pediatrics*. 2014;134(5):e1474–e1502.
50. Rosow LK, Strober JB. Infant botulism: review and clinical update. *Pediatr Neurol*. 2015;52(5):487–492.
51. Rubin G, Chezar A, Raz R, Rozen N. Nail puncture wound through a rubber-soled shoe: a retrospective study of 96 adult patients. *J Foot Ankle Surg*. 2010;49(5):421–425.
52. Saavedra-Lozano J, Falup-Pecurariu O, Faust SN, Girschick H, et al. Bone and joint infections. *Pediatr Infect Dis J*. 2017;36(8):788–799.
53. Sands A, Mulvey N, Iacono D, Cerise J, et al. Utility of methicillin-resistant *Staphylococcus aureus* nares screening in hospitalized children with acute infectious disease syndromes. *Antibiotics*. 2021;10:1434. https://doi.org/10.3390/antibiotics10121434.
54. Shah SN, Bachur RG, Simel DL, et al. Does this child have pneumonia? The rational clinical examination systematic review. *JAMA*. 2017;318(5):462–471.
55. Simonsen KA, Anderson-Berry AL, Delair SF, Davies HD. Early-onset neonatal sepsis. *Clin Microbiol Rev*. 2014;27(1):21–47.
56. Mattoo TK, Shaikh N, Nelson CP. Contemporary management of urinary tract infection in children. *Pediatrics*. 2021;147(2): https://doi.org/10.1542/peds.2020-012138. e2020012138.
57. Tian C, Jin S, Zhao Z, et al. Outcomes in pediatric patients with bacterial meningitis: a systematic review and meta-analysis of randomized controlled trials. *Clin Ther*. 2022;44(4):551–564.
58. Tunuguntla H, Jeewa A, Denfield SW. Acute myocarditis and pericarditis in children. *Pediatr Rev*. 2019;40(1):14–25.
59. US Department of Health and Human Services Centers for Disease Control and Prevention Sexually transmitted infections treatment guidelines, 2021. *MMWR Recomm Rep*. 2021;70(4):1–135.
60. Viscusi CD, Pacheco GS. Pediatric emergency noninvasive ventilation. *Emerg Med Clin N Am*. 2018;36:387–400.
61. Viscusi CD, Pacheco GS. Pediatric emergency noninvasive ventilation. *Emerg Med Clin N Am*. 2018;36:387–400.
62. Wald ER, Applegate KE, Bordley C, Darrow DH, et al. Clinical practice guideline for the diagnosis and management of acute bacterial sinusitis in children aged 1 to 18 years. *Pediatrics*. 2013;32(1):e262–280.
63. Wang CX. Assessment and management of acute disseminated encephalomyelitis (ADEM) in the pediatric patient. *Paediatr Drugs*. 2021;23(3):213–221.
64. Wasserman M, Chapman R, Lapidot R, Sutton K, et al. Twenty-year public health impact of 7- and 13-valent pneumococcal conjugate vaccines in US children. *Emerg Infect Dis*. 2021;27(6):1627–1636.
65. Wolff M, Bachur R. Serious bacterial infection in recently immunized young febrile infants. *Acad Emerg Med*. 2009;16:1284–1289.
66. Zwemer E, Stephens J. Things we do for no reason: blood cultures for uncomplicated skin and soft tissue infections in children. *J Hosp Med*. 2018;13(7):496–499.

CHAPTER 38

OPHTHALMOLOGIC EMERGENCIES

Katie Giordano

1. **What are the important components for triaging a patient with a chief complaint of eye problem?**

   Visual acuity is the "vital" sign for the eye. It is a very important piece of information when consulting an ophthalmologist. Some conditions preclude obtaining a visual acuity such as contamination with a caustic substance, acid, or alkali; sudden unilateral vision loss; or significant trauma. For these cases, perform a gross assessment of vision while other care is provided. Visual acuity at the time of presentation provides a baseline to follow for improvement or deterioration.

   The normal visual acuity of a toddler is 20/40 and improves gradually to the normal adult acuity of 20/20 by age 5 or 6 years.

2. **How should you check visual acuity?**

   Use a Snellen chart test at 20 feet (6 m) or a Rosenbaum chart at 14 inches. For younger patients who cannot read letters, you can use an Allen chart that depicts easily recognizable shapes. If the child wears glasses, corrective lenses should be worn for testing visual acuity. If the patient does not have their glasses, have them view the chart through a pinhole, which corrects most refractive errors. If no form of testing is available, visual acuity is recorded as being unable/able to count fingers, unable/able to perceive hand motion, or unable/able to perceive light.

3. **For patients presenting with a red or painful eye, what concerning findings on examination are associated with a serious diagnosis?**

   a. Severe ocular pain
   b. Persistently blurred vision
   c. Exophthalmos
   d. Decreased ocular light reflex
   e. Corneal epithelial defect or opacity
   f. Limbal injection (ciliary flush)
   g. Unreactive pupil
   h. Soft contact lens wearer
   i. Neonatal patient
   j. Immunocompromised patient
   k. Worsening signs after 3 days of treatment

4. **What is conjunctivitis?**

   Conjunctivitis, often called "pink eye," is an inflammation of the conjunctiva (the thin translucent membrane lining the anterior sclera and undersurface of the eyelids). In this condition, there is dilation of the conjunctiva vessels, which leads to hyperemia and edema. Viral conjunctivitis is the most common type overall and is seen more commonly in the summer. Bacterial conjunctivitis accounts for 50% to 75% of conjunctivitis in children and is more common from December through April. Both are typically self-resolving in 1 to 2 weeks. Typically patients will not have significant changes in vision due to conjunctivitis.

5. **How can you distinguish viral conjunctivitis from bacterial conjunctivitis?**

   Differentiating viral from bacterial conjunctivitis can be difficult. Both can be unilateral or bilateral. Viral conjunctivitis typically has a serous to mucoid discharge. The history of multiple sick contacts or the involvement of one eye after the other suggests a viral etiology. In patients older than 6 years, adenovirus is the most common cause. These children may also complain of a sore throat and have upper respiratory infection (URI) symptoms. There is often tearing of the eye (discharge is typically watery), and photophobia. This condition is highly contagious with an incubation period of 5 to 10 days. Epidemic keratoconjunctivitis, associated with adenoviral infection, can present with severe eyelid swelling, preauricular adenopathy, discharge, and a sandy foreign body sensation.

   Bacterial conjunctivitis is accompanied by purulent drainage. Lid edema, chemosis, and at times subconjunctival hemorrhage can be seen. *Staphylococcus* spp., *S. pneumoniae*, *Haemophilus influenza*, and *Moraxella* are common causes. About 60% of culture-proven bacterial conjunctivitis cases are self-limiting in 1 to 2 weeks. Severe bacterial conjunctivitis presenting with ocular discomfort, significant redness, and copious purulent drainage may be caused by *Neisseria gonorrhoeae*.

6. How is viral conjunctivitis treated?

Treatment of viral conjunctivitis is supportive with cool compresses and pain control. Strict handwashing is essential to prevent spread. Artificial tears may provide symptomatic relief.

7. What is the treatment for bacterial conjunctivitis?

About 60% of culture-proven bacterial conjunctivitis cases are self-limiting in 1 to 2 weeks. When antibiotics are prescribed, a broad-spectrum topical antibiotic can be used, such as erythromycin or trimethoprim/polymixin B. Ointment is preferred over drops as this is easier to apply in young children and requires less frequent dosing than drops. Avoid corticosteroids as these can cause serious complications, especially if herpes simplex virus (HSV) is the etiology of infection. Use of an antibiotic may shorten the course of disease, decrease transmissibility, and allow for a quicker return to school/daycare. The child can return to school after 24 hours of treatment. In a large Cochrane database analysis, there was no difference in outcomes between those treated and those given a placebo. Send a culture for those cases that are refractory to treatment. Neonates require special attention (see Question 8).

8. What are the special considerations for neonatal conjunctivitis?

Most hospitals apply erythromycin ointment or dilute betadine solutions to the eyes of newborns for prophylaxis against gonorrhea. However, prophylaxis does not completely eliminate the risk of chlamydial or gonococcal infection in the neonatal period.

Chlamydia and *N. gonorrhoeae* must be considered as possible pathogens in neonatal conjunctivitis. Gonorrhea usually occurs at 2 to 5 days of life and chlamydia at 5 to 14 days of life, but this is not a fixed timeline. A dramatically hyperemic conjunctiva with lid swelling and copious purulent drainage is characteristic of gonococcal infection. There is a high risk of corneal perforation with gonococcal infections, and therefore, you must presume the infant has this infection and treat it accordingly until proven otherwise. A Gram stain with the presence of gram-negative diplococci is helpful in determining the need to start treatment. Consider a sepsis workup for these infants. Admit patients for parenteral antibiotic therapy with ceftriaxone or ceftazidime and consult an ophthalmologist. Hourly saline lavage can limit the number of organisms that could penetrate the cornea. Gonococcal infections are rare outside of the neonatal period but should be considered in older children with severe conjunctivitis.

The examination of infants with chlamydial conjunctivitis usually reveals hyperemic conjunctiva, mucopurulent discharge, and lymphoid follicle formation (conjunctival stippling). Send a culture of the discharge. The majority of chlamydial conjunctivitis cases are unilateral. About 50% of neonates with chlamydial conjunctivitis have lung or nasopharynx infection. Treat with both topical and systemic oral antibiotics for culture-proven chlamydial conjunctivitis. The systemic treatment eradicates the carriage of *Chlamydia* in the nasopharynx and prevents the subsequent development of chlamydial pneumonitis.

HSV is another infection to consider. HSV can cause infection on the skin surrounding the eye but may involve the cornea and conjunctiva. The presence of vesicular skin lesions is a helpful clue to this infection.

9. What additional concerns should be considered in contact-wearing patients with conjunctivitis?

There is a high risk of bacterial keratitis in patients with conjunctivitis who wear contacts. Remove the contact lens immediately. Treat these patients with topical antibiotics and refer them to an ophthalmologist.

10. What is keratitis?

Keratitis is an inflammation of the cornea. Patients present with erythema of the perilimbal bulbar conjunctiva (limbal or ciliary flush) and pain. They may also complain of foreign body sensation, tearing, decreased vision, and photophobia. With fluorescein staining you may see pooling under a blue light examination. Ensure there is no corneal perforation. Relieve pain with a topical anesthetic. Diagnosis is made with the presence of corneal epithelial or stromal infiltrate, which is seen on slit lamp examination. If there is any concern about globe perforation, an immediate ophthalmology consult is warranted. Otherwise, follow up with ophthalmology in 1 to 2 days. Most patients with this condition can be discharged with topical antibiotics and oral nonsteroidal anti-inflammatory drugs for pain. Eye patching is not necessary.

11. What are the causes of preseptal (periorbital) cellulitis?

Preseptal cellulitis can occur after minor trauma or spread from local infections such as impetigo. Insect bites with local allergic reactions can mimic preseptal cellulitis as they cause significant redness and swelling of the eyelids, but usually without fever or tenderness, and they may have associated pruritis. Preseptal cellulitis is a bacterial infection, generally related to *Staphylococcus aureus*, including methicillin-resistant *S. aureus* (MRSA), or group A *Streptococcus*. These patients rarely have bacteremia. Culture of the blood is rarely needed and percutaneous aspiration of the cellulitis is unnecessary and difficult.

These children are generally younger than 2 years and typically present with swelling and redness of the eyelids. They may have fever. It may be difficult to see the eye (due to swelling), but the extraocular muscles are intact.

Preseptal cellulitis can also be a complication of paranasal sinusitis. *Streptococcus pneumonia* is commonly associated with these infections. Often the patient will be at least 2 years old, have URI symptoms, and a history of eye swelling in the morning, and on the day of presentation, the swelling did not subside. The edema and erythema of the eyelids can be very impressive and eversion and separation of the lids difficult, but pain and decreased range of motion of the extraocular muscle is not present.

12. **What is the treatment for preseptal (periorbital) cellulitis?**
Most cases can be treated with oral antibiotics such as cephalosporin. Consider coverage for MRSA if community prevalence is high. The patient should be reevaluated in 24 to 48 hours. Hospital admission for parenteral antibiotics is warranted if the patient is ill-appearing or the cellulitis is extensive.

13. **How can you distinguish preseptal (periorbital) cellulitis from orbital cellulitis?**
Orbital cellulitis is a vision-threatening condition so it is important to distinguish this from preseptal cellulits. This is not always easy with a young child. Both periorbital and orbital cellulitis may be associated with fever, pain, eyelid swelling, and eye redness. The hallmark signs of orbital cellulitis are decreased eye movement, proptosis, decreased vision, and signs of optic nerve involvement such as papilledema, decreased color vision, visual field deficits, or Marcus Gunn pupil.
Imaging studies are warranted to determine if orbital involvement is present and will determine the extent of infection and guide appropriate management. Computed tomography (CT) scanning is quick and provides distinct bony resolution. It can also be utilized in surgical image-guided procedures. Consider the use of magnetic resonance imaging (MRI) to avoid radiation exposure with CT. An abscess can potentially be seen on MRI without the use of contrast. The limitation of MRI is the length of the study and the potential need for sedation in younger children.

14. **What is the treatment for orbital cellulitis?**
Admit patients with orbital cellulitis to the hospital for intravenous (IV) antibiotics. Empiric antibiotics should cover typical skin, respiratory tract, and sinus pathogens. MRSA coverage should be considered. Blood cultures and cerebrospinal fluid (CSF) testing are rarely indicated. Loss of vision and extension of infection are complications of untreated orbital cellulitis.
Orbital cellulitis associated with subperiosteal or retrobulbar abscesses typically responds to IV antibiotics and does not require surgical management. Surgical intervention is necessary if there is a large, well-defined abscess, complete ophthalmoplegia, intracranial extension, or impairment of vision. Consult ophthalmology in all cases and involve otorhinolaryngology if sinusitis is associated.

15. **How do you test the afferent pupillary reflex? What will you see if the patient has an afferent pupillary defect?**
The pupillary light reflex is a reflex arc through the midbrain involving crossover innervation. It is assessed with the swinging light test: Shining a light in one eye should result in constriction of both pupils. No change in pupillary size should be noted when the light swings toward the other pupil. If a patient has an afferent pupillary defect, both pupils dilate when the light swings to the affected eye. The abnormal pupil, called a Marcus Gunn pupil, can result from a retinal artery or venous occlusions, retinal detachment, tumors, or ischemic optic neuropathy.

16. **What is the Bruckner test? How is it performed?**
The Bruckner test is a simultaneous bilateral red reflex test that elicits both a corneal light reflex and a red reflex. View the patient's eyes from about 2 feet away with a broad beam of light that encompasses both eyes. You should see both a red reflex and a small white light reflex in each eye. The key to a normal examination is symmetry. An absent or dull red reflex may indicate vitreous hemorrhage, cataract, hyphema, opacity of the cornea, enophthalmos, or misalignment of the globe.

17. **What can cause diplopia?**
- Blowout fractures
- Poisoning
- Central nervous system pathology: tumor, bleed, idiopathic intracranial hypertension (IIH)
- Shunt malfunction
- Arnold-Chiari malformation
- Head trauma

18. **What are the causes of papilledema?**
Papilledema is optic disk swelling. It is usually bilateral and is caused by anything that increases intracranial pressure. Unilateral papilledema suggests ipsilateral orbital trauma such as orbital hemorrhage, orbital tumor, or direct injury to the optic nerve. Ophthalmoscopic signs include blurring of the disk margins and disk edema. The disk

may be hyperemic due to telangiectasis of the capillaries and small hemorrhages. The patient may have visual field deficits. With acute papilledema, vision is maintained. Common causes of papilledema are the following:

- Increased or decreased CSF production
- Intracranial mass
- Obstruction of venous outflow
- Obstructive hydrocephalus
- Craniosynostosis
- Idiopathic intracranial hypertension (IIH)

19. **When should you be concerned about IIH?**
This condition (previously called pseudotumor cerebri) usually occurs in obese teenage girls who present with severe headache and papilledema on fundoscopic examination. The papilledema is usually bilateral. Some patients with this condition also have diplopia, visual field restriction, and abducens nerve (sixth cranial nerve) palsy (unilateral or bilateral). Neurological examination is otherwise normal.

Obtain neuroimaging when IIH is suspected. MRI (with and without contrast) is the imaging study of choice. The MRI shows normal brain parenchyma with no mass, hydrocephalus, or structural lesion. Perform a lumbar puncture after the MRI, unless there is a clear source of increased intracranial pressure. With IIH the lumbar puncture will show elevated opening pressure and CSF will be otherwise normal. Consult an ophthalmologist or a neurologist to help with visual field testing and management. Untreated IIH can result in vision loss.

20. **What makes up the orbit?**
- Frontal bone: Superior orbital ridge and the upper medial orbital ridge
- Zygoma: Lateral orbital rim
- Maxilla: Inferior and lower medial rim
- Maxillary sinus: Orbital floor
- Lacrimal bone: Separates the orbit from the nares
- Ethmoid bone: Medial wall and part of the posterior wall
- Sphenoid bone: Posterior wall

21. **What is the treatment for corneal abrasions?**
Corneal abrasions are very painful and treatment with oral analgesics is important. Topical nonsteroidal anti-inflammatory agents are used for pain control in adults but are not recommended for children. Some clinicians use topical antibiotics for the treatment of corneal abrasions. Ointments are more lubricating than drops, are better tolerated in young children, and do not need to be reapplied as often as drops. Antipseudomonal coverage is important for contact lens wearers, and they should discontinue lens use until the abrasion is healed and antibiotic therapy is complete. *Topical anesthetics are not indicated after the initial examination.* Continued use of topical anesthetics can predispose the patient to subsequent injury. Patching is not recommended, as it can increase moisture and increase the risk of infection. Randomized, controlled trials have shown that topical mydriatics give no improvement in pain control.

22. **What are the symptoms of retinal detachment?**
Retinal detachment is a separation between the sensory and pigment portions of the retina. Symptoms include "flashes," "floaters," and visual defects. Flashes of light are caused by traction on the peripheral retina. Floaters are caused by fibrous aggregates on the posterior portion of the vitreous that block light from reaching the retina. Retinal tears may be asymptomatic for years, but if the macula is involved, the visual loss is severe. Consult an ophthalmologist to evaluate all patients who report flashes or floaters to prevent the progression of partial retinal tears to complete detachment. Traumatic damage to the retina is often located at the periphery of the retina, an area that is not easily examined with a direct ophthalmoscope.

23. **How do you approach a child with a foreign body in the eye?**
Most foreign bodies can be removed after a thorough examination has been performed and visual acuity has been assessed. Patients are usually quite accurate in their localization of the foreign body based on sensation. Instill a topical anesthetic and fluorescein dye. Evert the upper eyelid while the patient looks down, and examine for foreign bodies. Shining the otoscope at an angle provides indirect lighting, and the foreign body may cast a shadow. Irrigation is often used to easily remove superficial foreign bodies. Use a premoistened cotton swab to remove the foreign body from the bulbar or palpebral conjunctiva. Corneal abrasions are common with a foreign body on the eyelid. Consult ophthalmology when the foreign body is embedded, removal attempts are unsuccessful, or there is a concern for a penetrating foreign body/ruptured globe.

24. **A teenager who was not wearing protective eyewear reports a "foreign body sensation" in his eye after hammering (metal on metal). How should this patient be managed?**
With this history, the emergency physician must be suspicious of an intraocular foreign body that has penetrated the cornea or sclera. The eye can heal quickly, and a laceration may not be visible. Subtle signs, such as red eyes,

pupil asymmetry, and decreased vision may be noted. However, small particles that rapidly penetrate the eye may produce few or no signs. Maintain a high index of suspicion. Consult an ophthalmologist.

25. **What is the differential for swelling of or around the eye?**
    - Blunt trauma
    - Tumor
    - Local edema-hypoproteinemia (nephrotic syndrome), congestive heart failure
    - Allergy
    - Infection
    - Insect bites

26. **Which tumors are associated with the eye?**
    Tumors that can involve the eye include metastatic neuroblastoma, which can present with periorbital ecchymosis and proptosis. This is sometimes misdiagnosed as child abuse. The "raccoon eyes" is due to periorbital bone and soft tissue involvement. Some children have Horner syndrome (ptosis, miosis, and anhidrosis). Retinoblastoma is a tumor that should be considered when a child presents with a white reflex pupil. This is known as leukocoria and can be seen with an otoscope. (Or parents may note this in their photos of the child.) Some have strabismus and poor visual acuity. Langerhans cell histiocytosis and granulocytic sarcoma can also involve the eye. Hemangiomas of the lid are also found at times.

27. **What are some infectious processes of the eyelid?**
    Bacterial, viral, and parasitic infections of the eyelid can occur. Bacterial infection of the lid margin is referred to as blepharitis. This is most commonly caused by *S. aureus* and *Staphylococcus epidermidis* and it can be acute or chronic. The presentation will include erythema and crusting of the lid margins especially upon awakening. The lid margins may become thickened. The child may be asymptomatic or complain of burning, itching, or a foreign body sensation. Gentle daily lid hygiene with soap and water can treat and prevent blepharitis. Topical application of antibiotics ointment can speed resolution.

    Molluscum contagiosum caused by the *Poxviridae* virus, can involve the eyelids. It is self-limiting over a few months except in immunocompromised hosts where treatment may be recommended to prevent autoinoculation. Lesions near the lid margin can cause conjunctival injection and can lead to corneal epithelial disease.

28. **What is the difference between a hordeolum (stye) and a chalazion?**
    A hordeolum is an acute inflammation of the sebaceous glands in the eyelid. This is usually sterile but can progress to infection, with *S. aureus* as the most common cause. Both internal and external hordeola (stye) have skin changes including edema and erythema, which can be tender along the eyelid. There is often a pustule or papule; one may need to evert the eyelid to see the pustule of an internal hordeolum. This condition will often spontaneously resolve in 5 to 7 days. Warm compresses for 10 to 15 minutes several times a day may hasten the course. Some advise applying baby shampoo to a washcloth and gently scrubbing the eyelashes when the eyes are closed. When significant blepharitis is also present, a course of topical antibiotics may reduce the recurrence rate of a hordeolum. Surgical intervention is rarely necessary.

    A chalazion also results from a blocked eyelid gland. It is a sterile lipogranulomatosis reaction and can occur spontaneously or after the resolution of an internal hordeolum. A chalazion presents as a nontender, localized bulge in the lid, and the overlying skin is normal. Smaller chalazions spontaneously resolve, but this can take months. Lesions 10 mm or larger often do not self-resolve and may need intervention such as surgical excision.

29. **What diagnosis would you suspect in an infant who presents with constant mucous crusting in the corner of the eye and tearing?**
    Nasolacrimal duct obstruction. This is often caused by incomplete canalization at the distal end of the nasolacrimal apparatus, which extends from the eyelid to the nose. It occurs in up to 20% of all normal newborns. Signs and symptoms include increased tear lake, mucopurulent discharge, and epiphora (excessive overflow of tears). The conjunctiva is not as erythematous as expected with an infection such as conjunctivitis. More than 90% spontaneously resolve during the first year of life. Treatment includes gentle lid hygiene and lacrimal duct massage (manual pressure over the lacrimal sac). Occasionally, topical antibiotics are needed and if resolution does not occur, surgical intervention may be warranted.

30. **A 17-day-old infant presents with redness and swelling below the inner corner of the left eye. What is the diagnosis, and what is the treatment?**
    This describes dacryocystitis, which is an emergency. This results from a congenital or acquired lacrimal outflow obstruction. There is usually acute erythema, pain, and swelling in the medial canthal region. Mucopurulent drainage can be noted from the lacrimal punctum. A fistula to the skin can also form; if this occurs it may need to be surgically removed after the infection clears. *S. aureus*, *S. epidermidis*, and alpha-hemolytic streptococci are likely causative organisms. Consult ophthalmology for these infants. A full sepsis workup should be considered if the neonate appears ill. Consider admission to the hospital for parenteral antibiotics.

KEY POINTS: EYE EMERGENCIES

1. Emergently treat neonatal conjunctivitis caused by *N. gonorrhoeae* with parenteral and topical antibiotics owing to the risk of corneal perforation.
2. Always attempt to document the visual acuity in assessing a patient with a complaint related to the eye.
3. The hallmark signs of orbital cellulitis are decreased eye movement, proptosis, decreased vision, and signs of optic nerve involvement.
4. Nasolacrimal duct obstruction occurs in up to 20% of all normal newborns. More than 90% will spontaneously resolve during the first year of life.

BIBLIOGRAPHY

1. Azari AA, Barney NP. Conjunctivitis: a systemic review of diagnosis and treatment. *JAMA.* 2013;310(16):1721–1729.
2. Bhatt A, et al. Ocular infections. In: Cherry JD, Harrison GJ, Kaplan SL, Steinbach WJ, eds. *Feigin and Cherry's Textbook of Pediatric Infectious Diseases.* 8th ed. Elsevier; 2019:578–597. e5.
3. Costakos DM. Eye disorders. In: Kliegman RM, Lye PS, Bordini BJ, Toth H, Base D, eds. *Nelson Pediatric Symptom-Based Diagnosis.* Elsevier; 2018:563–593. e2.
4. Dull KE. Visual disturbances. In: Shaw KN, Bachur RG, eds. *Fleisher & Ludwig's Textbook of Pediatric Emergency Medicine.* 8th ed. Wolters Kluwer; 2021:188–193.
5. Dupré AA, Wightman JM. Red and painful eye. In: Walls RM, Hockberger RS, Gausche-Hill M, eds. *Rosen's Emergency Medicine: Concepts and Clinical Practice.* 9th ed. Elsevier; 2018:169–183. e2.
6. Guluma K, Lee JE. Ophthalmology. In: Walls RM, Hockberger RS, Gausche-Hill M, eds. *Rosen's Emergency Medicine: Concepts and Clinical Practice.* 9th ed. Elsevier; 2018:790–819. e3.
7. Schonfeld D, Schnall BM. Ophthalmic emergencies. In: Shaw KN, Bachur RG, eds. *Fleisher & Ludwig's Textbook of Pediatric Emergency Medicine.* 8th ed. Wolters Kluwer; 2021:1392–1403.
8. Wald ER. Preseptal and orbital infections. In: Long SS, Prober CG, Fischer M, eds. *Principles and Practice of Pediatric Infectious Diseases.* 5th ed. Elsevier; 2018:517–522. e1.

CHAPTER 39

POISONINGS

Beverly Anderson, Brittney Russell and Kevin C. Osterhoudt

1. **How many poisonings occur in the United States each year? How many exposures involve children less than 6 years?**
   Over 2 million calls are made to regional poison control centers in the United States annually. Estimates suggest that 4 million people are poisoned each year, and not all poisonings are reported to the poison control center. Of the reported calls, 42% of cases involved children <6 years old.

2. **How often can poisonings be managed at home with the assistance of a regional poison control center?**
   The majority of calls to poison centers, around 70%, are managed outside of a healthcare facility, usually at the site of exposure, primarily the patient's own residence. Of the 30% managed at a healthcare facility, about 45% are treated and released.

3. **When was the first poison control center established and why?**
   Dr. Edward Press in Chicago established the first center in 1953 in response to an American Academy of Pediatrics study published in 1952, which found that 50% of all childhood injuries were due to potentially poisonous ingestions.

4. **What is the Poison Prevention Packaging Act and what impact did this have?**
   Passed in 1970, this act mandated safety packaging for pharmaceuticals. The frequency of poisoning and death due to poisoning in children decreased significantly in 1969, 1 year prior to the passage of the act. This effect was due to voluntary initiation of safety packaging (childproof caps) by manufacturers in anticipation of the law.

5. **What are the most common poisons to which young children are exposed?**
   In 2020, the top 10 exposures in young children from most frequent to least frequent were: cosmetics/personal care products, household cleaners, analgesics, foreign bodies (i.e., coins, toys, button batteries), dietary supplements, vitamins, topical preparations, antihistamines, pesticides, and plants.

6. **Who is more likely to ingest a poison: a 2-year-old boy or a 2-year-old girl?**
   Curiosity-driven toddler boys are slightly more likely to have reported poison exposures.

7. **Who is more likely to ingest a poison: a 15-year-old boy or a 15-year-old girl?**
   Adolescent girls are almost twice as likely than boys to have an intentional drug or chemical ingestion with the intent of self-harm.

8. **What is the typical setting for a pediatric poisoning incident?**
   The child is usually younger than 6 years and is at home. The poison is typically readily available to the child. Prescription medicines that children ingest frequently belong to a grandparent or older nonparent relative. In most cases, only one poison is ingested. Social history often discloses recent stress in the household, such as a recent move, a new baby, marital discord, visiting relatives, or distracting events (holidays, weddings).

9. **What are the three most common causes of fatality from pediatric poisonings?**
   The most common causes of fatality from pediatric poisonings include analgesics, gas/fumes, and cardiovascular drugs.

10. **What is the leading cause of death due to injury in the United States?**
    Poisoning! According to the U.S. Centers for Disease Control, there were 107,622 drug overdose deaths in the United States in 2021 and more than 70,000 of those deaths involved illegally manufactured fentanyl. Poisoning surpassed motor vehicle traffic fatalities as the leading cause of injury death in the United States in 2008.
    For children and teenagers, firearm-related injuries are the leading cause of death in the United States, surpassing car accidents in 2021. Drug poisoning ranks as the fourth leading cause of death for those under 18, with fatalities among youth increasing by 133.3% over the 10-year period of 2011-2021.

11. **Which medicinal drugs are often considered potentially life-threatening or fatal to a 10-kg toddler following ingestion of a single dose?**

    1. Opioids: fentanyl, methadone, oxycodone, hydrocodone buprenorphine, and codeine
    2. Cardiac medications:

a. Calcium channel blockers: verapamil and nifedipine
b. Beta blockers: propranolol and sotalol
c. Quinidine
d. Flecainide
e. Clonidine
3. Antidepressants and antipsychotics: imipramine, desipramine, chlorpromazine, clozapine, and thioridazine
4. Antimalarials: chloroquine, hydroxychloroquine, and quinine.
5. Theophylline
6. Sulfonylureas glyburide, glimepiride, glipizide, chlorpropamide, tolazamide
7. Antidiarrheal: diphenoxylate (Lomotil)
8. Topical products:
a. methyl salicylate: Ben-Gay, Icy Hot, and Oil of wintergreen liniment
b. camphor
c. benzocaine/topical anesthetics
d. lindane

KEY POINTS: POISONING EPIDEMIOLOGY

1. Nearly half of all poisoning exposures are reported among children younger than 6 years.
2. Natural exploratory behaviors of young children put them at risk for poisoning.
3. Substance use disorder, experimental risk-taking, and depression put adolescents at risk for poisoning.
4. Poisoning related to substance use disorder, largely associated with nonmedical use of opioids, and intentional large-dose drug ingestions have made it the leading cause of death due to injury in the United States.

12. **What are the most important actions that provide the best chance for recovery after poisoning?**
Most poisoned patients will do well with the provision of timely supportive care that ensures careful assessment and prompt management of airway, breathing, circulation, and neurologic disability.

13. **Which three antidotal drugs should be immediately considered in the resuscitation of the comatose child?**
Two are often not thought of as drugs per se, but they are essential substrates for brain function: oxygen and glucose. Administration of the opioid antagonist naloxone may also be warranted.

14. **What is a "toxidrome"?**
The word *toxidrome* can be thought of as a combination of the words "toxic" and "syndrome." Toxidromes are groupings of physical signs that may help to suggest the drug class responsible for poisoning. Note these signs in the examination of every potentially poisoned patient: mental status, vital signs, pupil size and reactivity, skin color and moisture, bowel sounds, and neuromotor exam.

15. **Describe the most common toxidromes.**
The most common toxidromes can be found in Table 39.1.

16. **How can the anticholinergic toxidrome be differentiated from the sympathomimetic toxidrome?**
Anticholinergic agents and sympathomimetic agents may both produce agitation and delirium, tachycardia, hypertension, hyperthermia, and mydriatic pupils, so distinguishing between these drugs is not easy. Look to the skin, the bowels, and the eyes for help. Anticholinergic poisoning is likely to produce flushed skin that is surprisingly dry to the touch, diminished or absent bowel sounds, and less reactive pupils. Many people remember the characteristics of the anticholinergic toxidrome with the mnemonic "mad as a hatter, blind as a bat (pupils do not accommodate well), red as a beet, dry as a bone, and hot as Hades."

17. **What would be the significance of a bitter almond smell to your morning coffee?**
Consider the possibility of cyanide in the coffee.

18. **Which toxicants are associated with characteristic odors?**
- Acetone, isopropyl alcohol, and phenol have the odor of acetone.
- Cyanide has the smell of almonds.
- Arsenic, thallium, organophosphates, and selenious acid have the odor of garlic.
- Chloral hydrate and paraldehyde have the scent of pears.

Table 39.1 Common Toxidromes

VARIABLE	SYMPATHOMIMETICS	ANTICHOLINERGICS	ORGANOPHOSPHATES	OPIATES/CLONIDINE	BARBITURATES/SEDATIVE-HYPNOTICS	SALICYLATES
Mental status	A, D, P, S	C, D, P, S	C, D, F, S	C	C	C, S
Heart rate	↑	↑	↓(↑)	↓	—	—(↑)
Blood pressure	↑	↑	—(↑)	↓	↓	—
Temperature	↑	↑	—	↓	↓	↑
Respirations	—	—	↑	↓	↓	↑
Pupil size	↑ (reactive)	↑ (sluggish)	↓	↓↓	↓	—
Bowel sounds	—	↓	↑	↓	—	—
Skin	Sweaty	Flushed/dry	Sweaty	—	Bullae (IV use)	Sweaty

A, agitation; C, somnolence/coma; D, delirium; F, fasciculations; IV, intravenous; P, psychosis; S, seizure.

- Hydrogen sulfide has the smell of rotten eggs.
- Methyl salicylate has the aroma of wintergreen.

19. **What is the gastrointestinal decontamination technique of choice for most poisonings?**
    Administration of activated charcoal is typically preferred to gastric emptying methods such as induced vomiting or gastric lavage, but most recently has only been used in <0.5% of pediatric poisoning cases.

20. **When is activated charcoal administration recommended?**
    Evidence suggests that patients who have ingested a substance known to bind well to activated charcoal, and who have an intact airway or have undergone endotracheal intubation, might benefit from activated charcoal if it can be administered early after ingestion (when the drug is likely to remain in the stomach). Children who would not otherwise require endotracheal intubation should not be intubated solely for the purpose of receiving activated charcoal.

21. **List common drugs and toxicants that are poorly adsorbed by activated charcoal.**
    - Ineffective: Alcohols, iron, lithium
    - Poorly effective: Hydrocarbons, metals
    - Contraindicated: Caustic corrosives

22. **What is whole-bowel irrigation?**
    Whole-bowel irrigation uses nonabsorbable polyethylene glycol solution (well known as a surgical bowel preparation) to wash intestinal contents through before absorption can take place. Typical administration is 500 mL/hour in a toddler and up to 2 L/hour in an adolescent, continued until the rectal effluent is clear and clinical signs of continued drug absorption have subsided.

23. **List the possible indications for whole-bowel irrigation.**
    Although not yet proven to improve patient outcomes, the use of whole-bowel irrigation has been advocated for the following situations (mnemonic—"LIMPS"):
    - Lithium
    - Iron
    - Metals
    - "Packers" (see Question 24)
    - Sustained-release drugs
        Some also consider whole-bowel irrigation for pharmaceutical patch ingestion, and treatment of massive drug ingestions or after ingestion of drugs known to cause concretions.

24. **What is a body packer or a body stuffer?**
    Body packers are smugglers who attempt to evade customs officials by swallowing packages (typically tied condoms) of drugs. Body stuffers are drug sellers or users who hurriedly ingest illicit substances to hide evidence from authorities. Because of the planning involved, packers are less likely to become toxic than stuffers; however, packers typically ingest more dangerous quantities of drugs.

25. **How often do poisoned patients require special therapy, such as antidote administration, elimination enhancement, or extracorporeal elimination?**
    Antidotes and elimination enhancement, such as urinary alkalinization or multiple-dose activated charcoal, are only performed in about 1% of all reported poisonings. Extracorporeal elimination (hemodialysis or hemoperfusion) is needed in less than 0.1%.

26. **Multiple doses of activated charcoal are believed to enhance clearance of what poison(s)?**
    Multiple-dose activated charcoal may be of benefit after ingestion of sustained-release compounds or after a toxic gastric concretion has formed. Charcoal may also be helpful to treat life-threatening poisoning caused by carbamazepine, dapsone, phenobarbital, quinine, and theophylline. Elimination of amitriptyline, dextropropoxyphene, digoxin, disopyramide, nadolol, phenylbutazone, phenytoin, piroxicam, and sotalol increases with multiple-dose activated charcoal; however, improved outcomes for ingestion of these poisons with respect to morbidity and mortality rates have not been shown in controlled trials.

27. **Are lipid emulsions helpful in some poisoned patients?**
    Lipid emulsions are intravenous (IV) preparations of fats primarily used medically to provide total parenteral nutrition. Administration of IV lipid emulsion therapy has been used in the treatment of patients with local anesthetic systemic toxicity. Animal studies and case reports have purported benefits from lipid emulsion therapy in cases of refractory cardiovascular toxicity associated with drugs such as amitriptyline, bupropion, and verapamil; however, the quality of evidence remains low and clinicians are encouraged to consult a medical toxicologist or a poison control center to determine if lipid emulsion therapy may be appropriate.

28. **What is extracorporeal removal?**
Extracorporeal removal refers to the elimination of poison from the blood after removing the blood or a portion of the blood from the body. The forms of extracorporeal elimination include hemodialysis, charcoal hemoperfusion, arteriovenous hemofiltration, venovenous hemofiltration, exchange transfusion, and plasmapheresis. Of these, hemodialysis is most commonly used.

29. **What factors predict adequate removal of a poison by hemodialysis?**
The substance should have the following characteristics: small volume of distribution, little protein binding, water solubility, low molecular weight, low endogenous clearance, and single-compartment kinetics.

30. **For which toxic agents is hemodialysis most commonly considered?**
    - Ethylene glycol
    - Lithium
    - Methanol
    - Salicylate
    - Theophylline

31. **When should hemodialysis be used?**
The decision to perform hemodialysis is based on clinical findings as well as drug levels. Always confirm an elevated level and check units of measurement before instituting hemodialysis. Toxicologists and nephrologists have worked together to provide consensus guidance on the use of extracorporeal treatments in poisoning: www.extrip-workgroup.org/recommendations.

32. **What is the rationale behind urinary alkalinization?**
Urinary alkalinization refers to the administration of sodium bicarbonate or sodium acetate to raise the urine pH to 8.0. This procedure converts renally excreted toxicants, which are weak acids, to their ionized form within the proximal renal tubules, and thereby prevents reabsorption in the distal tubules (ion-trapping). This technique is most useful for enhancing the excretion of salicylates and phenobarbital (but not other barbiturates). Urinary alkalinization may also be useful to protect the kidney during rhabdomyolysis.

33. **What are the pitfalls of urinary alkalinization?**
Urinary alkalinization is inhibited by the presence of hypokalemia. Urinary alkalinization has been associated with pulmonary and cerebral edema, and fluid administration must be monitored carefully. Electrolyte and acid-base disturbances can result from sodium bicarbonate administration and merit frequent monitoring.

34. **List some drugs that may lead to a delayed expression of clinical toxicity.**
    - Acetaminophen
    - Monoamine oxidase inhibitors
    - Oral hypoglycemic agents
    - Sustained-release drug formulations
    - Thyroid hormones
    - Warfarin

KEY POINTS: INITIAL POISONING MANAGEMENT

1. Toxidrome analysis is more clinically useful than toxicology urine analysis.
2. Prompt supportive care of airway, breathing, circulation, and neurological disability is key to good outcomes after pediatric poisonings.

35. **Describe the pathophysiology of acetaminophen poisoning.**
Acetaminophen is the drug most commonly administered to children. Toxicity may occur after an acute overdose of 150 to 200 mg/kg or after repeated supratherapeutic ingestions. Overdose of acetaminophen leads to increased production of an intermediate metabolite, *N*-acetyl-*p*-benzoquinone imine, via cytochrome oxidase (P-450) metabolism, which causes tissue damage once glutathione is expended. This metabolite binds to hepatocytes and causes centrilobular liver necrosis.

36. **What are the three stages of acetaminophen overdose poisoning?**
    - **Stage I** (30 minutes to 24 hours after ingestion): Often asymptomatic; occasionally nausea, vomiting, diaphoresis, and pallor

- **Stage II** (24 to 48 hours after ingestion): Nausea, vomiting, right-upper-quadrant abdominal pain, elevation of hepatic aminotransferase levels
- **Stage III** (72 to 96 hours after ingestion): Fulminant hepatic failure with jaundice, thrombocytopenia, prolonged prothrombin time, and hepatic encephalopathy. Renal failure and cardiomyopathy may occur. If the patient survives, complete resolution of liver abnormalities is possible.

37. How is acetaminophen intoxication diagnosed?

The potential for acetaminophen poisoning must be thoughtfully considered because most patients are initially asymptomatic. Measure the serum acetaminophen level in all patients with intentional drug overdose. After a single, acute drug ingestion at a known time, a serum acetaminophen level at 4 to 24 hours after ingestion can predict the potential for toxicity and determine the need for antidote administration based on the Rumack-Matthew nomogram.

38. What is the antidote for acetaminophen overdose? How does it work?

N-Acetylcysteine (NAC) is *antidotal* as it replenishes, and substitutes for, depleted glutathione stores in the liver and detoxifies the toxic metabolite. NAC also seems to be *supportive* and alleviates existing hepatotoxicity through antioxidant and procirculatory properties.

39. How is NAC administered?

Historically, NAC had been given orally with a loading dose of 140 mg/kg, followed by 17 doses of 70 mg/kg given every 4 hours. However, IV NAC is now U.S. Food and Drug Administration (FDA)–approved as a consecutive series of three infusions over 21 hours and avoids the problem of vomiting that is frequently encountered with oral administration. Experienced toxicologists are now tailoring the duration of NAC therapy, shorter or longer than 21 hours, based on clinical case criteria.

40. Does IV NAC have any particular risks?

The IV administration of NAC may cause a life-threatening anaphylactoid reaction, which most commonly occurs during the first, higher-dose infusion. Patients with asthma may be at the highest risk.

41. Off-label use of what antidote is now being investigated for the treatment of massive acetaminophen overdose?

Fomepizole, best known for inhibiting the enzyme alcohol dehydrogenase, inhibits the enzyme responsible for NAPQI (the byproduct of acetaminophen metabolism, which is toxic) formation and also supports hepatic mitochondria. Its potential role in the treatment of acetaminophen poisoning is currently being investigated.

42. Describe the treatment for acute salicylate poisoning.

Activated charcoal may be considered early after overdose. Achieve and maintain appropriate intravascular volume. Urinary alkalinization will enhance renal elimination and is appropriate for patients with symptoms and a peak serum salicylate concentration of more than 35 mg/dL (350 mg/L). Alkalemia, through ion-trapping, will reduce the passage of salicylate into the brain.

 Patients with unremitting metabolic acidosis, pulmonary edema, severe renal impairment, coma or seizures, liver impairment, and salicylate level greater than 70 mg/dL may meet criteria to warrant hemodialysis.

43. What hazard is associated with endotracheal intubation of salicylate-poisoned patients?

Salicylate-poisoned patients typically have profound respiratory alkalosis. This process is abruptly reversed by paralytic and sedative medications, and resulting acidemia may increase salicylate entry to the brain and cause seizures.

44. How does iron produce toxicity?

Iron acts as a gastrointestinal mucosal irritant and as an inhibitor of oxidative phosphorylation in the mitochondria. The body has no mode of excretion of excess iron.

45. What toxicity is expected from iron ingestion?

Expected toxicity can be estimated by the amount of elemental iron ingested (Table 39.2).

46. How much elemental iron is present in commonly available preparations?

- 65 mg (20% of tablet strength) is present in ferrous sulfate, 325 mg.
- 40 mg (12% of tablet strength) is present in ferrous gluconate, 325 mg.
- 105 mg (32% of tablet strength) is present in ferrous fumarate, 325 mg.
- 44 mg/5 mL is present in Feosol elixir (ferrous sulfate).
- 4 to 18 mg is present in children's chewable vitamins.
- 10 mg/mL is present in infant liquid vitamins.

Table 39.2 Expected Toxicity of Elemental Iron

DOSE INGESTED (MG/KG ELEMENTAL IRON)	TOXICITY
20-60	Mild gastrointestinal symptoms
60-100	Moderate toxicity
100-200	Serious toxicity
>200	Possibly lethal

47. **How has the epidemiology of childhood iron poisoning changed?**
From 1988 to 1998, iron poisoning was the leading cause of pediatric overdose death from pharmaceutical products, but this pattern abated with changes in iron formulations and packaging.

48. **What are the clinical manifestations of iron poisoning?**
Gastrointestinal irritation leads to vomiting, diarrhea, abdominal pain, melena, and hematemesis. Coma and shock are the hallmarks of severe mitochondrial poisoning. Multiorgan system failure may ensue. Patients recovering from severe iron poisoning may develop gastric scarring with pyloric obstruction 4 to 6 weeks later.

49. **What laboratory studies are helpful in the management of iron poisoning?**
An abdominal radiograph can confirm iron ingestion and give an impression of the amount of unabsorbed iron. However, a negative radiograph does not rule out iron ingestion, particularly more than 2 hours after ingestion, because dissolved or absorbed iron is *not* radiopaque. A serum iron level 4 to 6 hours after ingestion confirms and helps categorize iron poisoning:
   - Serum iron level less than 350 μg/dL is minimal toxicity.
   - Serum iron level 350 to 500 μg/dL is mild toxicity.
   - Serum iron level greater than 500 μg/dL is serious toxicity.
      The presence of metabolic acidosis may be the most telling indicator of cellular dysfunction from iron poisoning.

50. **What is the antidote for iron poisoning?**
Deferoxamine is an iron chelator that binds ferric iron (Fe^{3+}) in the blood. Typical dosing is 5 to 15 mg/kg/hour, up to 6 g/day intravenously. The use of deferoxamine has been associated with pulmonary fibrosis and acute respiratory distress syndrome in children given deferoxamine infusion for longer than 32 to 72 hours.

51. **List the major toxicities of cyclic antidepressants.**
   - Sodium channel blockade in the cardiac conduction system (dysrhythmia)
   - Seizures
   - α_1-Adrenergic blockade (hypotension)
   - Inhibition of norepinephrine reuptake
   - Anticholinergic toxicity

52. **What electrocardiographic findings correlate with potential toxicity from cyclic antidepressants?**
   - QRS complex longer than 0.1 second
   - Corrected QT interval prolonged for age
   - R wave height greater than 3 mm in lead aVR

53. **Why is sodium bicarbonate helpful for drug-induced ventricular dysrhythmias associated with a prolonged QRS interval?**
The QRS complex on an ECG correlates with ventricular repolarization through sodium channels. Many agents that cause ventricular tachycardia in overdose do so by blocking activated sodium channels, and then slow or prevent inactivation, which is essential to proper myocardial conduction. Sodium bicarbonate competitively inhibits this blockade by increasing available serum sodium. In addition, the modest serum alkalinization appears to promote, in a synergistic fashion, improved conduction that clinically appears as a narrowing of the QRS interval and cessation of ventricular tachycardia.

54. **What classes of drugs can typically induce bradydysrhythmias? What are some special considerations in terms of management for these types of dysrhythmias?**
Bradydysrhythmias commonly follow ingestion of beta blockers, calcium channel blockers, digitalis-containing compounds, and alpha-2-adrenergic agonists. These rhythm disturbances may not be amenable to standard therapy with atropine, epinephrine, and pacing.

55. How is high-dose insulin believed to ameliorate shock after calcium channel blocker poisoning?
High-dose insulin provides inotropic and vasodilatory support to cardiogenic shock:
- Improved myocardial cell calcium processing
- Improved cellular glucose transport
- Enhances endothelial nitric oxide

56. What are the manifestations of bupropion toxicity? How is this poisoning treated?
Pediatric bupropion poisoning has been increasing in recent years. Moderate toxicity can lead to tachycardia, agitation, and hallucination. Of note, bupropion ingestion was the leading cause (23%) of drug-induced seizures, which was most commonly seen after intentional overdoses in adolescents. Ventricular tachydysrhythmia and shock hallmark severe poisoning. Treatment is generally supportive, with benzodiazepines used for the neurologic symptoms.

57. What is flumazenil?
Flumazenil is a specific benzodiazepine-receptor antagonist that reverses benzodiazepine-induced central nervous system depression.

58. List problems that may be associated with flumazenil administration after a drug overdose.
- May precipitate benzodiazepine withdrawal
- May precipitate seizures and their complications
- Has a short duration of action compared with the duration of benzodiazepine toxicity

59. What are the most common medications responsible for pediatric drug-induced seizures? How are poison-induced seizures treated?
Antidepressants, particularly bupropion, are the most common medications causing drug-induced seizures in the United States. Benzodiazepines and barbiturates are the treatments of choice, regardless of the type of ingested drug. Seizures may recur and be difficult to treat. The cardiovascular effects of IV phenytoin may complicate cyclic antidepressant overdose. Pyridoxine is a specific antidote for seizures caused by isoniazid overdose. Drug-induced status epilepticus requires advanced modalities, such as pentobarbital coma or general anesthesia, more frequently than does status epilepticus complicating other types of seizure disorders.

KEY POINTS: PHARMACEUTICALS

1. Dangerous acetaminophen poisoning may be asymptomatic initially but can be predicted with serum levels.
2. Prevention of acidemia, maintenance of intravascular volume, and urinary alkalinization are key goals in the treatment of moderate aspirin poisoning.
3. Prevention strategies have reduced the pediatric mortality rate from ingestion of iron products.
4. Sodium bicarbonate therapy may be beneficial for toxic cardiac syndromes manifested by wide QRS tachycardia.

60. What signs and symptoms are expected after isolated benzodiazepine overdose in children?
The rate of pediatric benzodiazepine exposure has increased by over 50% between the years 2000 and 2015. Alone, benzodiazepines typically do not cause severe symptoms; they may lead to sedation, ataxia, and, in rare cases, respiratory depression. Ataxia without lethargy may occur in up to 30% of children after benzodiazepine ingestion. Apnea, deep coma, or cardiovascular instability suggests coingestion of another agent (e.g., ethanol, barbiturates, other sedative-hypnotics). In the adolescent age group, exposure is of particular concern; the severity of medical outcomes is increasing in recent years, intentional nonmedical use is becoming more common, and the rates of coingestion are high. Benzodiazepines have also been frequently implicated in child abuse by poisoning. Typically, the situation involves an elderly caretaker sedating a normally active toddler.

61. What is the mnemonic for the opioid toxidrome?
FAME: flaccid coma, **a**pnea, **m**iosis, and **e**xtraocular paralysis.

62. What substance is the leading cause of fatal poisonings in young children?
Opioids—In 2018, opioids accounted for more than 50% of fatal pediatrics poisonings (increasing from just 24% in 2005). In recent years, children are more often exposed to different forms of opioids, such as fentanyl, heroin, methadone, and buprenorphine. For example, fentanyl transdermal patches are an increasing concern for young children, as there have been more reports of accidental pediatric exposure to this type of patch. Many prescription opioids can cause life-threatening respiratory depression despite ingestion of only one pill or patch.

63. **Why do so many pediatric fentanyl poisonings get missed?**
Synthetic opioids, such as fentanyl, are not routinely tested on standard urinary drug screens. This is not because fentanyl does not have any metabolites; rather, its metabolites are not morphine or codeine. Further, the chemical structure of fentanyl is quite different from other opioids. Screening for fentanyl often requires specific urinary assays.

64. **How should a patient with fentanyl overdose be managed?**
Similar to other opioid poisonings! For respiratory depression, repeat naloxone as needed every few minutes until there is clinical improvement. However, is it important to note that a larger dose of naloxone may be needed with fentanyl overdoses, as it has a higher receptor affinity than morphine (fentanyl is about 100 times more potent than morphine!).

65. **What common pediatric drug toxicity closely mimics opioid intoxication but does not reliably respond to naloxone?**
The α_2-adrenergic agonist clonidine acts centrally to reduce sympathetic outflow, and its toxidrome may mimic opioid poisoning. Naloxone has been inconsistently reported to reverse coma and respiratory depression, and a trial of naloxone is reasonable in severely poisoned children presenting with marked CNS depression or apnea, with some experts suggesting high doses may be required. Tolazoline, a nonselective alpha-adrenergic antagonist, and yohimbine, an alpha-2-adrenergic antagonist, had previously been proposed as specific antagonists, however, they are available only in oral form and may cause clonidine withdrawal in patients receiving clonidine therapeutically. Therefore, their use in clonidine poisoning has been discouraged.

66. **Describe the typical findings after clonidine ingestion.**
As little as 0.1 mg (1 tablet) of clonidine has been associated with miosis, coma, apnea, bradycardia, and hypotension. Transient hypertension may also occur. More rare findings include modest hypothermia and pallor. These signs of toxicity are usually seen within 1 hour of ingestion, and new symptoms rarely arise more than four hours after exposure, except in the case of a clonidine patch.

67. **Are there any other distinguishing features between clonidine poisoning and opioid poisoning?**
Children with clonidine poisoning often have transient arousal and improvement in respiratory and hemodynamic instability with stimulation. Patients comatose from opioid poisoning are usually not arousable despite painful stimulation.

68. **Hallucinations or psychosis may be prominent with which psychoactive drugs?**
- Anticholinergics (antihistamines, Jimsonweed)
- Dissociatives (phencyclidine, ketamine, dextromethorphan)
- Hallucinogens (lysergic acid diethylamide, psilocybin, mescaline)
- Sympathomimetics (amphetamines, cocaine, 3,4-methylenedioxy-N-methylamphetamine [MDMA–ecstasy], synthetic cathinone [bath salts], synthetic cannabinoids [Spice, K2])
- High-dose THC use
- Withdrawal from ethanol or sedative-hypnotics

69. **What are the best agents for sedating patients with drug-induced agitation?**
Benzodiazepines are preferred. In addition to providing sedation, they also have anticonvulsant properties. Intramuscular or IV midazolam (0.05 to 0.1 mg/kg, maximum initial dose 5 mg) or IV lorazepam (0.1 mg/kg, maximum initial dose 2 to 4 mg, depending upon the degree of agitation) is often used. If intramuscular sedation is required, midazolam may be preferred because of its more rapid onset of action when compared to intramuscular lorazepam. Repeated doses may be given every few minutes until adequate sedation is achieved. In some patients with severe agitation caused by sympathomimetics or hallucinogens, the total dose necessary to achieve adequate sedation may be quite high.

70. **Why should neuroleptics, such as haloperidol, be used cautiously in the treatment of drug-induced psychoses?**
These agents may lower the seizure threshold of the overdose patient, may add to the cardiovascular toxicity of some drugs, and may limit the patient's ability to dissipate heat.

71. **What adverse effects are associated with cocaine intoxication?**
Cocaine abusers seek a pleasurable "rush" of euphoria and increased energy. However, intoxicating doses may produce agitation, tachycardia, hypertension, hyperthermia, mydriasis, and tremor. Altered judgment may lead to an increased incidence of accidents and interpersonal violence, and abusers may neglect societal obligations while engaging in high-risk behaviors. Seizures, intracranial hemorrhage, myocardial ischemia, rhabdomyolysis, pneumothorax, psychosis, and death may occur from cocaine abuse.

72. What is the treatment for the tachycardia, hypertension, and hyperpyrexia associated with cocaine overdose?

High doses of benzodiazepines are the most effective and safest pharmacotherapy for cocaine intoxication. Extreme hyperthermia may also warrant aggressive environmental cooling methods. Treat rhabdomyolysis with mechanical ventilation, paralysis, and bicarbonate infusion to reduce the chance of renal failure. Reserve sympatholytics for the most extreme cases. β-Adrenergic antagonist therapy may lead to detrimental unopposed α-adrenergic toxicity, leading to worsening coronary artery vasoconstriction and systemic hypertension; therefore, beta blockers are not routinely recommended in the acute setting. Persistent hypertensive crisis may respond well to nitroprusside infusion or phentolamine.

73. Name seven hyperthermic syndromes in toxicology.

1. Sympathomimetic poisoning
2. Anticholinergic poisoning
3. Neuroleptic malignant syndrome
4. Malignant hyperthermia
5. Serotonin syndrome
6. Uncoupling of oxidative phosphorylation (e.g., salicylate poisoning)
7. Acute withdrawal syndrome

74. Describe the serotonin syndrome.

The serotonin syndrome, or serotonin toxicity, is characterized by autonomic hyperactivity, increased neuromuscular tone (especially prominent in the lower extremities), hyperreflexia, and central nervous system depression after exposure to a drug or drugs with proserotonergic properties. In comparison to adult cases, pediatric patients exhibited a higher frequency of altered mental status, typically manifesting as agitation, poor cooperation, or confusion. The majority of these symptoms present within 24 hours of exposure. The diagnosis is clinical, and primarily based on a history of ingestion of a serotonergic drug.

75. Name some of the methods by which inhalants are used for inebriation.

- *Sniffing* describes direct inhalation of vapors from an open container.
- *Huffing* implies inhaling from a cloth soaked with the volatile substance.
- *Bagging* involves holding a volatile-containing bag over the nose.

76. Describe the most widely proposed mechanism for "sudden sniffing death."

Inhaled hydrocarbons are believed to potentiate the cardiovascular effects of catecholamines. Ventricular dysrhythmia may occur, especially if an inhalant abuser becomes surprised (perhaps by parents or police) or agitated. Another proposed mechanism is severe metabolic acidosis with lactate accumulation.

77. What are the most common presentations of electronic cigarette exposure?

In recent years, there has been a marked increase in pediatric exposure to electronic cigarettes (or "e-cigarettes"). Accidental exposure to electronic cigarettes, and subsequently liquid nicotine and the other fluids that go into the e-cigarette, may cause more severe effects compared to conventional cigarette exposure, particularly in patients younger than 6 years old. In the acute setting, the most common symptom is vomiting. Other clinical effects include nausea, coughing/choking, drowsiness, tachycardia, and agitation. Chronic exposure to some sources of e-cigarettes has been associated with the illness "EVALI," or e-cigarette or vaping-associated lung injury, a potentially life-threatening respiratory illness. Of note, liquid nicotine has a variable pH and may cause ocular irritation as well.

78. What are some of the symptoms noted after a child ingests an edible with tetrahydrocannabinol (THC)?

There has been an increase in the accessibility of THC edibles that appear similar to common children's snacks and desserts. US Poison Control centers have subsequently experienced an increase in reported cases of children ingesting large amounts of highly concentrated edible THC. Poisoning symptoms from THC edibles may be delayed and prolonged. Children <6 years old who have ingested THC may present with decreased mentation, extreme lethargy, ataxia, seizures, encephalopathy, coma, and respiratory depression.

Adolescents may have psychosis, ataxia, tremor, nystagmus, tachycardia, behavior changes, mydriasis, excessive motor activity, appetite changes, hypertension, and conjunctival injection.

79. What is the management of patients who ingest edibles with THC?

For young children <6 years old, supportive care, oxygen therapy, intubation, and critical care monitoring may be necessary, depending on the level of central nervous system (CNS) depression. For adolescents, primary management includes supportive care, decreasing environmental stimuli, and sometimes the treatment of agitation with benzodiazepines.

80. **What is cannabinoid hyperemesis syndrome (CHS)?**
    CHS has been increasingly diagnosed since it was first described in 2004. CHS is characterized by episodic vomiting associated with prolonged high-dose recreational cannabis use that resolves with cannabis cessation. Some authors describe CHS as a subset of cyclic vomiting syndrome and as a diagnosis of exclusion. Many reports on CHS discuss the role of hot showers being a key feature, which is thought to assist in stabilizing the hypothalamic thermostat and/or cutaneous steal syndrome. Hot showers are not sensitive or specific to CHS though it is often reported. One aspect of CHS that makes it difficult to research and evaluate is the different "formulations" of cannabis/marijuana.

81. **What medications can be used for treatment of CHS?**
    Haloperidol and topical capsaicin cream have been reported as effective treatments for CHS. Topical capsaicin 0.025% to 0.1%, which can be applied as a topical cream two to four times per day, or as a patch on the skin of the abdomen, may reduce the time in the ED and lead to fewer return visits to the ED. Parenteral haloperidol IM, IV 0.05 to 0.1 mg, max dose of 5 mg can be used for the treatment of CHS in cases that are refractory to other treatments. Monitor patients who receive haloperidol for side effects of extrapyramidal reactions including prolonged QTc.
    Conventional antiemetics such as ondansetron, metoclopramide, and promethazine are frequently ineffective when used alone to manage vomiting associated with CHS. IV benzodiazepines such as lorazepam have better efficacy in the control of pain and vomiting associated with CHS. IV lorazepam can be given every 4 to 6 hours in the ED and at discharge can be prescribed orally every 6 to 8 hours.

82. **What is Spice or K2?**
    These are just two of the names used by dealers selling synthetic cannabinoids. These substances contain analogs of naturally occurring cannabinoids, including THC, cannabidiol, and cannabinol. Unlike naturally occurring cannabinoids, synthetic cannabinoids often are not detected by urine tests for drugs of abuse.

83. **How does the toxicity of synthetic cannabinoids differ from that of marijuana?**
    Reports have described greater neurologic toxicity, including aggressive behavior, paranoia, dystonia, prolonged psychosis, and seizures. Synthetic cannabinoid use has also been associated with acute kidney injury and myocardial infarction. Chronic use can lead to more severe psychiatric and medical conditions, including death.

84. **What are "bath salts"? How does bath salt intoxication present?**
    Bath salts are synthetic cathinones that are related to the naturally occurring substance khat. Bath salt intoxication has many features of amphetamine overdose but is especially notable for causing prolonged agitation, aggressive and violent behavior, hallucinations, paranoia, and seizures. In severe cases, death may result from cerebral edema, myocarditis, or necrotizing fasciitis.

85. **Why have "bath salts" and "plant food" become popular drugs of abuse?**
    Bath salts and plant food are drugs of abuse—the names are just clever marketing. The Federal Analog Act that restricts drug sale, possession, and use has a loophole that a chemical has to be "for human consumption." By calling new synthetic drugs of abuse by names such as "bath salts," the drug dealers try to limit their legal liability.

KEY POINTS: "STREET DRUGS"

1. Naloxone dosing in patients who overdosed on heroin requires careful consideration of habituation to avoid precipitation of withdrawal.
2. Benzodiazepines are the most appropriate initial treatment for agitation caused by sympathomimetic and hallucinogenic drugs of abuse.
3. Malignant hyperthermia from overdoses of cocaine, amphetamines, or serotonergic drugs requires rapid treatment, including cooling measures, benzodiazepine administration, and mechanical ventilation with paralysis and bicarbonate infusion in the setting of rhabdomyolysis.
4. A wide variety of "novel psychoactive substance" drugs are created and marketed each year.

86. **What is the differential diagnosis for an increased anion gap metabolic acidosis?**
    One can make mountains out of the mnemonic MUDPILES:
    - **M:** Methanol, metformin
    - **U:** Uremia
    - **D:** Diabetic, alcoholic, or starvation ketoacidosis
    - **P:** Paraldehyde (and other aldehydes)

- **I:** Iron, isoniazid, inborn errors of metabolism
- **L:** Lactic acidosis
- **E:** Ethylene glycol
- **S:** Salicylates
    Others prefer the more physiologically based mnemonic KULTS (https://toxandhound.com/toxhound/kults-of-toxicology/): Ketonemia, Uremia, Lactatemia, Toxic alcohols, Salicylate.

87. **What is the differential diagnosis for hyperlactatemia with metabolic acidosis?**
    Lactic acidosis may be caused by sepsis, shock, seizures, anoxia, ischemia, or trauma. Toxic causes include poisoning from carbon monoxide (CO), cyanide, sodium azide, hydrogen sulfide, ibuprofen, adrenergic agents, isoniazid, and others.

88. **How is the osmolar gap calculated?**

$$\text{Osmolar gap} = \text{measured osmolality} - \text{calculated osmolarity}$$

$$\text{Calculated osmolarity} = 2([\text{sodium}]\,\text{mEq/L}) + ([\text{blood urea nitrogen}]\,\text{mg/dL})/2.8 \\ + ([\text{glucose}]\,\text{mg/dL})/18$$

89. **What is a "normal" osmolar gap?**
    Normal range is 7 to 10 mOsm.

90. **List the potential causes of a large osmolar gap.**
    - Acetone
    - Ethanol
    - Glycols
    - Isopropanol
    - Magnesium
    - Mannitol
    - Methanol
    - Renal failure
    - Severe ketoacidemia
    - Severe lactic acidemia

91. **How do toxic alcohols produce an increased osmolar gap?**
    Once absorbed into the bloodstream, alcohols are osmotically active. This principle explains why people have to urinate so frequently at Happy Hour. It is also the principle behind administering mannitol to head-injured patients.

92. **How can the osmolar gap be used to estimate the levels of toxic alcohols?**
    This calculation is based on the molecular weight of the alcohols:
    - **Methanol:** molecular weight = 32 mg/mmol; conversion factor = 3.2
    - **Ethanol:** molecular weight = 46 mg/mmol; conversion factor = 4.6
    - **Ethylene glycol:** molecular weight = 62 mg/mmol; conversion factor = 6.2
    - Alcohol level (mg/dL) = (osmolar gap) × (conversion factor)

93. **How does ethanol intoxication lead to life-threatening hypoglycemia in young children?**
    Ethanol is metabolized by the enzymes alcohol dehydrogenase and acetaldehyde dehydrogenase. This process involves the production of NADH (the reduced form of nicotinamide adenine dinucleotide [NAD]). An increased ratio of NADH to NAD inhibits gluconeogenesis and may lead to hypoglycemia in patients with insufficient stores of glycogen. Because of the depletion of glycogen, ethanol-induced hypoglycemia does not respond to glucagon administration. Hypoglycemia and hypoglycemic seizures are generally associated with poor nutritional status in adults, however, it is seen in adequately nourished pediatric patients.

94. **How quickly does an inebriated 14-year-old metabolize an ethanol level of 150 mg/dL to zero?**
    Ethanol is metabolized at a constant rate according to zero-order kinetics. The typical decrease is 15 mg/dL/hour in the noninduced (nonalcoholic) patient. Therefore, the level should be zero in 10 hours.

95. **How do some toxic alcohols lead to metabolic acidosis?**
    Early after methanol or ethylene glycol ingestion, there will be increased serum osmolality but little acidosis. The body subsequently metabolizes methanol to formic acid, and ethylene glycol to glycolic and oxalic acids.

The osmolar gap may drop, while the anion gap increases. Isopropyl alcohol is somewhat distinctive, as it is metabolized to acetone and typically does not lead to profound acidosis.

96. True or false: Ethylene glycol in the urine fluoresces when examined with a Wood lamp.
Generally false, but not entirely. The most common source of ethylene glycol exposure is automobile antifreeze. Some manufacturers put fluorescein in the antifreeze solution to allow detection of radiator leaks. Lack of fluorescent urine does not rule out ethylene glycol poisoning.

97. What is the physiologic basis for the treatment of methanol or ethylene glycol poisoning?
Formic acid is toxic to the retina, and glycolic and oxalic acids are toxic to the kidneys. The treatment goal is to prevent the metabolism of these toxic metabolites. Alcohol dehydrogenase is the enzyme responsible for this biotransformation, and inhibition of this enzyme will be protective.

98. What agents can be used to inhibit alcohol dehydrogenase in the setting of methanol or ethylene glycol poisoning?
- Fomepizole
- Ethanol

99. Do any vitamins or nutritional supplements have a role in the treatment of methanol or ethylene glycol poisoning?
Folic acid may promote the metabolic degradation of formic acid. Pyridoxine and thiamine may speed the transformation of glycolic acids to nontoxic metabolites.

100. When should an ingested disc or button battery be emergently removed?
Disc batteries (button batteries) may contain potentially toxic components, such as mercury or lithium, but are most dangerous as mucosal corrosives, leading to catastrophic hemorrhage. They are the most dangerous foreign body ingestion in pediatrics. Remove disc batteries lodged in the nares, ear canal, or esophagus immediately, within 2 to 4 hours if possible. Once in the stomach, they will almost always pass uneventfully. Of note, even after the removal of the battery, there is still a risk of aortoesophageal fistula formation and subsequent complications; consider ongoing evaluation for injury in these patients.

101. List some of the dangerous caustic agents frequently found in U.S. households.
Many cleaning products cause only mild irritation. Important exceptions include dishwashing detergent and laundry gel packets, which have caused serious caustic injuries. Hair-relaxing products typically have basic pH. Oven cleaners, toilet bowl cleaners, and drain products often contain hydrochloric acid or sodium hydroxide.

102. What characteristics of a caustic agent are most predictive of injury?
- pH
- Concentration
- Volume ingested
- Viscosity of product
- Manner of exposure
- Duration of exposure
  Therefore, thick hair-relaxer creams licked by an explorative child rarely lead to severe esophageal injury, but suicidal ingestions of liquid acids can be expected to lead to significant morbidity.

103. What are the complications of ingestion of caustic agents?
Acute complications:
- Upper airway obstruction
- Aspiration pneumonitis
- Gastrointestinal bleeding or perforation
- Systemic acidosis or disseminated intravascular coagulation
- Sepsis
Chronic complications:
- Esophageal stricture
- Impaired gastric function/pyloric obstruction
- Esophageal carcinoma (1000-fold increased risk for esophageal carcinoma; mean latency period is over 40 years.)

104. Which patients should be examined endoscopically, or by cross-sectional imaging, after caustic ingestion?
- Ingestion involving a concentrated, strong acid or base

- Suicidal ingestions
- Large-volume ingestions
- Patients with vomiting or two or more signs or symptoms of injury
    Note: The absence of oral burns is not a sensitive sign for excluding esophageal injury.

105. Give the advantages and disadvantages of using corticosteroids to palliate caustic esophageal burns.
Advantages:
- Anti-inflammatory
- May decrease tissue scarring and stricture
Disadvantages:
- May increase perforation risk
- May increase infection risk
- May mask signs of infection or perforation

106. When should steroids be used to palliate caustic esophageal burns?
Esophageal burns should be graded at endoscopy. First-degree burns do not lead to stricture formation, so steroids are not warranted. Third-degree burns will probably lead to stricture regardless of treatment, and the benefit is not likely worth the risk. Controversy surrounds the value of using steroids together with antibiotics to treat circumferential second-degree burns of the esophagus. Note that a less controversial indication for steroid therapy is the palliation of glottic edema and airway obstruction.

107. What are the indications for surgical exploration after caustic ingestion?
- Evidence of perforation
- Abdominal tenderness after acid ingestion
- Inability to evaluate injuries endoscopically
- Significant central nervous system depression
- Progressive metabolic acidosis
- Hypotension with tachycardia

108. Which characteristics of certain hydrocarbon products make them prone to aspiration?
- Low viscosity
- Low surface tension
- High volatility

109. Describe the time course of aspiration injury after hydrocarbon ingestion
Children may cough, gag, or sputter at the time of ingestion. A gradual evolution of radiographic findings occurs, but most children who develop pneumonitis have visible abnormality by 6 hours. More than 98% of children who develop clinical pneumonitis do so by 24 hours.

110. Do any hydrocarbons have serious systemic toxicity?
Central nervous system depression, seizures, hepatotoxicity, nephrotoxicity, and bone marrow toxicity are among the injuries that can occur after specific hydrocarbon ingestions. The hydrocarbons most noted for systemic toxicity can be remembered with this CHAMPion of mnemonics:
- **C:** Camphor
- **H:** Halogenated hydrocarbons (e.g., carbon tetrachloride, trichloroethane)
- **A:** Aromatic hydrocarbons (e.g., benzene, toluene)
- **M:** Metal-containing hydrocarbons
- **P:** Pesticide-containing hydrocarbons

111. List the clinical manifestations of organophosphate or carbamate insecticide poisoning.
These insecticides are examples of "cholinergic" poisoning.
1. **Muscarinic effects** (pre- and postganglionic parasympathomimetic)
    - **SLUDGE: s**alivation, **l**acrimation, **u**rination, **d**efecation, **g**astric cramping, **e**mesis
    - Bronchorrhea, bronchoconstriction
    - Bradycardia
    - Miotic pupils
2. **Nicotinic effect** (preganglionic sympathomimetic)
    - Tachycardia (often prominent early after exposure in children)
3. **Nicotinic effects** (neuromuscular end plate)
    - Muscle fasciculations
    - Muscle weakness

4. **Central nervous system effects**
   - Depressed consciousness
   - Seizures

112. **What antidotes are used to treat organophosphate poisoning?**
Atropine may be needed in large doses to reverse muscarinic toxicity. Pralidoxime regenerates active acetylcholinesterase, the enzymatic site of action of organophosphate insecticides. Diazepam can also be used to decrease neurocognitive dysfunction or to prevent convulsions.

113. **What is the appropriate response to an exploratory anticoagulant rodenticide ingestion by a toddler?**
Single exploratory ingestions by curious children have not been reported to produce dangerous bleeding diatheses. Some poison centers recommend decontamination with activated charcoal at the time of the event and evaluation of a prothrombin time 2 to 3 days afterward. Other poison centers recommend no treatment other than expectant observation at home. Note that suicidal ingestions of anticoagulant rodenticides have led to catastrophic consequences.

114. **How should coagulopathy from warfarin-like rodenticides be treated?**
These rodenticides inhibit hepatic production of the vitamin K–dependent coagulation factors II, VII, IX, and X. Acute bleeding can be palliated with transfusion of fresh frozen plasma. Administration of vitamin K_1 will restore the production of clotting factors with a lag time of approximately 6 hours. Prophylactic use of vitamin K_1 often complicates evaluation of the anticoagulant-poisoned patient. As the "superwarfarins" have a very long duration of effect, any patient treated with vitamin K_1 warrants monitoring for at least 5 days after the last dose.

115. **Describe the typical symptoms of CO poisoning.**
Typical symptoms are nonspecific and include malaise, nausea, lightheadedness, and headache, leading many children to be misdiagnosed with a viral illness. More severe poisoning may manifest as confusion, coma, syncope, seizure, or death. Survivors of acute intoxication are at risk of delayed neurologic sequelae, including cognitive deficits, personality changes, and movement disorders.

116. **Which member of the family is most likely to suffer the most from equivalent CO exposure?**
Infants and small children have higher oxygen consumption and a higher basal metabolic rate than adults. Therefore, they may be most susceptible to the effects of CO. This effect is the basic concept behind the "canary in a coal mine."

117. **Describe the pathophysiology of toxicity from CO exposure.**
   - CO displaces oxygen from the hemoglobin molecule, leading to decreased oxygen-carrying capacity. CO has an affinity for hemoglobin approximately 250 times that for O_2.
   - Allosteric inhibition of oxygen release to tissues occurs (displacement of the oxyhemoglobin dissociation curve to the left).
   - Cellular oxidative metabolism is reduced through inhibition of cytochrome oxidase enzyme systems.
   - Oxidative injury to the brain endothelium begins a cascade of leukocyte activation, lipid peroxidation, and impaired cerebral metabolism.

118. **How long does it take the body to eliminate carboxyhemoglobin?**
Carboxyhemoglobin elimination depends on inspired oxygen concentration.
   - **Room air:** 4 to 6 hours
   - **100% O_2:** 40 to 90 minutes
   - **Hyperbaric O_2 (3 atm):** 15 to 30 minutes

119. **When is hyperbaric oxygen therapy indicated for CO intoxication?**
Administer oxygen in the highest concentration to all symptomatic patients until CO levels are below 5% and symptoms subside. Hyperbaric oxygen therapy may prevent oxidative cerebral vasculitis and may prevent delayed neurologic injury. Proposed criteria for considering hyperbaric oxygen include syncope, confusion, central nervous system depression, and very high carboxyhemoglobin levels.

120. **Cyanosis that is unresponsive to supplemental oxygen therapy in the face of normal partial pressure of oxygen in arterial blood is characteristic of what physiologic abnormality?**
Poor response to oxygen therapy makes a pulmonary disorder unlikely. Normal partial pressure of oxygen rules out intracardiac shunting. This finding is the characteristic clinical scenario of abnormal hemoglobin, most commonly methemoglobinemia.

121. **What is methemoglobin?**
Hemoglobin is a heme (iron-containing) protein. Methemoglobin exists when the iron moiety is ferric (3^+) rather than ferrous (2^+). Methemoglobin is incapable of transporting oxygen.

122. **Describe the transient, illness-associated methemoglobinemia of infancy.**
Young infants have been found to be cyanotic with methemoglobinemia in conjunction with a number of illnesses, including diarrheal dehydration, metabolic acidosis, urinary tract infection, and others. Babies are uniquely susceptible to oxidant stress. Consider this condition in the evaluation of septic-appearing infants.

123. **What are some of the more common toxicants associated with the production of excessive methemoglobin?**
Many chemicals and pharmaceuticals can produce methemoglobinemia in susceptible people. Among the most commonly noted exposures are benzocaine, dapsone, some antimalarial agents, environmental (i.e., well water) nitrates, nitrites (i.e., amyl nitrite), phenazopyridine, and aniline dyes.

124. **What is the appropriate therapy for methemoglobinemia?**
Provide supplemental oxygen. Eliminate or treat the oxidative stress responsible for methemoglobin formation. Antidotal therapy with methylene blue (1-2 mg/kg of a 1% solution) is indicated in the presence of tissue hypoxia. Methylene blue is less likely to be effective and may worsen illness when administered to patients with severe forms of glucose-6-phosphate dehydrogenase deficiency. It may also precipitate serotonin syndrome in patients taking serotonergic medications.

125. **What historical feature often serves to differentiate "dangerous" toxic mushrooms from those that are only gastrointestinal irritants?**
The time course of vomiting. Delayed onset of vomiting (>5 hours) is an ominous symptom. See Table 39.3 for mushroom types and their toxicities.

126. **What are the most common toxic plant poisonings?**
Of the 20 most common plant exposures, the following toxic plants are most commonly encountered:
* The Arum family (*Dieffenbachia, Philodendron*), which may cause severe pharyngeal edema and possible airway obstruction through the elaboration of calcium oxalate crystals and proteolytic enzymes and direct mucosal irritation
* The *Taxus* species (yew), which cause gastrointestinal irritation, cardiac dysrhythmias, coma, and seizures if large amounts of leaves or seeds are ingested
* The *Solanum* family (Jerusalem cherry, black nightshade, climbing nightshade), which cause gastrointestinal effects, lethargy, or delirium

Table 39.3 Description of Toxic Mushroom Syndromes

MUSHROOM CLASS	TARGET TOXICITY
Severe Toxicity; Vomiting Typically Begins >5 Hours After Ingestion	
Gyromitra	Inhibits pyridoxine phosphokinase
Orellanine (*Cortinarius* spp.)	Nephrotoxic
Amanita + Galerina + Lepiota	Hepatotoxic (amatoxins inhibit RNA polymerase II)
Severe Toxicity; Vomiting Typically Begins <5 Hours After Ingestion	
Amanita smithiana	Nephrotoxic
Mild Toxicity; Vomiting or Symptoms Typically Begin <5 Hours After Ingestion	
Psilocybe	"Magic mushrooms" (serotonin)
Ibotenic acid (*Amanita muscaria*)	Ibotenic acid is glutamatergic; muscimol is GABA-like
Coprine ("inky cap")	Disulfiram-like
Emetogenic mushrooms (many types)	Gastric irritants
Muscarinic (*Clitocybe + Inocybe* spp.)	Cholinergic
Myotoxic (*Tricholoma* spp.)	Rhabdomyolysis

GABA, γ-aminobutyric acid.

- *Rhododendron* and *Azalea* spp., which cause gastrointestinal effects, bradycardia, lethargy, and paresthesias through elaboration of grayanotoxins

127. What other plants have potential for severe toxicity? Describe the treatment.
Categories of toxic plants and their potential treatments are listed in Table 39.4.

128. What venomous snakes are indigenous to the United States?
The Crotalinae family includes rattlesnakes, copperheads, and water moccasins. The Elapidae family includes coral snakes.

129. What are the clinical differences between bites from rattlesnakes and bites from coral snakes?
Rattlesnakes, copperheads, and water moccasins are long-fanged "pit vipers" whose bites produce significant local inflammation and may lead to shock, thrombocytopenia, and coagulopathy. The venom of coral snakes is less irritating locally and more typically produces neuromuscular paralysis. Of note, envenomation from the Mojave rattlesnake may more closely mimic that of coral snakes.

Table 39.4 Categories of Toxic Plants

SYMPTOM CLASS	PLANTS	POTENTIAL TREATMENT
Gastrointestinal irritants	Pokeweed Horse chestnut English ivy	Supportive care
Toxalbumin	Castor bean Rosary pea Autumn crocus (colchicine-containing)	Supportive care for multisystem organ failure
Digitalis-like toxin	Foxglove Oleander Lily of the valley	Digoxin Fab fragments
Other cardiac effects	Mistletoe Monkshood False hellebore Mountain laurel	Supportive care, standard treatment for dysrhythmias
Nicotinic effects	Wild tobacco Tobacco Poison hemlock	Atropine, supportive care for weakness, paralysis
Anticholinergic effects	Jimsonweed Angel's trumpet Matrimony vine Henbane Belladonna	Physostigmine for seizures, malignant hyperthermia Benzodiazepines for delirium
Seizures	Water hemlock	Anticonvulsants
Hallucinations	Morning glory Nutmeg Peyote	Sedation
Cyanogenic	Chokecherry Cherry (pit) Plum (pit) Peach (pit) Apple (seeds) Pear (seeds) Cassava Elderberry (leaves and shoots) Black locust	Cyanide antidote (rarely needed)

130. **When should a bystander use his or her mouth to suck the venom out of a snakebite site?**
Never! This practice is more likely to infect the wound than it is to reduce toxicity. The Sawyer extractor, a commercial suction device, is also of little value.

131. **What are the most important principles of first aid for a North American snakebite victim?**
Remove the victim from the snake and, if possible, wash the wound with soap and water. Keep the victim calm, as a hyperdynamic state may accelerate dissemination of the venom. Activate emergency medical systems to transport the victim to a hospital as soon as possible. Remove any potentially constricting apparel. Immobilize a bitten extremity well above the level of the heart. Tourniquets are more likely to increase injury to an extremity and are not routinely advised. Ice is not advised.

132. **What are the indications for the administration of antivenom to a patient following crotaline envenomation?**
Administer antivenom to most patients with progressive local injury, or those with systemic signs such as cardiovascular compromise, or coagulopathy.

133. **What antivenom products are available for treatment of North American pit viper envenomation?**
- Crotalidae polyvalent immune Fab (ovine).
- Crotalidae immune F(ab')2 (equine).

134. **Compare the toxic manifestations of bites from black widow spiders (*Latrodectus*) to those of brown recluse spiders (*Loxosceles*).**
The venom of black widow spiders leads to increased stimulation of the motor end plate. Restlessness, tachycardia, hypertension, muscular fasciculations, and muscle cramping are common signs and symptoms. In severe cases, black widow bites can mimic a surgical abdomen. In contrast, brown recluse spider venom is predominantly digestive in nature. Local inflammation may progress to tissue necrosis at the bite site. Systemic toxicity is possible but uncommon.

KEY POINTS: ENVIRONMENTAL POISONS AND VENOMS

1. Fomepizole is an antidote that inhibits alcohol dehydrogenase to provide protection against methanol and ethylene glycol poisoning.
2. After CO poisoning, hyperbaric oxygen is most beneficial in its ability to halt an inflammatory cascade in the brain.
3. The low surface tension and viscosity of hydrocarbons create a great risk for pulmonary injury after ingestion.

BIBLIOGRAPHY

1. Akakpo JY, Ramachandran A, Curry SC, et al. Comparing n-acetylcysteine and 4-methylpyrazole as antidotes for acetaminophen overdose. *Arch Toxicol.* 2022:453–465.
2. Allen JD, Casavant MJ, Spiller HA, Chounthirath T, et al. Prescription opioid exposures among children and adolescents in the United States: 2000-2015. *Pediatrics.* 2017;139(4):e20163382.
3. Vale JA, Krenzelok EP, Barceloux GD. Position statement and practice guidelines on the use of multi-dose activated charcoal in the treatment of acute poisoning. American Academy of Clinical Toxicology; European Association of Poisons Centres and Clinical Toxicologists. *Clin Toxicol.* 1999;37:731–751.
4. Brown KI, Crouch BI. Bupropion overdose: significant toxicity in pediatrics. *Clin Pediatr Emerg Med.* 2017;18(3):212–217. ISSN 1522-8401 https://doi.org/10.1016/j.cpem.2017.07.005.
5. Bruccoleri RE, Burns MM. A literature review of the use of sodium bicarbonate for the treatment of QRS widening. *J Med Toxicol.* 2016;12(1):121–129. https://doi.org/10.1007/s13181-015-0483-y.
6. Casavant MJ, Shah MN, Battels R. Does fluorescent urine indicate antifreeze ingestion by children? *Pediatrics.* 2001;107:113–114.
7. Cohen J, Morrison S, Greenberg J, Saidinejad M. Clinical presentation of intoxication due to synthetic cannabinoids. *Pediatrics.* 2012;129:e1064.
8. Cohen K, Weinstein AM. Synthetic and non-synthetic cannabinoid drugs and their adverse effects: a review from public health prospective. *Front Public Health.* 2018;6:162. https://doi.org/10.3389/fpubh.2018.00162.
9. Cole JB, Arens AM. Cardiotoxic medication poisoning. *Crit Care Clin NA.* 2022;40:395–416. https://doi.org/10.1016/j.emc.2022.01.014.
10. Finkelstein Y, Hutson JR, Freedman SB, Wax P, et al. Toxicology Investigators Consortium (ToxIC) Case Registry. Drug-induced seizures in children and adolescents presenting for emergency care: current and emerging trends. *Clin Toxicol.* 2013;51(8):761–766.
11. Fraser L, Wynne D, Clement WA, et al. Liquid detergent capsule ingestion in children: an increasing trend. *Arch Dis Child.* 2012;97:1007.
12. Friedrich JM, Christie S, Xue G, Diane P, et al. Child and adolescent benzodiazepine exposure and overdose in the United States: 16 years of poison center data. *Clin Toxicol.* 2020;58(7):725–731. https://doi.org/10.1080/15563650.2019.1674321.

13. Gaw CE, Osterhoudt KC. Legalization of marijuana in New Jersey: implications for pediatric injury prevention. *NJ Pediatr.* 2022:25–29. Summer.
14. Gaw CE, Osterhoudt KC. Ethanol intoxication of young children. *Pediatr Emerg Care.* 2019;35:722–732.
15. Gaw CE, et al. Characteristics of fatal poisonings among infants and young children in the United States. *Pediatrics.* 2023e2022059016.
16. Greene SL, Kerr F, Braitberg G. Review article: amphetamines and related drugs of abuse. *Emerg Med Austral.* 2008;20:391–402.
17. Gummin DD, Mowry JB, Beuhler MC, Spyker DA, et al. 2020 Annual report of the American Association of Poison Control Centers' National Poison Data System (NPDS): 38th annual report. *Clin Toxicol.* 2021;59(12):1282–1501. https://doi.org/10.1080/15563650.2 021.1989785. PMID: 34890263.
18. Henretig FM. Special considerations in the poisoned pediatric patient. *Emerg Med Clin North Am.* 1994;12:549–567.
19. Hoffman RS, Burns MM, Gosselin S. Ingestion of caustic substances. *N Engl J Med.* 2020;382(18):1739–1748. https://doi.org/10.1056/NEJMra1810769. PMID: 32348645.
20. Jolliff HA, Fletcher E, Roberts KJ, et al. Pediatric hydrocarbon-related injuries in the United States: 2000-2009. *Pediatrics.* 2013;131:1139.
21. Kichloo A, Albosta M, Aljadah M, El-Amir Z, et al. Marijuana: a systems-based primer of adverse effects associated with use and an overview of its therapeutic utility. *SAGE Open Med.* 2021;920503121211000909.
22. Klembczyck K, et al. Diagnosis and treatment of cannabinoid hyperemesis syndrome. *Contemp Pediatr.* 2022;39(3).
23. Leinwand K, Brumbaugh DE, Kramer RE. Button battery ingestion in children: a paradigm for management of severe pediatric foreign body ingestions. *Gastrointest Endosc Clin N Am.* 2016;26(1):99–118. https://doi.org/10.1016/j.giec.2015.08.003.
24. Levine M, Hoffman RS, Lavergne V, Stork CM, et al. Lipid Emulsion Workgroup. Systematic review of the effect of intravenous lipid emulsion therapy for non-local anesthetics toxicity. *Clin Toxicol.* 2016;54(3):194–221. https://doi.org/10.3109/15563650.2015.1126 286. Epub 2016 Feb 6. Erratum in: *Clin Toxicol (Phila).* 2016;54(3):297. PMID: 26852931.
25. Liebelt E, Ulrich A, Francis PD, Woolf A. Serial electrocardiogram changes in acute tricyclic antidepressant overdoses. *Crit Care Med.* 1997;25:1721–1726.
26. Martin JD, Osterhoudt KC, Thom SR. Recognition and management of carbon monoxide intoxication in children. *Clin Pediatr Emerg Med.* 2000;1:244–250.
27. Noble Matthew J. The new dangers of electronic cigarettes. *Clin Pediatr Emerg Med.* 2017;18(3):163–172. ISSN 1522-8401https://doi.org/10.1016/j.cpem.2017.07.004.
28. Mir A, Obafemi A, Young A, Kane C. Myocardial infarction associated with use of the synthetic cannabinoid K2. *Pediatrics.* 2011;128:e1622.
29. Osterhoudt KC. The toxic toddler: drugs that can kill in small doses. *Contemp Pediatr.* 2000;17(3):73–88.
30. Osterhoudt KC. No sympathy for a boy with obtundation. *Pediatr Emerg Care.* 2004;20:403–406.
31. Osterhoudt KC. Clonidine *and related imidazoline poisoning.* UpToDate; 2022 Accessed 12.07.22. https://www.uptodate.com/contents/clonidine-and-related-imidazoline-poisoning/print
32. Osterhoudt KC, Burns Ewald M, Shannon M, Henretig FM. Toxicologic emergencies. In: Fleisher GR, Ludwig S, Henretig FM, eds. *Textbook of Pediatric Emergency Medicine.* 6th ed. Wolters Kluwer/Lippincott Williams & Wilkins; 2010:1171–1223.
33. Osterhoudt KC, Cook MD. Clean but not sober: a 16-year-old with restlessness. *Pediatr Emerg Care.* 2011;27:892–894.
34. Osterhoudt KC, Durbin D, Alpern ER, et al. Activated charcoal administration in a pediatric emergency department. *Pediatr Emerg Care.* 2004;20:493–498.
35. Osterhoudt KC, Longo L. *Rise in child injury from cannabis: Not the high we wanted.* Center for Injury Research and Prevention; 2022. Available from: https://injury.research.chop.edu/blog/posts/rise-child-injury-cannabis-not-high-we-wanted
36. Palmer BF, Clegg DJ. Salicylate toxicity. *N Engl J Med.* 2020;382:2544–2555. https://doi.org/10.1056/NEJMra2010852.
37. Press E, Mellins RB. A poisoning control program. *Am J Public Health.* 1954;44:1515–1525.
38. Proudfoot AT, Krenzelok EP, Vale JA. Position paper on urine alkalinization. *J Toxicol Clin Toxicol.* 2004;42:1–26.
39. Raouf Mena, et al. A practical guide to urine drug monitoring. *Federal practitioner.* 2018;35(4):38–44.
40. Rumack BH, Bateman DN. Acetaminophen and acetylcysteine dose and duration: past, present and future. *Clin Toxicol.* 2012;50:91–98.
41. Seger DL, Loden JK. Naloxone reversal of clonidine toxicity: dose, dose, dose. *Clin Toxicol.* 2018;56(10):873–879. https://doi.org/10.1080/15563650.2018.1450986. Epub 2018 Mar 16. PMID: 29544366.
42. Seifert SA, Armitage JO, Sanchez EE. Snake envenomation. *N Engl J Med.* 2022;386:68–78. https://doi.org/10.1056/NEJMra2105228.
43. Thornton MD, Baum CR. Bath salts and other emerging toxins. *Pediatr Emerg Care.* 2014;30(1):47–52.10.1097/PEC.0000000000000069 quiz 53–5. PMID: 24378862.
44. Ting-Jang Guo. A rare but serious case of toluene-induced sudden sniffing death. *J. Acute Med.* 2015;5(4):109–111. ISSN 2211-5587https://doi.org/10.1016/j.jacme.2015.09.006.
45. Traub SJ, Hoffman RS, Nelson LS. Body packing: the internal concealment of illicit drugs. *N Engl J Med.* 2003;349:2519–2526.
46. Vardakou I, Pistos C, Spiliopoulou CH. Spice drugs as a new trend: mode of action, identification and legislation. *Toxicol Lett.* 2010;197:157.
47. Weaver LK. Carbon monoxide poisoning. *N Engl J Med.* 2009;360:1217–1225.
48. Wright RO, Lewander WJ, Woolf AD. Methemoglobinemia: etiology, pharmacology, and clinical management. *Ann Emerg Med.* 1999;34:646–656.
49. Xuev S, Ickowicz A. Serotonin syndrome in children and adolescents exposed to selective serotonin reuptake inhibitors: a review of literature. *J Can Acad Child Adolesc Psychiatry.* 2021;30(3):156–164.
50. Zimmerman JL. Cocaine intoxication. *Crit Care Med.* 2012;28:517–526. https://www.cdc.gov/nchs/nvss/vsrr/drug-overdose-data.htm.

PSYCHIATRIC EMERGENCIES

Arun Handa and Eron Y. Friedlaender

CHAPTER 40

1. **What constitutes a psychiatric emergency?**
   A psychiatric emergency is a dangerous, life-threatening situation in which a child needs immediate attention due to:
   - Risk of harm to self
   - Risk of harm to others
   - Changes in behavior or thinking

   Important immediate assessment of the following is recommended:
   - Is the patient acutely suicidal or homicidal?
   - Is the patient severely depressed, manic, psychotic, in delirium, or has significant intellectual disability, any of which may impair psychosocial functioning?
   - Does the patient have adequate insight, judgment, and impulse control to maintain safety?

2. **What is the epidemiology of psychiatric illness in children?**
   - The US Surgeon General estimates that as many as 1 in 10 children and adolescents in the United States suffers a serious psychiatric disturbance per year, whereas the National Institute on Mental Health has found that up to 1 in 5 children either currently or at some point during their life has a serious debilitating mental health disorder.
   - Only an estimated 20% of children in the United States with some form of mental health problem severe enough to require treatment are identified as such and are receiving mental health services.
   - Mental health conditions increased by 28% between 2011 and 2015. They account for 5% to 7% of all pediatric emergency department (ED) visits. Up to 31% to 54% of these encounters result in hospitalization.

3. **What was the impact of the COVID-19 pandemic on the incidence of psychiatric emergencies?**
   Adolescent ED visits for mental health increased dramatically during the pandemic (up 31% in 2020 compared to 2019). ED visits for suicide attempts in adolescent girls increased by 50% (Feb-Mar 2021 compared to 2019). The COVID pandemic resulted in school cancellation (or virtual format) and many children suffered from social isolation and interrupted service support. In addition, numerous children witnessed ill or dying family members. Furthermore, many families suffered economic hardship, which impacted children. Social media played a role in the significant increase in mental health issues during this time, as this was the only way some teens were able to stay connected with others.

4. **What are the most common psychiatric emergencies in children?**
   Mood (depression) and anxiety/panic disorders, psychosis, behavior problems, and substance use are common mental health concerns that are associated with significant impairment risk. These diagnoses are often complicated by suicidality, aggression, and impulsive behaviors that require intervention and/or deescalation. Children and adolescents with autism and related developmental disabilities represent a growing population of patients seeking emergency care for behavioral disruption and instability in the home environment.

5. **How common is suicide?**
   - Suicide is the second-leading cause of death for children, adolescents, and young adults from 15 to 24 years.
   - The suicide rate among adolescents and young children aged 10 to 24 years increased be 57.4% from 2007 to 2018.
   - From 2016 to 2018, suicide rates increased significantly in 42 US states.
   - In 2019, approximately one in six students reported making a suicide plan, a 44% increase since 2009.

6. **How common is depression?**
   The Centers for Disease Control and Prevention reports that a 2021 survey showed 57% of teen girls felt persistently sad or hopeless in the past year and 30% seriously considered suicide. About 18% experienced sexual violence. LGBTQ+ youths struggle with mental health and violence more than others.

KEY POINTS: EPIDEMIOLOGY OF PSYCHIATRIC EMERGENCIES

1. Up to 1 in 10 children and adolescents suffers from a serious emotional disturbance per year in the United States.
2. Psychiatric conditions account for 5% to 7% of all ED visits, and up to 50% of these encounters result in hospitalization.
3. Suicide is the second-leading cause of death in older adolescents.

7. **How should the initial approach be conducted when evaluating a child with a possible psychiatric emergency?**
   - Ensure safety of the patient, caregivers, and staff.
   - Clarify the psychiatric diagnoses (if any) contributing to the crisis and the patient's level of functioning at baseline.
   - Use simple language and approach the patient with compassion and utilize a nonjudgmental tone.
   - Obtain information to identify the relevant biological, social, and psychological factors influencing the patient.
   - Perform an acute medical evaluation: assess ABCs (see Question 8), vital signs, CNS function and stigmata of toxidromes.
   - Assess for possible toxic ingestion: identify possible toxidromes and obtain history of all possible medications in the home or accessible to the child.
   - Obtain a history of potential traumatic injury.
   - Evaluate past medical history that might indicate an organic cause of the acute psychiatric emergency.
   - Consider a focused medical assessment based on history and physical examination: electrolytes, glucose, thyroid function, blood gas, toxicological screen; electrocardiography; and cranial imaging with computed tomography or magnetic resonance imaging as clinically indicated.
   - Obtain a urine pregnancy test for all adolescent females.

8. **What are the ABCs of the mental status examination in the ER?**
   A: *Appearance/Affect:* appearance (distress, posture, dress/hygiene, grooming, eye contact, facial expression, body habitus, markings, areas of self-injury) affect (anxious, depressed, flat, hostile, euphoric, apathetic, appropriate or inappropriate, labile or nonlabile).
   B: *Behavior:* attitude (cooperative, manipulative, angry, violent, withdrawn) movement (agitation, fidgeting, tics, abnormal involuntary movements).
   C: *Cognition:*
   - Thought content (thematic)—suicidal or homicidal ideation; delusions; obsessions/compulsions; phobias; poverty of thought
   - Thought process (observed)—organization, goal-directedness, tangential, flight of ideas
   - Level of consciousness—orientation, attention, concentration

9. **List some of the medical considerations that can present as a psychiatric disorder or behavioral problem.**
   - *Neurological:*
     - Stroke/transient ischemic attack
     - Hemorrhage: subdural, subarachnoid, epidural
     - CNS vascular: aneurysms, ischemia, venous thrombosis, vasculitis
     - CNS malignancy/tumor
     - CNS trauma: primary injury, secondary injury, or sequelae of head injury
     - CNS infection: encephalitis, meningitis, brain abscess, syphilis, human immunodeficiency virus, malaria, Epstein-Barr virus
     - Seizures
     - Hydrocephalus
     - Congenital malformations
     - Migraine headache
     - Neurodegenerative disorders: Huntington chorea, multiple sclerosis
     - Tuberous sclerosis
   - *Toxin:* ethanol, benzodiazepines, barbiturates, cocaine, opiates, amphetamines, hallucinogens, marijuana, phencyclidine, anticholinergic medications (antihistamines, tricyclics), heavy metals, corticosteroids, neuroleptic medications, bath salts, synthetic cannabinoids, energy drinks, carbon monoxide
   - *Metabolic/endocrinological:* hypoglycemia, hypocalcemia, hypoglycemia, hyponatremia, hyperthyroidism or hypothyroidism, adrenal insufficiency, uremia, liver failure, diabetes mellitus, porphyria, Wilson disease

10. **How should the psychiatric evaluation be incorporated into the ED management of a child with a psychiatric emergency?**
    A psychiatric assessment follows treatment of active medical concerns and confirmation of medical stability. An effective relationship with a specialized mental health team is crucial. Engage the child and family in discussing the issues and develop trust. Attempt to minimize distractions during the assessment and offer privacy and quiet during interviews. Ensure continued monitoring of the patient for safety with constant supervision, visual or arms-length, in a room cleared of all potential safety hazards. Protect confidentiality and remain vigilant as a mandated reporter.

11. **What are the indications for the use of physical restraint in the ED setting?**
    - When the patient is an acute danger to themselves or others.
    - To prevent serious disruption of the treatment plan or significant damage to the physical environment.
    - When other less restrictive measures are not possible or have failed.

    Follow regulatory guidelines requiring monitoring when restraints are utilized.

12. **Describe the proper procedure in the use of physical restraint.**
    - Explain to the patient why physical restraint is necessary.
    - Use the least-restrictive age-appropriate method of restraint possible.
    - Nurses or physicians may initiate restraint.
    - Provide a physician's order specifying the specific type of restraint, the clinical indication, and document a face-to-face examination within 1 hour. Review this order every hour for patients 8 years old and younger and every 2 hours for patients 9 years and older.
    - Ensure supine positioning with the head of the bed elevated and free cervical range of motion.
    - Enlist five caretakers, one each to secure a limb and one for the head. Apply the restraint first to the extremity and then the restraint to the bed frame (avoid the handrails). Avoid pressure on the patient's throat or chest and keep hands away from the patient's mouth.
    - Closely supervise (1:1) the patient in physical restraints; assess restraints at least every 15 minutes and document findings.
    - Provide continuous vital sign monitoring and frequent evaluation of limb neurovascular status and assist with nutritional and bathroom needs while the patient is in restraints.
    - Minimize restraint for medically compromised or unstable patients.
    - Restrain for the least amount of time possible as appropriate for the clinical situation; ensure criteria for release.
    - Remove restraints only with adequate staff present, and when the patient has regained control.

KEY POINTS: PROPER ADMINISTRATION OF PHYSICAL RESTRAINTS

1. Explain to the patient why physical restraint is necessary.
2. Have at least five caretakers to apply restraints.
3. Avoid pressure on the patient's throat or chest.
4. Avoid placement of the restrained child in a prone position.
   a. Asphyxiation may occur with excess weight on the back of prone patients.
5. Provide constant supervision (1:1) while the patient is in physical restraints.
6. Assess restraints at least every 15 minutes and document the assessment.
7. Remove restraints only with adequate staff present, and when the patient has regained control.

13. **What is the difference between agitation and aggression?**
    - *Agitation* is generally considered excessive and aimless psychomotor activity typically in response to emotional/psychological trigger.
    - *Aggression* is generally considered impulsive or premediated behavior directed with the intent to cause harm.

14. **What are the drugs of choice to manage agitation and aggression?**
    - Many patients benefit from medications that may reduce agitation.
    - Medications are often used prior to the initiation of physical restraints although manual physical holds may be required for medication administration.
    - Chemical restraint is not practiced in the pediatric ED setting.
    - Consider:
      - Underlying etiology of agitation or aggression (anxiety, psychosis).
      - Previous medication trials that may have yielded a positive/negative response.
      - Current medication regimen; consider early or additional dose.
      - Onset of action and duration of effect based on route of administration; allow time for medication to take effect.
    - Common psychopharmacological interventions for acute agitation/anxiety are listed in Table 40.1.
    - Confirm with a pharmacist prior to mixing medications in the same syringe.
    - Nonemergent use of psychopharmacology for agitation/aggression requires parental consent.

15. **What are the extrapyramidal side effects of antipsychotic medications?**
    - **Acute dystonic reaction**: painful; muscular rigidity; commonly involves neck, jaw, back, extremities, etc.; often frightening for patients
      - Laryngeal/pharyngeal dystonia may be a medical emergency if the airway is compromised.
      - Oculogyric crisis involves prolonged involuntary upward deviation of the eyes.
    - **Akathisia**: feelings of internal motor restlessness; often manifests as an inability to sit still and desire to move lower extremities
    - **Pseudoparkinsonism**: symptoms include bradykinesia, resting tremors, cogwheeling, rigidity, masked facies, stooped posture, shuffling gait, sialorrhea
    - **Tardive dyskinesia**: involuntary muscle movement involving the face and/or extremities; chronic condition often associated with long-term use of antipsychotics
    - **Neuroleptic malignant syndrome**: acute, life-threatening reaction characterized by fever, muscle rigidity, autonomic instability, and mental status changes

Table 40.1 Common Psychopharmacological Interventions for Acute Agitation/Anxiety

DRUG	DOSE	COMMENT
Benzodiazepines		
Diazepam (Valium)	0.1 mg/kg PO or IM/IV	Usual dose, 2-10 mg Long duration of action with active metabolites Be mindful of delirium, respiratory depression, disinhibition
Lorazepam (Ativan)	0.05 mg/kg PO or IM/IV	Usual dose range, 0.5-2 mg Onset of action varies by route of administration Be mindful of delirium, respiratory depression, disinhibition
Midazolam (Versed)	0.25-0.5 mg/kg PO (max 15 mg) 0.035 mg/kg IV (max 2 mg) 0.07-0.08 mg/kg IM (max 5 mg) 0.2-0.4 mg/kg IN (max 10 mg)	Dose range, 2-15 mg Significantly shorter time to onset of sedation and a more rapid arousal
Typical Antipsychotics *High-potency*		
Haloperidol (Haldol)	0.025-0.075 mg/kg PO or IM/IV	Usual dose range, children: 0.5-2 mg/dose Usual dose range, adolescents: 2-5 mg/dose Increased risk of EPS particularly in young males Use IV formulation with caution outside of ICU due to QTc prolongation
Low-potency		
Chlorpromazine (Thorazine)	0.25-0.5 mg/kg PO or IM/IV	Maximum cumulative daily dose of 40 mg for children <25 kg and 75 mg for children 25-50 kg Be mindful of hypotension and reduction in seizure threshold Use IV formulation with caution outside of ICU due to QTc prolongation
Atypical Antipsychotics		
Risperidone (Risperdal)	0.25-0.5 mg PO (ODT starts at 0.5 mg)	Lower dose for patients 15-30 kg Can use 0.5 mg for >30 kg FDA indication for autism-related irritability/aggression
Olanzapine (Zyprexa)	2.5-10 mg PO (ODT starts at 5 mg)	Onset of action 15 min Lower dose for patients 30-60 kg Can use 10 mg for >60 kg Use with caution or avoid IM olanzapine and IM benzodiazepine combination given within 30 min of each other due to high risk of respiratory depression
Ziprasidone (Geodon)	10-20 mg PO/IM	For use in patients >60 kg Caution with use due to effects on QTc prolongation
Quetiapine (Seroquel)	6.25-25 mg PO	Oral tablets only formulation
Antihistamines		
Diphenhydramine (Benadryl)	0-5-1 mg/kg PO or IM/IV	Usually 12.5-50 mg Use with caution in children with delirium or with previous paradoxical reaction May be helpful when given in combination with antipsychotic to reduce EPS
Hydroxyzine (Atarax, Vistaril)	1-2 mg/kg PO or IM	Usually 12.5-50 mg Use with caution in children with delirium or with previous paradoxical reaction May be helpful when given in combination with antipsychotic to reduce EPS

Table 40.1 Common Psychopharmacological Interventions for Acute Agitation/Anxiety

DRUG	DOSE	COMMENT
Combination Therapy		
Haloperidol + Lorazepam		Results in a more rapid onset of sedation than single agent with a similar adverse effect profile
Haloperidol + Diphenhydramine		Results in a more rapid onset of sedation than single agent with a similar adverse effect profile Helpful if there is a history of EPS (acute dystonic reactions)
Antihypertensives		
Clonidine (Kapvay, Catapres)	0.05-0.1 mg PO	Useful in children with comorbid ADHD Monitor for hypotension
Propranolol (Inderal)	10 mg	Useful with akathisia

ADHD, attention deficit hyperactivity disorder; EPS, extrapyramidal symptoms; FDA, US Food and Drug Administration; ICU, intensive care unit; IM, intramuscularly; IN, intranasally; IV, intravenously; ODT, oral dissolving tablet; PO, per os (taken orally).

16. What is serotonin syndrome? How is it treated?

Given the high prevalence in use of selective serotonin reuptake inhibitors as well as the increased abuse of amphetamines such as ecstasy/MDMA (3,4-methylenedioxymethamphetamine), serotonin syndrome has become a more common toxicological emergency.

Although presentation varies, the common clinical triad includes autonomic instability (tachycardia, nausea, diarrhea, mydriasis, diaphoresis, hyperthermia), mental status changes (agitation, delirium, headaches), and neuromuscular symptoms (myoclonus, hyperreflexia, tremor). Treatment is generally supportive, with discontinuation of the offending agent. Benzodiazepines may assist with agitation and muscle rigidity.

17. What is catatonia? How is it diagnosed?
   - Complex syndrome characterized by aberrant motor and behavioral activity.
   - Pathophysiology is still poorly defined.
   - Catatonia may result from any medical or psychiatric etiology; consider thorough and broad workup.
     - Half of all cases are due to underlying medical etiology.
     - Mood disorders are the most common psychiatric etiology.
   - Clinical picture is diagnosed by three (or more) of the following symptoms:
     - Stupor (no psychomotor activity; not actively relating to the environment)
     - Catalepsy (passive induction of a posture held against gravity)
     - Waxy flexibility (slight, even resistance to positioning by examiner)
     - Mutism (no, or very little, verbal response)
     - Negativism (opposition or no response to instruction or external stimuli)
     - Posturing (spontaneous and active maintenance of a posture against gravity)
     - Mannerism (odd, circumstantial caricature of normal actions)
     - Stereotypy (repetitive, abnormally frequent, non-goal-directed movements)
     - Agitation
     - Grimacing
     - Echolalia (mimicking another's speech)
     - Echopraxia (mimicking another's movements)
   - There are multiple catatonia rating scales. Catatonia is a *clinical diagnosis* with no specific laboratory testing.

18. Identify risk factors for suicide attempts in children and adolescents.
   - Psychiatric disorder
     - Mood disorder
     - Substance use disorder
     - Personality disorder
     - Eating disorder
   - Previous suicide attempt

- Previous nonsuicidal self-injurious behavior
- Person/Personality characteristics
  - Male >> Female
  - 16 years and older
  - Impulsivity
  - Poor problem-solving skills
  - Substance use/abuse
  - Social isolation
  - Chronic pain
- Family factors
  - Mental health disorders in close family members, including suicide attempts
  - Poor communication
  - Direct conflicts
  - Violence
- Specific life events
  - Interpersonal loss
  - Trouble at school
  - Bullying
  - Abuse (physical, emotional, sexual)
  - Exploration of gender identity/gender dysphoria
  - Exposure to violence
  - Chronic medical conditions
- Contagion-imitation
  - Availability of means
  - Physical means/access to firearms
  Cognitive: sensationalized media, detailed internet information.

19. **Name some medications associated with depression?**
    See Table 40.2 for medications associated with depression.

20. **What questions can a clinician ask to help identify patients with depression and suicide risk?**
    - The Columbia-Suicide Severity Rating Scale (C-SSRS or Columbia Protocol) is a widely used, validated tool to support suicide risk assessment tool for individuals over the age of 11 (Table 40.3). It is a short questionnaire with utility in prehospital, hospital, and clinic settings and can be administered by providers as well as people without a medical background. An affirmative answer to any of the six questions prompts referral to a trained mental health professional for assessment. A response of "yes" to questions 4, 5, or 6 reflects a high risk for suicide.
    - The Patient Health Questionnaire-9 Item has specifically been validated to detect depression among adolescents. A score of 5 to 9 indicates mild depression, 10 to 14 moderate depression, and greater than 15 moderately severe to severe depression. A score of 11 or more has a sensitivity of 89.5% and a specificity of 77.5% of detecting depression in adolescents (Table 40.4).
    - The abbreviated (four-item) Suicide Ideation Questionnaire has high sensitivity (98%) and negative predictive value (97%) and can be used as a screening tool to detect suicidality in children and adolescents. Each of the four items listed in Table 40.5 when positive was individually predictive of suicidality and, therefore, can be effectively used to quickly assess mental health concerns in the busy ED.

21. **What is the role of the pediatric ED in identifying mental illness in children and adolescents?**
    Many vulnerable children with undiagnosed psychiatric illnesses seek care in the ED. The Joint Commission recommends a suicide risk assessment for any patient presenting with an emotional or behavioral disorder.

Table 40.2 Medications Associated With Depression

CATEGORY	SPECIFIC MEDICATIONS
Neuropsychiatric	Neuroleptics, barbiturates, benzodiazepines, carbamazepine, phenytoin, stimulants
Antimicrobial	Ampicillin, griseofulvin, metronidazole, trimethoprim
Anti-inflammatory/analgesic	Corticosteroids, opiates
Cardiovascular	Clonidine, propranolol
Miscellaneous	Chemotherapy, ethanol, caffeine, oral contraceptives

Table 40.3 Columbia-Suicide Severity Rating Scale Columbia-Suicide Severity Rating Scale

Screen with Triage Points for **Emergency Department**

Ask questions that are bolded and _underlined_.

Ask Questions 1 and 2

Past month

YES   NO

1) ***Have you wished you were dead or wished you could go to sleep and not wake up?***

2) ***Have you actually had any thoughts of killing yourself?***

If YES to 2, ask questions 3, 4, 5, and 6. If NO to 2, go directly to question 6.

3) ***Have you been thinking about how you might do this?***
E.g. "*I thought about taking an overdose but I never made a specific plan as to when where or how I would actually do it....and I would never go through with it.*"

4) ***Have you had these thoughts and had some intention of acting on them?***
As opposed to "*I have the thoughts but I definitely will not do anything about them.*"

5) ***Have you started to work out or worked out the details of how to kill yourself?***
Did you intend to carry out this plan?

6) ***Have you ever done anything, started to do anything, or prepared to do anything to end your life?***
Examples: Collected pills, obtained a gun, gave away valuables, wrote a will or suicide note, took out pills but didn't swallow any, held a gun but changed your mind or it was grabbed from your hand, went to the roof but didn't jump; or actually took pills, tried to shoot yourself, cut yourself, tried to hang yourself, etc.
If YES, ask: *Was this within the past three months?*

Lifetime

Past 3 Months

Item 1 Behavioral Health Referral at Discharge

Item 2 Behavioral Health Referral at Discharge

Item 3 Behavioral Health Referral at Discharge

Item 4 Immediate Notification of Physician and/or Behavioral Health and Patient Safety Precautions

Item 5 Immediate Notification of Physician and/or Behavioral Health and Patient Safety Precautions

Item 6 Over 3 months ago: Behavioral Health Referral at Discharge

Item 6 3 months ago or less: Immediate Notification of Physician and/or Behavioral Health and Patient Safety Precautions

■ High Risk ■ Medium Risk ▤ Low Risk

The US Preventive Services Task Force recommends screening all adolescents for depression if systems are in place to ensure accurate diagnosis and proper intervention. It is necessary to have efficient, culturally sensitive, developmentally appropriate, and preferably self-administered screening tools in place.
    Many adolescents who attempt suicide seek medical care before the event (50% the month before and 25% the week before). Good screening protocols may allow ED staff to intervene.

22. **Describe the specific ED management issues in the evaluation of a child with depression or suicidal ideation.**
First, assess the potential medical causes of the child's depression, with specific attention to evaluation of toxic ingestions. Maintain suicide precautions with 1:1 observation until the patient has been fully evaluated regarding this risk. Hospital staff, rather than family members, should provide this observation. Search the patient and his or her personal belongings for possible harmful objects and remove them. Remove items from the room that could cause strangulation such as medical tubing, electrical and equipment cords. Take all suicidal comments and acts seriously. A quiet, low-stimulation environment in the ED is ideal.

23. **List essential criteria for outpatient disposition of the suicidal child/adolescent.**
   • No requirement of inpatient medical care, including intoxication or delirium
   • No active suicide ideation
   • Presence in home of a supportive adult with a good relationship with child/adolescent
   • Adult agreement to safety plan with close observation of patient until scheduled outpatient follow-up appointment

Table 40.4 Patient Health Questionnaire-9 Item (PHQ-9)—Modified for Teens

Over the last 2 weeks, how often have you been bothered by any of the following problems?

	Not at all	Several days	More than half the days	Nearly every day
Little interest or pleasure in doing things	0	1	2	3
Feeling down, depressed, or hopeless	0	1	2	3
Trouble falling or staying asleep, or sleeping too much	0	1	2	3
Poor appetite or overeating	0	1	2	3
Feeling bad about yourself—or that you are a failure or have let yourself or your family down	0	1	2	3
Trouble concentrating on things, such as reading the newspaper or watching television	0	1	2	3
Moving or speaking so slowly that other people could have noticed—or the opposite, being so fidgety or restless that you have been moving around a lot more than usual	0	1	2	3
Thoughts that you would be better off dead or of hurting yourself	0	1	2	3
In the past year have you felt depressed or sad most days, even if you felt okay sometimes?	[ ] Yes			[ ] No
Has there been a time in the past month when you have had serious thoughts about ending your life?	[ ] Yes			[ ] No
Have you ever in your whole life tried to kill yourself or made a suicide attempt?	[ ] Yes			[ ] No
If you are experiencing any of the problems on this form, how difficult have these problems made it for you to do your work, take care of things at home, or get along with other people?	[ ] Not difficult at all	[ ]Somewhat difficult	[ ] Very difficult	[ ] Extremely difficult

Adapted from The REACH Institute. *Guidelines for adolescent depression in primary care—GLAD-PC tool kit, version 2*, 2010:71–73. Available at: http://www.glad-pc.org/. Accessed 18.07.13.

Table 40.5 Suicide Ideation Questionnaire

1. Are you here because you tried to hurt yourself?
2. In the past week, have you been having thoughts about killing yourself?
3. Have you ever tried to hurt yourself in the past other than this time?
4. Has something very stressful happened to you in the past few weeks?

- Adult agreement to remove or secure all lethal risks (firearms, medications, drugs, alcohol) in home
- Adult and patient are provided with indications to return to ED if condition deteriorates
- Follow-up arranged for additional evaluation and treatment
- Both patient and adult agree with plan and recommendations

24. After discharge from the ED for a mental health concern, do children get the help they need?
Unfortunately, children often do not get help they need after an ED visit. It is known that follow-up with a mental health provider lowers the risk of suicide, increases the likelihood of medication compliance, and reduces repeat visits to the ED. However, one study showed less than one-third of children had a mental health visit within

KEY POINTS: CRITERIA FOR OUTPATIENT MANAGEMENT OF THE PATIENT WITH SUICIDAL IDEATION

1. No inpatient medical care required
2. No active suicidal ideation
3. Presence in home of a supportive adult who agrees with safety plan and agrees to remove or secure all lethal risks (especially firearms)
4. Follow-up information provided
5. Agreement of both patient and adult with plan

7 days of discharge from the ED with a mental health issue. About 55% had a follow-up visit within 30 days. Black children are less likely to have a follow-up appointment. Children may not receive a follow-up mental health visit for a variety of reasons, including the lack of a supportive system with good capacity.

25. **In assessing the child with aggression, what key information is necessary to accurately evaluate the cause of this behavior?**
    - Onset of the symptoms and their severity
    - Use of weapons
    - Injury to self or others, including animals
    - Indications of intent to harm and lethality
    - Presence of other related symptoms
    - Presence of precipitants versus impulsive acts
    - Response to limit setting
    - Destruction of property, including fire setting

26. **What approach is suggested to address the child with aggression?**
    Avoid responding to the patient's aggression in a punitive manner. A respectful, nonjudgmental, and reassuring attitude helps the patient gain control and can reduce the aggressive behavior. Attempt to provide comfort and build rapport with the patient while simultaneously reassuring they are safe. Employ nonpharmacological interventions as first-line treatment (reduce lighting, limit people in the room, minimize ambient noise, engage child life specialists). Verbal deescalation techniques include the use of simplified language in a soft voice with slow movements. Space yourself from the patient and allow the patient space for pacing if possible. Offer food and drink in safe containers (aluminum cans may pose a safety hazard). Listen and empathize. Give the patient as much autonomy as possible, while setting limits to avoid damage to property and injury to staff and the patient. If pharmacological intervention is deemed to be helpful, offer medications early and discuss administration route with the patient (PO, SL, IV, IM) to avoid escalation to physical restraint. Aggression is common in the ED and accounts for 25% of adolescent emergency psychiatric presentations.

27. **Is it possible to provide oral medications to an agitated/aggressive child?**
    Most patients will cooperate with oral dosing of a medication, despite the belief that they may be too agitated and uncooperative. Aggressive behavior frequently causes shame and embarrassment to the child. Therefore actions that reflect a respectful, nonjudgmental, and reassuring attitude, such as offering the patient the option of oral medication versus "a shot," can accomplish much in reducing the agitation and additionally avoid any potentially punitive response. For some sedatives, oral administration can be as effective as intramuscular dosing to control agitation, and the onset of intramuscular dosing is not sufficiently more rapid to warrant its routine, first-line use.

28. **What are the three diagnostic criteria for anorexia nervosa?**
    - Restriction of energy intake relative to requirements leading to a significantly low body weight in the context of age, sex, developmental trajectory, and physical health. Significantly low weight is defined as a weight that is less than minimally normal or expected.
    - Intense fear of gaining weight or of becoming fat, or persistent behavior that interferes with weight gain, even though at a significantly low weight.
    - Disturbance in the way one's body weight or shape is experienced, or persistent lack of recognition of the seriousness of the current low body weight.

29. **What are some of the medical complications of starvation or persistent purging seen in anorexia nervosa or bulimia?**
    - Skeletal: marked loss of bone mineral density causing early osteopenia and osteoporosis
    - Cardiac: myocardial atrophy, mitral valve prolapse, pericardial effusion, profound sinus bradycardia and sinus node dysfunction, orthostatic hypotension, and sudden cardiac death
    - Pulmonary: spontaneous pneumothorax, aspiration pneumonia, and pneumomediastinum

- Neurological: cognitive changes due to generalized brain atrophy
- Psychiatrical: psychological functioning difficulties
- Gastrointestinal: gastroparesis, constipation, superior mesenteric artery syndrome, elevated transaminases
- Hematological: leukopenia, thrombocytopenia, normocytic anemia
- Endocrinological/metabolic: amenorrhea and infertility, hypoglycemia, hypokalemia, hyponatremia, and metabolic alkalosis in patients who purge by vomiting, laxative abuse, or diuretic abuse
- HEENT (head, ears, eyes, nose, and throat): dental erosion and enlarged salivary glands in patients with bulimia
- Dermatologic: acrocyanosis, lanugo hair growth, brittle nails and hair, and hypercarotenemia

30. **What is the initial medical evaluation for a patient with a suspected eating disorder?**
    - Weight and vital signs
    - Electrocardiogram and orthostatic vital signs
    - Pregnancy test and urinalysis
    - Complete blood count, electrolytes, blood urea nitrogen, creatinine, calcium (Ca), magnesium (Mg), phosphate (PO$_4$), glucose
    - Uric acid, cholesterol, triglycerides, liver transaminases
    - Thyroid function tests, celiac panel, prolactin, estradiol, testosterone, 25-vitamin D, follicle-stimulating hormone, luteinizing hormone, methylmalonic acid

31. **What is functional neurological symptom disorder (FND) (formerly, conversion disorder)?**
    This is a psychiatric illness in which physical symptoms are genuinely experienced and related to a functional rather than structural cause.
    DSM-5-TR Diagnostic Criteria:
    - One or more symptoms of altered voluntary motor or sensory function.
    - Clinical findings provide evidence of incompatibility between the symptom and recognized neurological or medical conditions.
    - The symptom or deficit is not better explained by another medical or mental disorder.
    - The symptom or deficit causes clinically significant distress or impairment in social, occupational, or other important areas of functioning or warrants medical evaluation.
    - Subtypes include:
      - Weakness or paralysis
      - Abnormal movements (tremor, dystonia, myoclonus, gait disorder)
      - Swallowing symptoms (dysphonia, slurred speech)
      - Attacks or seizure-like activity
      - Anesthesia or sensory loss
      - Special sensory symptoms (visual, olfactory, or hearing disturbance)
      - Mixed symptoms
      The most common presentations are motor dysfunction and functional seizures.
      This is a clinical diagnosis largely based on characteristic history and supported by positive signs including distractibility enhancement with attention, motor inconsistency, incongruency, suggestibility, absent pronator drift, variability, excessive slowness with neurological examination, knee-buckling, and tics. Diagnosis depends on familiarity with movement disorders and their common variants. It often co-occurs with other neurological conditions. Prevalence rates are unknown. Consider precipitating factors (injury, medical illness, emotional event) as well as perpetuating factors (pain, stress, anxiety, comorbid psychiatric illness) during evaluation. Symptoms typically present abruptly and may be constant or intermittent.

32. **Who is most likely to have a functional neurological symptom disorder?**
    FND may affect children as young as 6 years.
    - Predisposing factors:
      - Female
      - Emotional or personality disorders
      - Neurological disease
      - Comorbid health conditions
      - Difficulties in interpersonal relationships
      - Psychiatric illness
      - Trauma

33. **What is a psychogenic nonepileptic seizure (PNES)? How can you distinguish this from a true epileptic seizure?**
    PNES, previously called pseudoseizure, is a functional neurological symptom disorder (conversion disorder) in which the patient has seizure-like motor activity. These seizure-like movements are not rhythmic, unlike a true seizure. Occasionally the patient with a PNES may be moaning or even conversing and has purposeful movements

and may reach up to grab the examiner. The PNES may be prolonged, compared to most true seizures, and may continue even if anticonvulsants are administered. Urinary incontinence is rare with PNES, and the patient is unlikely to suffer an injury during the event. Occasionally, PNES may be coaxed by examiners at the bedside. Furthermore, a patient with a PNES rarely has autonomic changes, which is very different from a true seizure. Despite a prolonged episode, the postictal period after PNES may be very brief.

It is very important to recognize PNES and to avoid treatment with anticonvulsants, which could have serious side effects.

34. What is required for hospital admission of a minor with a psychiatric emergency?

For both involuntary and voluntary inpatient psychiatric admissions, most states require parental consent for commitment of a child under the age of 14 years. In children older than 12 to 16 years, many states require the consent of the minor. A legal process is required if the child does not consent to voluntary commitment. Most states allow some period of emergency involuntary admission, but this period varies greatly from state to state. Involuntary commitment requires physician (and/or designee) documentation of the patient's danger to self or others and can be in effect for several days without a court order (depending on state statutes).

35. What is the "Duty to Warn" or "Tarasoff Standard"?

The "Duty to Warn" in health law describes the physician's responsibility to warn an identifiable third party of an imminent serious threat of harm. This has been well recognized since *Tarasoff v. Regents of the University of California* (1976) and is one of the few exceptions to a patient's right to confidentiality. These standards may differ from state to state and should be verified prior to disclosure.

BIBLIOGRAPHY

1. Agarwal R, Gathers-Hutchins L, Stephanou H. Psychogenic non-epileptic seizures in children. *Curr Probl Pediatrc Adolesc Health Care*. 2021;51(7):101036.
2. American Academy of Child and Adolescent Psychiatry. *What Is a Psychiatric Emergency? AACAP Facts for Families*; 2018. Available from: https://www.aacap.org/AACAP/Families_and_Youth/Facts_for_Families/FFF-Guide/What_is_a_Psychiatric_Emergency_126.aspx
3. American Academy of Child and Adolescent Psychiatry. *Suicide in Children and Teens. AACAP Facts for Families*; 2021. Available from: https://www.aacap.org/AACAP/Families_and_Youth/Facts_for_Families/FFF-Guide/Teen-Suicide-010.aspx
4. American Psychiatric Association. *Desk Reference to the Diagnostic Criteria From DSM-5-TR*. American Psychiatric Association; 2022.
5. Centers for Disease Control and Prevention. *Youth Risk Behavior Surveillance Data Summary & Trends Report: 2009-2019*. U.S. Department of Health and Human Services; 2022. Available from:https://www.cdc.gov/healthyyouth/data/yrbs/pdf/YRBSDataSummaryTrendsReport2019-508.pdf
6. Chun TH, Mace E, Katz ER. American Academy of Pediatrics Committee on Pediatric Emergency Medicine, American College of Emergency Physicians. Evaluation and management of children with acute mental heath or behavioral problems Part II: recognition of clinically challenging mental health related conditions presenting with medical or uncertain symptoms. *Pediatrics*. 2016;138(3):e20161573.
7. Chun TH, Katz ER, Duffy SJ. Challenges of managing pediatric mental health crises in the emergency department. *Child Adol Psych Clin NA*. 2015;24(1):21–40.
8. Cost J, Krantz M, Mehler PS. Medical complications of anorexia nervosa. *Cleve ClinJ Med*. 2020;87:361–366.
9. Curtin SC. *State Suicide Rates Among Adolescents and Young Adults Aged 10-24: United States, 2000–2018. National Vital Statistics Reports*. Vol. 69, no. 11. National Center for Health Statistics; 2020.
10. Hill RM, Rufino K, Kurian S, Saxena J, et al. Suicide ideation and attempts in a pediatric emergency department before and during COVID-19. *Pediatrics*. 2021;147(3):e2020029280.
11. Kalb LG, Stapp EK, Ballard ED, Holingue C, et al. Trends in psychiatric emergency department visits among youth and young adults in the US. *Pediatrics*. 2019;143(4):e20182192.
12. Katz ER, Jhonsa A, Friedlander E, Fein JA, et al. Behavioral and psychiatric emergencies. In: Shaw KN, Bachur RG, eds. *Fleisher & Ludwig's Textbook of Pediatric Emergency Medicine*. 8th ed. Lippincott Williams & Wilkins; 2021:1427–1447. Chapter 126.
13. Office of the Surgeon General (OSG). *Protecting Youth Mental Health: The U.S. Surgeon General's Advisory [Internet]*. US Department of Health and Human Services; 2021.PMID: 34982518.
14. Pittsenbarger ZE, Mannix R. Trends in pediatric visits to the emergency department for psychiatric illnesses. *Acad Emerg Med*. 2014;21(1):25–30.
15. Posner K, Brown GK, Stanley B, Brent DA, et al. The Columbia-Suicide Severity Rating Scale: initial validity and internal consistency findings from three multisite studies with adolescents and adults. *Am J Psychiatry*. 2011;168(12):1266–1277.
16. Richardson LP, McCauley E, Grossman DC, et al. Evaluation of the Patient Health Questionnaire-9 item for detecting major depression among adolescents. *Pediatrics*. 2010;126(6):1117–1123.
17. Rufino KA, Kerr T, Beyene H, Hill RM, et al. Suicide screening in a large pediatric emergency department: results, feasibility and lessons learned. *Pediatr Emerg Care*. 2022;38(3):e1127–e1132.
18. Ruch DA, Sheftall AH, Schlagbaum P, Rausch J, et al. Trends in suicide among youth aged 10-19 years in the United States, 1975-2016. *JAMA Netw Open*. 2019;2(5):e193886.
19. Vassilopoulos A, Mohammad S, Dure L, et al. Treatment approaches for functional neurological disorders in children. *Curr Treat Options Neurol*. 2022;24:77–97.
20. Yard E, Radhakrishnan L, Ballesteros MF, Sheppard M, et al. Emergency department visits for suspected suicide attempts among persons aged 12-25 years before and during the COVID-19 pandemic—United States Jan 2019-May 2021. *MMWR Morb Mortal Wkly Rep*. 2021;70(24):888–894.

CHAPTER 41

RESPIRATORY EMERGENCIES

Sabina B. Singh and Stephen Sandelich

1. **What are the signs of respiratory distress in children with asthma?**
   - Increased work of breathing (retractions, accessory muscle use, nasal flaring)
   - Decreased breath sounds
   - Tachypnea
   - Prolonged expiratory phase
   - Wheezing

2. **How should pulse oximetry be interpreted in an acute asthma exacerbation?**
   Sao_2 (saturation of O_2 measured by pulse oximetry) of 95% correlates with Pao_2 of around 75 mm Hg, and Sao_2 of 90% is close to Pao_2 of 60 mm Hg, which is the top of the steep portion of the oxygen desaturation curve. Most clinicians set a cutoff point for normal somewhere in between. Asthma is primarily an obstructive disease and not one of diffusion, hence, more likely to present with hypercarbia than hypoxia.

3. **Why does hypoxemia sometimes occur paradoxically after treatment with inhaled bronchodilators?**
   Hypoxemia in asthma is due to ventilation-perfusion mismatch. The acute deleterious effects of bronchodilators on oxygenation are believed to be due to their effects on circulation rather than on airways. After treatment, particularly when administered with high concentrations of oxygen, there is improvement in local alveolar oxygenation. This, in turn, causes a reversal of hypoxia-induced pulmonary vasoconstriction, with the result that areas previously neither ventilated nor perfused are now perfused but not ventilated, increasing the mismatch.

4. **What is the value of a chest radiograph in the setting of an acute asthma exacerbation?**
   Chest radiography is of limited value in evaluation of acute asthma and is most beneficial in identifying complications such as an air leak (i.e., pneumothorax or pneumomediastinum) or a concomitant pneumonia. Routinely obtaining radiographs for acute asthma exacerbations, or for patients requiring hospital admission, rarely changes management. Limit chest radiographs to cases in which there is clinical suspicion of a radiographic abnormality, such as persistent rales or asymmetry of breath sounds, high fever, crepitus in the neck, very poor response to therapy, or deterioration after initial therapy.

5. **What is the value of radiography in children with a first episode of wheezing?**
   Similar to use in an asthma exacerbation, routine use of radiography in the first episode of wheezing is also of relatively low yield. Radiography is probably not necessary in children with clinical mild-to-moderate bronchiolitis, or with a history and clinical course highly suggestive of asthma (e.g., family history of asthma, personal history of atopy, good response to inhaled bronchodilator treatment). Some authorities recommend it as several conditions other than reactive airways disease may present with wheezing, which are important to exclude (Table 41.1). Radiography is of value if the diagnosis of asthma is in doubt, the history is suggestive of other causes (e.g., history of choking preceding).

Table 41.1 Causes of Wheezing Other Than Reactive Airways Disease

INFLAMMATORY/INFECTIOUS	INTRALUMINAL OBSTRUCTION	EXTRALUMINAL OBSTRUCTION
Bronchiolitis	Foreign body	Vascular ring
Aspiration (gastroesophageal reflux, tracheoesophageal fistula)	Tracheomalacia	Mediastinal mass
Bronchopulmonary dysplasia	Congestive heart failure	Cystic malformation of the lung
Cystic fibrosis	α_1-Antitrypsin deficiency cholinergic poisoning (e.g., organophosphate)	Congenital lobar emphysema

6. **What is the preferred initial treatment for children with acute asthma?**
   The mainstay of initial treatment is bronchodilators and these are tailored to severity of disease. For those with moderate to severe exacerbations, give three to four doses of an inhaled bronchodilator in the first hour of treatment until there is a good response; those with mild disease may require less aggressive treatment. Give systemic steroids early in the ED course for patients suffering from an acute asthma exacerbation or for those who remain symptomatic despite appropriate bronchodilator therapy at home.

7. **Is nebulization a more effective means of delivering inhaled β-receptor agonists than a metered dose inhaler (MDI)?**
   Several studies and meta-analyses have shown that nebulizer and MDI are clinically equivalent, provided that an appropriate dose is given and a spacer device is used. MDIs are also less expensive and lead to shorter ED stays. Standard doses of nebulized β-receptor agonist (0.15 mg/kg per dose, maximum 5 mg) are substantially higher than for MDI, however, the particles produced by the MDI deliver medication far more effectively to the lungs. Current recommendations of ED dosages of albuterol for acute asthma are for two to four puffs of albuterol for young children, four to six puffs for older children, and four to eight puffs for adolescents and adults. Spacer devices (e.g., Aerochamber) are available in a variety of sizes and configurations and can be used successfully even in young infants.

8. **What are adverse effects of albuterol?**
   - Tachycardia; tachyarrhythmias (rare)
   - Tremor
   - Central nervous system stimulation, hyperactivity
   - Hypokalemia
     Symptomatic hypokalemia requiring treatment is rare even with high-dose therapy, although mild degrees of hypokalemia are common (one-third of children in one study). For patients receiving high-dose continuous albuterol for more than 6 to 8 hours, monitor serum potassium.

9. **What is levalbuterol?**
   Racemic (standard) albuterol is a mixture of two isomers. Levalbuterol (Xopenex) is a pure R-isomer, which is responsible for bronchodilation. Most clinical evidence supports the notion that equipotent doses of albuterol and levalbuterol have similar bronchodilator efficacy and side effect profiles for acute use. There is evidence that the S-isomer may increase airway reactivity, suggesting that levalbuterol may be preferred for chronic use.

10. **What is the mechanism of action of ipratropium?**
    Ipratropium bromide binds to cholinergic receptors, located primarily in medium and large airways, leading to bronchodilation. Because vagally mediated bronchodilation is much less marked than that produced by adrenergic stimulation, ipratropium is a much less potent bronchodilator than albuterol and should not be used alone. Concomitant administration of both leads to a synergistic effect. Ipratropium is structurally related to atropine, it is a quaternary compound and therefore is poorly absorbed, thus, systemic side effects are minimal.

11. **Which patients should receive ipratropium?**
    Pediatric studies show that addition of ipratropium to albuterol leads to significant improvement in severe asthma exacerbation. Benefit in those with more moderate disease is less clear. Ipratropium has very little downside; costs and adverse effects are minimal. Give ipratropium to those with severe disease at presentation, and those who fail or have failed to respond well to β-receptor agonists alone.

12. **What is the optimal dose of ipratropium?**
    Standard individual dose is 0.5 mg regardless of weight. Although multiple doses have been shown to be better than a single dose, the optimal schedule is not known. Most authorities recommend adding ipratropium to two or three of the first three doses of albuterol given in the ED, then every 3 to 4 hours. There is no evidence that ipratropium has additional benefit after initial ED therapy in hospitalized patients.

13. **When should steroids be administered?**
    Asthma is an inflammatory disease. Bronchodilators control only the symptoms, not the underlying disease. Nearly all with acute asthma should receive systemic corticosteroids, preferably at the start of their ED treatment. That said, there is a trade-off in that too-frequent steroid administration may lead to complications. Patients with particularly mild disease, who require no or only a single treatment in the ED and have complete relief of symptoms with infrequent (no more than three to four times a day) treatments at home, may be managed without steroids with close outpatient follow-up.

14. **Which steroids should be administered?**
    Historically a 3- to 5-day course of oral prednisone was the steroid treatment of choice for status asthmaticus. In mild-to-moderate asthma a single- or two-dose regimen of dexamethasone is also efficacious. Studies have

shown that treating an asthma exacerbation with dexamethasone may increase compliance and decrease length of ED and overall hospital stays.

15. **What are the actions of corticosteroids in acute asthma?**
Steroids have multiple actions:
- Inhibition of mediator release and synthesis
- Interference with mediator action
- Upregulation of β-adrenergic receptors
 The last two help explain the observed onset of clinical effect within 2 hours of administration—during a typical ED visit. Peak effect of steroids requires interference with cellular synthetic pathways and occurs after 6 to 12 hours.

16. **When are intravenous (IV) steroids preferred over the oral route for asthma?**
There are several pediatric studies, and more from the adult literature, showing oral and IV corticosteroids to be equally effective, even among severely ill patients. Reserve the IV route for those unable to take oral medicine (persistent vomiting, severe respiratory distress) and those patients ill enough to be admitted to an intensive care unit (ICU).

17. **What are the contraindications to systemic steroids?**
- **Absolute contraindications:** Active varicella or herpes infection
- **Relative contraindication:** Exposure to varicella in an unprotected child
 Note that concomitant bacterial infection (e.g., otitis media, pneumonia) is *not* a contraindication to the use of steroids.

18. **Describe the role of magnesium sulfate in acute asthma.**
Magnesium sulfate produces bronchodilation via direct effect on smooth muscle because of calcium antagonism. It may provide added benefit when adrenergic and vagal receptors have been saturated. In severe exacerbations, the addition of magnesium sulfate to aggressive β-receptor agonist therapy and systemic steroids leads to greater clinical improvement and improved pulmonary function and Sao_2. The effectiveness in patients with less severe illness is equivocal. The dose of magnesium sulfate is 50 to 75 mg/kg (maximum 2 g) intravenously over 20 to 30 minutes.

19. **What are the indications for endotracheal intubation and mechanical ventilation in a patient with asthma?**
- Failure of maximal pharmacologic therapy
- Hypoxemia unrelieved by O_2 therapy
- Hypercarbia with rising Pco_2
- Deteriorating mental status
- Respiratory fatigue
- Respiratory arrest

20. **Which medications should be used during endotracheal intubation of an asthmatic patient?**
Use rapid sequence induction, including sedation and neuromuscular blockade. Ketamine is a good choice as a sedating agent because of its intrinsic bronchodilating properties and catecholaminergic response. However, because it also increases airway secretions, consider an anticholinergic agent such as atropine or glycopyrrolate as adjunct.

21. **What is the role of extracorporeal membrane oxygenation (ECMO) in the intubated asthmatic patient?**
Entotracheal intubation and mechanical ventilation are often challenging in asthmatics, it can often trigger further bronchospasm and worsening of underlying disease. ECMO can provide gas exchange and help prevent pulmonary barotrauma associated with mechanical ventilation in cases of severe asthma requiring intubation. There is no direct therapeutic effect on the lungs, however, given the bypass of the lungs, lungs are allowed to rest and improve with standard therapies. ECMO should be considered early in cases of severe status asthmaticus that is not responding to maximal pharmacological therapy.

22. **What are the two most common complications of mechanical ventilation?**
- **Air leak**, including pneumomediastinum, pneumothorax, due to barotrauma.
- **Hypotension** often occurs shortly after endotracheal intubation. It results from a combination of relative hypovolemia in severely ill patients and decreased venous return to the heart owing to positive intrapleural pressure.

KEY POINTS: TREATMENT OF ACUTE ASTHMA

1. Provide frequent (every 20 minutes) inhaled albuterol.
2. Provide early oral steroids (with or after first treatment).
3. Add ipratropium bromide to β-receptor agonists in case of incomplete response.
4. Monitor response to therapy with clinical assessment or peak expiratory flow rate.
5. Consider IV magnesium sulfate for severe or refractory cases.
6. Early consideration of ECMO in the most severe cases.

23. **What is bronchiolitis?**
    Bronchiolitis is a disease of lower airway inflammation and obstruction most often caused by a viral infection affecting mostly children younger than 2 years. Respiratory syncytial virus (RSV) accounts for approximately 80% of hospitalized cases; parainfluenza, human metapneumovirus, adenovirus, influenza virus, COVID-19, and other respiratory viruses are other common causes. Peak incidence is in winter, variations in seasonal timing were noted during the COVID-19 pandemic due to contact restrictions.

24. **Is there a test for RSV? How good is it?**
    RSV can be identified in nasal secretions by viral culture, antigen testing, and PCR. The sensitivity of the commercially available tests is generally in the range of 80% to 90%, and specificity is greater than 90%. Clinical utility of these tests is limited, because treatment is the same regardless of test results and is directed toward clinical manifestations.

25. **What are the clinical characteristics and natural history of bronchiolitis?**
    Bronchiolitis begins as an upper respiratory infection (URI), with coryza and cough. In adults, older children, and many infants, RSV infection remains confined to the upper respiratory tract. In some over a period of several days, lower tract becomes involved, with development of wheezing and rhonchi, as well as signs of respiratory distress. Typically, signs and symptoms peak in severity on the third to fifth days of illness and then begin to wane. The total duration of illness averages 14 to 15 days, although some may have a prolonged course. In one study, 25% of children were symptomatic at 3 weeks. Central apnea can occur in young infants usually at the onset of illness, before respiratory signs manifest.

26. **What is the role of albuterol in the management of bronchiolitis?**
    Most randomized controlled trials have shown no benefit to beta-adrenergic agents in the setting of bronchiolitis. While symptoms may transiently improve, there is no change in disease progression, resolution, hospitalization rate, or length of stay. Albuterol should not be given to infants and children with a diagnosis of bronchiolitis.

27. **Is there a role for corticosteroids in bronchiolitis?**
    Most studies to date have shown no benefit of corticosteroids, either systemic or inhaled, in the treatment of bronchiolitis. Steroids may be of benefit in selected infants with wheezing suspected of having intrinsic reactive airways disease, such as those with a prior history of wheezing, or strong family or personal history of atopy and good response to inhaled β-receptor agonists.

28. **What is the role of hypertonic saline (HTS) in acute bronchiolitis?**
    HTS may increase mucociliary clearance in the setting of acute bronchiolitis, which may be beneficial in decreasing mucous plugging. There is no clear evidence that HTS can reduce hospitalization rate and, as such, the current guideline is that clinicians may trial HTS on children who have been hospitalized with bronchiolitis.

29. **What is the role of high-flow oxygen therapy in infants with bronchiolitis?**
    High-flow oxygen can be delivered through a nasal cannula and can provide humidified and heated air and oxygen. Benefits include delivery of positive airway pressure and correction of hypoxia with a titratable FiO_2. High-flow nasal cannula can decrease work of breathing, improve oxygenation, and reduce the rate of intubation in infants with bronchiolitis.

30. **What are the best indicators of severe disease in bronchiolitis?**
    In several multicenter studies, initial pulse oximetry of less than 94% was the best predictor of need for admission. Other risk factors include age (<2 months), tachypnea, greater clinical severity (as indicated by greater work of breathing or higher Respiratory Distress Assessment Index), and inadequate oral intake. Although the need for supplemental oxygen would seem to mandate hospital admission, several studies support the use of home oxygen therapy.

31. **What is palivizumab? What is nirsevimab?**

    Palivizumab (Synagis) is a humanized mouse monoclonal antibody against RSV, administered as a monthly intramuscular injection. Prophylaxis has been shown to reduce the incidence and severity of bronchiolitis in high-risk patients. Nirsevimab is a new monoclonal antibody treatment for RSV, just approved by the US Food and Drug Administration in 2023. Administered as a single injection, it will hopefully provide infants born during or entering their first RSV season and toddlers up to 24 months with antibodies to protect against severe RSV illness.

KEY POINTS: MANAGEMENT OF BRONCHIOLITIS

1. Care is mainly supportive.
2. Inhaled β-receptor agonists do not improve disease course.
3. Use of corticosteroids for bronchiolitis is not supported by evidence.
4. Typical course is progression of symptoms over first 3 to 5 days, with resolution over 2 to 3 weeks.

32. **What is croup? How is it diagnosed?**

    Croup, or laryngotraceobronchitis, is a common pediatric condition. Parainfluenza virus can be recovered from the nasopharynx in over 90% of cases. Other cases are caused by influenza, RSV, measles, or adenovirus. Several cases related to COVID-19 infection have also been reported. It is most often seen in the fall months with a peak in October. It typically affects children between the ages of 6 to 36 months but can occur in older children as well. Patients classicly present with a harsh, barky, "seal-like" cough. There may be associated tachypnea, stridor, and subcostal retractions in more severe cases.

33. **What is the differential diagnosis of croup?**

    Differential diagnosis includes bacterial tracheitis, epiglottitis, and deep neck infections such as retropharyngeal abscess (Table 41.2). Epiglottitis is a much less common entity since 1990, with the introduction of the Hib vaccine. In a 6- to 24-month-old afebrile child, an index of suspicion should also be kept for an aspirated foreign body. Often a clear history of choking is not obtained. If a hemangioma is noted in the beard distribution, consider the possibility of a subglottic hemangioma causing airway obstruction and stridor.

34. **When are diagnostic tests indicated in croup?**

    Croup is a clinical diagnosis and children with characteristic signs and symptoms do not require further diagnostic testing. Anteroposterior and lateral radiographs of the neck may be indicated in children with atypical features (e.g., age less than 6 months, recurrent or prolonged croup, toxicity on examination). The typical radiographic findings are shown in Table 41.2.

35. **How do you assess severity of croup?**

    Several scoring systems have been devised to assess croup severity. The most used is the Westley score (Table 41.3). A score of less than or equal to 2 indicates mild disease, 3 to 7 indicates moderate disease, and a score of 8 and above indicates severe disease.

Table 41.2 Differential Diagnosis of Croup

VARIABLE	CROUP	EPIGLOTTITIS	RETROPHARYNGEAL ABSCESS	BACTERIAL TRACHEITIS
Anatomic area affected	Subglottic	Supraglottic	Retropharynx	Trachea
Age	6-36 months	Any	6 months-4 year	Any
Onset	Hours	1-3 days	1-3 days	3-5 days
Toxicity	None	Marked	Marked	Marked
Drooling	No	Yes	Yes	No
Voice	Hoarse	Muffled	Muffled	Normal
Cough	Barky	None	None	Painful
Radiographic finding	"Steeple" sign	"Thumb" sign	Widened retropharynx	"Shaggy" trachea

Table 41.3 Westley Croup Score

VARIABLE	0	1	2	3	4	5
Stridor	None	With stethoscope	At rest			
Retraction	None	Mild	Moderate	Severe		
Air entry	Normal	Mild decrease	Marked decrease			
Cyanosis					When agitated	At rest
Altered Mental Status						Disoriented

36. **What are indications for admission in a child with croup?**
Admission criteria include a croup score of 8, significant respiratory compromise, dehydration, an unreliable caretaker, or lack of adequate follow-up. For those severely ill patients not responding to therapy, an arterial blood gas may be helpful in deciding on admission to general ward versus pediatric ICU.

37. **Is there any scientific evidence that humidified air is beneficial in treatment of children with croup?**
No. In theory, the humidified air moistens secretions and soothes the inflammation of the mucosa. However, despite the ubiquitous recommendations for the use of "the steamy bathroom" and "misty ox," controlled trials have failed to demonstrate a clinical benefit.

38. **Is there any scientific evidence that steroids are beneficial in the treatment of croup?**
Yes. Treat patients with moderate to severe symptoms (e.g., a croup score = 1) with steroids. Although many randomized trials involving steroids use have relatively small numbers of patients, meta-analyses of these trials showed significant decreases in clinical croup scores and decreased the need for endotracheal intubation with steroid treatment. One study demonstrated that steroids reduce symptom duration even with mild disease.

39. **Which method of corticosteroid delivery is better: intramuscular or oral? What is the ideal dose?**
Dexamethasone (given orally or intramuscularly) is equally effective. The usual dose of dexamethasone for croup has traditionally been 0.6 mg/kg intramuscularly or orally, though doses of 0.15 and 0.3 mg/kg have been shown to be similarly effective.

40. **Is racemic epinephrine superior to "regular" L-epinephrine in the treatment of croup?**
Nebulized epinephrine has been shown to provide short-term benefits in the treatment of croup, presumably by reducing tracheal secretions and mucosal edema. Racemic epinephrine has been advocated traditionally, based on the belief that a mixture of D- and L-isomers would lead to less tachycardia. In randomized trials directly comparing the two drugs, they were equivalent in terms of efficacy and side effects. A dose of 5 mL of L-epinephrine 1:1000 is equal to 0.5 mL of the racemic (2%) mixture.

41. **Do patients who receive nebulized epinephrine in the ED require admission to the hospital?**
Because "rebound phenomenon"—tendency to return to baseline clinical picture after epinephrine wears off—administration of nebulized epinephrine to children with croup in the ED became a major reason for admission to the hospital in the 1980s and early 1990s. However, studies have demonstrated a lack of adverse outcome in children who are discharged after a period of observation (typically 2-4 hours) after epinephrine. To be safely discharged, it is recommended that the child remains clinically stable (no stridor at rest, normal air entry, and oxygen saturation) and receives a dose of dexamethasone prior to discharge.

42. **How reliable are signs and symptoms in diagnosing pneumonia in young children?**
Infants and young children with pneumonia often have subtle and nonspecific pulmonary findings. Several authors have found that the risk of pneumonia is very low in the absence of any findings, but they caution that tachypnea may be a sole finding. Tachypnea, in fact, has the greatest negative predictive value. A study of highly febrile children with leukocytosis (white blood cell count >20,000) found that 26% of such children in whom pneumonia was unsuspected clinically had infiltrates on chest radiograph. However, in this study, tachypnea was evaluated qualitatively.

Table 41.4 Most Common Bacterial Causes of Pneumonia in Children

NEONATE (0-2 MONTHS)	INFANT (2 MONTHS-3 YEARS)	PRESCHOOL/SCHOOL AGE (>3 YEARS)
Group B streptococci	*Streptococcus pneumoniae*	*Mycoplasma pneumoniae*
Gram-negative bacilli	*Staphylococcus aureus*	*S. pneumoniae*
S. aureus	*Haemophilus influenzae**	*Chlamydia pneumoniae*
Chlamydia trachomatis		
S. pneumoniae		

*In unimmunized populations.

43. **What are the most common bacterial causes of pneumonia in children?**
   The most common bacterial causes of pneumonia in children are listed in Table 41.4.

44. **Are blood cultures necessary for children with community-acquired pneumonia (CAP)?**
   There is no need for routine blood cultures in nontoxic, fully immunized children who will be managed as outpatients with CAP. Obtain a blood culture if there is no clinical improvement or deterioration after initiation of antibiotic therapy or complicated pneumonia, or if the child is ill enough to require hospital admission.

45. **What are the indications for admission to the hospital for an infant or child with CAP?**
   Admit if there is respiratory distress or hypoxemia (O_2 saturation <90%), infants younger than 3 to 6 months, and suspected infection due to community-associated methicillin-resistant *S. aureus* (CA-MRSA), noncompliant therapy, or when careful observation at home is unlikely.

46. **Which antibiotics are recommended for CAP in infants and children?**
   Use amoxicillin as first-line therapy for a previously healthy, appropriately immunized child with mild-to-moderate pneumonia suspected to be bacterial in origin. If the child is ill enough to be admitted to the hospital, use IV ampicillin when local epidemiologic data indicate lack of substantial high-level penicillin resistance for invasive *Streptococcus pneumoniae*. It is recommended to order a third-generation cephalosporin (ceftriaxone or cefotaxime) when the patient is not fully immunized or if there is suspected high-level penicillin resistance, or for those with life-threatening infection, such as empyema. Add a macrolide empirically for a hospitalized child if *Mycoplasma* or *Chlamydia* infection is suspected, and add vancomycin or clindamycin if infection with *S. aureus* is suspected.

47. **Can ultrasound (US) be used to diagnose pneumonia in children?**
   The standard imaging modality for diagnosing pneumonia is a chest radiograph, but there is emerging evidence that point-of-care US can be used to diagnose CAP. The benefits of US include decreased radiation exposure, decreased cost, and immediate bedside results. However, US may not be available in all settings and is operator dependent. A recent meta-analysis showed improved test characteristics for US versus chest x-ray (CXR).

48. **How does COVID-19 present in children?**
   Most children with severe acute respiratory syndrome coronavirus 2 infection are either asymptomatic or have mild symptoms. Common symptoms include fever, cough, headache, diarrhea and sore throat, myalgias, and shortness of breath. Severe disease requiring admission to a pediatric ICU with significant respiratory support is rare (<1% of cases) and is mostly seen in children with significant comorbidities. Complications to COVID infections in children include a multisystem inflammatory response (MIS-C), shock, myocarditis, and respiratory failure.

49. **What are radiological findings associated with COVID-19 infections?**
   In contrast to adult patients, pediatric patients will often have normal chest radiographs. When abnormal, a CXR will often appear with signs of a viral pneumonia. Chest CT scans will often show bilateral ground-glass opacification, however, this is less predominant than in adult patients.

50. **How should COVID-19 be treated in the pediatric population?**
   Most pediatric cases of COVID-19 are mild and present with URI symptoms and should be treated with supportive measures. While there is no large trial data, the American Academy of Pediatrics currently recommends targeted therapy against COVID-19 for specific high-risk patients at risk for severe disease progression. High-risk criteria include obesity, immunosuppressed patients, neurodevelopmental disorders, patients with medical-technology dependence, sickle cell disease, heart disease, chronic kidney disease, chronic liver disease, and diabetes.

51. **What is E-cigarette- or vaping use–associated lung injury (EVALI)?**

E-cigarette or vaping product use–associated lung injury is an acute lung injury initially recognized in 2019. Consider this serious condition when an adolescent presents with significant respiratory symptoms such as shortness of breath, chest pain, cough, and possibly fever and chills. Many also have gastrointestinal symptoms such as nausea, vomiting, or diarrhea. History reveals recent use of an e-cigarette or vaping product. A CXR shows diffuse hazy opacities. A CT scan shows the classic bilateral opacities, typically ground glass in density. A urine drug screen is frequently positive for terahydrocannabinol. These patients are often hypoxic and require hospital admission. Treatment with systemic glucocorticoids leads to clinical improvement in most patients.

BIBLIOGRAPHY

1. Aregbesola A, Tam CM, Kothari A, Le ML, Ragheb M, Klassen TP. Glucocorticoids for croup in children. *Cochrane Database Syst Rev.* 2023;1(1):CD001955. https://doi.org/10.1002/14651858.CD001955.pub5. PMID: 36626194; PMCID: PMC9831289.
2. Alsohime F, Temsah MH, Al-Nemri AM, Somily AM, Al-Subaie S. COVID-19 infection prevalence in pediatric population: etiology, clinical presentation, and outcome. *J Infect Public Health.* 2020;13(12):1791–1796. https://doi.org/10.1016/j.jiph.2020.10.008.
3. American Academy of Pediatrics. *Management Strategies in Children and Adolescents with Mild to Moderate COVID-19.* https://www.aap.org/en/pages/2019-novel-coronavirus-covid-19-infections/clinical-guidance/outpatientcovid-19-management-strategies-in-children-and-adolescents/.
4. Balk DS, Lee C, Schafer J, Welwarth J, Hardin J, Novack V, Yarza S, Hoffmann B. Lung ultrasound compared to chest X-ray for diagnosis of pediatric pneumonia: a meta-analysis. *Pediatr Pulmonol.* 2018;53(8):1130–1139. https://doi.org/10.1002/ppul.24020. Epub 2018 Apr 26. PMID: 29696826.
5. Bradley JS, Byington CL, Shah SS, et al. The management of community-acquired pneumonia in infants and children older than 3 months Wegener: Clinical Practice Guidelines by Pediatric Infectious Diseases Society and Infectious Diseases Society of America. *Clin Infect Dis.* 2011;53:e25–e376.
6. Corneli HC, Zorc JJ, Holubkov R, et al. The Bronchiolitis Study Group for Pediatric Emergency Care Applied Research Network: bronchiolitis: clinical characteristics associated with hospitalization and length of stay. *Pediatr Emer Care.* 2012;28:99–103.
7. Expert Panel on Management of Asthma. *Guidelines for Diagnosis and Management of Asthma: Clinical Practice Guidelines.* Available from: http://www.nhlbi.nih.gov/guidelines/asthma/asthgdln.htm.
8. Franklin D, Babl FE, Schlapbach LJ, Oakley E, Craig S, Neutze J, Furyk J, Fraser JF, Jones M, Whitty JA, Dalziel SR, Schibler A. A randomized trial of high-flow oxygen therapy in infants with bronchiolitis. *N Engl J Med.* 2018;378(12):1121–1131. https://doi.org/10.1056/NEJMoa1714855. PMID: 29562151.
9. Halstead S, Roosevelt G, Deakyne S, Bajaj L. Discharged on supplemental oxygen from an emergency department in patients with bronchiolitis. *Pediatrics.* 2012;129:e605–e610.
10. Hemani SA, et al. Dexamethasone versus prednisone in children hospitalized for acute asthma exacerbations. *Hosp Pediatr.* 2021;11(11):1263–1272.
11. Keahey L, Bulloch B, Becker AB, et al. Initial oxygen saturation as a predictor of admission in children presenting to emergency department with acute asthma. *Ann Emerg Med.* 2002;40:300–307.
12. Mansbach JM, Clark S, Christopher NC, et al. Prospective multicenter study of bronchiolitis: predicting safe discharges from emergency department. *Pediatrics.* 2008;121:680–688.
13. National Institute for Health and Care Excellence. *Bronchiolitis: Diagnosis and Management of Bronchiolitis in Children. Clinical Guideline NG 9*; 2015.
14. Nelson K, Hirsch A, Nagler J. Pulmonary emergencies. In: Bachur R, Shaw K, eds. *Fleischer and Ludwig's Textbook of Pediatric Emergency Medicine.* 8th ed. Wolters Kluwer; 2021:946–964.
15. Petruzella FD, Gorelick MH. Duration of illness in infants with bronchiolitis evaluated in the emergency department. *Pediatrics.* 2010;126:e285–e290.
16. Ralston SL, et al. Clinical practice guideline: the diagnosis, management, and prevention of bronchiolitis. *Pediatrics.* 2014;134(5):e1474–e1502. https://doi.org/10.1542/peds.2014-2742.
17. Rao DR, Maple KL, Dettori A, Afolabi F, et al. Clinical features of E-cigarette or vaping product use: associated lung injury in teenagers. *Pediatrics.* 2020;146(1):e20194104.
18. Wilkinson M, Bulloch B, Garcia-Filion P, Keahey L. Efficacy of racemic albuterol versus levalbuterol used as a continuous nebulization for the treatment of acute asthma exacerbations: a randomized, double-blind, clinical trial. *J Asthma.* 2011;48:188–193.
19. Yeo HJ, Kim D, Jeon D, et al. Extracorporeal membrane oxygenation for life-threatening asthma refractory to mechanical ventilation: analysis of the Extracorporeal Life Support Organization registry. *Crit Care.* 2017;21:297. https://doi.org/10.1186/s13054-017-1886-8.

CHAPTER 42

TECHNOLOGY-ASSISTED CHILDREN— ACUTE CARE

Jill C. Posner and Ellen G. Szydlowski

1. **How should practitioners approach children with technology-assisted devices?**
   Up to one-quarter of pediatric ED visits are represented by children with complex medical conditions, many of whom utilize devices such as tracheostomy tubes, gastrostomy tubes, cerebrospinal fluid (CSF) shunts, and venous catheters. Practitioners should familiarize themselves with the child's medical history and technology dependence while partnering with the family to understand concerns and goals of the ED visit.

2. **What are the most common reasons for tracheostomy tube placement in a child?**
   In children, tracheostomies are indicated for respiratory insufficiency due to a variety of causes, most commonly bronchopulmonary dysplasia and airway anomalies (e.g., congenital anomalies and subglottic stenosis). Other indications are neuromuscular disorders or central disorders, such as brain tumor or Chiari malformation. A child with a tracheostomy may or may not require additional ventilatory assistance.

3. **How do I determine the appropriate tracheostomy tube size?**
   A tracheostomy tube is sized by three dimensions: inner diameter, outer diameter, and length. Check the flanges of the tube where the inner diameter, and in some cases the outer diameter, is imprinted. Many caretakers of technology-assisted children become experts in their child's technology and are excellent resources for medical personnel. Often, children will travel with emergency boards or "go bags," which contain all the equipment necessary to change a tracheostomy tube, including a replacement tube. If a patient presents without a tube in place and no replacement tube on hand, a reasonable estimate would be to use the formula for sizing an uncuffed endotracheal tube: $(16 + \text{age})/4$ or $4 + (\text{age}/4)$.

KEY POINTS: THREE DIMENSIONS OF A TRACHEOSTOMY TUBE

1. ID (inner diameter)
2. OD (outer diameter)
3. L (length)

4. **What are the immediate management priorities for a child with a tracheostomy in respiratory distress?**
   Assume this patient has an inadequate airway until proven otherwise. The tracheostomy tube may be obstructed or malpositioned. Assess airway patency and the adequacy of breathing through a detailed physical examination. Administer supplemental oxygen. Suction the tracheal tube to evaluate patency and to clear secretions, as this may help to alleviate symptoms. Do not be falsely reassured by a tube entering into the stoma, because it may actually descend into the soft tissues of the neck rather than into the trachea, especially if a prior tracheostomy tube change was attempted and unknowingly resulted in a false passage. An emergent tracheostomy tube change may be indicated if respiratory distress persists, or the cannula is clearly dislodged.

5. **What are the most common causes of respiratory distress in a child who has a tracheostomy tube?**
   Mechanical failure (cannula obstruction or dislodgement), infectious causes (pneumonia, tracheitis, viral respiratory infections), asthma, or reactive airway disease.

6. **What are the causes of bleeding from the tracheostomy tube?**
   The most common cause of bleeding from the tracheostomy tube is drying and friability of the tracheal mucosa due to inadequate humidification. Anatomically, the tracheostomy tube inserts into the airway below the vocal cords. Therefore inspired air bypasses the natural warming and humidification processes of the upper airway. Humidification is an important component of the ventilator circuit for patients with mechanical ventilation. For those patients who breathe independently from the ventilator, a heat-moisture exchanger device is attached at the opening of the tube. This plastic device contains a hydrophilic substance that captures the patient's own heat and humidity on exhalation so that it can be inhaled on inspiration. Other causes of bleeding include granuloma formation, infection (i.e., tracheitis), and erosion of the tube tip into a blood vessel.

7. How should I manage bleeding from the tracheostomy tube?
First, ensure the adequacy of the airway, breathing, and circulation. Suction frequently to avoid aspiration of blood. Minor bleeding usually indicates the need to increase inspired humidification. Evaluation by an airway specialist (e.g., otorhinolaryngologist) may be indicated for persistent minor bleeding to assess for intratracheal granuloma formation. A larger amount of blood may indicate that the tip of the tube has eroded into a blood vessel. Treat this as a surgical emergency with immediate notification of surgical, anesthesia, and operating room personnel. Obtain intravenous (IV) access with two large-bore catheters and initiate resuscitation with isotonic fluids or blood products. Overinflating the tracheostomy tube may tamponade the bleeding vessel, thereby providing a temporizing measure. Importantly, leave the tracheostomy tube in place, as this may be the only way to ensure airway patency.

8. What can I do if I am unable to replace a dislodged tracheostomy tube?
When a tracheostomy tube becomes dislodged, there is a tendency for the stoma to constrict, making it difficult to replace the tube. If stomal constriction prevents insertion of the replacement tube, several options are available: (1) insert a smaller tracheostomy tube; (2) insert a smaller endotracheal tube (being careful not to advance it into a mainstem bronchus), and then slowly dilate the stoma by inserting tubes of successively increasing size; (3) cover the stoma and use a bag-valve-mask device to ventilate by using traditional methods via the patient's upper airway; and (4) insert an oral tracheal tube. Oral intubation may be exceptionally difficult, especially if the original indication for tracheostomy was to overcome an airway anomaly. Therefore use neuromuscular blocking agents with great caution and consider consulting specialists from anesthesiology or otolaryngology early.

9. What are the indicators for placement of a gastrostomy tube in a child?
Enteral feeding may be indicated for patients who have impaired swallowing or motor function, excessive metabolic demand, or impaired absorption or digestion.

10. What is the difference between a percutaneous endoscopic gastrostomy (PEG) tube and a surgically placed gastrostomy tube?
A *PEG* procedure may be performed under sedation or general anesthesia. An endoscope is inserted into the esophagus, and a light source indicates the appropriate location on the stomach wall. An incision is made on the external abdominal wall, and the tube is placed via this aperture. A *surgical or open gastrostomy tube* is placed via laparotomy or laparoscopy under general anesthesia. A purse-string suture is made in the stomach to secure the tube, and the stomach is then sutured to the abdominal wall.

11. What are some of the complications of gastrostomy tubes in children?
Complications can be divided into mechanical tube-related problems and problems with the stoma. The most common complication is dislodgement of the gastrostomy tube. Other mechanical complications include clogging of the tube, leaking around the tube, gastric outlet obstruction, gastric ulceration, and worsening gastroesophageal reflux. Stomal complications include skin irritation, cellulitis, bleeding, and granulation tissue.

12. How is dislodgement of a gastrostomy tube managed in the emergency department (ED)?
The first step is to determine the age of the stoma. If the stoma is older than 6 weeks and has already been replaced previously, the ED clinician should feel comfortable replacing the tube. If the stoma is less than 6 weeks or if the gastrostomy tube has not been replaced yet, contact the gastroenterologist or surgeon for input. The first tube replacement should be performed by the service that created the tract. As soon as possible, stent the stoma open with a temporizing device, such as a similarly sized Foley catheter, placed with lubricant. When the replacement gastrostomy tube is located, remove the Foley catheter and replace it with the gastrostomy tube. Apply gentle, but steady pressure perpendicular to the abdominal wall. If the tube has been dislodged for an extended period of time (hours), smaller Foley catheters may be initially required to dilate the stoma. Always check the balloon's function before replacing the tube. Fill the balloon with water (amount indicated on tube) and check to ensure that it is snug.

KEY POINTS: STEPS TO REPLACE A DISLODGED GASTROSTOMY TUBE

1. Determine the age of the stoma and seek advice if the tube was recently placed.
2. Consider analgesics or anxiolytics.
3. Stent the stoma open with a temporary device.
4. Check the balloon of the new gastrostomy tube.
5. Remove the temporary tube.
6. Place the new gastrostomy tube using lubricant.
7. Fill the balloon and check for adequate fit and location.
8. Aspirate stomach contents to confirm accurate placement.

13. **What is the danger of inserting a tube into a stoma that has recently been placed?**
The stomach wall may not have adhered to the peritoneal lining and skin. The fistula tract can be disrupted, and a false lumen into the peritoneum may be formed. Formula inserted through the tube can lead to chemical or bacterial peritonitis.

14. **Is it necessary to perform a dye study in order to verify gastrostomy tube location after replacement?**
Not usually. Aspiration of stomach contents after the gastrostomy tube is replaced, which confirms that the tube is in the stomach. Listening over the stomach for borborygmi when 15 mL of air is inserted into the tube's lumen is also confirmatory. If in doubt after these actions, take a plain radiograph before and after radiopaque contrast material is inserted through the tube. One may also consider obtaining a dye study in the case of significant trauma to the tract when the tube was dislodged, or difficulty in replacing the gastrostomy tube.

15. **What is the best treatment for a clogged gastrostomy tube?**
Crushed tablets, especially potassium and iron supplements, can cause tube blockage. Warm water has been shown to be superior to vinegar, soda, and juices. Repeated flushing using a small syringe is advised to unblock the tube. Prevention is best accomplished with regular flushing before and after each gastrostomy tube use.

16. **What are some complications that can occur in relation to the stoma?**
Stomal complications include peristomal infections (bacterial and fungal), irritant dermatitis, bleeding, stretching, and hypergranulation tissue.

17. **How is a stomal granuloma treated?**
Application of silver nitrate to the granuloma is most often successful. Use caution to avoid touching the surrounding skin, causing a chemical burn. Consider applying petroleum jelly in a wide radius to protect the peristomal skin.

18. **How common are CSF shunt–related complications?**
In the United States, approximately 15,000 patients/year are admitted to hospitals for complications related to CSF shunt placement including infection, obstruction, and overdrainage.

19. **Name the most common symptoms associated with CSF shunt obstruction.**
Typical symptoms frequently include headache, vomiting, and some alteration of mental status. However, parents' descriptions of "the last time the shunt was obstructed" can be quite reliable. Papilledema and/or vital sign changes (i.e., Cushing triad) are late findings and may reflect significantly increased ICP. Seizures are rarely the only manifestation of increased ICP and more likely represent an underlying seizure disorder.

KEY POINTS: SYMPTOMS OF VENTRICULOPERITONEAL SHUNT OBSTRUCTION

1. Headache
2. Vomiting
3. Change in mental status (may be subtle)
4. Alteration of vital signs

---

20. **What is the best study to diagnose shunt malfunction?**
It has been suggested that easy depression of a shunt reservoir bubble signifies that the distal end is patent, and rapid refilling of this bubble signifies that the proximal shunt is patent. In reality, pumping the shunt identified <40% of obstructed shunts, and "normal filling" missed 10% to 35% of shunt obstructions. Many shunts have no reservoir that can be pumped. Computed tomography (CT) is an adjunct to diagnose shunt obstruction or, when available, rapid T2-weighted magnetic resonance imaging (MRI) is a reasonable alternative. Consider consultation with neurosurgical colleagues early in management to ensure selection of the best imaging study based on MRI capability and programmability.

21. **When should shunt infection be suspected? How can I differentiate CSF shunt infection from obstruction?**
Suspect shunt infection in any febrile child with a shunt. However, in one series, fever was present in fewer than half of the patients with shunt infection. A history of surgical manipulation of the shunt in the prior 2 months

should increase suspicion of infection; infections rarely occur more than 6 months after surgery. An age of less than 6 months at initial shunt placement or having had one or more revisions significantly increases the rate of subsequent infection. CSF shunt infection can lead to obstruction and therefore the symptoms often overlap considerably. Keep in mind that for ventriculoperitoneal shunts, the CSF fluid drains into the abdomen and therefore abdominal pain may be a symptom of shunt infection and/or obstruction.

22. **What studies are helpful in diagnosing CSF shunt infections?**
    CSF culture is the most accurate method of diagnosing a shunt infection. The shunt fluid white blood cell count and a Gram stain are helpful but not foolproof methods of determining if a shunt is infected. The Gram stain is positive in a little more than half of all shunt infections. CSF that is aspirated from an infected shunt usually reveals a moderate pleocytosis but can be misleadingly normal, as can the CSF glucose level. Peripheral white blood cell counts and blood cultures are frequently normal in the presence of a shunt infection. Consult neurosurgery before tapping the shunt as the neurosurgeon may prefer that the procedure not be done by ED personnel due to the risk of introducing infection during the procedure.

23. **What techniques can an emergency medicine practitioner use to treat a critically ill patient with a CSF shunt obstruction?**
    When a child with a suspected CSF shunt obstruction is critically ill with signs of increased intracranial pressure (ICP), emergent action is required. Hyperventilation and hypertonic saline administration may be used but, if possible, relieve the pressure by accessing the shunt. If there is a distal obstruction or partial proximal obstruction, withdraw fluid from the shunt reservoir in a sterile fashion using a 23-gauge butterfly needle and 20-mL syringe. This potentially lifesaving procedure is usually done by a neurosurgeon, but do not delay if the patient's condition is deteriorating—the procedure is well described in pediatric emergency procedure textbooks.

24. **What is the role of an endoscopic third ventriculostomy (ETV)?**
    ETV allows for management of pediatric hydrocephalus without the utilization of an indwelling catheter, thus minimizing the risk of infection and shunt disconnection. In brief, the endoscopic neurosurgical procedure creates fenestrations at the base of the third ventricle, allowing for drainage to the basal cisterns. These patients are at risk of restenosis and obstruction and should be evaluated promptly for shunt failure in the same fashion as those patients with CSF shunts.

25. **What are the indications for a central venous catheter (CVC)?**
    CVCs may be indicated in patients with limited or difficult peripheral access, need for parenteral nutrition, chemotherapy, or apheresis. The most common types of CVCs seen in the ED are tunneled catheters (e.g., Broviac or Hickman) and totally implantable venous access devices, also known as ports.

26. **What are some tips for accessing a tunneled catheter?**
    Use an aseptic technique whenever you access an indwelling venous device. Do not use clamps or hemostats with teeth because they may damage the device. Use povidone-iodine or 2% chlorhexidine and clean the hub for at least 15 seconds. Use a 5 to 10 mL syringe as smaller syringes can generate significant pressure and cause the catheter to break. Flush the entire IV circuit before accessing the system. Discard the first 3 to 5 cc of blood before sending your samples for the most accurate results. Always close the clamps when the system is open, and do not infuse medications or fluid until patency of the system has been established. Flush the catheter with 10 mL of saline between medications to reduce the chance of occlusion and flush the cap or reservoir with heparin when the procedure is completed.

27. **What are some tips for accessing a port?**
    Apply topical anesthetic cream if possible. After the allotted time, wipe off and clean the skin with povidone-iodine or 2% chlorhexidine. Using a sterile technique, insert a Huber noncoring needle into reservoir diaphragm. Aspirate and flush to confirm patency. After use, flush with heparin.

KEY POINTS: COMPLICATIONS FROM ACCESSING A CVC

1. Occlusion of the catheter that can be positional or due to precipitate
2. Air embolus
3. Break in the catheter
4. Displacement of the catheter
5. Infection

BIBLIOGRAPHY

1. Ares G, Hunter C. Central venous access in children: indications, devices and risks. *Curr Opin Pediatr.* 2017;29:340–346.
2. Duhaime AC. Evaluation and management of shunt infections in children with hydrocephalus. *Clin Pediatr.* 2006;45(8):705–713.
3. Fleet S, Duggan C. *Overview of Enteral Nutrition in Infants and Children.* UpToDate; 2021. https://www.uptodate.com/contents/overview-of-enteral-nutrition-ininfants-and-children.
4. Fuchs S. Gastrostomy tubes, care and feeding. *Pediatr Emer Care.* 2017;33:787–793.
5. Hasanain AA, Abdullah A, Alsawy MFM, et al. Incidence of and causes for ventriculoperitoneal shunt failure in children younger than 2 years: a systematic review. *J Neurol Surg A.* 2019;80:26–33.
6. Kohna J, McKeona M, Munhallb D, Blanchettea S, Wells S, Watters K. Standardization of pediatric tracheostomy care with "Go-bags". *Int J Pediatr Otorhinolaryngol.* 2019;121:154–156.
7. Lee P, DiPatri Jr. AJ. Evaluation of suspected cerebrospinal fluid shunt complications in children. *Clin Pediatr Emerg Med.* 2008;9(2):76–82.
8. Mitchell RB, Hussey HM, Setzen G, Jacobs IN, Nussenbaum B, Dawson C, Brown CA, Brandt C, Deakins K, Hartnick C, Merati A. Clinical consensus statement: tracheostomy Care. *Otolaryngol Head Neck Surg.* 2013;148(1):6–20.
9. Posner JC. Acute care of the child with a tracheostomy. *Pediatr Emerg Care.* 1999;15:49–54.
10. Posner JC, Cronan K, Badaki O, Fein JA. Emergency care of the technology-assisted child. *Clin Pediatr Emerg Med.* 2006;7:38–51.
11. Sandberg F, Viktorsdottir M, Salo M, et al. Comparison in major complications in children after laparoscopy-assisted gastrostomy and percutaneous endoscopic gastrostomy placement: a meta-analysis. *Pediatr Surg Int.* 2018;34:1321–1327.
12. Simon TD, Whitlock KB, Riva-Cambrin J, et al. Revision surgeries are associated with significant increased risk of subsequent cerebrospinal fluid shunt infection. *Pediatr Infect Dis J.* 2012;31(6):551–556.
13. Sivaganesan A, Krishnamurthy R, Sahni D, et al. Neuroimaging of ventriculoperitoneal shunt complications in children. *Pediatr Radiol.* 2012;42(9):1029–1046.
14. Szydlowski E, Cronan K, Fein J, Posner J. Technology-assisted children. In: Shaw KN, Bachur RG, eds. *Fleischer and Ludwig's Textbook of Pediatric Emergency Medicine.* 8th ed. Wolters Kluwer; 2021:E135-1-E135-23. eBook.
15. Townley A, Wincentak J, Krog K, et al. Paediatric gastrostomy stoma complications and treatments: a rapid scoping review. *J Clin Nurs.* 2018;27:1369–1380.
16. Walters KF. Tracheostomy in infants and children. *Respir Care.* 2017;62(6):799–825.
17. Wiley JF, II Duhaime AC. Ventricular puncture. In: King C, Henretig FM, eds. *Textbook of Pediatric Emergency Procedures.* 2nd ed. Lippincott Williams & Wilkins; 2008:527–530.

DENTAL/PERIODONTAL EMERGENCIES

Thomas M. Kennedy

CHAPTER 43

1. **Does teething cause fever in infants?**
   Teething has been blamed for several symptoms in infants throughout time, ranging from fever, congestion, diarrhea, and rashes to seizures and death. A prospective descriptive study of 475 tooth eruptions in 89 infants looked at parental reports of 18 "teething symptoms" daily for 8 months. Symptoms that were statistically associated with the eruption of a tooth included low-grade fever (temperature <102°F), irritability, increased biting, drooling, gum-rubbing, sucking, wakefulness, ear-rubbing, facial rash, and decreased appetite for solid foods. Symptoms that were *not* associated with teething include high-grade fever, congestion, cough, loose stools, sleep disturbance, decreased appetite for liquids, and rashes other than facial rash. Do not assume teething is the cause of fever in an ill-appearing young infant.

2. **Can children and adolescents develop fever from the eruption of teeth?**
   A localized, acute infection surrounding an erupting tooth, known as pericoronitis, can cause fever in children and adolescents. It is most often associated with the eruption of the third molars, or "wisdom teeth," in adolescence, but a milder form can also be seen with the eruption of the first permanent molar in children 6 to 7 years old. Symptoms include pain, erythema, and edema localized to the gingiva in the retromolar area. Fever, painful lymphadenopathy, dysphagia, and trismus may also be present. The cusp of the erupting tooth is usually visible or palpable, and exudate may be expressed from beneath the infected flap of gum tissue.

3. **What is the cause of this black-blue cystic lesion on the alveolar ridge of an 8-year-old child?**
   An eruption cyst, associated with the eruption of a primary or permanent tooth, may arise from the pre-eruptive dental sac (Fig. 43.1). It appears as swelling of the alveolar ridge. Occasionally, it can fill with blood and is then referred to as an eruption hematoma. Treatment is unnecessary because the erupting tooth usually emerges within several days.

4. **Why does this dental abscess emerge from the labial aspect of the gingiva rather than the lingual aspect?**
   Infection travels along the planes of least resistance, which is predetermined by anatomic barriers such as muscles, bones, and fascia (Fig. 43.2). Pus perforates bone where it is thinnest and weakest. Therefore abscesses form on the buccal or labial surface of the gingiva in the mandible. In the maxilla, they form on the lingual aspect of the molars and the labial aspect of the anterior teeth. If the infection does not drain intraorally, it can rapidly progress along the fascial planes of the face or neck.

5. **When should you consider hospital admission for a patient with a dental abscess?**
   Most dental abscesses can be managed on an outpatient basis with oral antibiotics and close dental follow-up for drainage or extraction of the affected tooth. Analgesics and warm compresses over the area on the face are helpful. Amoxicillin, or clindamycin for penicillin-allergic patients, is the preferred oral antibiotics. Consider hospitalization for parenteral antibiotics if there is a high fever or secondary facial cellulitis, to halt the potentially dangerous spread. Also, consider admission if the degree of swelling compromises the airway or ability to drink fluids, if the patient is toxic-appearing or lacks appropriate social support for follow-up. Consult a dentist for drainage of the abscess.

6. **How do you manage persistent hemorrhage after tooth extraction?**
   An extraction site may normally ooze for 8 to 12 hours after the procedure. Persistent oozing beyond 12 hours or frank bleeding warrants intervention. A home remedy that can be effective is the application of a moistened tea bag over the socket because tannic acid in tea may initiate or accelerate coagulation. If this is ineffective, having the patient bite down on folded gauze placed directly over the open socket for 30 to 60 minutes is indicated. If bleeding continues despite direct pressure, consider the application of a topical hemostatic or antifibrinolytic agent such as tranexamic acid. Alternatively, you can close the socket with a 4-0 or 5-0 chromic gut suture after administering local anesthesia.

7. **What is "dry socket"?**
   "Dry socket" refers to a condition known as alveolar osteitis. This is a postoperative complication that usually presents 72 hours after mandibular wisdom tooth extraction and results in severe pain. The exact pathogenesis of this condition is not well understood, but it is thought to result from early disintegration of the blood clot within the

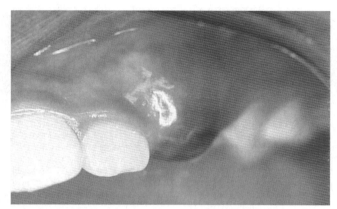

Fig. 43.1 Eruption hematoma. (From Baumhardt H, Chapman M, D'Alesio A, et al. Oral disorders. In: Zitelli BJ, McIntire SC, Nowalk AJ, et al., eds. *Zitelli and Davis' Atlas of Pediatric Physical Diagnosis.* 8th ed. Elsevier; 2023.)

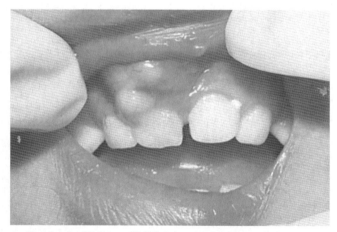

Fig. 43.2 Dental abscess. (From Baumhardt H, Chapman M, D'Alesio A, et al. Oral disorders. In: Zitelli BJ, McIntire SC, Nowalk AJ, et al., eds. *Zitelli and Davis' Atlas of Pediatric Physical Diagnosis.* 8th ed. Elsevier; 2023.)

alveolar socket and exposure of the underlying bone. Examination reveals a "dry socket." Alveolar osteitis differs from the rare postextraction infection, where examination reveals pus within the alveolar socket. Patients with alveolar osteitis should be referred to a dentist for debridement and packing of the socket with local anesthesia. Antibiotic therapy is not indicated.

8. **What are the most common causes of stomatitis in young children?**
   Stomatitis is most commonly caused by viral infections in young children less than 6 years old. Herpes simplex virus causes a syndrome of very painful vesicles and gingival inflammation, sometimes to the point of bleeding, in the anterior mouth and tongue. Herpes stomatitis is often associated with high fever (temperature of 39°C-40°C), headache, and cervical lymphadenopathy. Coxsackie viruses usually cause a vesicular eruption on the posterior pharynx. Also known as herpangina, this infection causes pain, low-grade fever, and drooling. An acral viral exanthem (hand, foot, and mouth disease) is seen with some strains of coxsackie virus.

9. **Which treatments are effective for viral stomatitis?**
   Acyclovir has benefits for immunocompetent patients with herpes stomatitis if given within 96 hours of symptom onset and at any time, regardless of symptom onset, for immunosuppressed patients.
   "Magic mouthwash," which is usually made as a combination of aluminum hydroxide and magnesium hydroxide suspension (Maalox) and diphenhydramine (Benadryl) with or without viscous lidocaine, lacks evidence

of benefit and has potential harm due to toxicity from systemic absorption of the medications. A randomized, blinded, and placebo-controlled trial showed no improvement in oral fluid intake among children presenting to an emergency department with infectious oral ulcers 1 hour after the administration of viscous lidocaine versus placebo.

Oral analgesics and antipyretics are helpful. Ensure hydration. Intravenous fluids may be needed for some patients with stomatitis who refuse to drink.

10. How can you distinguish aphthous stomatitis from herpes stomatitis?

Aphthae are recurrent, circular, shallow, small (2-4 mm), painful ulcers with a yellowish floor and sharply defined red margins (Fig. 43.3). They often start in childhood or adolescence and peak in early adulthood before spontaneously resolving. In contrast to herpes stomatitis (Fig. 43.4), they are never preceded by vesicles and only occur on nonkeratinized areas of the mouth, such as the tongue, cheek, or vestibule. If the hard palate or gingival margins are affected, it is unlikely to be aphthous stomatitis. Treatment of aphthous ulcers with medication is usually unsatisfactory, and the best recommendation may simply be to eat a bland, nonacidic diet to avoid irritating them.

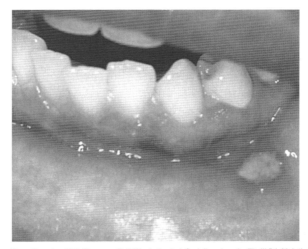

Fig. 43.3 Aphthous ulcer. (From Baumhardt H, Chapman M, D'Alesio A, et al. Oral disorders. In: Zitelli BJ, McIntire SC, Nowalk AJ, et al., eds. *Zitelli and Davis' Atlas of Pediatric Physical Diagnosis.* 8th ed. Elsevier; 2023.)

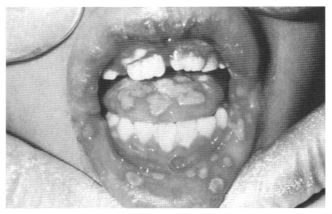

Fig. 43.4 Herpes simplex virus stomatitis. (From Neville BW, Damm DD, Allen CM, et al. Viral infection. In: *Oral and Maxillofacial Pathology,* 4th ed. Philadelphia, PA: Elsevier, 2016, Fig. 7.1 (Courtesy of Dr. David Johnsen)).

11. **What causes acute necrotizing ulcerative gingivitis (ANUG)?**
This condition, also known as Vincent disease or trench mouth, results from increases in fusiform bacillus and *Borrelia vincentii*, a spirochete, which usually coexist in a symbiotic relationship with other oral flora. Risk factors include emotional stress, immunosuppression, malnutrition, and poor oral hygiene. ANUG is typically seen in adolescents and young adults. Patients complain of gingival pain with a wedging sensation as if something is stuck between their teeth and a metallic taste. They may have hyperemic gingivae, and the gingivae between teeth are usually missing or "punched out" (Fig. 43.5). Treat this condition with amoxicillin or metronidazole for 7 to 10 days and 0.12% chlorhexidine (Peridex) rinses. Refer the patient to a dentist after the acute phase is over for debridement.

12. **Are dental caries contagious?**
In a sense, yes. The disease of dental caries is multifactorial in origin, and *Streptococcus mutans* has been shown to be involved in its pathogenesis. This bacterium can be transmitted both vertically and horizontally. It can colonize the mouths of infants even prior to the eruption of teeth. Thus practices such as the premoistening of a pacifier with maternal saliva before insertion into the infant's mouth should be strongly discouraged.

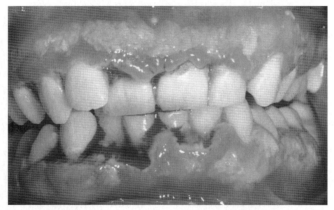

Fig. 43.5 Acute necrotizing ulcerative gingivitis. (From Neville BW, Damm DD, Allen CM, et al., eds. Periodontal diseases. In: Neville BW, Damm DD, Allen CM, et al., eds. *Oral and Maxillofacial Pathology.* 4th ed. Elsevier; 2016.)

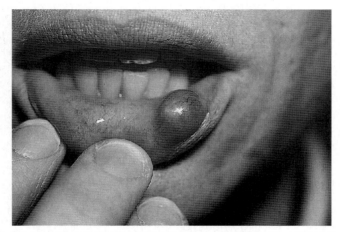

Fig. 43.6 Mucocele. (From Swartz MH. *Textbook of Physical Diagnosis: History and Examination.* 7th ed. Philadelphia, PA: Saunders, 2014, Fig. 9.13.)

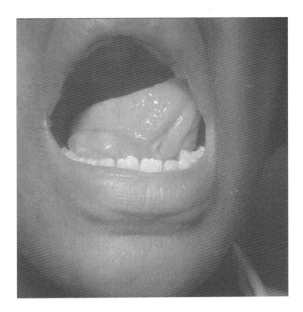

Fig. 43.7 Ranula.

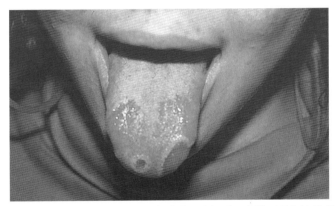

Fig. 43.8 Geographic tongue. (From James Fitzpatrick, Joseph Morelli: *Dermatology Secrets*, 6th ed. Philadelphia, PA: Mosby, 2020, Fig. 57.6.)

13. **How does a ranula differ from a mucocele? What is a plunging ranula?**

A mucocele is a mucous retention cyst usually located in the mucosa of the lower lip (Fig. 43.6). A ranula is a mucous retention cyst on the floor of the mouth, under the tongue (Fig. 43.7). Both are painless and thought to be due to trauma to minor salivary gland ducts. A plunging ranula occurs when fluid from the obstructed gland dissects between the fascial planes and muscles of the base of the tongue to the submandibular space, causing bulging of the soft tissues in the submandibular area. Treatment includes excision for mucoceles and marsupialization for a ranula.

14. **What is meant by the term geographic tongue?**

Geographic tongue, or benign migratory glossitis, is a painless condition of erythematous "islands" of denuded papillae surrounded by elevated whitish borders (Fig. 43.8). The islands appear to migrate over the surface of the tongue over time, akin to the movement of continents on the globe. The etiology is unknown, with allergy, infection, and stress all implicated as potential contributors. It generally resolves without treatment over a period of weeks to months.

15. **What is Ria-Fede disease?**
    It is a condition seen in infants with a natal or neonatal tooth characterized by ulcerations on the ventral surface of the tongue from irritation caused by the edges of the lower incisor during nursing or suckling. Treatment is rarely required but is indicated in two scenarios. If there is bleeding and pain from the irritation, the tooth can be smoothed off in the dental office. If the tooth interferes with feeding, extraction may be necessary.

16. **What is Ludwig angina?**
    This is a life-threatening, rapidly progressive cellulitis of the sublingual and submandibular spaces. Patients will have high fever, erythema of the surrounding skin, and trismus. The infection can spread to the neck and cause airway obstruction. Treatment involves broad-spectrum antibiotics and surgical drainage.

KEY POINTS: CONDITIONS FOR WHICH TEETHING SHOULD NOT BE BLAMED

1. High-grade fever
2. Nasal congestion
3. Cough
4. Diarrhea

KEYPOINTS: AREAS INTO WHICH UNTREATED DENTAL ABSCESSES CAN EXTEND

1. Sinuses
2. Orbits
3. Brain
4. Airway
5. Mediastinum

BIBLIOGRAPHY

1. Fida Z., Chase I.I. Dental Emergencies. In Shaw K.N., Bachur R.G., ed. *Fleischer and Ludwig's Textbook of Pediatric Emergency Medicine*, 8th ed. Philadelphia, PA: Wolters Kluwer; 2021: 1313–1318.
2. Hopper S.M., McCarthy M., Tancharoen C., et al. Topical lidocaine to improve oral intake in children with painful infectious mouth ulcers: a blinded, randomized, placebo-controlled trial. *Ann Emerg Med*. 2014;63(3):292–299.
3. Markman L. Teething: facts and fiction. *Pediatr Rev* 2009; 30 (8): e59–64.

GENERAL SURGERY EMERGENCIES

Louise Malburg and Dee Hodge

CHAPTER 44

1. **What is the most common acute surgical condition of the abdomen?**
   Appendicitis.

2. **What is the classic presenting history in a child with suspected appendicitis?**
   If you are lucky, the child will have a history of periumbilical pain that migrated to the right lower quadrant (RLQ). However, pediatric patients rarely read the textbook. Usually, the child presents with a history of diffuse abdominal pain, possibly associated with vomiting or anorexia, and a low-grade fever. Diarrhea may also be present and is a common cause of misdiagnosis in patients <3 years of age. Unlike with adults, it is often hard to obtain an accurate history and to reliably examine children. The presenting symptoms of appendicitis are similar to those of many other childhood diseases. Gastroenteritis, urinary tract infections, streptococcal pharyngitis, constipation, and pneumonia are some of the illnesses that mimic appendicitis. Once peritoneal inflammation occurs, most older children with appendicitis will complain of pain in the RLQ.

3. **Where else might a child with appendicitis localize pain?**
   If the appendix is located in the lateral gutter, the child may have tenderness in the lateral abdomen or flank. An appendix pointing toward the pelvis might cause pubic pain and diarrhea. A retrocecal appendix causes pain on deep palpation. This information is important because not all children with appendicitis present with RLQ pain. In addition, it is important to consider the presentation of perforated appendicitis. These children often have fever, muscle guarding, and a longer duration of pain, and they tend to be younger.

4. **Does a white blood cell (WBC) count of only 11.5 WBCs/mm^3 rule out appendicitis?**
   No. A child with a nonperforated appendicitis usually has a WBC count of 11,000 to 15,000 WBCs/mm^3 in the first 1 to 2 days of illness. A higher WBC count with a left shift may be found later in the course, as the appendix undergoes further degeneration, or if the appendix has ruptured. Although laboratory values may help to support your clinical diagnosis, they should not replace a good history and physical examination.

5. **What laboratory findings are suggestive of appendicitis?**
   The two tests that should be done on all patients who are suspected of having appendicitis are a complete blood count (CBC) with differential and urinalysis (UA). Elevated leukocyte counts and a left shift appear to be highly associated with both uncomplicated and complicated acute appendicitis and are a good tool to aid in diagnosis. Although a normal or low WBC count may still be found in patients with appendicitis, this combination has been found to have a high negative predictive value. The UA may show ketosis due to decreased oral intake. If the inflamed appendix lies near the bladder or ureter, sterile pyuria may be seen as well. However, a normal CBC and a normal UA do not rule out appendicitis.

6. **Is C-reactive protein (CRP) helpful in diagnosing appendicitis?**
   Greatly elevated CRP levels (e.g., >50 mg/L) have been found to be associated with perforated appendicitis. A patient with a normal leukocyte count and a normal CRP level is unlikely to have appendicitis. Although many institutions do not routinely measure CRP in the diagnostic workup of appendicitis, there is increasing evidence that it may be an important consideration in assigning a clinical relative risk.

7. **What is the pediatric appendicitis score (PAS)?**
   The use of clinical scoring systems can help to risk stratify patients with suspected appendicitis and determine the need for advanced imaging or surgical consultation. The most widely used tool in the pediatric population is the PAS (Table 44.1), which uses a combination of three symptoms, three physical signs, and two laboratory findings. A point value is assigned to each feature with a maximum score of 10. Scores of 6 or higher are generally considered high risk for acute appendicitis.

8. **What are the pros and cons of ultrasound (US) in the diagnosis of appendicitis?**
   Appendiceal US is the diagnostic test of choice in the evaluation of pediatric appendicitis because it is noninvasive, quick, and does not expose patients to ionizing radiation. The appearance of a thickened, noncompressible appendix greater than 6 mm in diameter confirms the diagnosis. The sensitivity and specificity vary by institution but generally range between 44% and 88% and 90% to 97%, respectively. However, there are limitations to this technology:

Table 44.1. Pediatric Appendicitis Score

FEATURE	SCORE
Fever	1
Anorexia	1
Nausea/vomiting	1
RLQ tenderness	2
Migration of pain	1
Pain with cough/hop/percussion	2
Leukocytosis (WBC >10,000/mm³)	1
Neutrophilia (ANC >7500/mcL)	1
Total score	10

ANC, absolute neutrophil count; RLQ, right lower quadrant; WBC, white blood cell.

- It requires an experienced technician.
- It may be uncomfortable and difficult to perform on a crying, uncooperative child due to a need for graded compression of the overlying bowel.
- It has low sensitivity in identifying perforated appendicitis.
- The appendix may not be fully visualized in cases of a retrocecal orientation, obesity, or an inexperienced technician.

9. **How should a patient with an equivocal US be managed?**
A US may be equivocal or nondiagnostic if the appendix is not visualized or only partially visualized. Typically, in cases of appendicitis, secondary signs may be seen, such as surrounding free fluid, echogenic fat, and/or regional lymphadenopathy. If these signs are present, or if the patient's PAS is in the high-risk category, you should consider additional testing with computed tomography (CT) or magnetic resonance imaging (MRI) or surgical consultation. Low- or intermediate-risk patients may be discharged with strict return precautions and reexamination in 24 hours, or admitted for observation and serial abdominal examinations. Parental comfort, local resources, and their ability to return to the emergency department (ED) if needed should all be considered prior to discharge.

10. **What are the pros and cons of CT in the diagnosis of appendicitis?**
CT has a sensitivity of about 94% and a specificity of about 95% for the diagnosis of appendicitis. Drawbacks for CT include higher cost, the need for contrast, and a longer preparatory period prior to the study. However, radiation exposure is the greatest concern. In an effort to reduce the exposure to unnecessary radiation, many institutions have initiated protocols for the evaluation of appendicitis, and there are several studies describing the protocols and outcomes. In most studies, when imaging is needed in the evaluation, the US is the first choice. If the US is equivocal or if it is negative and there is still a concern for appendicitis, most authors recommend either a CT scan or admission for serial abdominal examinations.

11. **Is oral or intravenous (IV) contrast needed to diagnose acute appendicitis on abdominal CT?**
For the evaluation of acute appendicitis, CT should be completed with IV contrast. Oral contrast is not necessary as it takes longer to complete and often causes the patient to vomit. Additionally, neither rectal nor oral contrast has been shown to increase the diagnostic accuracy of CT. Noncontrast abdominal CTs have a slightly lower sensitivity and specificity for acute appendicitis and are much less accurate in characterizing complications such as perforation or abscess. When available, MRI without contrast is a better choice for a patient with no IV access.

12. **Can MRI be used instead of an abdominal CT scan to diagnose appendicitis?**
Yes. MRI is an alternative to abdominal CT in children suspected of appendicitis when the patient has an inconclusive US. It has the advantage of not exposing patients to radiation and maintains a high sensitivity and specificity of approximately 94% when performed either with or without contrast. MRI is limited by cost and the need for children to remain still for an extended period, which can be achieved with swaddling or sedation. However, some institutions offer rapid protocols that eliminate this concern.

13. **Why does the pain of appendicitis typically start centrally (periumbilically) and then localize to the RLQ?**
The initial pain of appendicitis is visceral: a dull, aching pain localized to the mid- or lower abdomen. Visceral or splanchnic pain originates in those abdominal organs, such as the appendix, that have visceral peritoneum. Increased hollow viscus wall tension and ischemia cause impulses to be sent from the organ to the spinal cord. In the case of the appendix, visceral afferent autonomic nerves enter the spinal cord from T8 to T10. These segments supply the periumbilical area, which explains the initial, poorly localized pain associated with appendicitis.
    As the appendix becomes more inflamed, it causes inflammation of the serosa and parietal peritoneum. The inflammation triggers local somatic pain fibers. Somatic pain is mediated by afferent nerve fibers in segmental spinal nerves. Thus, the pain is sharper and more localized, usually to the RLQ.

14. **Describe the pathophysiologic mechanism that leads to appendicitis.**
The appendix contains increasing amounts of lymphatic tissue as a child ages. Acute appendicitis occurs when the lumen of the appendix becomes obstructed. Sources of obstruction include fecaliths, lymphatic hypertrophy, worms, vegetable matter, and tumors. The appendix continues to secrete mucosal fluid, leading to distention of the viscus.

15. **Which of these patients with appendicitis is most likely to present with a perforation? Why?**
    - A 2-year-old boy with abdominal pain and diarrhea for a few days
    - A 12-year-old girl with severe pain for 24 hours
    - An 8-year-old boy with a temperature of 40°C
    - A 16-year-old with a WBC count of 18,000/mm^3
        Although any one of the patients could present with a perforated appendix, the 2-year-old boy with pain for a few days and diarrhea is statistically most likely to have a perforation at presentation. The rates of perforation are higher in younger children because of several factors: (1) the appendix is more thin-walled, predisposing them to early perforation, (2) younger children are less able to communicate clearly, resulting in prolonged symptoms before diagnosis, (3) the level of suspicion for appendicitis is often lower in younger age groups, leading to a delay in diagnosis, and (4) the signs and symptoms of appendicitis are often nonspecific in the younger child.

16. **Why does perforated appendicitis progress to peritonitis more quickly in infants and children than in adults?**
The omentum is not as well developed in infants and children as it is in adults. Because the omentum is primarily responsible for walling off the infection in a perforated appendix, its insufficiency contributes to the development of peritonitis. This complication of perforated appendicitis may play a role in the increased mortality risk in young children with appendicitis.

17. **What conditions must be considered in a teenage girl with symptoms of appendicitis?**
Gynecologic conditions and emergencies should be considered in the differential diagnosis of any teenage girl with RLQ pain. Specifically, ovarian cysts, corpus luteal cysts, mittelschmerz, tubal pregnancy, ovarian torsion, and salpingitis can all present similarly to appendicitis.

18. **Your 10-year-old patient with presumed appendicitis is in extreme pain. His tearful mother is asking if there is anything you can give him to make him feel better. The surgeons will not be available to examine him for another hour. What should you do?**
Provide pain relief for this patient! Studies in both children and adults have shown that the administration of opiates decreases pain scores but does not hide evidence of peritoneal irritation. In the pediatric patient, adequate pain control can even improve your ability to obtain an accurate abdominal examination.
    Despite the growing evidence that opiate administration will not affect diagnostic accuracy, some surgeons still prefer to examine patients prior to the administration of pain medication. It is important to respect the practice in your institution while remaining aware of the current literature. Reassure your patient's mother that you will address the issue and give your surgical colleagues a call to let them know your plan.

19. **Can acute appendicitis be managed nonoperatively?**
The traditional treatment for acute appendicitis is surgical appendectomy. In recent years, there has been an increasing body of evidence supporting nonoperative treatment with a course of antibiotics only. Small, prospective pediatric trials have shown early treatment success in 90% of patients with uncomplicated appendicitis without an appendicolith after 24 to 48 hours of broad-spectrum IV antibiotics, which is typically transitioned to oral antibiotics to complete a course of 7 days. Recurrence of appendicitis within 1 year occurs in roughly 20% of patients, ultimately requiring surgical treatment. Although these preliminary studies show that nonoperative management may be a valid alternative for uncomplicated appendicitis more large, controlled trials are needed.

20. **What is the most common cause of acute pancreatitis in children?**
Abdominal trauma.

21. **What are the radiographic findings in a child with acute mechanical bowel obstruction?**
Multiple dilated loops of the bowel and an air-fluid level visible in the upright or lateral decubitus views on plain films are common.

22. **What is the most common cause of acute intestinal obstruction in a child between 3 and 12 months of age?**
Intussusception. This occurs when a proximal segment of the bowel telescopes into a distal segment. It is commonly ileocolic, but the small bowel may also telescope into itself.

23. **Define "lead point."**
The lead point is the area that is thought to initiate the intussusceptum. The causes of lead points differ by age. In infants, lead points are often hypertrophied Peyer patches. In older children, there are many possibilities for focal lead points, including intestinal polyps, Meckel diverticulum, and a tumor.

24. **What causes intussusception?**
There is no definitive cause, though there is an association between intussusception and a history of a preceding viral illness, diarrhea, or, perhaps, Henoch-Schönlein purpura (HSP). The association between the rotavirus vaccine and increased frequency of intussusception led to the recall of the original rotavirus vaccine.

25. **How does the child with intussusception present?**
The classic history is that the patient has crampy abdominal pain. Because this is a disease that mostly occurs in preverbal children, the parent may give the history that the child behaves normally or is slightly irritable but has episodic bouts of severe abdominal pain characterized by drawing the knees to the chest, laying still, or screaming inconsolably. Some children may present with profound lethargy. Intussusception should be a strong consideration in the differential diagnosis of any infant or toddler presenting with lethargy. Vomiting may become bilious as the small bowel becomes completely obstructed. There may be a history of rectal bleeding or bloody stool. On physical examination, the child's abdomen may be distended due to the partial or complete obstruction of the bowel. You may be able to palpate a sausage-like mass, typically in the right upper quadrant (RUQ).

26. **What is the origin of pain in intussusception?**
Intussusception is the result of invagination of a portion of the proximal intestine into the distal intestine. The intussuscepted mass can obstruct the intestinal lumen. Abdominal pain is due to distension and peristaltic rushes against the mass.

27. **If there is no abdominal tenderness on examination, can you dismiss intussusception in the differential diagnosis?**
No. Because intussusception is a dynamic process, that is, the bowel can telescope in and out, and abdominal pain may be intermittent. The classic signs and symptoms of intussusception—abdominal pain, palpable abdominal mass, and red currant jelly stool—are found in fewer than 50% of cases.

28. **What is "currant jelly" stool?**
Currant jelly is made from a small, round, acidic berry that may be black or red. This term is used to describe the reddish, heme-positive stool of mixed mucus and blood associated with intussusception. It occurs when the edematous bowel causes compression of the mesenteric veins. It is a late sign of intussusception indicating mucosal damage and is present in only about one-third of patients. Do not rule out the possibility of intussusception in the absence of currant jelly stool.

29. **How do you diagnose intussusception?**
Have a high index of suspicion for lethargic infants and toddlers and take a detailed history and physical examination! The US is the diagnostic test of choice for intussusception and is highly sensitive and specific. The classic appearance of the transverse view is a "target" or "doughnut sign" with concentric bowel loops that are hyperechoic centrally and hypoechoic externally due to edema of the bowel wall. Obtaining these diagnostic views is simple and may be accomplished by emergency medicine providers with training in point-of-care US.

30. **How does intussusception appear on a radiograph?**
A positive finding on an obstruction series includes the target or crescent sign. The target sign is a mass in the RUQ that may have a target-like appearance or may just resemble a solid mass. The crescent sign is caused by the lead point protruding into a gas-filled pocket, which may result in a crescent-shaped finding on a radiograph. However, these signs are not present in most cases of ileocolic intussusception and should not be relied upon to either rule in or out the diagnosis.

The main role radiographs play in the evaluation of intussusception is to rule out an associated bowel perforation.

31. **What is the only absolute contraindication to enema in the diagnosis of intussusception?**
The presence of free air or signs of peritoneal irritation is the only absolute contraindication.

32. **How do you treat intussusception?**
This is a trick question, as the diagnostic test (enema) is usually therapeutic as well. Intussusception can be reduced by either air or hydrostatic enema in about 85% of cases. The reduction should only be performed in a facility where pediatric surgery is immediately available, due to the risk of perforation of potentially gangrenous bowel. Prophylactic antibiotics prior to reduction are no longer recommended as it has not been shown to decrease postreduction complications.

33. **Do all patients with intussusception require hospitalization?**
Overall recurrence rates are 7.5% to 15% after a successful enema reduction of intussusception, regardless of the technique. However, recent evidence suggests that early recurrence within 24 to 48 hours is much lower, ranging from 0.6% to 2.45%, and is unlikely to occur during a hospital or ED observation stay. The American Pediatric Surgical Association recommends ED observation for 4 hours postreduction then discharge to home with ensured follow-up and return precautions.

34. **How do you explain intussusception to the parents of the child you just diagnosed?**
Visual descriptions are helpful for families. One way to explain it is the sock model. In other words, if you want turn a sock inside out, you pull the toe of the sock through the cuff. This is similar to what the bowel does.

35. **Why are inguinal hernias usually repaired when detected in young infants?**
There is a high risk of intestinal incarceration in male infants and adnexal entrapment in female infants. Hernias that reduce spontaneously are generally repaired electively soon after detection. Those that require sedation and manual reduction are usually repaired 24 to 48 hours after reduction.

36. **Is an incarcerated hernia more common in girls or boys?**
Contrary to what you might think, it is more common in girls and usually involves the ovary rather than the intestine.

37. **What is the difference between an incarcerated and a strangulated hernia?**
Incarceration means that the intestine or ovary is nonreducible but not necessarily gangrenous. However, if the hernia is not reduced, it can become strangulated. Once strangulated, venous and lymphatic obstruction occur, leading to the occlusion of arterial supply. This sets the stage for necrosis and possible perforation.

38. **On examination of a 3-month-old child brought in for a minor complaint, you notice a large umbilical hernia. The mother asks you what she should do about it. What do you tell her?**
Umbilical hernias are common in infants and young children, especially African Americans. Incarceration of an umbilical hernia is rare. Your best advice is to reassure the parents (and often the grandparents, aunts, and uncles) that most of these hernias reduce spontaneously. If there is a large ring that has not diminished by age 2, or if incarceration has occurred, the defect should be closed operatively. Otherwise, the hernia can be closed electively at age 5 or 6 if it persists.

39. **A 3-week-old infant presents with bilious vomiting. What diagnostic study should be ordered first?**
Upper gastrointestinal (UGI) series. Bilious emesis in an infant is due to malrotation with volvulus until proven otherwise! UGI has a sensitivity of 93% to 100% for malrotation and a positive predictive value of 90%. You may notice an abnormal configuration of the duodenum on the UGI and if volvulus is present, this will show a corkscrew pattern with signs of obstruction and absence of the ligament of Treitz. The accuracy of a UGI series to identify volvulus relies heavily on technique and should be performed and read by a specialized radiologist. In facilities without this resource or in unstable patients, abdominal radiographs may be performed first. Radiographs may also help evaluate for complications such as bowel perforation or pneumatosis.

40. **The 3-week-old infant undergoes UGI and radiographs. The UGI study reveals the absence of the ligament of Treitz. The upright film shows a "double-bubble" sign. What should you do next?**
You should call a surgeon and reserve the operating room ASAP! The "double-bubble" sign on the upright abdominal radiograph represents partial obstruction of the duodenum, causing distention of the stomach and the first part of the duodenum. This is highly suggestive of malrotation with volvulus, which is further supported by the UGI findings. This is a true surgical emergency.

41. **When does intestinal malrotation present?**
    Intestinal malrotation is a rare congenital anomaly that results in the bowel not being fixed properly in place, predisposing it to twist on itself, and causing bowel ischemia. The majority (90%) of cases present within 1 year of age, and 75% present within 1 month of age. The most common presentation is bilious emesis in early infancy, but patients may also present with nonbilious emesis, abdominal pain and distention, and profound shock. Patients presenting later in life may have chronic or episodic symptoms due to intermittent volvulus.

42. **How is malrotation with volvulus treated?**
    The ED management of patients with malrotation and volvulus should include medical resuscitation and urgent surgical consultation for a corrective Ladd procedure.

43. **What is the most common surgically correctable cause of vomiting in infants?**
    Pyloric stenosis. This condition is estimated to occur in about 1 in 400 births.

44. **What is pyloric stenosis? How does it present?**
    Pyloric stenosis is a narrowing of the outflow tract of the stomach due to hypertrophy of the pyloric musculature. Pyloric stenosis is often found among first-born males, and males predominate by a factor of 4 to 5. There may be a family history for this condition. The infants are usually clinically normal at birth. In the typical history, the infant does well for the first few weeks of life, usually regaining birth weight. At about the third week of life, the infant starts to vomit, usually at the end of feedings. The vomiting eventually becomes projectile or "shoots across the room." It is typically nonbilious, though blood may be seen if there is an associated gastritis or esophagitis. Most patients present between 2 and 6 weeks of age. The infant is often described as hungry all the time, eating even after vomiting, because the infant cannot achieve adequate nutrition. In time, the infant may become profoundly dehydrated and emaciated.

45. **How do you examine an infant with suspected pyloric stenosis?**
    Examine the infant on his or her back, preferably on the parent's lap, and while he or she is quiet. Hold the infant's legs and flex them to 90 degrees at the hips to help relax the abdominal musculature. A bit of sugar or juice on a pacifier may help to relax the child even more. Begin the examination from below the liver, palpating in a rocking motion. A firm, ballotable mass may be felt in the region of the pylorus. This is the classic physical finding of pyloric stenosis—the "olive." If you cannot palpate an olive and still have a high suspicion of pyloric stenosis, US is the test of choice.

46. **Where is the "olive" usually found?**
    Usually it is found on abdominal examination in the right upper quadrant, just below the xiphoid.

47. **What US findings are associated with pyloric stenosis?**
    UGI tract examination has long been used to diagnose pyloric stenosis. The diagnosis is made by documentation of delayed gastric emptying and visualization of a long pyloric channel. You cannot see the hypertrophied pylorus muscle. US, however, is quickly becoming the favored radiologic test for diagnosing pyloric stenosis. The reasons are that there is no radiation and no need to introduce barium into the GI tract of a potential surgical candidate who is at high risk for aspiration. Additionally, US allows visualization of the hypertrophied pylorus muscle. If the pyloric canal lengthening is greater than 16 mm and the wall thickness is more than 4 mm, suspect pyloric stenosis.

48. **What is the classic laboratory finding in a child with pyloric stenosis?**
    The classic finding is hypochloremic, hypokalemic metabolic alkalosis. This is a result of vomiting gastric fluids containing potassium and hydrogen chloride, contraction alkalosis from volume loss, and a failure of compensatory mechanisms. Serum bicarbonate may be as high as 65 to 75 mEq/L. Acidosis usually signifies a more dangerous metabolic state due to extreme dehydration. With early diagnosis of pyloric stenosis, neither alkalosis nor acidosis is found.

49. **How is pyloric stenosis treated?**
    Initially, correct the infant's fluid and electrolyte status with IV fluids. Once the infant is euvolemic and the electrolytes have returned to normal, a surgeon should perform a pyloromyotomy.

50. **What are the most common surgically correctable causes of vomiting in the following infant age groups: First week of life? First month of life? After the neonatal period?**
    In the *first week of life*, consider anatomic malformations. Esophageal atresia, duodenal or jejunal atresia, duodenal stenosis, midgut malrotation, ileal atresia, and meconium ileus are the most common causes.
    In the *first month of life*, consider pyloric stenosis and gastroesophageal reflux. As a general rule, gastroesophageal reflux can be managed medically. However, if medical management fails and the infant is failing to gain weight, bleeding, or aspirating, a surgical antireflux operation, such as fundoplication, may be warranted.

Other causes of vomiting in babies this age include Hirschsprung disease, esophageal or intestinal webs, infection, increased intracranial pressure, and metabolic defects.

Beyond the neonatal period, consider intussusception, appendicitis, and bowel obstruction caused by malrotation, incarcerated or strangulated hernia, duplication cysts, or Meckel diverticulum.

51. **What are the common causes of rectal bleeding in the pediatric age group? How do they present?**
    1. **Fissures**. Fissures are probably the most common cause. Often there is a history of constipation or passing a large, hard stool. The blood typically is bright red and found in streaks on the outside of the stool or on the toilet tissue. The diagnosis can be made by anal examination under a good light source. Treatment consists of sitz baths and lubrication of the rectal area with petroleum jelly. If the child suffers from constipation, address this as well.
    2. **Juvenile polyps**. Polyps occur in older infants and children in the lower part of the colon. They may be palpated on digital rectal examination and may bleed, especially if they break free. They are not premalignant, but they may serve as a lead point for intussusception.
    3. **Meckel diverticulum**. Remember the rule of 2's! Two percent of the population is born with a Meckel diverticulum. It is usually located about 2 feet proximal to the terminal ileum. And only 2% of people with a Meckel diverticulum have any clinical problems. Meckel diverticuli usually contain ectopic gastric mucosa, and the acid secretion produces erosion at the junction of the normal ileal mucosa and the Meckel mucosa. It may present with painless rectal bleeding, perforation with peritonitis, diverticulitis, or intussusception.
    4. **HSP**. This vasculitis can cause symptoms ranging from painless rectal bleeding to abdominal pain and hematuria. The associated submucosal hemorrhage may also serve as a lead point for intussusception.
    5. **Other causes**. Intestinal vascular malformations, intussusception, inflammatory bowel disease, duplications, swallowed blood, bleeding peptic ulcer disease, bleeding varices, and trauma can cause rectal bleeding.

52. **A 3-year-old child swallowed a safety pin that she found on the floor. You have located the object in her stomach on plain films, and the pin appears to be open. What do you do now?**
    Most foreign bodies that reach the stomach will pass completely through the GI tract and be evacuated in the stool. Occasionally, a foreign body may get stuck at the junction of the duodenum and jejunum at the ligament of Trietz. This is more likely to occur in objects that exceed 6 cm in length or 2.5 cm in width, or in sharp-pointed objects, as described in the case above. Because perforation may occur, close interval imaging to ensure passage is recommended. Prompt surgical removal of objects that "catch" beyond the pylorus should be arranged. Obtain a radiograph in all children who have a history of swallowing a foreign body, both for the already mentioned reasons and to make sure that it is not lodged above the level of the thoracic inlet, where it could be aspirated if the child coughs. Rates of nonoperative intervention vary from 10% to 20% across all age groups. Less than 1% require surgery.

53. **Two months later, the same 3-year-old child swallows a button battery from a toy. Should this child be managed differently?**
    Button batteries present a special hazard. The 3-V lithium batteries have an increased risk compared to alkaline batteries. Injury occurs when the battery becomes embedded in tissue on both sides, creating an electrical current. This activation causes a rapid increase in pH at the negative pole resulting in caustic injury. To avoid missing the battery, obtain radiographs of the neck, esophagus (chest), and abdomen. Most ingested batteries are 20 mm in diameter and can be differentiated from coins by their "double-ring" or "halo" appearance on radiographs. Batteries in the esophagus can cause significant erosive damage within 2 hours and warrant immediate removal. Temporizing measures such as giving the patient honey or sucralfate orally may slow the rate of injury in acute ingestion but should not delay definitive management. If the battery is in the stomach and the child is asymptomatic, daily radiographs may be obtained to ensure passage. Management and identification help is available by consulting the National Battery Ingestion Hotline at 800-498-8666 or www.poison.org/battery/guideline.asp.

54. **Does the ingestion of magnets cause serious problems? Do they need to be retrieved urgently?**
    The ingestion of multiple magnets can cause significant complications. The strong attraction force of the magnets can occur across the mucosal folds of the stomach or between loops of the bowel, leading to bowel perforation, volvulus, ischemia of the bowel wall, and death. It may be difficult to determine if the attached magnets are across the bowel wall. Surgical consultation is required.

55. **What is a vascular ring?**
    A vascular ring is a congenital condition that causes airway or esophageal obstruction. The obstruction is usually at the level of the trachea, but a ductus arteriosus or a pulmonary artery sling can also compress the bronchi. Many of these rings are caused by the failure of involution of various segments of the six embryologic aortic

arches. Infants who present with stridor, recurrent pneumonia, or a history of noisy breathing since birth should prompt consideration of this diagnosis.

56. **What is the difference between a pilonidal dimple and a pilonidal sinus?**
Both are located in the midline of the sacrococcygeal area. Close inspection reveals that the dimple does not have a central pore, but the sinus does. The sinus is a tract lined by stratified squamous epithelium that extends toward the spinal canal, but not into it. The sinus is asymptomatic until it becomes infected or obstructed, usually in adolescence. Predisposing factors are male gender, being overweight or hirsute, and a sedentary lifestyle. Once infection occurs, an abscess forms and expands deep to the skin's surface. Patients usually complain of low back pain that is worse with sitting. They may also complain of localized tenderness. On examination, you will note a tender, indurated area in the sacrococcygeal region.

57. **How is a pilonidal abscess treated?**
Because these lesions typically expand inward, they must be incised and drained. Probe the abscess cavity to break up any loculations and remove hair because it acts as a foreign body. Following incision and drainage, begin sitz baths and oral antimicrobial therapy (targeting *Staphylococcus*, anaerobes, and fecal flora). Once the inflammation has resolved, arrange elective incision of the entire cyst and its sinus tracts.

58. **What is omphalitis?**
Omphalitis is an infection of a newborn's umbilical cord stump and the surrounding tissues, usually occurring in the first 2 weeks of life. The infant initially presents with purulent, foul-smelling drainage from the umbilical stump and surrounding abdominal erythema, indicative of cellulitis. If the infection is not diagnosed and treated early, it can lead to more serious problems, such as peritonitis, liver abscess, or sepsis. The usual bacterial pathogens are *Streptococcus pyogenes*, *Staphylococcus aureus*, group B streptococcus, and Gram-negative rods.

59. **How is omphalitis treated?**
If the infant has obvious signs of omphalitis, or appears toxic, presume a serious systemic infection. Obtain appropriate laboratory evaluation for sepsis, admit, and treat with IV antibiotics.
    If the findings are not clearly suggestive of omphalitis, that is, there is minimal drainage or erythema, the infant can be treated at home with good skin/cord care (cleaning the cord with each diaper change and using topical antibiotics). Reevaluation in 24 hours is recommended. Instruct parents to return for reexamination if the child has a change in feeding, activity, or disposition.

KEY POINTS: COMMON FINDINGS IN ACUTE APPENDICITIS

1. Diffuse or periumbilical abdominal pain
2. Low-grade fever
3. Vomiting or diarrhea
4. Anorexia

KEY POINTS: CLASSIC FINDINGS IN INTUSSUSCEPTION

1. Severe, intermittent abdominal pain
2. Currant jelly stool
3. Irritability
4. Vomiting
5. Lethargy

KEY POINTS: WHICH TEST IS BEST?

1. Appendicitis: US (CT and MRI are also useful)
2. Pyloric stenosis: US
3. Intussusception: Air contrast enema (many use US initially for diagnosis)
4. Malrotation: UGI series

KEY POINTS: FINDINGS THAT REQUIRE IMMEDIATE SURGICAL CONSULTATION

1. Strangulated hernia on physical examination
2. Distended abdomen and "double-bubble" sign on upright abdominal radiograph
3. Bilious emesis, especially in the first few months of life
4. Absence of the ligament of Treitz on upper GI study
5. Ultrasonography findings consistent with ovarian torsion

BIBLIOGRAPHY

1. Abuzneid YS, Alzeerelhouseini HIA, Rabee A, et al. Double magnet Ingestion causing intestinal perforation with peritonitis: case report and review of the literature. *Case Rep Surg.* 2022;2022:4348787. https://doi.org/10.1155/2022/4348787.
2. Arroyo AC, Zerzan J, Vazquez H, et al. Diagnostic accuracy of point-of-care ultrasound for intussusception performed by pediatric emergency medicine physicians. *J Emerg Med.* 2021;60(5):626–632. https://doi.org/10.1016/j.jemermed.2020.11.030.
3. ASGE Standards of Practice Committee Management of ingested foreign bodies and food impactions. *Gastrointest Endosc.* 2011;73(6):1085–1091. https://doi.org/10.1016/j.gie.2010.11.010.
4. Choi G, Je BK, Kim YJ. Gastrointestinal emergency in neonates and infants: a pictorial essay. *Korean J Radiol.* 2022;23(1):124–138. https://doi.org/10.3348/kjr.2021.0111.
5. Expert Panel on Pediatric Imaging Koberlein GC, Trout AT, et al. ACR appropriateness criteria suspected appendicitis-child. *J Am Coll Radiol.* 2019;16(5 Suppl):S252–S263. https://doi.org/10.1016/j.jacr.2019.02.022.
6. Gavriilidis P, de'Angelis N, Tobias A. To use or not to use opioid analgesia for acute abdominal pain before definitive surgical diagnosis? A systematic review and network meta-analysis. *J Clin Med Res.* 2019;11(2):121–126. https://doi.org/10.14740/jocmr3690.
7. Gudjonsdottir J, Marklund E, Hagander L, Salö M. Clinical prediction scores for pediatric appendicitis. *Eur J Pediatr Surg.* 2021;31(3):252–260. https://doi.org/10.1055/s-0040-1710534.
8. Harel S, Mallon M, Langston J, Blutstein R, Kassutto Z, Gaughan J. Factors contributing to nonvisualization of the appendix on ultrasound in children with suspected appendicitis. *Pediatr Emerg Care.* 2022;38(2):e678–e682. https://doi.org/10.1097/PEC.0000000000002394.
9. Hartford EA, Woodward GA. Appendectomy or not? An update on the evidence for antibiotics only versus surgery for the treatment of acute appendicitis in children. *Pediatr Emerg Care.* 2020;36(7):347–352. https://doi.org/10.1097/PEC.0000000000002157.
10. He K, Rangel SJ. Advances in the diagnosis and management of appendicitis in children. *Adv Surg.* 2021;55:9–33. https://doi.org/10.1016/j.yasu.2021.05.002.
11. Kelley-Quon LI, Arthur LG, Williams RF, et al. Management of intussusception in children: a systematic review. *J Pediatr Surg.* 2021;56(3):587–596. https://doi.org/10.1016/j.jpedsurg.2020.09.055.
12. Li XZ, Wang H, Song J, Liu Y, Lin YQ, Sun ZX. Ultrasonographic diagnosis of intussusception in children: a systematic review and meta-analysis. *J Ultrasound Med.* 2021;40(6):1077–1084. https://doi.org/10.1002/jum.15504.
13. Lu YT, Chen PC, Huang YH, Huang FC. Making a decision between acute appendicitis and acute gastroenteritis. *Children (Basel).* 2020;7(10):176. https://doi.org/10.3390/children7100176.
14. Painter K, Anand S, Philip K. *Omphalitis.* StatPearls Publishing; 2022.<https://www.ncbi.nlm.nih.gov/books/NBK513338/>[Updated May 1, 2022] StatPearls [Internet].
15. Plut D, Phillips GS, Johnston PR, Lee EY. Practical imaging strategies for intussusception in children. *Am J Roentgenol.* 2020;215(6):1449–1463. https://doi.org/10.2214/AJR.19.22445.
16. Sethia R, Gibbs H, Jacobs IN, Reilly JS, Rhoades K, Jatana KR. Current management of button battery injuries. *Laryngoscope Investig Otolaryngol.* 2021;6(3):549–563. https://doi.org/10.1002/lio2.535.
17. Svetanoff WJ, Srivatsa S, Diefenbach K, Nwomeh BC. Diagnosis and management of intestinal rotational abnormalities with or without volvulus in the pediatric population. *Semin Pediatr Surg.* 2022;31(1):151141. https://doi.org/10.1016/j.sempedsurg.2022.151141.
18. Zvizdic Z, Golos AD, Milisic E, et al. The predictors of perforated appendicitis in the pediatric emergency department: a retrospective observational cohort study. *Am J Emerg Med.* 2021;49:249–252. https://doi.org/10.1016/j.ajem.2021.06.028.

CHAPTER 45

NEUROSURGICAL EMERGENCIES

Meghan Meghpara and Jillian Stevens Savage

1. **How does the Monro-Kelli doctrine explain increased intracranial pressure (ICP)?**
   The cranium functions as a rigid compartment housing mainly brain tissue but also blood and cerebrospinal fluid (CSF). Based on the Monro-Kellie doctrine, any abnormal increase in the volume of one of these components, without a corresponding decrease in one or both of the others, will result in increased ICP. In a healthy individual, the ICP will remain relatively stable with minor changes in volume. Once a critical ICP is reached, it becomes significantly more sensitive to even the smallest increase in volume.

2. **How does increased ICP lead to cerebral ischemia?**
   Cell survival depends on oxygen delivery through adequate cerebral blood flow (CBF). Cerebral perfusion pressure (CPP) is the pressure gradient that generates CBF, thereby perfusing the brain. CPP is influenced by changes in mean arterial pressure (MAP) and ICP (CPP = MAP − ICP). CPP maintains adequate CBF only when the MAP is greater than 60 mm Hg and the ICP is less than 40 mm Hg. Outside these limits, CBF drops, resulting in suboptimal oxygen delivery, cell injury, and brain ischemia.

3. **What are the symptoms of increased ICP?**
   Symptoms vary by age and timing (acute versus chronic). Neonates and infants may be noted to have irritability, altered mental status, and persistent vomiting. In older children, presenting symptoms are typically headache, nausea, and vomiting.

4. **What are the signs of increased ICP?**
   In infants, the fontanel may be full or bulging. On ophthalmologic examination, papilledema, optic nerve atrophy, or retinal hemorrhages may be appreciated. Look for cranial nerve (CN) deficits; specifically, deficits of CN IV and CN VI may produce head tilt and sunset eyes, respectively. Additional neurologic sequelae of increased ICP include change in mental status, hemiparesis, decorticate or decerebrate posturing, and meningismus. Be aware that a normal examination does not reliably rule out increased ICP; a strong clinical suspicion warrants consideration of neuroimaging, inpatient observation, and serial examinations.

5. **What is Cushing triad?**
   Cushing triad—bradycardia, systemic hypertension, and irregular respirations—is highly suggestive of increased ICP and is a late sign of impending herniation.

6. **How will you recognize the patient who is herniating?**
   Transtentorial herniation is the most common type of herniation. Initially, there will be headache, vital sign changes, decreasing level of consciousness, and ispsilateral pupil dilation (anisocoria) from a third nerve palsy. You may note contralateral hemiparesis and posturing. As herniation progresses, there may be alteration of respirations, pupils will become midposition and fixed. The patient will have decerebrate or decorticate posturing. If not treated, bradycardia and cardiac arrest will follow.

7. **What are the causes of increased ICP?**
   Increased brain volume or cerebral edema
   - Vasogenic causes: Tumor, abscess, hemorrhage
   - Cytotoxic causes: Hypoxia, ischemia, infections
   - Interstitial causes: Blockages in CSF absorption, shunt malfunction
     Increased CSF or hydrocephalus
   - Congenital causes: Dandy-Walker cyst, Arnold-Chiari malformation, vein of Galen arteriovenous malformation
   - Acquired causes: Meningitis, tumor, leukemia, inflammatory response to hemorrhage
     Increased blood volume
   - Subdural or epidural hematoma
     Idiopathic
   - Idiopathic intracranial hypertension (previously called pseudotumor cerebri)

8. **Describe the initial management of increased ICP.**
   - Emergent stabilization of airway, breathing, circulation

- Prevention of hypoxemia, hypercarbia, and systemic hypotension
- Immobilization of the cervical spine in patients with suspected cervical spine trauma or unknown cause of increased ICP

9. **What are the benefits and drawbacks of intubation in a patient with increased ICP?**
   - Early endotracheal intubation allows for airway stabilization and regulation of ventilation, limits aspiration, and optimizes oxygenation.
   - Laryngoscopy alone can cause hypertension and bradycardia secondary to vagal response as well as increased ICP. Rapid sequence intubation (RSI) can help prevent these side effects.

10. **Discuss pharmacologic considerations in RSI in patients with increased ICP.**
    The choice of sedative in the setting of increased ICP is based on cardiovascular status. Ketamine can be beneficial in patients with hemodynamic instability. Previously, ketamine was thought to increase ICP; however, its effect on ICP is variable and has been shown to be beneficial in improving CPP and systemic arterial pressure. Etomidate is another excellent choice, noting the risk of adrenal suppression, even with one dose. In patients with hemodynamic instability, midazolam is a safe sedative choice. Rocuronium is typically the paralytic of choice in pediatrics due to the risk of rhabdomyolysis with succinylcholine.
    Lidocaine has traditionally been used as an RSI premedication to prevent the vagal responses of ICP associated with laryngoscopy and intubation. Evidence on the efficacy of lidocaine is limited and primarily exists in the adult literature. The clinician should use clinical judgment when considering this adjunctive agent.

11. **What nonpharmacologic treatments should be considered in the management of increased ICP?**
    - **Elevate the head of the bed** to 15 to 30 degrees to lower ICP without compromising CPP. Keep the patient's head in the midline position to promote venous drainage.
    - **Hyperventilation** is recommended only for impending herniation. Hyperventilation generates cerebral vascular constriction, which in turn lowers CBF and therefore may lead to cerebral ischemia. In nonemergent situations, maintain the $PaCO_2$ at 35 to 38 mm Hg.
    - Seek **early neurosurgery consultation**. Consider CSF drainage in cases of increased ICP refractory to pharmacologic treatment.

12. **What pharmacologic treatments are considered in the management of increased ICP?**
    - **Hypertonic saline** is a hyperosmolar treatment option. This treatment is favored over mannitol in hypovolemic patients, as its diuretic properties are more attenuated. Other benefits include increased cardiac output and antiinflammatory effects. Cautious use is advocated in patients with renal insufficiency.
    - **Mannitol** reduces ICP by two mechanisms. First, it immediately but transiently reduces blood viscosity. Onset of the effect is rapid (1-5 minutes), and the peak of the effect ranges from 20 to 60 minutes after administration. Second, mannitol acts more slowly as an osmotic diuretic with onset of effect in 15 to 30 minutes and duration of effect up to 6 hours. It is contraindicated in patients with hypovolemia. Use it judiciously in patients with renal insufficiency.
    - **Corticosteroids** are not indicated to treat increased ICP in the setting of infarction, hemorrhage, or head trauma, as multiple studies have been unable to show benefit from therapy. However, in the setting of vasogenic edema from mass effect (e.g., abscess or tumor), steroids may be indicated for an antiinflammatory effect.
    - Use **sedation, antipyretics, and analgesics** aggressively if agitation, fever, and pain are present, respectively. All three states increase cerebral metabolism, which in turn increases CBF and ICP. See prior discussion on sedative choice in the setting of increased ICP.
    - **Antiepileptics** may be indicated in patients who are at increased risk for seizure in order to prevent an increase in ICP associated with seizure activity. Levetiracetam is an acceptable option and typically easier to administer than phenytoin. Benzodiazepines are recommended in the setting of breakthrough seizures.
    - **Barbiturate coma** is a therapeutic modality used in the intensive care unit for patients with increased ICP refractory to conventional nonpharmacologic and pharmacologic treatments. By decreasing cerebral metabolism, this state decreases ICP. Barbiturates can depress cardiac function and cause hypotension. Judicious fluid management is indicated.

13. **What imaging modalities can be utilized in the evaluation of increased ICP?**
    - Computed tomography (CT) is indicated for emergent detection of intracranial injury and masses.
    - Magnetic resonance imaging (MRI) is considered superior to CT in detecting intracranial pathology and is the imaging modality of choice if the patient is stable.

KEY POINTS: INCREASED INTRACRANIAL PRESSURE

1. Regardless of the cause, the first and most important step in the treatment of increased ICP is the maintenance of the child's airway, circulation, and breathing.
2. Endotracheal intubation allows for airway protection. Rapid sequence induction medications will limit further ICP elevation during intubation.
3. Reserve hyperventilation for cases of impending herniation.
4. Early consultation with the neurosurgery service is imperative.

---

14. **Define hydrocephalus.**

    Hydrocephalus is the presence of an increased volume of CSF resulting in ventricular dilatation. It may result from overproduction or decreased absorption of CSF. A new diagnosis of hydrocephalus in the emergency department (ED) is rare. However, patients with hydrocephalus treated with the placement of a ventricular shunt will often present to the ED with shunt complications and require immediate attention.

15. **What treatments are used for hydrocephalus?**

    - Benign and stable hydrocephalus does not need treatment. Ventricular shunts remain the gold standard for the treatment of progressive hydrocephalus. Most shunts have three components: a ventricular catheter, a unidirectional valve (including a reservoir system), and a distal catheter. The distal catheter is most commonly placed such that it drains into the peritoneum, but in select cases it will be placed to drain into the right atrium or lung pleura.
    - Endoscopic third ventriculostomy is a treatment option developed as an alternative to shunt placement. In this procedure, a small hole is made in the floor of the third ventricle, allowing continuous drainage of CSF into the basal cisterns, bypassing the obstructed or stenosed aqueduct of Sylvius. As there is no indwelling catheter, this procedure limits long-term complications, specifically infection. Short-term complications of malfunction are still possible, and approximately 35% of patients will ultimately still require shunt placement.

16. **What are the potential complications of CSF shunt placement in pediatric patients?**

    - **Shunt malfunction** is the most common complication of shunt placement. This is often a problem of decreased drainage due to obstruction, but increased drainage can also occur. The shunt can also malfunction secondary to valve dysfunction, catheter disconnection, or catheter migration.
    - **Shunt infection** occurs in 5% to 10% of shunt placements, usually within the first 6 postoperative months. Eighty percent of infections occur within the first 3 months and 90% occur within the first 6 months after shunt placement.
    - **Other complications** include scrotal or inguinal migration, small bowel obstruction, intussusception, omental cyst torsion, persistent hiccup, abdominal CSF collection or pseudocyst, volvulus, colon perforation, shunt nephritis, diaphragm perforation, intra-abdominal organ perforation, and subdural hemorrhage (from increased drainage and tearing of bridging veins or as a surgical complication).

17. **How does a shunt infection occur, and what are the respective signs and symptoms?**

    - Colonization of the shunt: This is the most common type of shunt infection and results in nonspecific symptoms in children with ventriculoperitoneal (VP) shunts such as lethargy, headache, nausea or vomiting, bulging fontanel, fever, or abdominal pain. Typically, this occurs within months of surgery. Ventriculoatrial (VA) shunts can result in septic pulmonary emboli or infectious endocarditis.
    - Complication of local wound infection: Typically, this occurs within weeks of surgery and results from an overlying wound infection along the shunt, followed by signs of shunt infection.
    - Infection of the distal shunt results in peritonitis: This presents with abdominal complaints consistent with peritonitis (tenderness and guarding) in the setting of a VP shunt. VA shunt infection may present with fever or chest discomfort.

18. **How common is shunt failure?**

    Mechanical shunt failure or shunt failure from an infection is quite common, occurring in up to 35% to 40% of shunt placements within the first postoperative year. About 15% will fail in the second postoperative year. Although rates decrease to less than 7% thereafter, failure remains a risk.

19. **What are the signs and symptoms of shunt malfunction?**

    The most common symptoms include nausea, vomiting, irritability, altered mental status, and a bulging fontanel if age applicable.

20. **What imaging studies may be utilized in the evaluation of shunt malfunction?**

    - **SSFSE MRI** (single-shot fast spin-echo MRI), also referred to as "fast spin MRI," is increasingly used over CT scan as the imaging method of choice to assess shunt position and the size of fluid-filled structures (e.g., ventricles).

This minimizes radiation and scanning time and eliminates the need for sedation or anesthesia in young or behaviorally challenged children. Proponents of this technology also laud its ability to detect vascular anomalies missed by other imaging modalities. However, some researchers caution that poor contrast resolution and the use of only one type of pulse sequence may limit the detection of bleeding and abnormalities such as venous sinus thrombosis. The provider must also be aware if the shunt is a programmable shunt—as MRI can affect these devices and a programming magnet must be immediately available upon completion of the study.

- **Noncontrast head CT** may be utilized when MRI is unavailable. CT shows brain anatomy, ventricle size, and shunt position. The availability of previous head CT scans is important for comparison purposes.
- **Shunt survey** may be used to evaluate the integrity of the entire length of the shunt with plain radiography. This is now an infrequently ordered study but may be utilized to supplement MRI or CT in the assessment of shunt connectivity.
- **Ultrasound** of the abdomen should be employed for patients with VP shunts and abdominal pain to evaluate for the presence of a pseudocyst or intussusception.

21. What is the treatment for CSF shunt malfunction?

Definitive treatment of shunt malfunction is surgical shunt revision. Temporizing bedside procedures include CSF shunt tap (effective for distal obstruction only) and burr hole puncture (effective for proximal obstruction refractory to medical management and for life-threatening symptoms). Temporizing medical management includes acetazolamide, dexamethasone, and hyperventilation, with the latter only considered in unstable patients.

22. What is the treatment of shunt infection?

Neurosurgical and infectious disease resources recommend combined surgical and medical treatment. Seek early consultation with a neurosurgeon, as the infected device may need to be removed or at least temporarily externalized until CSF cultures are negative and the patient shows clinical improvement. Treat the infection empirically with broad-spectrum antibiotics, which can later be tailored when susceptibilities are available. In the ED, it is reasonable to start with cefepime and vancomycin to cover for *Staphylococcus epidermidis*, *Staphylococcus aureus*, and Gram-negative organisms as well as *Pseudomonas aeruginosa*.

23. What are some historical clues to identifying a patient with a brain tumor?

Brain cancers are the most common solid tumor in childhood and the second most common pediatric cancer overall, making up about 25% of all childhood neoplasms. Initial symptoms can be nonspecific resulting in diagnostic delays. Complaints include irritability, increasing head circumference, listlessness, failure to thrive, behavioral disturbances, vomiting, and anorexia. Later, these children have more classic symptoms of a space-occupying intracranial mass. Historical clues that should prompt neuroimaging include vomiting (especially without fever, abdominal pain, or alteration in the stooling pattern), persistent headache, vision changes (blurred, loss, diplopic), regression of developmental milestones, seizures, neuroendocrine dysfunction (e.g., new-onset diabetes insipidus), focal weakness, sensory change(s), neck pain, and acquired torticollis.

KEY POINTS: CHARACTERISTICS OF BRAIN TUMOR HEADACHES

1. Recurrent morning headaches
2. Prolonged incapacitating headaches
3. Changes in headache quality, frequency, and pattern

24. What clues from the physical examination suggest a brain tumor?

Cranial nerve deficits, visual abnormalities (loss of visual acuity, visual field loss, afferent papillary defect, or nystagmus), ataxia, loss of coordination or balance, and upper motor neuron signs. The latter include hyperreflexia, clonus, paraparesis, weakness, decreased or abnormal sensation, fundoscopic evidence of increased ICP, and macrocephaly. These are important clues to recognize, and any one of them warrants investigation.

25. Which two specific syndromes should raise concern for intracranial disease?

- **Parinaud syndrome** suggests the presence of a tumor in the pineal region. Symptoms include vertical gaze limitation, pupillary dilatation reactive to accommodation but not to light, convergence-retraction nystagmus (on the attempt of upward gaze, eyes move medially, and globes retract), and eyelid retraction.
- **Diencephalic syndrome** raises concern for a tumor in the suprasellar or third ventricular region (diencephalon), typically involving the hypothalamus and thalamus. Symptoms include failure to thrive with emaciation, euphoria, and emesis.

26. What are the predisposing factors that may lead to brain abscess?

There are two pathophysiologic mechanisms behind the development of a brain abscess. The most common is hematogenous spread of infection in children. Predisposing conditions or factors include cyanotic congenital heart disease (up to 6%), endocarditis (especially left sided), jugular venous thrombophlebitis associated with parapharyngeal infection (Lemierre syndrome), pulmonary arteriovenous malformation, cystic fibrosis, and recent endoscopy leading to spinal venous plexus bacterial infection.

Less common is a brain abscess that can arise from the contiguous spread of infection from the oropharynx, middle ear, paranasal sinuses, or orbits. Risk factors for abscess formation by this mechanism are trauma (face, skull), recent neurosurgery, intracerebral hematoma, and neoplasm.

27. **What are some of the clues that can help identify brain abscesses?**
Unfortunately, the early presentation of brain abscess in children is often nonspecific and fever is present in only 50% of patients, headache in 60% to 70%; 50% have a focal neurological deficit on examination. Later, brain abscesses may manifest as seizures, mental status change, coma, focal neurologic deficits, papilledema, meningeal signs, and hemiparesis. A unilateral headache in a febrile child should raise concern for the presence of a brain abscess.

28. **What is the diagnostic modality of choice for focal, suppurative central nervous system (CNS) infections?**
Contrast-enhanced CT or MRI is indicated if the clinician suspects a focal suppurative CNS infection. In the setting of an unstable patient, CT scan is preferred. Consult with a radiologist to help choose the correct study for a given patient.

29. **What is the treatment for focal suppurative CNS infections?**
A multidisciplinary approach including infectious disease, neurosurgery, radiology, and critical care services is critical to the prompt and successful treatment of a child with a suppurative CNS infection. As always, patient stabilization takes precedence in the management of increased ICP. Ideally, obtain cultures prior to the initiation of antibiotics and do not delay treatment if surgery is not imminent. It may be necessary to initiate antibiotic treatment prior to surgery (where the culture will be obtained). The choice of antibiotics should be guided by the clinician's knowledge of the patient's risk factors, as this can determine the likely pathogens involved. In the absence of such information, a reasonable choice is the combination of a third-generation cephalosporin, metronidazole, and vancomycin. Surgical treatment will be determined by the site of the infection. Corticosteroids are indicated only if cerebral edema has resulted in increased ICP or neurologic deterioration. Also consider administration of antiepileptics.

30. **Compare hemorrhagic and ischemic strokes.**
Contrary to the adult population, hemorrhagic strokes are more common in pediatrics than ischemic strokes. Hemorrhagic stroke refers to spontaneous intraparenchymal bleeding and nontraumatic subarachnoid hemorrhage. The most common risk factor is arteriovenous malformation. Other common risk factors of hemorrhagic stroke include coagulopathies (vitamin K deficiency, clotting factor deficiency, and thrombocytopenia), hemorrhage into a tumor, vascular malformations (sickle cell disease, berry aneurysms), and arterial hypertension secondary to renal disease, coarctation of the aorta, pheochromocytoma, or sympathomimetic drug use. Ischemic stroke refers to a focal reduction in CBF leading to hypoxic damage to the brain.

31. **Name some underlying risk factors that predispose a pediatric patient to a stroke.**
The most common risk factor is congenital heart disease (up to 25% of patients). Other risk factors include hypercoagulability, hyperviscosity, certain medications (e.g., oral contraceptive pills), acquired valvular defects, and vascular disease (sickle cell, homocystinuria, moyamoya, migraine).

32. **How may stroke present in the pediatric ED?**
Fortunately, stroke is an uncommon diagnosis in the pediatric ED but requires a high index of suspicion. As with many early presentations of neurosurgical conditions, stroke may present in a nonspecific fashion. Ischemic strokes often present with a focal neurologic deficit (e.g., hemiplegia), whereas hemorrhagic strokes may present with a variety of vague symptoms including headache, seizure, and change in mental status. With nonverbal children (e.g., infants, toddlers, children with special needs), diagnosis is even more challenging.

33. **What is the initial radiographic evaluation for a suspected stroke?**
The most sensitive imaging is MRI with diffusion-weighted studies. However, noncontrast head CT is a reasonable first study in the ED because it will identify hemorrhage if there are limitations to obtaining MRI, such as timeliness and need for sedation. Unfortunately, CT may not detect an ischemic event in its early stages (12-24 hours after the event) and provides a limited evaluation of the posterior fossa.

34. **What are the next steps in the diagnostic workup for stroke?**
The workup that follows emergent neuroimaging is directed at identifying the cause of the hemorrhage or ischemia. Such an evaluation may include vascular studies (magnetic resonance angiography, magnetic

resonance venography, transfontanel Doppler), cardiac evaluation (electrocardiography, chest radiography, echocardiography with or without bubble contrast), and laboratory evaluation (complete blood count, electrolytes, drug screen, prothrombin time/partial thromboplastin time/international normalized ratio, anticardiolipin antibodies, lupus anticoagulants, erythrocyte sedimentation rate, antinuclear antibody, and screening for antithrombin III, protein C and protein S deficiencies, and factor V Leiden mutation).

35. **What is the treatment for stroke?**
Cardiorespiratory stabilization is the priority in acute management. Obtain a dextrose level immediately and treat abnormalities aggressively, as both hypoglycemia and hyperglycemia can worsen ischemic stroke. Antipyretics are recommended, as hyperthermia can increase metabolic demand. Treat seizures with antiepileptics. In the case of hypotension, give fluids judiciously to avoid cerebral edema. Keep the head of the bed flat to avoid postural perfusion fluctuations. Hypertension should not be treated aggressively as this can affect CPP and blood pressure should be lowered cautiously.

    Additional treatment depends on the type of stroke and identified cause. Ischemic strokes may be treated with anticoagulation after consultation with hematology and neurosurgery. At this time, further research is needed to determine evidence-based guidelines on tissue plasminogen activator use and endovascular therapies in children. Hemorrhagic strokes may require neurosurgical intervention if there is evidence of rapid hematoma expansion.

36. **What are the common causes of nontraumatic spinal cord compression?**
Nontraumatic spinal cord compression may be caused by primary neoplasms, vertebral metastases, abscesses, epidural hematomas, disk herniation, or tethered cord.

37. **What are the signs and symptoms of nontraumatic spinal cord compression?**
Back pain. This is a rare complaint in children and therefore should never be discounted without the performance of a careful and thorough history and physical examination. Weakness, increased or absent tendon reflexes, presence of a Babinski reflex, symmetric loss of sensation, and sphincter abnormalities are concerning signs of spinal cord compression that prompt urgent evaluation. Conus medullaris and cauda equina compression are present in a similar fashion.

38. **What is the approach to suspected nontraumatic spinal cord compression?**
Emergent imaging with MRI is the cornerstone of the initial evaluation of such patients. Early consultation with a neurosurgeon is imperative. If a tumor is identified and there has been a rapid progression of symptoms or there is a clear cord-level deficit, administer intravenous high-dose corticosteroids without delay and consult an oncologist immediately.

39. **What are the signs and symptoms of concussion?**
The symptoms of concussion can be nonspecific but can include headache, photophobia, phonophobia, dizziness, disorientation, amnesia, mood changes, and visual changes. Patients with concussions have a normal physical examination. Any focal neurological deficits should prompt neuroimaging to assess for traumatic brain injury.

40. **What is the typical management for a concussion?**
After 24 to 48 hours, patients may gradually return to activity, while limiting themselves to stay below their symptom threshold. The exact amount of rest recommended requires further research. Typical recommendations include starting with light aerobic exercise and progressively building up to full practice in a stepwise fashion.

41. **What type of skull fracture requires immediate surgical consultation?**
Neurosurgical consultation is required for open, basilar, and burst fractures as well as skull fractures with greater than 1 cm of depression and diastatic fractures greater than 3 mm. Children with fractures that are nondepressed, linear, and unilateral without any additional intracranial injuries, and a normal neurological examination, can typically be managed with supportive care. One must consider nonaccidental trauma prior to the discharge of infants and young children with a skull fracture.

42. **What clinical decision tool can be utilized to determine the need for head imaging after a traumatic head injury in children?**
Pediatric Emergency Medicine Collaborative Research Network developed a clinical decision tool to assess the need for head imaging after traumatic head injury. The tool divides history and clinical findings by age less than 2 and age 2 and greater. Red flag symptoms in which CT head is recommended include abnormal score on the Glasgow Coma Scale, signs of basilar skull fracture, and altered mental status. In children not imaged, observation for 4 to 6 hours to assess for deterioration in clinical status is recommended.

BIBLIOGRAPHY

1. Chinta SS, Gray MP. Neurologic emergencies. In: Shaw KN, Bachur RG, eds. *Textbook of Pediatric Emergency Medicine*. 8th ed. Lippincott Williams & Wilkins; 2021:881–900.
2. Kochanek P, Tasker R, Bell M, et al. Management of pediatric severe traumatic brain injury: 2019 consensus and guidelines-based algorithm for first and second tier therapies. *Pediatr Crit Care Med*. 2019;20(3):269–279.
3. Kristopher TK, Abhaya VK, David DL, Benjamin CW. Hydrocephalus in children. *Lancet*. 2016;387(10020):788–799.
4. McCrory P, Meeuwisse WH, Dvorčák J, et al. Consensus statement on concussion in sport: the 5th International Conference on Concussion in Sport Held in Berlin, October 2016. *Br J Sports Med*. 2017;51(11):838–847.
5. McManemy J, Jea A, Ducis K. Neurotrauma. In: Shaw KN, Bachur RG, eds. *Textbook of Pediatric Emergency Medicine*. 8th ed. Lippincott Williams & Wilkins; 2021:1254–1262.
6. Nagler J, Donoghue AJ, Yamamoto LG. Airway. In: Shaw KN, Bachur RG, eds. *Textbook of Pediatric Emergency Medicine*. 8th ed. Lippincott Williams & Wilkins; 2021:34–42.
7. Piatt JH, Garton HJ. Clinical diagnosis of ventriculoperitoneal shunt failure among children with hydrocephalus. *Pediatr Emerg Care*. 2008;24(4):201–210.
8. Prusseit J, Simon M, Brelie C, et al. Epidemiology, prevention and management of ventriculoperitoneal shunt infections in children. *Pediatr Neurosurg*. 2009;45:325–333.
9. Schutzman S, Mannix R. Head. In: Shaw KN, Bachur RG, eds. *Textbook of Pediatric Emergency Medicine*. 8th ed. Lippincott Williams & Wilkins; 2021:268–274.
10. Szydlowski EG, Cronan KM, Fein JA, Posner JC. Technology assisted children. In: Shaw KN, Bachur RG, eds. *Textbook of Pediatric Emergency Medicine*. 8th ed. Lippincott Williams & Wilkins; 2021:E135-2–E135-20.
11. Wolf J, Flynn PM. Infection associated with medical devices. In: Kliegman RM, ed. *Nelson Textbook of Pediatrics*. 21st ed. Elsevier; 2020:1410–1413.
12. Weinberg GA. Brain abscess. *Pediatr Rev*. 2018;39:270–272.

CHAPTER 46

ORTHOPEDIC EMERGENCIES

Christopher J. Russo

1. **Describe the presentation of osteomyelitis.**
   Patients with osteomyelitis classically demonstrate fever and pain at the affected site. The absence of fever does not rule out osteomyelitis. Other signs of systemic illness, such as anorexia, malaise, and vomiting, may be present. Infants often exhibit decreased feeding, irritability, or listlessness. When an extremity is involved, pain may manifest as pseudoparalysis. Examination findings typically include focal swelling, warmth, tenderness, or erythema, often metaphyseal in location. Neonates and younger children are more prone than older patients to present with secondary joint involvement. Some patients present with symptoms of severe illness, including signs of generalized sepsis and shock.

2. **How are most cases of osteomyelitis acquired?**
   Hematogenous spread is the most common source of osteomyelitis in children. It is believed that there is a transient bacteremia and bacteria then enter the bone at the metaphysis, the site of the predominant blood supply. Less commonly, direct inoculation into the bone or local invasion from a contiguous infection or trauma can occur. Infection due to vascular insufficiency is rare in children.

3. **What laboratory tests are helpful in the diagnosis of osteomyelitis?**
   Diagnosis of osteomyelitis rests primarily on clinical findings; laboratory results and diagnostic imaging help confirm the diagnosis. The erythrocyte sedimentation rate (ESR) and C-reactive protein (CRP) are more sensitive indicators than peripheral white blood cell (WBC) count, which is unreliable and elevated only 20% of the time. ESR is elevated in up to 90% of cases of hematogenously acquired osteomyelitis. CRP is elevated in up to 98% of cases. Obtain a blood culture, though it may not identify a causative organism. The highest yield for isolating a causative organism is achieved when bone aspirate, joint aspirate, and blood are collected for culture. Together these cultures can establish a microbiologic diagnosis 50% to 80% of the time. With the exception of patients who are clinically unstable, obtain these cultures before initiation of parenteral antibiotics.

   Polymerase chain reaction (PCR) may be helpful in identifying infections secondary to *Bartonella henselae* and *Kingella kingae*. Although more rapid and sensitive, PCR does not provide information regarding antibiotic sensitivity and resistance.

4. **Which imaging studies are indicated when osteomyelitis is suspected?**
   - **Plain radiography** is a reasonable initial imaging choice in the emergency department (ED) for a patient with suspected osteomyelitis. Plain films can rule out fracture or bone malignancy. Bone abnormalities in osteomyelitis (lytic lesions, periosteal elevation, and periosteal new bone formation) may not appear until 10 to 20 days after symptoms begin. Changes to adjacent soft tissue (deep soft tissue swelling and loss of normal tissue planes) may occur much earlier, as early as several days after symptoms begin.
   - **Technetium-99 bone scanning** is more sensitive in the early diagnosis of osteomyelitis than plain radiography, with reported sensitivities of 80% to 100%. It is useful when osteomyelitis is suspected but the site cannot be localized by physical exam or multiple foci of infection are considered.
   - **Magnetic resonance imaging (MRI)** (Fig. 46.1B) is the imaging study of choice for evaluating a patient with suspected osteomyelitis. Sensitivity ranges from 92% to 100%. MRI helps differentiate osteomyelitis from cellulitis and can demonstrate myositis or pyomyositis contiguous to the site of bone involvement. As with bone scanning, malignancy, fracture, and infarction can appear similar to osteomyelitis on MRI.

5. **Which organisms are commonly seen in osteomyelitis?**
   Staphylococcus aureus is the most common causative organism. Other common organisms include *Streptococcus pneumoniae*, *Streptococcus pyogenes*, and *K. kingae*. In addition to *S. aureus*, group B streptococci and enteric gram-negative organisms are important organisms to consider in the neonatal period.

   Consider *Neisseria gonorrhoeae* in sexually active adolescents. Anaerobic bacteria may be found in cases associated with sinusitis, mastoiditis, or dental abscesses. *Serratia* and *Aspergillus* species are found in patients with granulomatous disease. Consider coagulase-negative staphylococci in patients who have undergone medical procedures. *Salmonella* species and gram-negative enteric organisms are found in patients with hemoglobinopathies. *Pseudomonas aeruginosa* is a pathogen found in puncture wounds to the foot, classically a nail penetrating a sneaker. Exposure to kittens should prompt consideration of *B. henselae*, and *Coxiella burnetii* should be considered in cases of exposure to farm animals. *Haemophilus influenzae* type B is only rarely seen since the advent of the *H. influenzae* type B vaccine but remains a consideration in an unimmunized child.

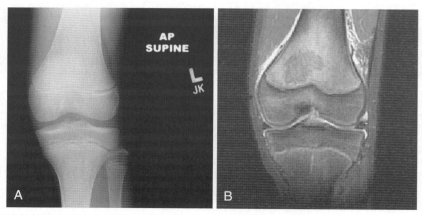

Fig. 46.1 A, Plain radiograph of a knee with bone that registers as normal. **B**, Magnetic resonance image of the same knee with a positive reading of osteomyelitis.

The increasing prevalence of methicillin-resistant *S. aureus* (MRSA) is worthy of particular attention and concern. Osteomyelitis caused by MRSA can be particularly virulent and is associated with multiple sites of bone involvement, myositis, pyomyositis, intraosseous and subperiosteal abscess formation, pulmonary involvement, and vascular complications (such as deep vein thrombosis and septic pulmonary emboli). These patients may be quite ill and require admission to the intensive care unit.

Mycobacterial and fungal infections are rare causes of osteomyelitis.

6. **What historical features should raise suspicion for osteomyelitis (or septic arthritis) from *K. kingae*?**

K. kingae is a gram-negative bacillus that colonizes the upper respiratory tract and plays an important role in osteomyelitis and septic arthritis in children. Infection with this organism typically occurs in children younger than 2 years of age and often follows an upper respiratory tract infection, pharyngitis, or stomatitis. It may be seasonal in occurrence (late summer through winter). Typically, the course of illness for osteomyelitis is more subacute and may lead to delays in diagnosis. Fever is less common in bone and joint infections from *K. kingae*; CRP and peripheral WBC counts are typically lower. Outbreaks of invasive infections from this organism have been reported in daycare populations.

7. **How should bone aspirate or synovial fluid be handled to improve isolation of *K. kingae*?**

Recovery of *K. kingae* is improved when synovial fluid aspirate or bone aspirate is collected in an aerobic blood culture medium. PCR assays substantially improve the detection of this organism.

8. **How is osteomyelitis treated?**

Initiate antibiotic treatment as soon as appropriate cultures have been collected. Regardless of the patient's age, treatment should address the likelihood of infection with *S. aureus*. Given the increasing prevalence of MRSA in many communities, coverage of MRSA is very important. Many MRSA isolates are susceptible to clindamycin. In children, adolescents, and infants over 2 months of age, clindamycin is a good choice for initial antimicrobial coverage. Isolate testing for resistance to clindamycin should be performed. Vancomycin provides excellent coverage for MRSA. However, because of concerns about the widespread use of vancomycin resulting in increasing antimicrobial resistance, reserve this for patients who are moderately to severely ill or who live in communities where significant resistance to clindamycin has been demonstrated. In infants younger than 2 months of age, additional antimicrobial coverage for group B streptococcus and enteric gram-negative bacteria is important. In this age group, clindamycin or vancomycin plus cefotaxime or gentamycin are appropriate initial antimicrobial choices.

Special circumstances warrant consideration of antimicrobial coverage specific to the likely pathogens in such cases. For example, when considering infection with *K. kingae*, the addition of a third-generation cephalosporin is prudent.

It is wise to consult your local antibiogram because the prevalence of community-acquired MRSA varies by geographic location and sensitivities to antibiotics vary as well.

Involve an orthopedic surgeon in cases of suspected or confirmed osteomyelitis. Surgical treatment is indicated in a number of circumstances; chronic osteomyelitis is typically managed surgically while acute osteomyelitis generally responds well to antibiotic therapy alone. Moreover, surgical tissue is often helpful in identifying a causative organism to guide antimicrobial treatment.

9. **Describe the signs and symptoms of septic arthritis.**
Pain, fever, and decreased use of the involved limb are common symptoms of septic arthritis. Hip, knee, and ankle joints account for about 80% of cases of septic arthritis. Fever, malaise, and anorexia are seen in most patients. The involved joint is often held in a position of comfort. In the knee this is usually flexion. The hip is typically held in flexion, abduction, and external rotation. Passive range of motion away from the position of comfort is painful. In joints other than the hip, tenderness, swelling, warmth, and erythema may be seen and an effusion may be palpable. As in osteomyelitis, neonates may present with pseudoparalysis and tenderness of the affected limb.

   Other diagnoses to consider in the patient with suspected septic arthritis include traumatic joint pain, transient synovitis ("toxic synovitis"), reactive arthritis, Lyme arthritis, juvenile rheumatoid arthritis, acute rheumatic fever, osteomyelitis, pyomyositis, necrotizing fasciitis, tumor, slipped capital femoral epiphysis (SCFE), and Legg-Calvé-Perthes disease.

10. **What laboratory tests help diagnose septic arthritis?**
ESR and CRP levels are usually elevated in cases of septic arthritis. The WBC count appears to be less useful than ESR in differentiating septic arthritis from transient synovitis. A child with an ESR less than 20 mm/hour and CRP less than 2 mg/dL is very unlikely to have septic arthritis, but if either of these values is increased, consider arthrocentesis.

    Blood culture and synovial fluid analysis (cell count, Gram stain, and culture) are essential in the evaluation of children with suspected septic arthritis. Ideally, perform these tests before the administration of antibiotics. Blood culture yields an organism in up to 40% and synovial fluid in up to 50% to 60% of cases. When combined, they yield an organism in up to 60% to 70% of cases. The yield of synovial cultures may be improved by inoculation of the fluid into blood culture media. The typical synovial fluid WBC count is over 50,000 cells/mm^3, with a predominance of polymorphonuclear cells (>75%-90%). However, cell counts less than 50,000 cells/mm^3 can be seen in cases of septic arthritis, and counts over 50,000 cells/mm^3 are seen in juvenile rheumatoid arthritis. Synovial fluid glucose and protein levels are not reliable enough to differentiate septic arthritis from other infectious or inflammatory processes.

11. **Which imaging studies can help make the diagnosis of septic arthritis?**
The initial imaging choice in the ED is plain radiography. Soft tissue swelling, joint space widening, and changes suggestive of osteomyelitis may be seen. In the hip, capsular swelling and loss of the gluteal fat planes may be seen as early evidence of infection in the joint. If hip infection is suspected, consider ultrasonography followed by joint aspiration. MRI is a sensitive modality for detecting joint infection and is useful for delineating changes in the adjacent soft tissues and bone.

12. **Which organisms are commonly seen in septic arthritis?**
The organisms commonly responsible for septic arthritis are much the same as those commonly associated with osteomyelitis (see Question 5). Consider *N. gonorrhoeae* in neonates and in sexually active patients, especially those with multifocal joint involvement. Also consider *Candida* species in neonates.

13. **What is the treatment for septic arthritis?**
Optimal treatment involves antibiotics and joint drainage. See Question 8 for a discussion of antibiotics. Early consultation with an orthopedic surgeon is mandatory. Emergent surgical drainage of infected hip and neonatal shoulder infections is appropriate, whereas repeated nonsurgical aspiration may be reasonable for other joints.

14. **Reactive arthritis is in the differential diagnosis for the patients described earlier. What are the common organisms responsible for reactive arthritis?**
Salmonella, Shigella, Campylobacter species, and *Yersinia enterocolitica* from the gastrointestinal tract; *N. gonorrhoeae* and *Chlamydia trachomatis* from the genitourinary tract; and *S. pyogenes, Mycoplasma pneumoniae,* and *Neisseria meningitidis* from the blood. Both *Neisseria* species and *S. pyogenes* can also cause septic arthritis.

15. **Describe the typical presentation and evaluation of suspected pyomyositis.**
Unfortunately, the diagnosis of pyomyositis is often not made until symptoms have been present for several weeks. Initial symptoms include crampy local muscle pain, most commonly involving large muscle groups like the thigh, calf, buttock, upper extremity, and iliopsoas muscles. Early in the course of the infection local edema is present, although the overlying skin is often normal. Over time, induration, edema, erythema, and tenderness increase. Fever, increasing constitutional symptoms, toxicity, and signs of sepsis may develop if the infection progresses and is untreated. Presentation is often subacute. Pyomyositis is more common in tropical climates.

    Laboratory test results are often nonspecific. Peripheral leukocytosis, elevated CRP levels, and elevated ESR may develop as the infection progresses. Collect blood cultures. Creatine kinase level is often normal.

Ultrasonography remains a quick and inexpensive way to demonstrate pyomyositis. CT and MRI may demonstrate the presence of pyomyositis. MRI is the most common imaging modality used to make the diagnosis and is more sensitive than CT.

16. **How is pyomyositis treated?**
The organisms most commonly responsible for pyomyositis are *S. aureus* and *S. pyogenes* (often associated with varicella infection). As is the case in osteomyelitis and septic arthritis, MRSA must be considered in these patients and antimicrobial treatment directed appropriately. When an identifiable abscess is present, drainage is indicated. In the interest of isolating an organism, consider delaying the initiation of antibiotics until drained fluid can be collected for culture in stable patients. More extensive surgical intervention may be necessary if there is muscle necrosis.

17. **Describe the typical presentation and evaluation of suspected necrotizing fasciitis.**
Necrotizing fasciitis is a rare, but rapidly progressive and potentially fatal, bacterial infection of the subcutaneous tissue and superficial fascia. Patients with necrotizing fasciitis often have soft tissue swelling and pain near a site of trauma. Initially, pain with manipulation may be out of proportion to the skin findings. Induration and edema follow, then blistering and bleb formation. The skin can become dusky or drain fluid. Subcutaneous pain and tenderness become severe—again, often out of proportion to the appearance of the overlying skin. There is often a high fever and signs of systemic illness. The process may be quite fulminant, accompanied by toxic shock syndrome and multiorgan failure.
　　Laboratory evaluation and imaging, particularly MRI, may be helpful in establishing the diagnosis. However, because of the rapidly progressive nature of necrotizing fasciitis, do not delay surgical consult and initiation of treatment while obtaining laboratory studies and imaging. Collect wound, tissue, and blood cultures (aerobic and anaerobic).

18. **What is the treatment for necrotizing fasciitis?**
The most important aspect of treatment for necrotizing fasciitis is immediate surgical debridement. Seek surgical consultation as soon as possible. Direct antibiotic treatment at the likely causative organisms, including *S. pyogenes* and *S. aureus* (including MRSA). A reasonable antibiotic choice would be clindamycin plus oxacillin. Many recommend vancomycin in patients who are very ill and in areas where MRSA is prevalent. Ampicillin-sulbactam and piperacillin-tazobactam are other possible antimicrobial choices. It cannot be overemphasized, however, that antibiotic treatment alone is insufficient for this severe, rapidly progressive, and often life-threatening infection. Antibiotic delivery to the affected tissues is often limited, and surgical debridement remains essential.

19. **What concerns should the ED physician have when a child younger than 4 years presents with back pain?**
Back pain is not common in young children, nor is it a particularly common expression of functional pain in young children. Concerning signs and symptoms in a young child with back pain include refusal to walk, limited range of motion in the back, persistent or increasing pain despite rest and analgesics or antiinflammatory agents, fever, weight loss, signs of systemic illness, and abnormal neurologic signs. Consider serious causes in the young child including diskitis, vertebral osteomyelitis, and tumors.

KEY POINTS: ORTHOPEDIC EMERGENCIES

1. MRSA is an important organism to consider in bone, joint, and soft tissue infections. Provide adequate antimicrobial coverage if it is prevalent in your area. Consult your local antibiogram.
2. Overlying skin findings may not be very remarkable early in the course of pyomyositis and necrotizing fasciitis.
3. Surgical debridement without delay is the most important aspect of treating necrotizing fasciitis.
4. Back pain in a young child warrants serious consideration.
5. Compartment syndrome is an orthopedic emergency requiring prompt decompression.

20. **How do children with SCFE present?**
SCFE is the most common hip disorder in children. SCFE usually occurs during the rapid growth phase of adolescence and tends to occur more often in obese children. Males are affected almost twice as often as females. Black adolescents are affected about twice as often as white adolescents. SCFE may be chronic, acute, or acute superimposed on chronic in its presentation. Most (90%) are stable—those who are unable to bear weight are considered unstable. The presentation of SCFE is bilateral in approximately 20% of cases. Patients with SCFE often have pain in the anterior hip, groin, medial thigh, or knee and will also demonstrate limitation of hip motion. Because pain is often localized to the distal thigh or knee, the presence of knee pain in a child or adolescent mandates a thorough examination of the hip. Patients who are ambulatory may have an antalgic gait

with external rotation of the affected leg. Passive internal rotation of the hip is painful, and passive hip flexion is associated with compensatory external rotation.

21. **How can the diagnosis of SCFE be confirmed?**
    Plain radiography is the first step in the evaluation of patients with suspected SCFE. Films show displacement of the femoral capital epiphysis from the metaphysis through the growth plate (see Fig. 46.2). If the slip is chronic, metaphyseal remodeling may be seen. The anteroposterior view often demonstrates the presence of the slip. A line drawn tangent to the superior femoral neck should intersect the lateral aspect of the femoral head (Klein's line). In SCFE this line passes more lateral to the capital epiphysis. Cross-table lateral radiography of the hip can help define the extent of posterior epiphyseal displacement. Although a frog-leg view of the pelvis may reveal a subtle slip, avoid movement of the hip for radiography as it may cause further slippage. Although a slip may be symptomatic on one side only, radiographs often show bilateral SCFE. Because as many as 40% of patients have bilateral slips, comparing sides on plain films may give false reassurance and result in failure to diagnose both slips.

22. **What is the approach to the patient with suspected SCFE in the ED?**
    Once the diagnosis is strongly suspected, obtain urgent orthopedic consultation. Do not allow the patient to bear weight. Most patients are admitted to the hospital for urgent surgical management.

23. **What are the features of "growing pains"?**
    - Pain occurs most commonly in the lower extremities and is bilateral.
    - Pain occurs in the evening hours and is *better by morning.*
    - Pain can become severe and is relieved by acetaminophen or ibuprofen.
    - The physical examination is normal.
    - There is often a family history of growing pains.
    - Pain is chronic and may last for years.

24. **What is the cause of growing pains?**
    The cause of growing pains remains unknown. Many causes have been suggested. Typically, growing pains are not associated with fever or joint inflammation. Growing pains do not correlate with growth spurts and do not affect growth. They do not occur at the growth plate regions. Possible causes include fatigue, abnormal posture, restless legs syndrome, and overuse. Psychological stress and decreased pain threshold have been postulated as contributory. Growing pains are often seen in children with other types of recurrent pain, such as headaches and abdominal pain. They are slightly more common in girls.

25. **What are some "red flags" to consider that suggest a disease other than growing pains?**
    - Pain that is persistent and unilateral (Consider imaging to rule out malignancy or fracture.)
    - Fever and weight loss; hepatosplenomegaly or lymphadenopathy (Consider blood work to rule out an oncologic process.)

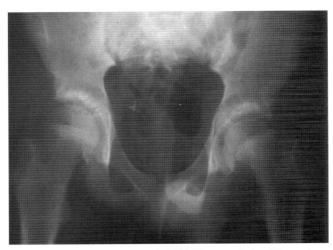

Fig. 46.2 Slipped capital femoral epiphysis, more prominent on the left hip ("ice cream slipping off the cone.)

- Morning stiffness, back or groin pain, synovitis (Consider inflammatory joint disease.)
- Rashes suggesting vasculitis, systemic lupus erythematosus, or psoriasis
- Limp or abnormal gait are unusual in growing pains.

26. **When should one suspect sacroiliitis in children?**
Consider sacroiliitis in a child with fever and hip, back, or gluteal pain. Sacroiliitis is relatively uncommon, accounting for approximately 1.5% of all cases of septic arthritis in children. These children are often initially misdiagnosed owing to the condition's rarity, low suspicion on the part of the diagnostician, and rare abnormal findings on plain radiographs. The clinical presentation varies widely, and the condition mimics other, more common disorders (septic arthritis of the hip, diskitis, and even appendicitis). Infection is thought to arise from hematogenous spread or, less commonly, from direct extension from adjacent joints or soft tissue.
      Incidence is highest in the second decade of life, presumably because the blood supply to the sacroiliac joint peaks at that time.

27. **How is the diagnosis of sacroiliitis made?**
High clinical suspicion based on physical examination should prompt further investigation. The **FABER** (**f**lexion, **ab**duction, **e**xternal **r**otation) test or Patrick test can be helpful in diagnosis. The patient is placed supine; the hip is flexed, abducted, and externally rotated until the limit of passive motion is reached. The sacroiliac joint is then compressed by downward pressure on the medial aspect of the knee while stabilizing the pelvis. When this causes pain, the test is reported as positive. Also, straight leg raising as well as lateral compression of the pelvis often induces pain.
      Laboratory testing is nonspecific: ESR and CRP are often elevated. Peripheral leukocytosis may be seen. Plain radiographs are usually not diagnostic. MRI is the mainstay of diagnosis for these patients.

28. **What are the features of compartment syndrome?**
Compartment syndrome is caused by rapid fluid influx into a closed fascial compartment. An increase in tissue pressure results in decreased perfusion and can lead to muscle and nerve ischemia. Most cases are caused by fractures but soft tissue injuries can cause compartment syndrome as well.
      Look for the 5 Ps: pain, paresthesis, paralysis, pallor, and pulselessness. Pain out of proportion to injury and pain with passive stretch are often the first signs. Also look for the 3 As (agitation, anxiety, analgesia need), though this pain assessment is less reliable.
      Compartment syndrome is a clinical diagnosis; measurement of compartment pressures need only be done as a confirmatory test.

29. **When should one suspect the presence of compartment syndrome in children?**
Specific injuries associated with compartment syndrome in children include supracondylar humerus fractures, tibial tubercle fractures, forearm fractures, and so-called "floating elbow" fractures—fractures of the humerus and forearm. Fractures of the tibia or fibula are responsible for 60% to 70% of cases. Snakebite injuries are also at risk for causing compartment syndrome.

30. **What is the treatment for compartment syndrome?**
Emergent fasciotomy and decompression are indicated when the diagnosis of compartment syndrome is made. Timely diagnosis is of the essence.

31. **What is a felon?**
A felon is an abscess that occurs in the fingertip pad. Pressure from the abscess causes pain; prompt drainage can help prevent such complications as digital pad necrosis, osteomyelitis, or flexor tenosynovitis. Typically related to puncture wounds, these infections are most commonly caused by *S. aureus*.

BIBLIOGRAPHY

1. Castillo C, Mendez M. Slipped capital femoral epiphysis: a review for pediatricians. *Pediatr Ann*. 2018;47(9):e377–e380.
2. Dodwell ER. Osteomyelitis and septic arthritis in children. *Curr Opin Pediatr*. 2013;25:58–63.
3. Gornitzky AL, Kim AE, O'Donnell JM, et al. Diagnosis and management of osteomyelitis in children: a critical analysis review. *JBJS Rev*. 2020;8(6):e1900202.
4. Grippi M, Zionts LE, Ahlmann ER, et al. The early diagnosis of sacroiliac joint infections in children. *J Pediatr Orthop*. 2006;26(5):589–593.
5. Haidar R, Saad S, Khoury N, Musharrafieh U. Practical approach to the child presenting with back pain. *Eur J Pediatr*. 2011;170:149–156.
6. Hosseinzadeh P, Hayes CB. Compartment syndrome in children. *Orthop Clin N Am*. 2016;47:579–587.
7. Jamal N, Teach S. Necrotizing fasciitis. *Pediatr Emerg Care*. 2011;27:1195–1202.

8. Joffe MD, Loiselle JM. *Musculoskeletal emergencies*. In: Shaw KN, Bachur RG, eds. *Fleisher & Ludwig's Textbook of Pediatric Emergency Medicine*. 8th ed. Wolters Kluwer; 2021:1358–1381.
9. Lehman PJ, Carl RL. Growing pains. *Sports Health*. 2017;9(2):132–138.
10. Montgomery NJ, Epps HR. Pediatric septic arthritis. *Orthop Clin NA*. 2017;48:209–216.
11. Ohns MJ, Walsh ME, Douglas Z. Acute compartment syndrome in children: don't miss this elusive diagnosis. *J Nurse Pract*. 2019;16:19–22.
12. Quick RD, Williams J, Fernandez M, et al. Improved diagnosis and treatment of bone and joint infections using and evidence-based treatment guideline. *J Pediatr Orthop*. 2018;38(6):e354–e359.
13. Saavedra-Lozano J, Falup-Pecurariu O, Faust SN, et al. Bone and joint infections. *Pediatr Infect Dis J*. 2017;36(8):788–799.
14. Schmitt SK. Osteomyelitis. *Infect Dis Clin North Am*. 2017;31:325–338.
15. Taylor ZW, Ryan DD, Ross LA. Increased incidence of sacroiliac joint infection at a children's hospital. *J Pediatr Orthop*. 2010;30(8):893–898.
16. Vij N, et al. Primary bacterial pyomyositis in children: a systematic review. *Pediatr Orthop*. 2021;41(9):e849–e854.

CHAPTER 47

OTORHINOLARYNGOLOGY EMERGENCIES

Megan Lavoie and Frances M. Nadel

1. **From what part of the nose do most nosebleeds originate?**
   Most nosebleeds in children arise anteriorly (90%). On the anterior part of the septum, many capillaries converge, giving rise to Kiesselbach plexus. Anterior nosebleeds tend to be slow and persistent. Posterior nosebleeds usually originate from branches of the sphenopalatine artery and ethmoidal arteries. As a result, posterior nosebleeds are more profuse.

2. **What factors often contribute to nosebleeds in otherwise normal children?**
   Desiccation of the fragile nasal mucosa makes the tissue more friable. Inflammation from a viral upper respiratory tract infection or allergies may also make the mucosa more likely to bleed. Finally, local trauma from nose picking is often a major contributor.

3. **How can one elicit a truthful answer about nose picking?**
   Ask the child which finger she uses to pick her nose!

4. **Though most nosebleeds occur from the benign local conditions listed previously, what else should be considered in the differential diagnosis of nosebleeds?**
   See Table 47.1 for a differential diagnosis of nosebleeds.

5. **What factors make one suspicious of a systemic cause of a nosebleed?**
   Children with a history of bleeding from other sources, easy bruising, weight loss, or other constitutional symptoms; a family history of a bleeding disorder; and severe or recurrent nosebleeds may need a more extensive workup or subsequent follow-up. Children with abnormal vital signs, those who are pale, have diffuse adenopathy, nasal mass, or suspicion of a posterior source of the bleeding, will likely need a more extensive evaluation as well.

6. **What is the most common age of children who present to the emergency department (ED) with nosebleeds?**
   Nosebleeds requiring an ED visit occur most commonly in children between the ages of 2 and 10 years old, and most have a readily identifiable local cause for their bleeding. Nosebleeds in children less than 1 year old are rare. In this age group, consider more serious illness or injury, including child abuse.

7. **What steps should be taken for a patient who has a nosebleed in the ED?**
   Calming the patient and family is often the first and most important step. Parents or the child can squeeze the soft part of the nose below the nasal bridge (the nasal alae) together for 10 minutes continuously, while tilting the head forward to avoid swallowing blood. If this is not enough to stop the bleeding, for an anterior bleed, you may then insert a roll of cotton saturated with a topical decongestant (oxymetazoline or adrenaline) in the affected side and squeeze the nose gently for 5 minutes to compress the cotton against the septum. If the bleeding site is visible, cauterize it with silver nitrate. Add a topical anesthetic to the cotton ball to greatly decrease the amount of discomfort of cautery. If the bleeding cannot be stopped with cautery, then pack the nose. Have bleeding that cannot be stopped with these measures evaluated by an otolaryngologist without delay.

8. **What findings would make you more suspicious of a posterior nosebleed?**
   Though rare in children, suspect a posterior nosebleed when no obvious site is visible anteriorly. Bleeding from both nostrils and blood in the posterior pharynx suggest a posterior nosebleed but can occur from brisk anterior epistaxis. Continued bleeding despite adequate anterior pressure is also concerning. Posterior bleeding may present more subtly in the form of hematemesis, hemoptysis, or melena.

9. **A teenage boy presents with recurrent, profuse unilateral epistaxis. Over the last 2 months, he has had difficulty breathing through the same side of his nose. What other diagnosis should you consider?**
   Teenage males may develop *juvenile nasopharyngeal angiofibroma*. These uncommon tumors arise from the sphenopalatine region and can present with severe epistaxis. The diagnosis is made with nasal endoscopy or

Table 47.1 Differential Diagnosis of Epistaxis

Local Predisposing Factors

Trauma

Facial trauma

Direct nasal trauma

Nose picking

Local inflammation

Acute viral upper respiratory tract infection (common cold)

Bacterial rhinitis

Nasal diphtheria (rare),* usually a blood-tinged discharge

Congenital syphilis

Hemolytic streptococci

Foreign body

Acute systemic illnesses accompanied by nasal congestion: measles, infectious mononucleosis, acute rheumatic fever

Allergic rhinitis

Nasal polyps (cystic fibrosis, allergic, generalized)

Staphylococcal furuncle

Sinusitis

Rhinitis sicca

Cocaine or heroin sniffing

Lobular capillary hemangioma (pyogenic granuloma)

Telangiectasias (Osler-Weber-Rendu disease)

Juvenile angiofibroma*

Other tumors, granulomatosis (rare)*

Systemic Predisposing Factors

Hematologic diseases*

Platelet disorders

Quantitative: idiopathic thrombocytopenic purpura, leukemia, aplastic anemia

Qualitative: von Willebrand disease, Glanzmann disease, uremia

Other primary hemorrhagic diatheses: hemophilias

Clotting disorders associated with severe hepatic disease, disseminated intravascular coagulopathy, vitamin K deficiency

Anatomic: pseudoaneurysm of the major vessel from infection/trauma

Drugs: aspirin, nonsteroidal anti-inflammatory drugs, warfarin, rodenticide, valproate

Vicarious menstruation

Hypertension*

Arterial (unusual cause of epistaxis in children)

Venous: superior vena cava syndrome or paroxysmal coughing is seen in pertussis and cystic fibrosis

*Life-threatening condition.
Adapted from Delgado EM, Nadel FM. Epistaxis. In: Shaw K, Bachur RG, eds. *Textbook of Pediatric Emergency Medicine*, 8th ed. Wolters Kluwer; 2021:167.

computed tomography (CT). These patients need a referral to an otolaryngology specialist for further surgical management.

10. **A teenager presents with her fifth nosebleed in as many months. Her history and physical examination are otherwise unremarkable. What additional information regarding her nosebleeds may be helpful?**
Ask her about the timing of nosebleeds in relation to her menstrual cycle. Some girls may experience "vicarious menstruation" in which they have a nosebleed at the same time as their menses.

11. **Who should be tested for group A streptococcus (GAS) pharyngitis with a throat swab?**
Children with a sore throat and fever, lymphadenopathy, palatal petechiae, and tonsillar exudate should be tested for GAS. Those with rhinorrhea, cough, hoarse voice, and other symptoms indicating a more likely viral cause need not be tested. Also, those younger than 3 years old typically do not need to be tested, as they are more likely to be carriers of GAS than to have true streptococcal pharyngitis, and the occurrence of acute rheumatic fever is rare in this age group.

12. **What are the common signs and symptoms of a retropharyngeal abscess (RPA)?**
Commonly, there is a recent history of an upper respiratory tract infection, fever, and poor oral intake. Patients may be drooling, have a stiff neck (refusal to extend the neck) or torticollis, and have tender cervical adenopathy. Respiratory symptoms of stridor, stertor, or dyspnea are usually late findings and are rarely described in the most current series of patients. A midline oropharyngeal mass can sometimes be seen in the posterior pharynx.

13. **Why is it unusual to see RPA in children older than 4 years of age?**
The retropharyngeal nodes of Rouvière usually involute around 5 years of age, making RPA a rare disease in older children.

14. **What is a parapharyngeal abscess?**
A parapharyngeal or lateral space infection develops in the lateral aspect of the neck. This space is shaped like an inverted cone. It is divided into two compartments: (1) the anterior compartment contains no vital structures and is closely related to the tonsillar fossa; (2) the posterior compartment contains some of the cranial nerves and the carotid sheath. Infection in the lateral space results from dental infection, pharyngitis, tonsillitis, parotitis, and mastoiditis.
Parapharyngeal abscesses are less common than RPA, but symptoms are very similar.

15. **What are the mechanisms of infection of the retropharyngeal space?**
Retropharyngeal abscesses usually occur as bacteria in the nasopharynx spread via lymphatic channels to the nodes of Rouvière, where they multiply and suppurate. Other possible mechanisms include oral trauma (causing a mucosal tear), hematogenous spread during bacteremia, or, rarely, extension from vertebral osteomyelitis. About half of the children with an RPA had a preceding upper respiratory infection.

16. **Which pathogens are common in RPA?**
RPA is usually a polymicrobial infection and may include *Streptococcus* spp., *Staphylococcus aureus* (including methicillin-resistant strains), and anaerobes. *Haemophilus influenzae* type b has become a less common pathogen since the introduction of the Hib vaccine. Pathogens such as *Klebsiella* and *Salmonella* spp., *Candida*, and *Mycobacterium tuberculosis* have also been reported.

17. **How wide is the normal retropharyngeal space on a lateral neck radiograph in children?**
Radiologist will measure the prevertebral space at the level of C2 and C6, with values over 7 mm and 14 mm, respectively, indicating a widening of the prevertebral space and concern for RPA. As a general rule of thumb often used by emergency medicine providers, the prevertebral soft tissues at the level of C3 should measure less than two-thirds of the anteroposterior width of the body of the third cervical vertebrae. This space is markedly widened in a child with RPA (Fig. 47.1).

18. **List the causes of a false-positive lateral neck radiograph for RPA.**
   - Neck not in full extension
   - Radiography done during expiration
   - Not a true lateral position
   - Crying child

19. **How does CT scan assist in RPA management?**
A hypodense region with rim enhancement and scalloping of the wall suggests an abscess, but a more heterogeneous mass without rim enhancement suggests retropharyngeal cellulitis only. However, the CT scan

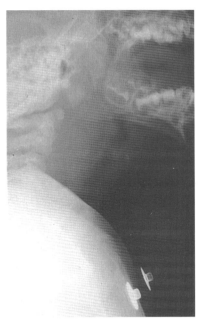

Fig. 47.1 Widened retropharyngeal space on a lateral neck radiograph of a child with a retropharyngeal abscess.

results should be clinically correlated, as the accuracy of CT scans reported in the literature varies greatly. CT scans can help demonstrate the extent of infection and the potential for airway compromise. The scan also helps the otolaryngologist decide whether intraoral drainage is feasible or whether an external approach is necessary.

Point-of-care ultrasound (US) is increasingly used as an alternative to CT scans to identify RPA. Findings on bedside US include a hypoechoic or anechoic collection in the prevertebral space, as well as irregular or poorly defined borders around that collection and possible thickening of the tissue surrounding the fluid collection.

In children with the clinical diagnosis of retropharyngeal infection without evidence of extension of infection beyond the retropharyngeal space, no signs of respiratory compromise, and a lateral neck consistent with a retropharyngeal process, a CT scan may not be necessary for the initial evaluation.

20. **Do most patients with RPA require surgery?**
    The management of RPA varies greatly in the literature and by the surgeon. Though it was previously the standard to drain all abscesses, more clinicians are willing to attempt a trial of intravenous (IV) antibiotics alone. Children more likely to need surgical management of their RPA include those with abscesses larger than 2.5 cm, persistent fever after 24 to 48 hours of IV antibiotics, and older age, as well as those with multiple abscesses, airway compromise, or signs of mediastinitis or meningitis.

21. **How far inferiorly does the retropharyngeal space extend in the neck?**
    The retropharyngeal space extends from the base of the skull to the level of the second thoracic vertebra. An RPA can rupture into the prevertebral space, which communicates with the mediastinum and descends as far as the psoas muscles.

22. **What are some of the complications of RPA?**
    Earlier recognition and treatment and improved diagnostic strategies have greatly reduced the morbidity and mortality risks of RPAs. However, a large RPA may obstruct the airway at the pharyngeal, laryngeal, or tracheal level, and a tracheostomy may be necessary. Aspiration of purulent fluid may occur from the rupture of the abscess. Sepsis, mediastinitis, jugular vein thrombosis, Lemierre syndrome, and carotid arteritis with subsequent rupture are rare complications.

23. **Define mastoiditis.**
    Mastoiditis is an infection of the temporal bone mastoid air cells. Technically, a simple case of acute otitis media leads to some inflammation of the air cells, but true coalescent mastoiditis implies bony destruction. In younger children, mastoiditis may develop via hematogenous spread, not as a complication of acute otitis media.

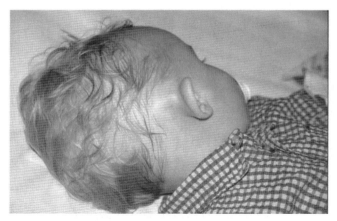

Fig. 47.2 Protruding ear in a child with acute mastoiditis.

24. **How does a patient who has acute mastoiditis present?**
    Patients commonly present with persistent symptoms of acute otitis media, such as ear pain or drainage. Fever is common. The ear may protrude away from the head, and in younger children, the ear is pushed down and out (Fig. 47.2). The postauricular skin is often tender, erythematous, fluctuant, or edematous. Otoscopy shows findings consistent with acute otitis media. One may see sagging of the posterosuperior external ear canal due to periosteal thickening.

25. **What are the common pathogens seen in acute mastoiditis?**
    Streptococcus pneumoniae, *Streptococcus pyogenes*, and *Streptococcus aureus*. *Haemophilus influenzae* is a rare pathogen. Anaerobic enteric bacteria and *Pseudomonas* spp. are more often seen in subacute or chronic disease and should be suspected if the child is not responding to therapy.

26. **Does every child with acute mastoiditis need a CT scan for diagnosis?**
    No. If the clinical examination is sufficient to make the diagnosis and there are no concerns for associated complications, a CT scan may not be necessary. However, a CT scan with contrast or magnetic resonance imaging may confirm the diagnosis in less obvious presentations, as well as show whether there is a subperiosteal abscess, intracranial extension, or sigmoid sinus thrombosis.

27. **What are some of the central nervous system complications of mastoiditis?**
    The temporal bone's proximity to many important intracranial structures can lead to serious complications including meningoencephalitis and intracerebral, epidural, or subdural abscesses. Progressive thrombophlebitis may lead to sigmoid or lateral sinus thrombosis. Any child with mastoiditis with focal neurologic symptoms should receive an immediate evaluation for intracranial spread. Other concerning findings include a toxic appearance, stiff neck, persistent fever despite adequate antibiotic treatment, headache, vomiting, and unusual behavior.

28. **Your patient with classic findings for acute mastoiditis also has a torticollis and not well-circumscribed swelling, redness, and tenderness on the same side of the neck. What rare extracranial complication must you consider?**
    Bezold abscess. This infection erodes the distal tip of the mastoid and ruptures into the space between the digastric and sternocleidomastoid muscles. Children may feel better after rupture of the mastoid.

29. **What is Lemierre syndrome?**
    Lemierre syndrome is a septic thrombophlebitis of the internal jugular vein. Pharyngitis and PTAs are the most common initial sites of infection, but it is also seen after other local infections such as otitis media, mastoiditis, or sinusitis.

30. **What is the most common pathogen in Lemierre syndrome?**
    Fusobacterium necrophorum.

31. **Wait. How do differentiate tender neck mass of Bezold abscess from Lemierre syndrome?**
    Though both may present with a tender lateral tender neck mass, children with Lemierre syndrome are usually older (teens) with a recent history of sore throat, high spiking fevers and rigors, and often look toxic with

accompanying respiratory symptoms from septic emboli to the lungs. The neck swelling is along the tender thrombosed internal jugular vein.

32. **What is Gradenigo syndrome?**
Gradenigo syndrome occurs from inflammation of the petrous apex of the temporal bone (petrositis), affecting cranial nerves V and VI. Children present with suppurative otitis, have pain around the eye and ear, abducens nerve paralysis (inability to move the eye laterally), and diplopia. Additional symptoms are facial paresis, vertigo, and fever.

33. **When do children usually present to the ED with postoperative tonsillectomy bleeding?**
They usually present 7 to 10 days after surgery, but bleeding can occur as early as 3 days and as late as 21 days.

34. **How does the normal healing eschar of oropharyngeal tissue look after tonsillectomy?**
The healing operative site will be covered with a grayish-white exudate. Beneath the exudate, there is usually beefy red granulation tissue. A blood clot will appear dark red, purple, or black and may be located inferiorly near the tongue.

35. **What is the significance of seeing a clot on inspection of the oropharynx after tonsillectomy?**
A blood clot not only shows you where the offending vessel is located but also indicates that the vessel is in the earliest stages of hemostasis and may continue to bleed if provoked. *Never remove this blood clot in the ED, as brisk bleeding and loss of the airway can ensue!.*

36. **Why do children die from postoperative bleeding?**
The usual mechanism of death is aspiration of blood, though some may die from hemorrhagic shock.

37. **How should you manage a patient who is actively bleeding after tonsillectomy in the ED?**
Assess the ABCs (airway, breathing, and circulation), with particular attention to obstruction of the airway due to blood, as well as circulatory compromise due to blood loss. It is important to calm the patient and the family. Assess for any active bleeding. Leave any clot in the tonsillar fossa undisturbed! For severe, active bleeding, tamponade the site with gauze and digital pressure until the otolaryngologist arrives. Anticipate a difficult airway if the patient requires tracheal intubation.

KEY POINTS: MANAGEMENT OF BLEEDING AFTER TONSILLECTOMY AND ADENOIDECTOMY

1. Attend to the ABCs.
2. Restore intravascular volume.
3. If there is a clot, leave it alone.
4. For severe active bleeding, tamponade the site with gauze and digital pressure.

38. **Define the classic presentation of PTA, also known as quincy.**
A muffled (hot potato) voice, trismus, and odynophagia. Other symptoms may include fever, worsening sore throat, ear pain, and neck pain.

39. **Which way does the uvula point when there is a PTA?**
The abscess pushes the uvula away to the contralateral side of the oropharynx.

40. **How do you distinguish a PTA from a peritonsillar cellulitis (PTC) by physical examination?**
In both, the tonsils and pharynx will be erythematous and often have an exudate. One tonsil may be larger than the other, but by itself this asymmetry does not confirm an abscess. With a PTA, the soft palate ipsilateral to the larger tonsil is red and bulging, and the uvula is deviated to the contralateral side. Often there is trismus and ipsilateral cervical adenopathy. If there is tonsillar asymmetry without palatine or uvular changes, a PTC is more likely.

41. **What are the sonographic differences seen in a PTC compared to a PTA?**
A US of a PTC will show tonsil parenchymal heterogeneity and surrounding increased perifocal echogenicity due to soft tissue edema. A PTA US will show a hypoechoic or anechoic fluid-filled cavity of the tonsil with irregular borders.

42. **Why should a child see their regular provider in about a month after the diagnosis of a PTA?**
Rarely, lymphoma may present as an asymmetric tonsillar enlargement, so it is important to make sure the asymmetry has resolved with long-term follow-up.

43. **What are the indications for a surgical intervention or bedside drainage of a PTA?**
PTA treatment varies greatly based on the severity of illness, a child's ability to cooperate with a painful procedure, confidence in diagnosis, and the practitioner's judgment. For patients with impending airway compromise, immunodeficiency, sepsis, or other complications prompt surgical intervention is indicated. For patients without an urgent surgical need, a drainage procedure usually done by an otolaryngologist may offer immediate symptomatic relief and confirm the diagnosis. Some practitioners prefer a course of IV antibiotics, with aspiration reserved for treatment failures. Once drained, treat a PTA just like acute tonsillitis: with antibiotics, hydration, and analgesics.

44. **What are the best antibiotic choices in a PTA?**
Ampicillin-sulbactam or clindamycin are good initial parenteral options. Vancomycin or linezolid should be considered in those who present with more severe disease or are not responding to first-line therapy. Oral amoxicillin-clavulanate and clindamycin are appropriate for children who are well-appearing and able to swallow. The route of administration will depend on the patient's general appearance and ability to swallow.

KEY POINTS: DANGERS OF DEEP NECK INFECTIONS

1. Localized infections in the head and neck can spread regionally.
2. Intracranial extension may present with prolonged symptoms, change in mental status, or focal neurologic deficit.
3. Mediastinal extension can be associated with prolonged symptoms, poor response to therapy, respiratory symptoms, and sepsis syndrome.

BIBLIOGRAPHY

1. Akhavan M. Ear, nose, throat: beyond pharyngitis: retropharyngeal abscess, peritonsillar abscess, epiglottitis, bacterial tracheitis, and postoperative tonsillectomy. *Emerg Med Clin N Am*. 2021;39:661–675. https://doi.org/10.1016/j.emc.2021.04.012.
2. Bandarkar AN, Adeyiga AO, Fordham,et al. Tonsil ultrasound: technical approach and spectrum of pediatric peritonsillar infections. *Pediatr Radiol*. 2016;46:1059–1067. https://doi.org/10.1007/s00247.015-3505-7.
3. Cassano P, Ciprandi G, Passali D. Acute mastoiditis in children. *Acta Biomedica*. 2020;91:54–59. https://doi.org/10.23750/abm. v91i1-S.9259.
4. Homme JH. Acute otitis media and group a streptococcal pharyngitis: a review for the general pediatric practitioner. *Pediatr Ann*. 2019;48:e343–e348. https://doi.org/10.3928/19382359-20190813-01.
5. Krulewitz NA, Fix ML. Epistaxis. *Emerg Med Clin N Am*. 2019;37:29–39. https://doi.org/10.1016/j.emc.2018.09.005.
6. Liu JH, Anderson KE, Willging JP, et al. Posttonsillectomy hemorrhage: what is it and what should be recorded? *Arch Otolaryngol Head Neck Surg*. 2001;127:1271–1275.
7. Malia L, Sivitz A, Chicaiza H. A novel approach: point-of-care ultrasound for the diagnosis of retropharyngeal abscess. *Am J Emerg Med*. 2021;46:271–275. https://doi.org/10.1016/j.ajem.2020.07.060.
8. Marom T, Roth Y, Boaz M, et al. Acute mastoiditis in children: necessity and timing of imaging. *Pediatr Infect Dis J*. 2016;35:30–34. https://doi.org/10.1097/INF.0000000000000920.
9. McLaren J, Cohen MS, El Saleeby CM. How well do we know Gradenigo? A comprehensive literature review and proposal for novel diagnostic categories of Gradenigo's syndrome. *Int J Pediatr Otorhinolaryngol*. 2020;132:109942. https://doi.org/10.1016/j. ijporl.2020.109942.
10. Osborn AJ, Blaser S, Papsin BC. Decisions regarding intracranial complications from acute mastoiditis in children. *Curr Opin Otolaryngol Head Neck Surg*. 2011;19:478–485. https://doi.org/10.1097/MOO.0b013e32834b0d92.
11. Patel PN, Levi JR, Cohen MB. Lemierre's syndrome in the pediatric population: trends in disease presentation and management in literature. *Int J Pediatr Otorhinolaryngol*. 2020;136:110213. https://doi.org/10.1016/j.ijporl.2020.110213.
12. Send T, Bertlich M, Eichhorn KW, et al. Etiology, management, and outcome of pediatric epistaxis. *Pediatr Emerg Care*. 2021;37:466–470. https://doi.org/10.1097/PEC.0000000000001698.
13. Svider P, Arianpour K, Mutchnick S. Management of epistaxis in children and adolescents: avoiding a chaotic approach. *Pediatr Clin North Am*. 2018;65:607–621. https://doi.org/10.1016/j.pcl.2018.02.007.
14. Toppozada H, Michaels L, Toppozada M, et al. The human nasal mucosa in the menstrual cycle. *J Laryngol Otol*. 1981;95:1237–1247.
15. Virk JS, Pang J, Okhovat S, et al. Analysing lateral soft tissue neck radiographs. *Emerg Radiol*. 2012;19:255–260.
16. Wong D, Brown C, Mills N, et al. To drain or not to drain: management of pediatric deep neck abscesses: a case-control study. *Int J Pediatr Otorhinolaryngol*. 2012;76:1810–1813.

CHAPTER 48

UROLOGIC EMERGENCIES

Kate M. Cronan

1. **How is the diagnosis of testicular torsion made?**
   - **Symptoms:** Scrotal pain. Pain may be referred to the abdomen. Other symptoms may include nausea, vomiting, and diaphoresis.
   - **Physical examination:** A torsed testis is typically swollen and tender and lies higher in the scrotum than that on the contralateral side. Erythema of the scrotal skin may or may not be present. Edema increases with time. In the case of complete torsion, the cremasteric reflex is absent. The presence of a brisk cremasteric reflex with a 2- to 3-cm testicular shift makes the diagnosis of testicular torsion very unlikely.
   - **Studies:** Doppler ultrasonography is the imaging study of choice. However, no clinical findings, laboratory tests, or radiographic studies can approach the sensitivity of surgical exploration. On occasion, the urologist will explore based on the history even if the Doppler shows arterial flow.

2. **Can testicular torsion be intermittent?**
   Yes. With intermittent testicular torsion, the patient has symptoms compatible with testicular torsion. This may include acute scrotal pain and swelling and in some cases nausea and vomiting. However, the pain is intermittent with quick resolution. The clinical assessment may be normal, or there may be findings on physical examination such as swelling of the spermatic cord, mobile testes, or an anterior epididymis (if there is a 180-degree twist). Ultrasound results will show arterial flow to both testes.

   Those patients with a normal physical examination and ultrasound may be discharged with comprehensive instructions and a referral for follow-up with a urologist.

3. **What is the presentation in a patient with torsion of the appendix testis?**
   Although it can happen at any age, torsion of the appendix testis is most common from ages 7 to 12 years. The pain arises because of the ischemia and inflammation resulting from the torsed appendage. This results in a red hemiscrotum and boys often walk with a wide gait. The pain is not as severe as that felt in testicular torsion. Classically, the *blue dot sign* on the scrotum indicates the site of the infarcted appendage. As edema increases, this may become obscured. Doppler ultrasonography reveals normal or increased blood flow to the affected testis in the case of torsion of the appendix testis, whereas arterial blood flow is absent or diminished in the case of testicular torsion. Treatment of a torsed appendix includes analgesics or anti-inflammatory medications, scrotal support (snug underwear), and rest. Pain usually resolves in 2 to 5 days.

4. **Why does epididymitis occur more frequently in adolescent males?**
   Epididymitis is inflammation of the epididymis. It usually results from infection, which may lead to an enlarged and tender epididymis on palpation. Patients may also have symptoms of urinary tract infection (UTI), including dysuria and frequency. Most cases in young men are caused by sexually transmitted organisms, predominantly *Chlamydia trachomatis*, followed by *Neisseria gonorrhoeae* and *Ureaplasma urealyticum*. These organisms are common among adolescent boys. Treat patients for both chlamydial infection and gonorrhea. Epididymitis is extremely rare among prepubertal boys; if it is diagnosed, further investigation is warranted to rule out structural abnormalities of the urinary tract.

5. **How is epididymitis treated?**
   Outpatient therapy is appropriate. Treatment for sexually transmitted disease–related epididymitis includes a single dose of ceftriaxone, 250 mg intramuscularly, and doxycycline, 100 mg orally twice daily for 7 to 10 days. Azithromycin can be used as an alternative. Make sure the patient is aware that the sexual partner(s) need to be treated as well. Only treat prepubertal children if there is evidence of a UTI. Appropriate antibiotics include trimethoprim-sulfamethoxasole or cephalosporin. Scrotal support and nonsteroidal anti-inflammatory drugs (NSAIDs) are also helpful to relieve pain.

   Admit patients who are febrile and toxic-appearing for treatment with intravenous (IV) antibiotics, and possibly for further diagnostic tests (e.g., testicular ultrasonography) to exclude a scrotal or testicular abscess.

6. **What is the difference between phimosis and paraphimosis?**
   Both of these conditions are diagnosed in the uncircumcised male. *Phimosis* occurs when the distal foreskin is too tight to retract over the glans penis. *Paraphimosis* occurs when the foreskin left in the retracted position, becomes swollen, and is then not able to be reduced (Fig. 48.1). Phimosis is generally not a problem in children and is normal in boys younger than 6 months. Retraction of the foreskin should not be attempted routinely in infants.

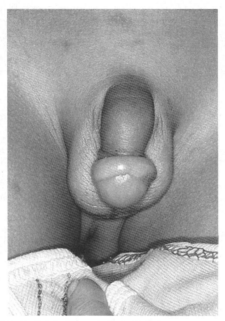

Fig. 48.1 Paraphimosis. (Photograph by John Loiselle, MD; used with permission.)

In contrast, paraphimosis should be reduced in the emergency department (ED). In general, this is accomplished by applying lidocaine gel to the swollen foreskin, followed by steady pressure on the glans, and then pulling the foreskin forward while pushing the glans backward with the thumb. A dorsal penile block with local anesthetic may make the patient more comfortable but is generally not needed.

7. **Describe balanoposthitis.**
Balanoposthitis is an inflammation of the foreskin and may affect the glans penis. It occurs in uncircumcised boys. If the foreskin is irritated as the result of poor hygiene, a break in the skin may occur, allowing bacteria to establish a skin infection. If there is true cellulitis, treatment with cephalexin will cover typical skin flora. Voiding may be more comfortable while the patient is sitting in a tub of warm water. True phimosis may occur as a complication, resulting from scarring after the inflammatory reaction. Circumcision may be necessary to avoid recurrent infections. The term *balanitis* is used to describe an infection involving only the glans penis.

8. **What are other causes of penile swelling in children?**
Penile swelling is usually painful and results from infection, sickling of red blood cells (boys with hemoglobin SS), or trauma. Other considerations in the presence of isolated, nontender penile swelling include insect bite (look for the lesion), allergic reaction, idiopathic penile edema, or more generalized edematous states, including renal, cardiac, or hepatic problems.

9. **How do a "communicating" and a "noncommunicating" hydrocele differ?**
A hydrocele is an accumulation of fluid within the tunica vaginalis, which surrounds the testis. Infants are often left with a simple noncommunicating hydrocele because fluid is trapped around the testis. This happens after the processus vaginalis closes during development with testicular descent. The baby presents with painless scrotal swelling of constant size. Management consists of observation only, as most are resorbed by the age of 12 to 18 months.

If the history is of scrotal swelling that "waxes and wanes" especially with crying or exertion, the processus vaginalis may not have closed. This allows "communication" of fluid between the scrotum and the abdominal cavity. Treatment in this case is a surgical exploration with ligation of the processus vaginalis and drainage of the hydrocele.

10. **How can a hydrocele be differentiated from an inguinal hernia in an infant?**

    The infant with an inguinal hernia presents with nonerythematous inguinal and scrotal swelling in males, and inguinal swelling in females. This swelling typically worsens if the baby is crying or straining. Occasionally bowel sounds may be heard over the swelling if enough intestine has prolapsed into the hernia sac. In young females with tender inguinal swelling, consider the possibility that the ovary may have herniated into the hernia sac and may be ischemic. This would be detected by ultrasound and would constitute emergency grounds for emergency exploration if the hernia cannot be reduced. The hydrocele lacks inguinal swelling.

    Transillumination with a high-intensity light does *not* definitively make the distinction. Although the mass of a hydrocele generally does transilluminate, transillumination of a hernia can be variable.

11. **What should be done to reduce an inguinal hernia?**

    Make sure the testes are descended and then apply steady gentle pressure to the mass up into the direction of the internal ring. Typically, the mass will slip back into the abdominal cavity making a very characteristic gurgling sound though this may take several minutes of steady pressure. If the hernia remains difficult to reduce one can rely on sedation with midazolam and placing the patient in a Trendelenburg position. This is also the time to consult general surgery to evaluate the child because a hernia that cannot be reduced constitutes a surgical emergency as the intestine can become ischemic.

12. **What is a ureterocele?**

    A ureterocele is a dilation of the distal ureter that produces a cystic structure within the obstruction. In a female, a ball-valving ureterocele is the most common cause of bladder outlet obstruction. These patients will present with a painless pink cystic structure that is bulging out between the labia. This can be reduced by placing a feeding tube within the bladder. Ureteroceles should be managed by urologists, who will usually opt to carry out an endoscopic puncture and decompression of the obstructed system.

13. **How can one distinguish between a prolapsed ureterocele and a prolapsed urethra?**

    The differentiation between a prolapsed ureterocele and urethral prolapse can usually be made by physical examination. A urethral prolapse appears as a red or purplish doughnut-shaped mass; typically the parent notes blood in the diaper. It is usually not tender and is 1 to 2 cm in diameter (Fig. 48.2). A small central dimple indicates the lumen of the urethra. Rarely, there may be a dark ring of necrotic tissue around the edge of the prolapse. In contrast, the prolapsed ureterocele is a cystic swelling of the terminal ureter and appears as a pink cystic mass protruding from the urethra.

14. **What is the most common cause of severe obstructive uropathy in children?**

    Posterior urethral valves are most common and occur only in boys. If the condition is not diagnosed in utero, the child presents with a palpably distended bladder, a weak urinary stream and occasionally a UTI. Urgent urologic consultation is indicated.

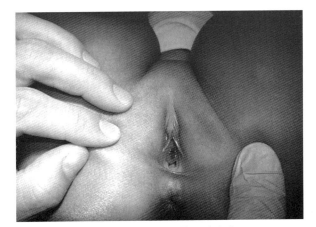

Fig. 48.2 Urethral prolapse. (Photograph by Steven M. Selbst, MD; used with permission.)

15. **What is the first evaluation to do for a patient with "blood in the urine"?**
It is important to first confirm that the red urine actually contains blood. Urine can appear red as the result of ingestion of a number of foods (blackberries, beets, red Kool-Aid drink, or popsicles, Fruit Loops cereal), substances (aniline dyes, urates), or drugs (phenazopyridine, phenolphthalein).
A urine dipstick test can determine whether blood is present. If the result is positive, microscopic analysis is needed to determine the presence or absence of red blood cells. Myoglobin will also give a positive result for blood on the dipstick. Consider the presence of more than 5 to 10 red blood cells per high-power field to be hematuria. This may warrant further work-up.

16. **Describe the differences among bacteriuria, cystitis, pyelonephritis, and urethritis.**
Bacteriuria refers to the presence of bacteria anywhere in the urinary tract. It may or may not cause symptoms.
Cystitis and pyelonephritis are part of the continuum of UTIs. *Cystitis* is bacteriuria with invasion of the bladder mucosa. Patients with cystitis typically have urgency, frequency, and dysuria and may occasionally develop a low-grade fever. *Pyelonephritis* occurs when the UTI has localized within the renal parenchyma and causes systemic symptoms. This is the most serious of UTIs. Children present with fever (temperature often >39°C), pyuria, and bacteriuria. They may have nausea, vomiting, leukocytosis, flank pain, and tenderness.
Urethritis indicates inflammation or infection localized to the urethra. There is usually a discharge. In adolescents, urethritis generally is a manifestation of a sexually transmitted disease (*C. trachomatis* or *N. gonorrhoeae* infection). Urethritis can also result from noninfectious causes, including local irritation from detergents, fabric softeners, soaps, or bubble baths, as well as minor injury.

17. **What are the most common organisms in UTI?**
Escherichia coli is isolated in about 90% of cases. Other less common organisms include *Enterobacter*, *Klebsiella*, and *Proteus* spp., and *Enterococcus* sp. occasionally is isolated from patients of any age. *Staphylococcus saprophyticus* and *Staphylococcus epidermidis* are seen in adolescents, and group B streptococci are found in infants and during pregnancy. In immunocompromised and chronically ill patients, as well as patients with anatomic abnormalities or indwelling catheters, *Pseudomonas aeruginosa*, *Candida albicans*, and *Staphylococcus aureus* account for a small percentage of UTIs. Cystitis may be caused, in addition, by adenoviruses.

18. **Which age groups most commonly get UTIs?**
Overall, UTIs are more common in neonates and infants and in sexually active adolescent females. As many as 3% to 5% of febrile young infants presenting to the ED have a UTI. In neonates and infants under the age of 6 months, males have a higher incidence. By age 1 year, girls are more likely to have a UTI than boys. This continues through childhood and the teen years. In contrast, girls have a rate of UTI as much as 10-fold higher than that of boys between the ages of 6 months and 2 years, with the risk being greater in the first year than in the second.

19. **How does the clinical presentation of UTI vary with the age of the patient?**
   - *Neonates and very young infants* with UTI may present with fever or with nonspecific symptoms, including poor feeding, vomiting, diarrhea, irritability, jaundice, and rarely seizures. This is clearly why assessment of the urine is an integral part of the "full sepsis work-up" performed on infants with any of these presenting symptoms.
   - *Older infants and children* up to the age of 2 years often have fever, and parents may notice such urinary symptoms as a change in voiding pattern or foul-smelling urine.
   - *Preschool and school-age children* describe specific urologic symptoms, such as frequency, urgency, dysuria, and enuresis. They may have fewer specific symptoms, including abdominal pain and vomiting.
   - *Children older than 6 years* may have fever, vomiting, dysuria, enuresis, and incontinence.

KEY POINTS: CLINICAL PRESENTATION OF URINARY TRACT INFECTIONS BY AGE

1. **Neonates:** Nonspecific symptoms, fever
2. **Infants up to age 2 years:** Fever, voiding issues, foul-smelling urine
3. **Preschool and school-age children:** Dysuria, frequency, urgency, abdominal pain

---

20. **When should one get a catheterized urine specimen as opposed to a "clean-catch" specimen?**
If the patient is ill-appearing or needs antibiotics promptly, obtain a catheterized urine specimen in any patient who lacks bladder control (e.g., infants and toddlers), has evidence of vaginitis, or is unable to provide an adequate midstream specimen. Putting a urine "bag" on an infant or toddler may not be helpful if the specimen is collected for culture, because the urine will probably be contaminated with perineal flora no matter how much preparation is done. In the febrile infant who does not need immediate antibiotics, urine could be obtained by a catheter or through the most convenient means to perform a urinalysis (UA). If the UA suggests a UTI (positive

leukocyte esterase or nitrite test) or microscopic analysis results for leukocytes or bacteria, then a urine specimen for culture should be obtained by catheterization.

21. **What is the significance of a positive test result for nitrites on the urine dipstick?**
Most urinary pathogens (with the exception of *Enterococcus*) are able to reduce urine nitrates to nitrite. Hence, a positive test result may indicate the presence of pathogenic bacteria.

22. **How should dipstick indicators be used to screen for UTI?**
Many studies have been published regarding the usefulness of these tests in diagnosing UTI. Most of the studies have been performed in adult patients, and the results of studies in children frequently differ. A meta-analysis by Gorelick and Shaw concludes that the presence of nitrites or leukocyte esterase or both on a dipstick test is almost as sensitive as a Gram stain in detecting UTI in children.

KEY POINTS: SCREENING FOR INFECTION VIA URINE DIPSTICK

1. **Nitrite positive:** Indicates probable pathogenic bacteria (does not screen for *enterococcus*)
2. **Leukocyte esterase positive:** Specific for pyuria

23. **Do white blood cells in the urine always signify a UTI?**
No, not always. Pyuria can be found in the absence of bacteriuria (i.e., "sterile pyuria"). Inflammatory process in the abdomen (e.g., appendicitis, inflammatory bowel disease, pelvic inflammatory disease) or Kawasaki disease can cause white blood cells to appear in the urine. Vaginitis can cause the leukocyte esterase test result to be positive, but this does not necessarily mean the patient has a UTI. A recent meta-analysis shows that the presence of white blood cells in the urine (either spun or unspun) is only about 75% sensitive for UTI.

24. **How accurate are dipsticks in predicting a positive urine culture?**
A dipstick test is sensitive in predicting whether a urine culture will show positive growth. This is dependent upon the accuracy of the sample collection. The dipstick indicators for nitrites (triggered by bacteria) and leukocyte esterase (triggered by white blood cells) are in the 70% range as individual parameters but rise to 93% when both are positive. The specificity for both parameters is 70%. Taken together this means that when evaluating a symptomatic child, a positive dipstick for leukocytes and nitrates allows one to begin treating for a presumptive UTI.

25. **Which factors in patients with UTI indicate they should be admitted for parenteral antibiotics?**
   - Age younger than 2 months
   - Toxic appearance; signs of shock
   - Immunocompromised patient
   - Vomiting or not being able to tolerate oral medication
   - Suspicion for lack of adequate outpatient follow-up
   - Failure of outpatient therapy
   - Anatomic factors that may cause an obstruction to urinary flow
   - Culture positivity for a pathogen known to be resistant to oral antibiotics

26. **A newborn boy presents to the ED 2 days after circumcision. He has had prolonged bleeding from the incision site onto the diaper. What are the steps you would take?**
First, put a pressure dressing on and if the bleeding continues, consult Urology and Hematology and order a complete blood count (CBC), prothrombin time (PT), partial thromboplastin time (PTT), and factor levels. Ask about the family history of bleeding disorders. Keep in mind that von Willebrand disease and the hemophilias can arise from denovo mutations meaning there will be a negative family history. Bleeding from a circumcision site or from the umbilicus after the cord has separated are two ways in which such coagulopathies can present in early life.

27. **Does circumcision offer a health care benefit?**
Uncircumcised boys are more likely to present with a febrile UTI relative to circumcised boys. This is due, in part, to the mucosal surface of the foreskin. It binds uropathogenic bacteria on a circumcised penis. Also, partial obstruction of the urethral meatus due to tight foreskin could explain higher numbers of UTIs in uncircumcised boys. This effect is even more pronounced in boys with an underlying obstructive uropathy, like posterior urethral valves, where circumcision was proven superior in a randomized clinical trial. In another randomized clinical trial circumcision was also shown to lower the chances of HIV seroconversion.

28. **What causes urinary retention in infants?**
In the infant, most urinary retention is the result of obstruction. In males, the most common cause is obstruction of posterior urethral valves; other causes include urethral polyps, strictures, diverticula, trauma, infection, and, rarely,

meatal stenosis. Urinary retention has been noted as a complication of the Plastibell device used for circumcision. Female infants may experience a prolapsing ureterocele, urethral prolapse, trauma, infection, or a foreign body. Neurologic urinary retention may result from a spinal cord lesion.

29. **How can sexual abuse contribute to urinary retention?**
Always be aware that urinary retention or dysfunctional voiding may on rare occasions be the presenting symptom of sexual abuse. Children who have been sexually abused are often very fearful of any processes involving the genitalia and seek to avoid that portion of their anatomy. Furthermore, abusive acts may result in genital or urethral trauma or infection. Ask appropriate questions if no other cause for urinary retention can be found.

30. **What should be done in the ED about urinary retention?**
The approach depends on the cause. Newborn infants with ineffective voiding should be referred to a urologist for further evaluation. Consider obtaining a basic metabolic panel to check electrolytes, blood urea nitrogen (BUN), and creatinine. A bladder scan can quickly determine how much urine is in the bladder. A suprapubic tap may be necessary to obtain a specimen for UA. Consult a neurologist if a spinal cord lesion is suspected on examination. Older children who have previously voided normally may be catheterized for UA if they are unable to void. Treat infections with appropriate antibiotics. Treat patients with retention from trauma to the urethra with frequent sitz baths (at least three times per day). Discontinue medications causing retention if possible. Refer patients with urinary retention suspected to be of psychosomatic origin or as the result of sexual abuse to psychiatric and sexual abuse management specialists as appropriate. If the patient is unable to void, catheterization may be necessary.

31. **What causes renal stones in children?**
Renal stones (calculi) are less common in children and adolescents than in adults. Seven percent of urinary calculi occur in children younger than 16 years. The cause of calculi depends in part on geography. In the United States, most stones are attributed to metabolic causes, and most contain calcium. Infectious stones are more common in European children, and uric acid stones occur in Southeast Asian children. Boys and girls are equally likely to be affected, and 94% of stones occur in white persons.

32. **What are the symptoms of urolithiasis in children?**
The classic presentation is that of excruciating abdominal pain. However, approximately 15% to 20% are without symptoms. The patient may appear uncomfortable and may report flank pain, abdominal pain, or costovertebral angle tenderness. Almost all children have some degree of hematuria, which may be microscopic or macroscopic. They may also have symptoms of dysuria, urinary frequency, or urinary retention. The cause of these symptoms needs to be distinguished from UTI.

33. **How is the diagnosis of urolithiasis confirmed?**
The first test to obtain is a UA, to look for hematuria and for crystals in the urinary sediment. In recent years, ultrasound has become the first diagnostic test because this avoids radiation exposure. If the ultrasound is inconclusive, spiral, noncontrast computed tomography (CT) can be done.

34. **What treatment for urolithiasis should be initiated in the ED?**
The foremost issue that must be addressed in the ED is pain management. NSAIDs and opioids are used to treat pain associated with acute nephrolithiasis. If the pain is not relieved, administer further pain medication intravenously and give IV fluids. Obtain a urologic consultation for any patient with evidence of obstruction, because endoscopic stenting may be indicated.

35. **Which patients with urolithiasis need to be admitted?**
Admit a patient with urolithiasis if there is
- Evidence of obstruction for urologic consultation, because immediate intervention (e.g., endoscopic stenting or ureteroscopy with stone extraction) is necessary to relieve the obstructing stone.
- Severe pain requiring parenteral analgesia.
- Vomiting, dehydration, or inability to tolerate oral hydration.
- Renal insufficiency, structural abnormalities of the genitourinary tract, or a solitary kidney.
- Fever, indicating possible impending sepsis due to infection above the obstructing stone.

36. **What are the presenting symptoms of ureteropelvic junction (UPJ) obstruction in older children?**
Children with UPJ obstruction will have a history of episodic pain that can occur in the abdomen, flank, or back. Nausea and vomiting may occur. The episodes of pain last from 30 minutes to several hours. UPJ obstruction presents more commonly on the left side and is bilateral in 10% of cases. The male-to-female ratio is 2:1. Examination may reveal an enlarged kidney and tenderness.

37. **Is imaging needed for UPJ in the ED?**
Yes, it is crucial to image the kidneys with an ultrasound or CT scan at the time they are having pain. *This is because often the imaging reverts to normal once the symptoms resolve.*

38. **What is the most common cause of acute glomerulonephritis (AGN)?**
There are numerous causes of AGN, but in children the most common is *postinfectious* or *poststreptococcal nephritis.* This syndrome occurs predominantly in school-age children. It is characterized by the sudden appearance of either grossly bloody or tea-colored urine, peripheral edema, and decreased urine output. Patients typically present 1 to 2 weeks after having had a sore throat. Rarely it can occur 2 to 3 weeks after a case of impetigo. Other infectious causes include viral upper respiratory tract infections and mononucleosis.

39. **What are the physical findings in AGN?**
Children with AGN can develop peripheral edema. The edema is firm and initially appears around the eyes. Other symptoms may include lethargy, headache, weight gain, reduced urine output, rash, and joint pain. Patients may have mildly elevated blood pressure. Some children have no symptoms other than abnormally colored, dark, or bloody urine. In others, hypertension can be significant and lead to complications requiring emergency intervention.

40. **What laboratory tests should I order for suspected AGN?**
The most important test is the UA, with a microscopic examination of the urine. Dysmorphic red blood cells and casts are diagnostic of AGN. Significant proteinuria is also characteristic. White blood cells may be present. Because hematuria and proteinuria may be presenting signs of a UTI, order a urine culture in the initial evaluation.
   Other studies include CBC with differential, platelet count, erythrocyte sedimentation rate, serum electrolytes, calcium, BUN, creatinine, total protein, albumin, and complement (C3 and C4). Also, test for antistreptolysin O titer if poststreptococcal AGN is considered; antinuclear antibody and anti-double-stranded DNA should be done in the case of systemic lupus erythematosus. Order PT and PTT if there is concern about a bleeding diathesis. A throat culture may reveal group A streptococcal infection, and chest radiography may be important to evaluate heart size and to look for signs of congestive heart failure (CHF) in a hypertensive patient.

41. **What are the goals of ED management of AGN?**
The goal is aggressive treatment of life-threatening complications, particularly hypertension, CHF, and hyperkalemia. If the blood pressure is elevated but the patient is asymptomatic, oral antihypertensives (sublingual nifedipine or captopril) may be adequate. In the patient with acute neurologic changes, give antihypertensives (diazoxide or hydralazine) intravenously. Treat CHF by keeping the head of the bed elevated, providing supplemental oxygen, and promoting diuresis with furosemide (0.5–1.0 mg/kg via IV route). Restrict fluid volume and sodium and replace only insensible losses plus urine output. Do not give potassium until the patient's urine output is established and hyperkalemia is resolved. Admit children with AGN to the hospital.

42. **What are the clinical findings of nephrotic syndrome in children? What are the most common causes?**
Nephrotic syndrome occurs as a constellation of findings:
- Edema—often facial (and scotal edema in males)
- Proteinuria
- Hypoalbuminemia
- Hyperlipidemia
   Nephrotic syndrome can occur in children as a primary renal disorder or secondary to systemic disease, environmental toxins (heavy metals, bee venom), or medications.

43. **How is the diagnosis of nephrotic syndrome made?**
Check the patient's urine for protein. Measure total serum protein, albumin, and cholesterol levels. Usually, values in nephrotic syndrome are as follows: a urinary protein of 3 to 4+ on dipstick, serum albumin level lower than 3 g/dL, and elevated cholesterol level. Other values that may be important for management include the hematocrit (which may be elevated secondary to intravascular volume depletion), electrolytes (sodium is often low), and BUN/creatinine (BUN level may initially be elevated, reflecting the lowered intravascular volume; creatinine level may be normal or elevated depending on whether there is primary renal damage).

44. **What are the five important complications of idiopathic nephrotic syndrome?**
- Infection
- Thromboembolism
- Renal insufficiency
- Anasarca
- Hypovolemia

45. In a child with nephrotic syndrome, what management decisions need to be made in the ED?

Complications requiring urgent management include the progression from hypovolemia to shock, hypercoagulability, and pleural effusions and ascites leading to difficulty walking, abdominal pain, or respiratory distress.

The child must be evaluated for peritonitis, usually due to *Streptococcus pneumoniae*. Consider antibiotics if the child is febrile, or if peritonitis is otherwise suspected, after obtaining a blood culture. If restoration of circulation is needed, begin normal saline boluses (20 mL/kg). For symptomatic massive edema, give furosemide orally, or in extreme cases, albumin followed by IV furosemide. Rarely is paracentesis necessary. Avoid deep venipunctures because of the increased risk of thromboembolic events.

46. Should all patients with nephrotic syndrome be admitted?

Admit those with the following:
- Newly diagnosed patients
- Patients in whom there is a possibility of infection
- Any who are symptomatic from dehydration or edema
    Contact a pediatric nephrologist regarding steroid therapy and indications for renal biopsy.

BIBLIOGRAPHY

1. Cristoforo TA. Evaluating the necessity of antibiotics in the treatment of acute epididymitis in pediatric patients: a literature review of prospective studies and data analysis. *Pediatr Emerg Care.* 2021;37(12):e1675–e1680.
2. Liebelt EL, Davis VA. Hematuria. In: Shaw KL, Bashur RG, eds. *Fleisher & Ludwig's Textbook of Pediatric Emergency Medicine.* 8th ed. Wolters Kluwer; 2021:235–239.
3. Mattoo TK, Shaikh N, Nelson CP. Contemporary management of urinary tract infections in children. *Pediatrics.* 2021;147(2):e2020012138.
4. Miah T, Kamat D. Pediatric nephrolithiasis: a review. *Pediatr Ann.* 2017;46(6):e242–e244.
5. Roberts K, Wald E. The diagnosis of UTI: colony count criteria revisited. *Pediatrics.* 2018;141(2):e20173239.
6. Upsal NG. Urethral prolapse. In: Hoffman RJ, Wang VJ, eds. *Fleisher & Ludwig's 5-Minute Pediatric Emergency Medicine Consult.* 2020:966–967.
7. Weiss DA, Jacobstein CR. Genitourinary emergencies. In: Shaw KL, Bashur RG, eds. *Fleisher & Ludwig's Textbook of Pediatric Emergency Medicine.* 8th ed. Wolters Kluwer; 2021:1533–1541.

Section V   TRAUMA

ABDOMINAL TRAUMA

Deborah L. Hammett and Margarita S. Lorch

1. **What are the most common mechanisms of injury for pediatric patients with abdominal trauma?**
   In the United States, blunt mechanisms account for 90% of abdominal trauma in children. The most common causes are motor vehicle collisions (as passengers or pedestrians) and falls.

2. **What makes children more prone to blunt abdominal injury compared to adults?**
   Compared to adults, children have compact torsos with a larger organ-to-body mass ratio. Forces delivered to the abdomen dissipate over a smaller area leading to an increased risk of injury. Infants and toddlers have a larger portion of the liver and spleen exposed below a more flexible rib cage, placing those organs at greater risk for injury. In addition, young children involved in automobile crashes may have injuries related to lap belts if they are improperly restrained.

3. **What is the "lap belt complex" seen with motor vehicle crash victims?**
   This complex refers to injuries sustained during a motor vehicle crash when the seat belt rides up from the pelvic bones and compresses the softer abdominal viscera against the spine in an improperly restrained child. This may result in soft tissue injury to the abdomen, Chance fractures (compression fractures of the lumbar spine), and intra-abdominal injury. The seat belt sign specifically refers to a linear bruise or mark across the abdomen in patients restrained by a lap belt in a motor vehicle collision and is associated with a higher likelihood of significant intra-abdominal injuries, such as solid-organ injury, bowel perforations, mesenteric injury, or bladder injury.

4. **What is the significance of a blow to the abdomen from the handlebars of a bicycle?**
   A direct blow to the abdomen of a child from the handlebars of a bicycle can result in significant injury, often with limited external physical findings. Common injuries are solid-organ injury, intestinal perforation, and abdominal wall hernia. Children presenting with abdominal pain, fever, vomiting, and/or a handlebar imprint on their abdomen or chest should undergo additional diagnostic work-up due to concern for serious underlying injury. Diagnosis of these injuries is sometimes delayed, and a high proportion of those who returned for worsening symptoms required a surgical procedure.

5. **When is abdominal injury suspicious of physical child abuse?**
   While no intra-abdominal injury is pathognomonic for abuse, it is important to consider the possibility of physical child abuse as a potential mechanism of injury in the pediatric patient presenting with abdominal trauma. Solid-organ injuries are the most common abdominal injuries resulting from accidental trauma and abusive trauma, yet hollow viscus and pancreatic injuries are more commonly found in victims of abuse. Abusive abdominal injuries have been shown to account for a large proportion of abdominal trauma among infants and toddlers. Consider child abuse in patients who have delayed presentation or an unwitnessed traumatic event.

6. **What physical examination findings are useful for identifying abdominal injuries?**
   Physical findings, including absent or diminished bowel sounds, evidence of peritoneal irritation with involuntary guarding or rebound, abdominal distention or rigidity, abdominal wall abrasions or bruising, abdominal or flank tenderness, lower chest wall injury, or unexplained hypotension may indicate the presence of an abdominal injury. Evaluation for tenderness or instability of the pelvic bones is necessary because pelvic fractures have been associated with an increased risk of intra-abdominal injury. Perform a rectal examination in patients with a significant injury to assess for palpable mass, lacerations, pelvic brim fracture, or blood.

7. **Which laborory studies are useful for evaluating patients with abdominal trauma?**
   Complete blood counts, transaminases, and urinalysis are useful in identifying possible injury. Serial blood counts in patients with abdominal pain or tenderness may be useful in identifying acute blood loss. Elevation of serum transaminases has been shown to be associated with an increased risk of intra-abdominal injury, however, aspartate aminotransferase/alanine aminotransferase (AST/ALT) thresholds to prompt further abdominal imaging are not clearly understood. A study completed by Bevan et al. found an ALT value above 104 IU/L was 96% sensitive for identifying liver injury following blunt abdominal trauma. Alternatively, higher cut-off levels of AST >200 IU/L and ALT >125 IU/L have been proposed by Holmes et al. to have an increased odds ratio (17.4; 95% confidence interval 9.4-32.1) of serious intra-abdominal injury in pediatric blunt abdominal trauma. Unexplained

anemia, gross or microscopic hematuria (>5 red blood cells [RBCs]/high-power field), or elevated serum transaminases may indicate the presence of intra-abdominal injury even in the absence of other findings. The utility of pancreatic enzymes is unclear but may be helpful in assessing for intra-abdominal injury.

8. **What is the treatment for a child with an apparent abdominal injury and clinical instability?**
The initial care for the unstable pediatric patient with abdominal trauma must begin with the ABCs (airway, breathing, circulation). Once the airway and breathing are secure and the cervical spine is stabilized, address circulation with an initial infusion of an isotonic crystalloid solution (normal saline or lactated Ringer solution) of 20 mL/kg via the intravenous route. For patients who continue to be hemodynamically unstable, consider RBC transfusion. Blood transfusion should be strongly considered in hemodynamically unstable trauma patients receiving greater than 40 mL/kg of crystalloid. Transfusion of 1:1:1 of RBCs, plasma, and platelets is advised during initial resuscitation efforts.

9. **Is there a role for the use of tranexamic acid (TXA) for the treatment of pediatric intra-abdominal hemorrhage?**
The use of TXA for the treatment of pediatric hemorrhagic shock remains unclear and additional research is needed to determine its utility. Early operative intervention should be considered in patients with persistent hemodynamic instability due to ongoing blood loss.

10. **What is the role of computed tomography (CT) in pediatric abdominal trauma?**
For the clinically stable pediatric patient with blunt trauma, CT continues to be the gold standard for abdominal injury diagnosis. CT is both sensitive and specific for the diagnosis of liver, spleen, and retroperitoneal injuries. Disadvantages include limited utility in the clinically unstable patient, radiation exposure, and limited sensitivity for the diagnosis of bowel injury. If the decision is made to proceed with CT imaging to evaluate for underlying organ injury, radiation level should be kept As Low as Reasonably Achievable (ALARA) in the pediatric trauma patient.

11. **Are there any evidence-based clinical decision tools in identifying children at low risk of clinically significant abdominal injury?**
Several tools have been developed and studied to evaluate children at low risk of clinically significant injuries following blunt abdominal trauma. The Pediatric Emergency Care Applied Research Network group identified seven clinical features including Glasgow Coma Score (GCS) >13, lack of abdominal trauma or seat belt sign, not reported abdominal pain, absence of abdominal tenderness, no vomiting, absence of thoracic wall trauma, and presence of normal breath sounds, which were associated with low risk of clinically significant abdominal injury (negative predictive value [NPV] of 99.9%).

Using clinical, laboratory, and radiographic factors, Streck et al. suggest with their prediction model that abdominal CT is not needed in children with a reliable physical examination who present with the following: normal systolic blood pressure for age, normal abdominal examination, AST <200 U/L, hematocrit >30%, and normal chest x-ray. Finally, the blunt abdominal trauma in children (BATiC) score looks at the following 10 radiographic, laboratory, and clinical features to identify children who need not receive abdominal CT as part of their evaluation of blunt abdominal trauma. The BATiC score assigns the following points to each criterion: abnormal abdominal Doppler ultrasound (4), signs of peritoneal irritation (2), hemodynamic instability (2), AST >60 IU/L (2), ALT >25 IU/L (2), white blood cells >9.5 g/L (1), lactate dehydrogenase >330 IU/L (1), lipase >30 IU/L (1), and creatinine >50 μg/L (1). The risk of serious intra-abdominal injury is low in patients with BATiC scores ≤7 (NPV 97%); CT abdomen and hospitalization may be avoided in these low-risk patients.

12. **Can patients who meet the criteria for CT imaging following blunt abdominal trauma be safely discharged from the emergency department (ED)?**
Patients with negative CT imaging may be considered safe for discharge home if they have no abdominal pain, no seat belt sign, the ability to tolerate oral fluids, and no concern for any other serious traumatic injuries. Additionally, if there is a concern for physical abuse, a safe-discharge plan must be arranged with child protective services or the patient should be observed in the hospital setting. When discharging patients home from the ED, it is important to provide clear discharge instructions including reasons to return to care.

13. **What is the role of the FAST examination in the evaluation of pediatric abdominal trauma?**
The focused abdominal sonography for trauma (FAST) examination is helpful to identify intra-abdominal free fluid and parenchymal injury by rapidly imaging the right and left upper quadrants, subxiphoid region, and pelvis. It is advantageous because it is a rapid, convenient, inexpensive tool that does not expose a child to radiation. Also, it can be done at the bedside, so the patient does not need to be transported.

In the unstable patient, a positive FAST examination may be an indication for operative intervention. In a stable patient, identification of intra-abdominal fluid on FAST examination indicates the need for an abdominal CT. A negative FAST, however, does not exclude intra-abdominal injury.

14. **What is the sensitivity and specificity of the FAST examination in children? Which patients would benefit most from a FAST examination?**

Limited studies evaluating the utility of the FAST examination in children have been performed. A 2022 meta-analysis evaluating the FAST examination in children presenting with blunt abdominal trauma found only a 35% sensitivity, but a 96% specificity of the FAST examination in the pediatric population. Thus a positive FAST examination in children suggests that intra-abdominal injury is likely, but a negative FAST does not rule out the need for additional diagnostic testing if otherwise clinically indicated.

However, a study looking specifically at ED ultrasonography in hypotensive children with blunt abdominal trauma found a sensitivity of 100% and specificity of 100%. Therefore, although not necessarily recommended for routine use, there may be a role for FAST in the rapid evaluation of unstable patients with concern for intra-abdominal injury.

15. **What is the recommended ED management of splenic injury in children?**

All children with splenic injury will require admission to the hospital and those with hemodynamic instability should be admitted to the pediatric intensive care unit (ICU). The majority (90%-95%) of patients are managed nonoperatively with monitoring of vital signs, hematocrit, and urine output. Transfuse packed RBCs as necessary for hemodynamic changes or significant anemia. Operative intervention should be dictated by clinical course rather than the grade of injury. For those who are hemodynamically stable but requiring multiple transfusions, arterial embolization may provide an alternative to operative intervention. Arterial embolization has been used frequently in adults but there is limited experience with this procedure in children.

The American Pediatric Surgery Association has established guidelines for resource utilization (including length of ICU and hospital stay as well as activity restriction) based on the grade of injuries as seen on CT. However, at least one recent study has shown shorter length of stay and decreased resource use when hemodynamic stability and hematocrit were used as the basis for clinical decision-making.

16. **What are the indications for emergent laparotomy or laparoscopy for pediatric abdominal trauma?**

See Table 49.1 for the indications for emergency laparotomy or laparoscopy.

17. **What is the clinical approach to penetrating abdominal trauma?**

Because of their high velocity and penetrating ability, more than 90% of gunshot wounds to the abdomen will result in organ injury requiring laparotomy. Stab wounds are typically of lower velocity, with less penetrating ability, and can be managed more selectively. Triple-contrast CT, laparoscopy, clinical observation, or local wound exploration have all been advocated to identify peritoneal penetration or intra-abdominal organ injury in stable stab wound victims. Clinicians should start broad-spectrum antibiotics for all patients with penetrating abdominal trauma. Findings of clinical instability, peritoneal irritation, pneumoperitoneum, hematuria, or rectal blood are all absolute indications for laparotomy in patients with gunshot or stab wounds.

18. **Do children with blunt abdominal trauma have good outcomes with nonoperative management?**

Despite the long list of indications for laparotomy/laparoscopy mentioned above, operative intervention is infrequently required for pediatric blunt abdominal trauma, and nonoperative management is the current standard of care for the majority of patients. With few exceptions, the need for an operation rests entirely with the patient's clinical condition, rather than with specifics of the intra-abdominal organ injuries or the grade or severity of organ injury. Studies indicate that appropriately selected patients (i.e., those without surgical indications) have excellent overall outcomes, low transfusion rates, and few complications.

19. **What traumatic abdominal injuries are typically associated with a late presentation?**

Pancreatic pseudocyst (presenting with epigastric pain, abdominal mass, and hyperamylasemia), duodenal hematoma (presenting with symptoms of intestinal obstruction), and hematobilia (presenting with abdominal pain and upper gastrointestinal bleeding) often have a delayed presentation after injury. These injuries may present days to weeks after abdominal trauma.

Table 49.1 Indications for an Emergent Laparotomy for the Pediatric Trauma Patient

- Evidence of abdominal injury and persistent hemodynamic instability
- Penetrating abdominal trauma
- Pneumoperitoneum
- Multisystem injuries requiring craniotomy with intraperitoneal blood identified, or strong history or physical findings to indicate intra-abdominal injury
- Abdominal distention with associated hypotension

KEY POINTS: ABDOMINAL TRAUMA

1. The finding of a seat belt sign should prompt higher suspicion for significant intra-abdominal injury.
2. Laboratory tests (hematocrit, urinalysis, AST, ALT) are excellent adjuncts to the physical examination to screen for an abdominal injury in a stable pediatric patient.
3. Patients with no abdominal or thoracic bruising or tenderness, a GCS >13, a normal lung examination, and no vomiting, are at low risk for significant abdominal injury and may not require CT scan.
4. A negative FAST study does not exclude intra-abdominal injury.
5. Clinical instability is the most important indication for an emergent laparotomy in a child with an abdominal injury.

Acknowledgment
The authors wish to thank Dr. Ronald Funival for his contributions to this chapter in previous editions.

BIBLIOGRAPHY

1. Bevan CA, Palmer CS, Sutcliffe JR, et al. Blunt abdominal trauma in children: how predictive is ALT for liver injury? *Emerg Med J.* 2009;26(4):283–288.
2. Borgialli DA, Ellison AM, Ehlrich P, et al. Association between the seat belt sign and intra-abdominal injuries in children with blunt torso trauma in motor vehicle collisions. *Acad Emerg Med.* 2014;21:1240.
3. Cheung R, Shukla M, Akers KG, Farooqi A, Sethuraman U. Bicycle handlebar injuries: a systematic review of pediatric chest and abdominal injuries. *Am J Emerg Med.* 2022;51:13–21.
4. Christian CW, Committee on Child Abuse and Neglect American Academy of Pediatrics The evaluation of suspected child physical abuse. *Pediatrics.* 2015;135(5):e1337–1354.
5. Cotton BA, Beckert BW, Smith MK, et al. The utility of clinical laboratory data for predicting intra-abdominal injury among children. *J Trauma.* 2004;56:1068–1074.
6. Davies KL. Buckled-up children: understanding the mechanism, injuries, management, and prevention of seat belt related injuries. *J Trauma Nurs.* 2004;11(1):16–24.
7. Holmes JF, Sokolove PE, Brant WE, Palchak MJ, Vance CW, Owings JT, Kuppermann N. Identification of children with intra-abdominal injuries after blunt trauma. *Ann Emerg Med.* 2002;39(5):500–509.
8. Holmes JF, Lillis K, Monroe D, et al. Identifying children at very low risk of clinically important blunt abdominal injuries. *Ann Emerg Med.* 2013;62:107.
9. Karam O, Sanchez O, Chardot C, La Scala G. Blunt abdominal trauma in children: a score to predict the absence of organ injury. *J Pediatr.* 2009;154(6):912–917.
10. Kerrey BT, Rogers AJ, Lee LK, et al. Pediatric Emergency Care Applied Research Network A multicenter study of the risk of intra-abdominal injury in children after normal abdominal computed tomography scan results in the emergency department. *Ann Emerg Med.* 2013;62(4):319–326.
11. Lane WG, Dubowitz H, Langenberg P, Dischinger P. Epidemiology of abusive abdominal trauma hospitalizations in United States children. *Child Abuse Negl.* 2012;36(2):142–148.
12. Liang T, Roseman E, Gao M, Sinert R. The utility of the focused assessment with sonography in trauma examination in pediatric blunt abdominal trauma: a systematic review and meta-analysis. *Pediatr Emerg Care.* 2021;37(2):108–118.
13. McVay M, Kokoska E, Jackson R, et al. Throwing out the "grade" book: management of isolated spleen and liver injury based on hemodynamic status. *J Pediatr Surg.* 2008;43(6):1072–1076.
14. Nance ML, Holmes JH, Wiebe DJ. Timeline to operative intervention for solid organ injuries in children. *J Trauma.* 2006;61(6):1389.
15. Ozcan A, Ahn T, Akay B, Menoch M. Imaging for pediatric blunt abdominal trauma with different prediction rules: is the outcome same? *Pediatr Emerg Care.* 2022;38(2):e654–e658.
16. Merrick C, Exec. ed. Pediatric trauma. In: *Advanced Trauma Life Support (ATLS) for Doctors: Student Course Manual.* 10th ed. American College of Surgeons; 2018:187.
17. Saladino RA, Gaines BA. Abdominal trauma. In: Shaw KN, Bachur RG, eds. *Fleisher & Ludwig's Textbook of Pediatric Emergency Medicine.* 8th ed. Wolters Kluwer; 2021:1084–1094.
18. Sharma OP, Oswanski MF, Kaminski BP, et al. Clinical implications of the seat belt sign in blunt trauma. *Am Surg.* 2009;75(9):822–827.
19. Streck Jr CJ, Jewett BM, Wahlquist AH, Gutierrez PS, Russell WS. Evaluation for intra-abdominal injury in children after blunt torso trauma: can we reduce unnecessary abdominal computed tomography by utilizing a clinical prediction model? *J Trauma Acute Care Surg.* 2012;73(2):371–376.

BURNS AND SMOKE INHALATION

David Bergamo and John M. Loiselle

1. **How common are burns and fire-related deaths among children?**
   Injury-related deaths are the leading cause of death in children ages 1 to 14 years. Centers for Disease Control and Prevention statistics published in 2019 rate fire- or burn-related injuries as the third leading cause of injury-related deaths in this age group, behind motor vehicle–related deaths, and drownings. (In 2021, firearm-related deaths eclipsed motor vehicle-related deaths.) In the United States, an average of 300 children die from burns annually, and more than 100,000 children are treated in hospitals or emergency departments. Globally, burns are the 11th leading cause of death in children aged 1 to 9 and the fifth most common cause of nonlethal injury.

2. **What functions of the skin do burns affect?**
   - Temperature control
   - Protection from infection
   - Pain and sensation
   - Fluid homeostasis

3. **How are different depths of burns classified?**
   Such a classification is mentioned in Table 50.1.

4. **How do age and developmental abilities influence the epidemiology of burns in children?**
   The majority of burn victims are less than 5 years old. According to the National Burn Repository, scald burns are the most common type of burn injury and account for two-thirds of all burns in this age group. Most of these occur when the child pulls over a hot liquid from the surface of a table or stove. Nonaccidental burns account for up to 14% of burns in children less than 1 year of age. In children between 5 and 16, fire or flames account for approximately half of the burns, with only one-third due to scalds (Table 50.2).

   About 90% of burns occur in the home, but adolescents are more likely to sustain burns outside of the home. Adolescents are more likely to start and play with fires, while toddlers are more likely to spill or touch hot surfaces. More than a third of all pediatric burn injuries occur in the kitchen. This has important implications for preventive measures.

5. **How long must the skin be in contact with hot water to cause a burn?**
   The actual duration of contact and water temperature required to cause a partial-thickness burn depends on the location and thickness of the skin. Partial-thickness burns on the soles of the feet require a longer period of contact with the water because of the thick layer of skin. Scald burns occur more rapidly on the skin of young children than in adults, and partial- or full-thickness burns can occur in less time than listed below. Of note, hot chocolate and hot tea are often served at 160°F to 180°F.

Table 50.1 Classification of Burn Depth

WOUND DEPTH	LAYER INVOLVED	CLINICAL FINDINGS	COMMON CAUSES
Superficial	Epidermis	Erythema	Sun exposure
Superficial partial thickness	Dermis	Erythema, blistering	Hot liquids
Deep partial thickness	Deeper dermis	Dry to waxy, blister, capillary burst	Scald, oil, flame
Full thickness	Subcutaneous tissue	Pale/charred, waxy or leathery, does not bleed, insensate	Flame
Fourth degree	Fascia, muscle, or bone	Deep visualized structures	Flame or high-voltage electricity

Table 50.2 Common Sources of Burns in Children			
HOSPITALIZED PATIENTS	**%**	**EMERGENCY DEPARTMENT PATIENTS**	**%**
Flames	36	Contact	43
Scald	35	Scald	34
Immersion	14	Flame	11
Contact	9	Cigarette	5.5
Chemical	3.5	Electrical	2.8
Electrical	1.5	House fire	0.9
Other	2.7		

Fluid temperature and immersion time necessary to cause a partial thickness burn.
160°F—1 second
150°F—2 seconds
140°F—5 seconds
130°F—30 seconds
120°F—300 seconds

6. **Why is it important to interview the paramedics who arrive with fire victims?**
Paramedics can provide the answers to questions that influence therapy as well as prognosis. Important questions include the following:
- Did the fire occur in an open or enclosed area?
- Where was the child found?
- What was the duration of exposure to smoke?
- Did the child lose consciousness?
- How long was the transport?
- What therapy was instituted?
- Is trauma, any other injuries, identified?
- What materials were at the fire scene?
- Is additional toxic fume exposure a concern?

7. **Name the methods commonly used to estimate the percentage of body surface area (BSA) damaged by burns in a child.**
In both children and adults, BSA is calculated by including partial-thickness and full-thickness burns. Superficial or first-degree burns are excluded. The distribution of BSA is different in children and adults. The standard "rule of nines" used in adults is not as accurate in children. The young child has a greater proportion of the BSA in the head and less in the lower extremities. Nagel and Schunk demonstrated that the entire palmar surface of a child's hand (including the fingers) is approximately 1% of BSA. The Lund and Browder chart (Fig. 50.1) provides useful estimates of larger contiguous burn areas in children younger than 10 years of age.

8. **What is the initial treatment of major burns in a child?**
   1. Address and stabilize the airway, breathing, and circulation using proper cervical spine precautions and apply 100% oxygen by rebreather mask if concerned about smoke exposure.
   2. Remove clothing and any remaining hot or burning material.
   3. Obtain IV access and begin fluid resuscitation for severe burns.
   4. Administer pain medication.
   5. Monitor and maintain core temperature.
   6. Assess the extent and depth of burns.
   7. Irrigate burns with lukewarm sterile saline.
   8. Gently remove devitalized tissue with sterile gauze.
   9. Perform escharotomies, for full-thickness circumferential burns with evidence of compartment syndrome.
   10. Apply topical antibiotics or appropriate dressings to partial-thickness burns except when transferring to the burn center.
   11. Cover large burn areas with sterile sheets.
   12. Administer tetanus prophylaxis as indicated.
   13. Consider transfer to a burn center.

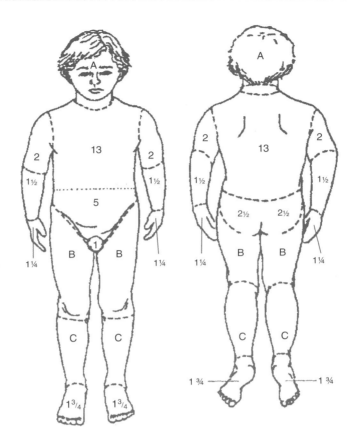

Lund and Browder Chart

Age (years)	0	1	5	10	15	Adult
A: Half of head	9 ½	8 ½	6 ½	5 ½	4 ½	3 ½
B: Half of thigh	2 ¾	2 ¼	4	4 ¼	4 ½	4 ¾
C: Half of leg	2 ½	2 ½	2 ¾	3	3 ¼	3 ½

Total area burned = second-degree surface area and third-degree surface area

Initial fluid maintenance: Ringer's lactate solution* given at:

$$\frac{\text{Surface area burned} \times \text{weight (kg)}}{4} = \text{mL/hr}$$

*Some authors recommend adding sodium bicarbonate or 5% albumin to the solution.

Fig. 50.1 Lund and Browder charts are somewhat more accurate in estimating the percentage of body surface burn than the rule of nines. Compared with adults, children have larger heads and smaller legs. Other areas are relatively stable throughout life. (From Roberts JR, Hedges JR. *Clinical Procedures in Emergency Medicine.* 2nd ed. W.B. Saunders; 1991:614–615.)

9. **Name some recommended topical therapies for burns.**
   Multiple creams and ointments are appropriate for the treatment of most small burns. They should perform several functions, including minimizing bacterial colonization, preventing desiccation, and reducing pain. Superficial burns require only a moisturizer. Gauze or other dressing is then used to cover the burn to absorb excess moisture. The "ideal" dressing, as characterized internationally by global experts, should (1) lack adhesion

to matrix, (2) offer pain-free dressing change, and (3) require fewer dressing changes. The application of a long-term dressing has also been shown to decrease overall cost.

Commonly used topical therapies include:

- Bacitracin ointment, or bacitracin—polymyxin B sulfate (polysporin)—for burns on the face and perineum.
- Erythromycin or neomycin ophthalmic ointment—for burns around the eye.
- 1% silver sulfadiazine cream—for burns on the body.
- 11.1% mafenide acetate (Sulfamylon)—for burns on the external ear. Mafenide acetate penetrates the burn eschar to reach and protect the cartilage of the ear.
- Synthetic membranes and other long-lasting silver-impregnated wound dressings have been implemented in the management of partial-thickness burns.

10. **How should blisters be treated?**
Management of blisters is controversial. Intact blisters maintain a sterile environment below the surface while unroofing the blisters allows for easier cleaning. Nonviable skin from a ruptured blister that is allowed to remain in the burn provides a medium for bacterial growth. Blisters should never be aspirated as this predisposes to infection by disrupting the sterile environment and can introduce bacteria into the wound. In general, small blisters should be allowed to remain intact. Open blisters, large blisters likely to rupture, and those crossing joints should be unroofed and debrided. The burn is then cleaned with mild soap and water.

11. **What is the approach to fluid management of a child with severe burn injuries?**
Fluid resuscitation is typically required in children with partial- or full-thickness burns covering 15% or more of the total BSA. The use of lactated Ringer's is preferred over normal saline due to the risk of hyperchloremic metabolic acidosis. Early initiation of a bolus of 20 mL/kg of isotonic fluid is recommended during the assessment of the extent of burns. Fluid replacement can be estimated by following one of two formulas. The Parkland formula dictates that 4 mL/kg/% BSA burned be administered over the first 24 hours. Half of the total volume is infused over the first 8 hours and half over the next 16 hours. Add maintenance requirements for children younger than 5 years of age in the form of 5% dextrose in normal saline.

The Galveston Shriners formula uses BSA rather than weight to calculate fluid therapy. Galveston Shriners recommends 5,000 mL/m²/% of BSA in the first 24 hours with half during the first 8 hours and half over the next 16 hours. An additional 2000 mL/m²/day is added as maintenance. Initial resuscitation is followed by fluids titrated to maintain urine output at 0.5 to 1 mL/kg/hour. Overhydration is poorly tolerated and may contribute to the development of acute pulmonary edema. Consider placement of a central venous pressure monitor in severe cases.

12. **What are the criteria for outpatient management of burns?**
Institutions may have varied practices, however, generally acceptable discharge criteria include:

- Involvement of less than 10% of the BSA in children over 10 years of age or less than 5% in children less than 10 years of age.
- No airway or pulmonary involvement
- Noncircumferential burn
- Not involving face, hands, feet, major joints, perineum, or genitals
- Abuse not suspected
- The presence of an adult capable of managing wound cleaning and dressing changes

13. **What are the indications for referral to a regional burn center?**
- Burns accompanied by respiratory injuries or major trauma
- Major chemical or high-voltage electrical burns
- Partial-thickness and full-thickness burns covering over 5% BSA in children under 10 years of age or over 10% in children older than 10 years
- Full-thickness burns over 5% BSA
- Burns that involve the face, eyes, ears, hands, feet, genitalia, perineum, or major joints
- Burn injury in patients with preexisting medical conditions affecting management or prognosis
- Burn injury in patients requiring special social, emotional, or long-term rehabilitative intervention

14. **Describe the patterns of burns commonly associated with child abuse.**
- **Immersion burns**. This pattern of injury occurs as the result of a body part being submerged in a hot liquid. These burns are often circumferential with a sharply demarcated border. Burns in a glove-and-stocking distribution is a classic example.
- **Doughnut burn**. This term describes the sparing of the central area of the buttocks when it is held in contact with the cooler ceramic surface of the bathtub floor. The surrounding areas of skin remain in contact with the water and sustain more severe burns. Burns involving the genitals, the buttocks, or perineum are unlikely to be accidental.
- **Contact burns on the dorsum of the hands**. Children are more likely to sustain accidental burns by reaching for hot objects and grasping them with the palmar surface.

- **Burn patterns consistent with an object**, such as a cigarette or an iron, held to the skin.

      In addition, burns that are inconsistent with the history, associated with additional injuries such as bruising or fractures, or are reportedly attained in a manner beyond the developmental capacities of the child deserve further investigation. The majority of children with nonaccidental burns are under 2 years of age.

15. **A 4-year-old boy sustains burns on the tip of his index finger and thumb when he places a bobby pin in an electrical outlet. What is the recommended management?**
    Household electrical outlets in the United States are generally 120 or 240 V. These rarely result in serious injuries or cardiac arrhythmias. Studies suggest that a patient who has not suffered an arrhythmia or cardiac arrest at the scene and is asymptomatic at presentation to the ED is safe to discharge to home. These patients do not require an electrocardiogram (ECG) or inpatient monitoring. ECGs that are normal on presentation do not develop late-onset arrhythmias.

16. **What is appropriate pain management for the pediatric burn patient?**
    - Intranasal fentanyl or IV morphine works well as initial pain control
    - A clean sheet placed over large surface burns prevents pain from air passing over burn areas
    - Application of topical ointments and dressings protects the area and provides additional pain relief
    - Child Life team intervention and distraction techniques are important adjuncts to assist the child with burn-related anxiety and pain.
    - Oral ibuprofen in appropriate weight-based doses is helpful.
    - Diphenhydramine can alleviate itching, which typically occurs a few days after the burn as part of the healing process.
    - In extensive burns requiring hospitalization, sedation is necessary for debridement and dressing changes.

17. **What are the indications for intubation of the trachea of a fire victim?**
    - **Early-onset stridor**. The presence of stridor or hoarseness suggests upper airway injury is likely to progress. Laryngeal edema does not peak until 2 to 8 hours after exposure. Intubation for this cause frequently requires an endotracheal tube with a smaller internal diameter than standard calculations suggest because of airway swelling.
    - **Severe burns of the face or mouth**. These patients are at significant risk for upper and lower airway injury. The presence of soot in the nares or carbonaceous sputum in isolation is not an indication of intubation.
    - **Progressive respiratory insufficiency**. Respiratory insufficiency may be diagnosed clinically or by finding a widening arterial-alveolar gradient or rising levels of partial pressure of carbon dioxide. Hypercarbia may result from depressed mental status, pain associated with chest wall movement, restriction of chest wall movement secondary to burns, pulmonary restrictive or obstructive injury, or upper airway swelling and obstruction.
    - **Inability to protect the airway** due to coma or profuse tracheobronchial secretions.
    - **Carboxyhemoglobin levels >50**. Intubation and active ventilation provide increased oxygen concentrations and help to decrease levels more rapidly.

18. **What considerations are necessary when intubating the trachea of a pediatric burn victim?**
    Rapid sequence intubation medications:
    - Rocuronium or succinylcholine are appropriate paralytics.
    - Succinylcholine can be used for paralysis up to 48 hours after acute burns without risk of hyperkalemia.
    - Sedative agents such as ketamine or etomidate will not suppress blood pressure.
    Endotracheal tube:
    - Airway edema secondary to thermal injury may reduce the diameter of the trachea making a smaller size endotracheal tube necessary.
    - The use of a cuffed endotracheal tube is recommended as decreased pulmonary compliance in smoke inhalation victims may require higher ventilator pressures.
    - Securing the endotracheal tube in a patient with extensive facial burns can be challenging. Cotton tracheotomy tape can be wrapped behind the head and then used to tie the endotracheal tube in place or orthodontic attachments to the teeth may be necessary.

19. **What acute findings are common on the chest radiograph of a child with smoke inhalation?**
    Initial chest radiographs are usually normal. Radiographic findings lag behind physiologic symptoms. Chest radiographs are thus an insensitive means of determining lung injury and rarely dictate ED management.

      Early findings suggest severe injury. Diffuse interstitial infiltrates are consistent with significant smoke inhalation. Focal infiltrates in the first 24 hours indicate atelectasis. Bronchopneumonia as the result of smoke inhalation does not typically occur until 3 to 5 days after injury. Pulmonary edema typically follows aggressive fluid resuscitation and does not appear until 6 to 72 hours after exposure. Pneumothorax is often the result of barotrauma after intubation and positive-pressure ventilation.

20. **Describe the classic presentation of a patient with carbon monoxide (CO) toxicity.**
    Patients with CO poisoning typically complain of a dull headache, dizziness, weakness, vomiting, and confusion. Often, other household contacts are reported to have similar symptoms. The symptoms can be vague, however, a history of fire/smoke exposure when paired with these symptoms is highly suggestive.

21. **Describe the pathophysiologic effects of carbon monoxide toxicity**
    Carbon monoxide binds hemoglobin with 240 times the affinity of oxygen. The production of carboxyhemoglobin significantly reduces the oxygen-carrying capacity of blood. The binding of carbon monoxide to the hemoglobin molecule shifts the oxygen dissociation curve to the left. This shift inhibits the release of oxygen at the tissue level. Carbon monoxide also has toxic effects on the cellular level. Carbon monoxide binds cytochrome oxidase and effectively blocks cellular respiration. This blockade facilitates free radical production and disrupts mitochondrial function. The results are tissue hypoxia and metabolic acidosis despite adequate oxygen delivery.

22. **How is the half-life of carboxyhemoglobin affected at different oxygen concentrations?**
    - **Room air (21%, 1 atmosphere [atm])**: Half-life of 4 hours
    - **100% O_2 1 atm**: Half-life of 60 to 90 minutes
    - **Hyperbaric oxygen (100% oxygen, 2.5 atm)**: Half-life of 15 to 30 minutes

23. **How is a pulse oximeter reading affected by the presence of carboxyhemoglobin?**
    The pulse oximeter measures the absorption of two separate wavelengths of light. These wavelengths correspond to the peak absorption spectra of oxygenated and deoxygenated hemoglobin. Carboxyhemoglobin absorbs light at a wavelength similar to oxygenated hemoglobin and therefore does not affect the overall reading. The result is a falsely high oxygen saturation reading. Standard pulse oximeter readings are unreliable measures of true oxygen saturation in patients with smoke inhalation. Pulse CO-oximeters have been developed to determine carboxyhemoglobin levels but are not as accurate as laboratory measurements.

24. **When is hyperbaric oxygen therapy indicated?**
    The use of hyperbaric oxygen in the setting of smoke inhalation is highly controversial. Studies have not demonstrated reduced mortality or improved neurologic outcome with treatment after smoke inhalation. When indications for a particular patient remain unclear, seek further consultation from hyperbaric experts. To be considered a candidate for hyperbaric oxygen therapy, the patient must be deemed stable enough for transport. The potential benefits should outweigh the risks of transferring the patient to the chamber, especially when long distances are involved. Active resuscitation is not possible in single-occupancy chambers.

25. **What are the criteria for hyperbaric oxygen therapy?**
    Generally accepted criteria include:
    - Syncope
    - Severe neurologic symptoms on presentation (seizures, focal neurologic findings, coma)
    - Myocardial ischemia diagnosed by history of electrocardiography
    - Cardiac dysrhythmias (ventricular, life-threatening)
    - Persistent neurologic symptoms and signs after several hours of 100% oxygen therapy at ambient pressure (mental confusion, visual disturbance, ataxia)
    - Pregnancy (symptomatic, carboxyhemoglobin level > 15%, evidence of fetal distress)
    - Severe metabolic acidosis pH < 7.1

    Criteria for consideration:
    - Carboxyhemoglobin level >20% to 25%
    - Abnormal results on neuropsychological examination
    - Age <6 months with symptoms (lethargy, irritability, poor feeding) or involved in same exposure as adults with any of the above criteria
    - Children who have underlying diseases (i.e., sickle cell anemia) for whom hypoxia may have deleterious effects

26. **What is the evidence for cyanide toxicity in relation to house fires?**
    The most common cause of cyanide poisoning in pediatric patients arises from exposure to fires, especially with high temperatures leading to incomplete combustion of materials such as plastics, vinyl, wool, or silk. A study performed in France measured cyanide concentrations in blood samples obtained from fire victims by ambulance physicians at the scene. Cyanide levels were found to be significantly higher than those in one control group of patients with no fire exposure and a second control group with isolated carbon monoxide poisoning. Mean cyanide levels in fire victims declared dead at the scene were over 110 μmol/L. Mean cyanide levels in survivors were 21.6 μmol/L. Lethal cyanide levels are generally considered those exceeding 40 μmol/L.

27. **How might a patient with cyanide toxicity present?**
    Similar to CO toxicity, symptoms are vague and nonspecific including headache, nausea, or vomiting. Occasionally, patients with cyanide toxicity are reported to have "cherry-red" flushed cheeks. Altered mental status and

metabolic acidosis are highly suggestive of cyanide toxicity. Serum cyanide levels are unreliable and generally not rapidly available and should not be used to aid in treatment decisions.

28. **What are the indications for treatment of cyanide poisoning in fire victims?**
Cyanide levels are not immediately available and the administration of antidote cannot be delayed. Treatment for cyanide poisoning is indicated in fire victims with evidence of significant smoke inhalation, such as carbonaceous material in oropharynx or altered neurologic status. Elevated lactate levels (>8 mmol/L) and metabolic acidosis correlate with the presence of cyanide and are typically available sooner than a cyanide level.

29. **What treatments are available for cyanide poisoning?**
    - **Decontamination**—the patient must be rapidly removed from the source and clothing must be removed and discarded.
    - **Hydroxocobalamin** binds cyanide to form cyanocobalamin (vitamin B$_{12}$), which is excreted in the urine and should be the *first-line treatment as it is safe and effective*. Hydroxocobalamin is administered intravenously in a dose of 70 mg/kg to a maximum dose of 5 g over 10 minutes. It has a rapid onset of action without serious adverse effects.
    - **Sodium thiosulfate** can be administered intravenously as an infusion of a 25% solution of sodium thiosulfate at a dose of 1.65 mL/kg administered over 10 minutes. The maximum dose is 12.5 g or 50 mL of a 25% solution. It is the rate-limiting compound in the conversion of cyanide to thiocyanate, which is excreted harmlessly in the urine. It has a slow onset of action. If hydroxocobalamin is unavailable, consider the administration of both sodium thiosulfate and sodium nitrate.
    - **Sodium nitrate** converts hemoglobin to methemoglobin, which preferentially binds cyanide in the form of cyanmethemoglobin. This therapy is generally not recommended for CO-exposed patients because it further reduces the level of normal hemoglobin in fire victims who already have a significant amount of dysfunctional hemoglobin.

30. **What preventive measures will reduce morbidity and mortality from burns and smoke inhalation?**
Anticipatory guidance and preventive care have the greatest potential to reduce deaths from burns and house fires. Over 90% of childhood deaths from fires occur in homes without properly functioning smoke detectors, and most children in house fires die from smoke inhalation rather than burns. Smoke detectors should be installed on every level of the house and tested regularly. Batteries should be replaced twice a year. Families should be educated about escape routes, evaluating fire risks in the house, and in the use and storage of fire extinguishers. Careless (or any) cigarette use should be avoided. Lowering the setting on the water heater to deliver water at a maximum temperature of 120°F (48.8°C) substantially increases the time it takes for direct exposure to induce a full-thickness burn (see question 5). Boiling liquids should be placed on the back burners of the stove where they are out of the reach of young children. Children should not be allowed to operate or remove objects from microwave ovens. Children should be dressed in flame-retardant sleepwear.

KEY POINTS: MAJOR THREATS TO CHILDREN WITH EXTENSIVE BURN INJURIES

1. Hypothermia
2. Hypovolemia
3. Infection

KEY POINTS: PATHOPHYSIOLOGIC EFFECTS OF SMOKE INHALATION

1. Airway burns and edema from superheated gases and particles
2. Hypoxia due to carbon monoxide
3. Disruption of cellular respiration by carbon monoxide and cyanide
4. Bronchospasm from gases and particulate matter

BIBLIOGRAPHY

1. American Burn Association. *National Burn Repository 2019 Update: Report of Data from 2009-2018*; 2019.
2. Buboltz JB, Robins M. *Hyperbaric treatment of carbon monoxide toxicity. StatPearls [Internet]*. StatPearls Publishing; 2022.
3. Buckley NA, Juurlink DN, Isbister G, et al. Hyperbaric oxygen for carbon monoxide poisoning. *Cochrane Database Syst Rev.* 2011:CD002041.
4. Brown F., Diller K. Calculating the optimum temperature for serving hot beverages. *Burns.* 2008;34(5):648–654.
5. Chen EH, Sareen A. Do children require ECG evaluation and inpatient telemetry after household electrical exposures? *Ann Emerg Med.* 2007;49:64–67.

6. Karl SR. Trauma. In Fuchs S, Yamamoto L, eds. *The Pediatric Emergency Medicine Resource*. 5th ed. Boston: Jones and Bartlett Publishers; 2012:204–261.
7. D'Souza AL, Nelson NG, McKenzie LB. Pediatric burn injuries treated in US emergency departments between 1990 and 2006. *Pediatrics*. 2009;124:1424–1430.
8. Fidkowski CW, Fuzaylov GM, Sheridan RL, et al. Inhalation burn injury in children. *Pediatr Anesthesia*. 2009;19:147–154.
9. Hodgman EI, Pastorek RA, Saeman MR, et al. The Parkland Burn Center experience with 297 cases of child abuse from 1974 to 2010. *Burns*. 2016;42(5):1121–1127.
10. Lanham JS, Nelson N, Hendren B, Jordan T. Outpatient burn care: prevention and treatment. *Am Fam Physician*. 2020;101(8):463–470.
11. Lawson-Smith P, Jansen EC, Hyldegaard O. Cyanide intoxication as part of smoke inhalation—a review on diagnosis and treatment from the emergency perspective. *Scand J Trauma Resusc Emerg Med*. 2011;19:14.
12. Lund C, Browder N. The estimation of areas of burns. *Surg Gynecol Obstet*. 1944;79:352–358.
13. *Mayo Clinic Staff. Infant and Toddler Health*. Burn safety: protect your child from burns. <https://www.mayoclinic.org/healthy-lifestyle/infant-and-toddler-health/in-depth/child-safety/art-20044027> Accessed 07.08.22.
14. McLeod JS, Maringo AE, Doyle PJ, et al. Analysis of electrocardiograms associated with pediatric electrical burns. *J Burn Care Res*. 2018;39(1):65–72.
15. Mintegi S, Clerique N, Tipo V, et al. Pediatric cyanide poisoning by fire smoke inhalation: a European expert consensus. *Pediatr Emer Care*. 2013;29(11):1234–1240.
16. Nagel TR, Schunk JE. Using the hand to estimate the surface area of a burn in children. *Pediatr Emerg Care*. 1997;13:254–255.
17. Nischwitz SP, Luze H, Popp D, et al. Global burn care and the ideal burn dressing reloaded—a survey of global experts. *Burns*. 2021;47(7):1665–1674.
18. Partain KP, Fabia R, Thakkar RK. Pediatric burn care: new techniques and outcomes. *Curr Opin Pediatr*. 2020;32:405–410.
19. Romanowski K, Palmieri T. Pediatric burn resuscitation: past, present, and future. *Burns Trauma*. 2017;5:26.
20. Sen S. Pediatric inhalation injury. *Burns Trauma*. 2017;5:31.
21. Strobel AM, Fey R. Emergency care of pediatric burns. *Emerg Med Clin North Am*. 2018;36(2):441–458.
22. https://www.cdc.gov/injury/wisqars/index.html

CHAPTER 51

CHILD ABUSE

Stephen Ludwig

1. **What four elements should you consider in making a diagnosis of suspected child abuse?**
   1. Detailed history of injury
   2. Physical findings and their correspondence with the history
   3. Laboratory and radiographic information
   4. Observed interaction between parent-child and health care team members
      Combining these four elements should help to determine whether you have sufficient grounds to institute a report of suspected abuse.

2. **What forms of abuse are defined by most state child abuse laws?**
   - Physical abuse
   - Physical neglect
   - Sexual abuse
   - Psychological/emotional abuse

3. **Which form of abuse is reported most often? What form occurs most often?**
   Child neglect is most common, accounting for 76% of reported cases of abuse. Psychological abuse occurs most often and has the most disabling long-term consequences, though it is not often reported. Physical abuse accounts for about 17% of cases. Sexual abuse accounts for about 9% of cases.

4. **How common is child abuse?**
   Child protective service agencies investigate more than 2 million reports of suspected child maltreatment each year. After investigation, more than 650,000 children are substantiated as victims of maltreatment.

5. **How many abuse victims are killed each year in the United States?**
   Approximately 1800 children die from child abuse annually. This rate has been fairly constant from year to year.

6. **What injury accounts for most deaths due to child abuse?**
   Head injury accounts for most child abuse–related deaths. Abdominal trauma causes most other child abuse–related deaths. Most maltreatment fatalities are attributed to neglect, with or without physical abuse.

7. **What are common characteristics of child homicide cases?**
   Most victims of child homicide are known to child protective services. They have been involved in prior Emergency Medical Services calls for a wide range of conditions. The victims tend to be older than children who died of natural causes. The chief causes are trauma, malnutrition, neglect, toxicological, and environmental issues. The victim of a male perpetrator is likely to have a more severe injury and a worse outcome.

8. **Abuse occurs most often in which ethnic group?**
   The rate of abuse by ethnic groups roughly matches the ethnic distribution in the general population. Thus White children are abused most often.

9. **Who is required to report a case of suspected child abuse?**
   The mandate to report varies by state and local jurisdictions. Most states require physicians, nurses, and mental health care providers to report suspected abuse. Teachers and others who work with children and are responsible for their care are also mandated to report a case that is suspicious. Social workers and law enforcement personnel are also considered mandated reporters in most locations. Most cases are reported by nonphysicians and non-health care institutions. Abuse is rarely reported by primary care physicians (probably less than 2% of reported cases nationwide). A report should be made if the provider has a reasonable suspicion of abuse. The reporter need not be certain but just have a reasonable suspicion of abuse. If a mandated reporter fails to report a case of suspected abuse, they can be charged with a misdemeanor. More importantly, the child may suffer future abuse leading to additional injury and death.

10. **What factors place a child at greater risk for abuse?**
    Stress in the family is a major factor leading to child abuse. Poverty is known to be a great stressor, and therefore this is a risk factor for child abuse. Alcoholism occurs in all socioeconomic groups, and this also places a

Table 51.1 Factors That Place a Child at Risk for Abuse

CHILD	PARENT/CARETAKER
Young child, infant, or toddler	Young parent
Unwanted/unplanned child	Poor knowledge of child development
Twin/multiple siblings	Single parent
Behavioral problem/hyperactive	Depressed/mental illness
Chronically ill or disabled	Alcoholism/substance abuse
Poverty	Unemployed/poverty
	Abused as child
	Low self-esteem
	Poor impulse control
	Not biologically related to child

child at risk for abusive injury. See Table 51.1 for a list of risk factors attributed to the child and the parent or caretaker.

11. **What has happened to the rates of hospitalization for child abuse over the past 15 years?**
The rates of hospitalizations have remained the same, but rates of abuse such as abusive head trauma (AHT) increased in the midst of the economic crisis from 2007 to 2009.

12. **How did the COVID-19 pandemic impact the rates of child abuse?**
The national number of children who received a child protective services investigation decreased from 3,476,000 in 2019 to 3,145,00 in 2020. One multicenter study showed pediatric emergency department (ED) encounters concerning child physical abuse decreased by 19% during the pandemic. The reduction was mostly due to low-severity clinical encounters. It is unclear whether this represents a true decrease in child physical abuse or lack of recognition during the pandemic. It is known that school encounters are extremely important for recognition of abuse. Many cases of abuse may not have been reported because children were not in school during the pandemic and teachers are often the ones who recognize abuse. Similarly, a decrease in in-person health care visits during the pandemic may have contributed to reduced diagnosis of child abuse.

13. **When should the history make you suspicious of child abuse?**
It is wise to consider abuse whenever a child presents with an injury. In particular, be suspicious when:
- There is no history to explain a significant injury.
- The history is not consistent with the injury (e.g., a serious injury from a shortfall).
- The history changes when the caretaker is interviewed.
- The history is not consistent with the age or developmental ability of the child.
- There is an unexplained or unexpected delay in seeking care for the injury.
- The caretaker giving the history seems unconcerned.

14. **What findings on the physical examination of an injured child should make you suspicious of abuse?**
- The injury does not fit the story given by the caretaker.
- There are multiple injuries in various stages of healing.
- Particular patterns of injury (loop marks, slap marks, bites).
- Certain anatomical locations of injury (ear, neck, face, abdomen, back, buttocks, and genitalia).

15. **What is the TEN-4 FACES bruising rule?**
This rule describes bruises that should raise concern for physical child abuse:

Bruising to the:
T = Torso
E = Ear
N = neck for a child 4 years or younger

Any bruising to a child 4 months or younger
F = frenulum
A = auricular
C = cheek
E = eyelid
S = sclera

These bruises increase concern but are not diagnostic of abuse. They must be interpreted with other findings of the history and examination.

16. **Can the color of bruises on a child's body be used to date the injury definitively?**
No. The color of a bruise is determined by location, nature of the traumatic force, amount of subcutaneous tissue, and other factors. Aging of bruises based on color is highly unreliable.

17. **How does a victim of abusive head injury present?**
These victims are usually young, often less than 1 year old. The history may be that of sudden deterioration. The child may present with a seizure, coma, or respiratory arrest. The infant may have a full fontanel; there is rarely a bruise on the head. Retinal hemorrhage is found in 85% of cases. These infants have severe morbidity (70%), and death is likely in 11% to 36%.

18. **Why is AHT sometimes missed?**
AHT peaks at 8 to 12 weeks of age and is most common in infants. Many of these infants may present with nonspecific symptoms such as vomiting or fussiness. They may not have any evidence of trauma on examination. Occult injuries, including fractures, are common with AHT.

19. **Why is it difficult to diagnose abusive abdominal trauma?**
This can be a difficult diagnosis because children with abdominal injury from abuse may have a misleading history of an accidental mechanism. They may present with nonspecific findings of vomiting, lethargy, or shock. Abdominal bruising is present in less than 50% of cases and even abdominal tenderness may be absent. Elevated liver and pancreatic enzymes can help identify a child with abdominal injury. An abdominal CT scan with IV contrast should be performed if abusive abdominal injury is suspected.

20. **In a child with multiple bruises and a normal neurological examination, is computed tomography (CT) of the head indicated?**
There is a high yield of positive CT findings, even in children with normal neurological examinations. CT screening appears to be more helpful than routine ophthalmological examinations. AHT may be found in 30% of infants who have facial bruising or multiple fractures, yet have no neurological symptoms.

21. **What are the most common skin lesions mistaken for abuse?**
Congenital dermal melanocytosis (previously called Mongolian spots), which most commonly occur on the back, at the base of the spine, and on the buttocks is often mistaken for abuse. However, they may also occur on other skin surfaces. Also, areas of denuded skin that result from drug reactions such as toxic epidermal necrolysis are often misinterpreted as scald burns. There are many other acute dermatological conditions that may mimic signs of abuse.

22. **What conditions may lead to easy bruisability?**
Ehlers-Danlos syndrome and other connective tissue disorders may lead to easy bruisability. Hemophilia usually results in deep soft tissue and joint bleeding rather than superficial skin bruises. Idiopathic thrombocytopenia purpura and other platelet abnormalities lead to petechiae and mucous membrane bleeding rather than bruises. Henoch-Schönlein purpura also may be initially confused with bruising.

23. **What developmental skill is associated with bruising?**
Walking or learning to walk may be associated with bruises. However, bruises found on children who have not yet learned to walk should be considered a sign of possible abuse. Children who do not cruise or walk generally do not bruise.

24. **A 2-week-old infant, seen in the ED for crying, has several fractures at varying stages of healing. What may you conclude from these findings?**
Although this scenario may indicate abuse, the young age of the infant and the possibility that fractures may have occurred in utero make a metabolic bone disease more likely.

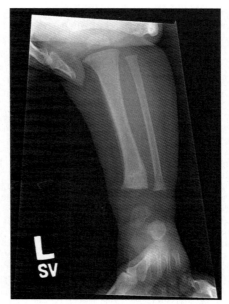

Fig. 51.1 Metaphyseal chip fracture.

25. **What findings make osteogenesis imperfecta more likely than child abuse?**
    Blue sclera, dental abnormalities, hearing loss, wormian bones, and radiographs showing osteopenia and healing with abundant callus formation.

26. **Which specific fractures have a high probability of being caused by child abuse?**
    Rib fractures, metaphyseal chip fractures (Fig. 51.1), spine and scapula fractures, and complex skull fractures. Child abuse is the most common cause of rib fractures in children younger than 12 months. They are rarely accidental and are most likely due to squeezing of the child's chest.
    Any fracture in a nonambulatory child is suspicious.

27. **Which specific fractures have a low specificity for abuse?**
    Linear skull fractures, clavicle fractures, single-bone transverse fractures, and spiral fractures of the tibia (toddler's fracture).

28. **What type of force is consistent with the finding of a metaphyseal fracture?**
    Metaphyseal fractures occur when an extremity is pulled in the direction of its long axis. Stress on the tight periosteal attachments along the metaphysis results in a chip or corner fracture (Fig. 51.1).

29. **In evaluating child abuse, a skeletal survey is required for which children?**
    According to the American Academy of Pediatrics clinical report on the Evaluation of Suspected Child Physical Abuse, a skeletal survey is mandatory in all cases of suspected physical abuse in children younger than 2 years. This should also be obtained in infants and siblings <2 years old who are household contacts of an abused child. In one study, 29% of skeletal surveys were positive in a cohort of witnessed abused patients with absent physical findings. Occult fractures are found in up to 42% of children less than 2 years old with concerns for AHT, so skeletal surveys are very helpful in this population. A repeat skeletal survey 2 weeks after the initial evaluation may increase the diagnostic yield.

30. **What tests should be used to differentiate rickets from child abuse as the cause of skeletal abnormality?**
    - Bone density (appearance of bones)
    - Serum calcium and phosphorus
    - Serum alkaline phosphatase
    - X-rays—the best radiograph to demonstrate rickets is that of the distal radius and ulna (wrist)

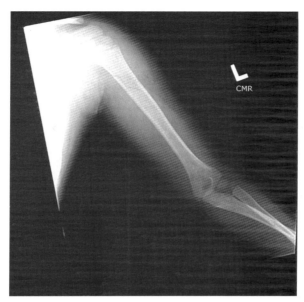

Fig. 52.2 Spiral fracture of humerus.

31. What history of injury matches a spiral fracture?
    A spiral injury is caused by torque or twisting (Fig. 51.2). The extremity is twisted, or the child's body is twisted while the extremity is held in a fixed position. If the mechanism of injury does not match the nature of the injury, suspect abuse.

32. What study has the highest sensitivity and specificity for diagnosing a suspected skull fracture?
    A skull radiograph best shows a skull fracture, although a CT scan of the head often reveals a fracture. If the fracture line is horizontal, it may be missed by the horizontal cuts of the CT scan.

33. What is the preferred imaging technique for acutely injured children suspected to have neurotrauma as the result of abuse?
    The head CT is the preferred modality, as it is readily available in most centers and will identify most significant injuries. The CT should be followed by an early magnetic resonance imaging (MRI). Recent studies show a fast MRI is a reasonable alternative to CT to identify traumatic brain injury in hemodynamically and neurologically stable children who do not need sedation, and this eliminates radiation exposure. Noncontrast MRI is superior to CT to identify the pattern, extent, and timing of head injuries. CT may be more likely to identify skull fractures and acute subarachnoid or subdural hemorrhage.

34. Can shaking an infant lead to serious head injury?
    The term "shaken baby syndrome" has become a subject of debate by lawyers defending alleged perpetrators in child abuse cases. Some early biomechanical models raised concerns about the ability of shaking alone to generate sufficient forces to induce serious brain injuries in infants. They implied that impact was a necessary prerequisite to result in a head injury. However, subsequent studies have highlighted the limitations of that earlier work and validated shaking alone as a mechanism for inducing infant brain injury. Bony, soft tissue, or spinal cord injury is not always present in cases of AHT. Unfortunately, legal challenges to the term "shaken baby syndrome" can distract from the more important questions of accountability of the perpetrator. It is therefore advised to use the term "abusive head trauma" rather than a term that implies a single injury mechanism, such as shaken baby syndrome, in the diagnosis and communication about infants with head injury.

35. A 6-month-old boy is brought to the ED for new onset of seizures. You note retinal hemorrhages. A CT scan of the brain is read as normal. What is your conclusion?
    CT may not pick up all central nervous system (CNS) injuries. Your next step is to order an MRI of the brain. MRI may detect small punctate hemorrhages or subdural collections that are isodense on CT. A new onset of seizures and retinal hemorrhages has a high probability of being caused by child abuse.

36. **What preimaging signs may be clues to AHT?**

Retinal hemorrhages are present in 75% to 80% of cases. Signs of external trauma are minimal or absent. The child may present with hypothermia or respiratory difficulties. Xanthochromic fluid may be present in the cerebrospinal fluid obtained to rule out sepsis. Bruising may be seen on the upper extremities or chest wall in the place where the child was grasped and shaken.

37. **True or false: In a comparison between inflicted head trauma and noninflicted head trauma, the neurological findings are similar.**

False. Children with inflicted head trauma have more severe head injury, which requires more ED management and longer hospital stays and is associated with poorer outcomes.

38. **How often have children with head trauma due to child abuse been injured only once?**

Rarely. Studies demonstrate that by the time head trauma due to child abuse is diagnosed, many earlier episodes probably have gone undiagnosed and unreported. Chronic effusions from old blood or cerebral atrophy may be present.

39. **Which retinal hemorrhages are concerning for AHT?**

Nonabusive head injury may result in retinal hemorrhages. However, retinal hemorrhages that are too numerous to count in one or both eyes, those present in all layers of the retina, and those extending into the periphery, are more common in AHT than in accidental head injury.

40. **What are the classic CT findings in AHT?**

The classic findings are subdural hemorrhage, particularly in the intrahemispheric fissure; injury to the frontal or occipital lobe; loss of gray-white matter differentiation; and basal ganglia injury. Evidence of an old CNS injury is another alerting sign.

41. **Which metabolic disease is associated with CNS hemorrhage?**

Glutaric acidemia has the features of CNS hemorrhage and retinal hemorrhage. Usually, other signs of metabolic derangement and mental retardation are present. Glutaric acidemia is extremely rare, unlike abuse.

42. **A child is taken to a babysitter. Six hours later the child collapses, has seizures, and is brought to the ED, where a serious head injury is found. The babysitter claims that the injury occurred at home before the parent dropped off the child. What is the likely determination?**

With the exception of an epidural hematoma, symptoms develop just after the trauma is inflicted. There is no lucid or normal interval. The findings suggest that the babysitter or someone in the babysitter's house inflicted the trauma.

43. **Raccoon eyes are a sign of what kind of injury?**

Raccoon eyes are consistent with basilar skull fracture. More common than true raccoon eyes is bilateral infraorbital ecchymosis due to a midline forehead hematoma and tracking of blood into the infraorbital position.

44. **If a child is slapped forcefully, what skin finding is typical?**

A slap mark shows the outline of the shape of the fingers in petechiae or bruise lesions—not the imprint of the fingers themselves.

45. **What does a cigarette burn look like?**

Cigarette burns are often talked about but rarely seen. When a cigarette is extinguished on a child's skin, the mark is usually circular and the width is slightly larger than the cigarette (roughly 0.8-1 cm). The second-degree burn should be uniform throughout the circular lesion, and the edges of the circle should be raised by 1 to 2 mm. Inadvertent contact between a child and a cigarette (nonintentional) produces a simple partial-thickness bullous lesion.

46. **What factors help to differentiate an inflicted bathtub scald burn from an accidental burn?**

If the child is of toilet-training age, if there was a delay (>1-2 hours) in seeking care, and if the person who brings the child to the ED is not the person who was supervising the child when the burn occurred, the likelihood of abuse increases. Inflicted injuries are often deeper. When a child is immersed in hot bathwater, there may be well-demarcated lines of injury ("stocking-glove" distribution). Other injuries may also be present as the child may have been beaten before being placed in hot water. Scald burns of the buttocks or perineum from immersion should raise concern for abuse.

47. If a child is immersed in hot water while wearing some articles of clothing, what might a physical examination of the burn reveal?
The clothed areas have increased burn severity because clothes hold the hot water closer to the skin. On the other hand, areas of thicker skin (e.g., palms and soles) may be relatively spared.

48. What is a "boxed ear"? How do you recognize it?
A boxed ear is a common injury caused by abuse. It results when the child receives a blow to the side of the head, including the ear. The finding to look for is ecchymosis on the inside surface of the pinna. This area is not exposed to other forms of injury.

49. What is the significance of a duodenal hematoma in the evaluation of child abuse?
A duodenal hematoma in children younger than 2 years is highly suspicious for abuse. Other causes such as handlebar injuries and lap belt trauma do not occur in children this young.

50. What is "bottle-jamming"?
Trauma to the upper gum line and frenulum, which results when a frustrated parent forcefully jams a bottle into the child's mouth. These injuries are sometimes disregarded, and the child may return to the ED with additional injuries. Accidental injuries to the frenum may be seen in older children who are learning to walk (8-18 months old), but these are very concerning for abuse in younger infants.

51. A child with multiple bruises is brought to the ED. Other than documentation of normal coagulation, what laboratory studies should be obtained?
Assess amylase, lipase, and liver enzymes. Studies have shown that the rate of intraabdominal injury is higher than what may be apparent. Also, order a urinalysis to look for signs of renal bleeding.

52. A 10-month-old baby is brought to the ED, essentially dead on arrival. No marks, bruises, or ecchymoses are found on the child's body, and there is no history of illness. Is sudden infant death syndrome (SIDS) the most likely diagnosis?
SIDS is one of several causes of sudden unexplained infant deaths. These cases usually occur at ages 2 to 5 months. Once a child is older than 6 months, you should be highly skeptical. Accurate diagnosis of SIDS requires a complete autopsy and death-scene investigation.

KEY POINTS: SUSPECTED CHILD ABUSE

1. Child abuse occurs frequently. Consider child abuse as a possible mechanism in every traumatic injury.
2. Physicians and nurses are mandated to report the suspicion of abuse.
3. A level of suspicion is built by compiling elements of history, physical examination, laboratory and radiographic data, and observed interactions of the family.
4. Injuries that kill children are head injuries from both direct trauma and shaking and abdominal injuries.
5. The more similar the family is to you in such characteristics as age, race, socioeconomic status, and education level, the more difficult it will be to suspect abuse.

53. What are the characteristics of a parent who may be involved in medical child abuse (previously called Münchausen syndrome by proxy)?
- Mother
  - Has a medical background or experience as a patient
  - Is articulate and cooperative
  - Asks you to diagnose an unusual or unexplainable disorder
  - Is always present when the episode, event, or finding is discovered
  - May be overly involved in the child's care
  - Has a distant relationship with the child's father

54. A child is brought to the ED for spitting up blood. The mother brings in a bib with a large blood spot. She reports that it has happened before, and the child underwent an extensive workup at a nearby medical center. What should you do?

Check the type of blood on the bib to confirm that it is the same as the baby's blood. Get the records from the other hospital to see what the physician's impressions were. Check with the child's primary care physician. Collect as much background data as possible.

55. What chief complaint is associated most often with medical child abuse?

The complaint of apnea, sometimes needing resuscitation, has been documented in many case series. The child often presents with recurrent problems and has been evaluated in several EDs. Poisoning, induced sepsis, factitious fever, hematuria, and GI bleeds are also frequently found in cases of medical child abuse.

56. What features of medical history indicate an increased risk for intentional suffocation?
- Recurrent cyanosis, apnea, and BRUEs occurr only while in the care of the same person
- Age at death older than 6 months
- Previous unexplained death of a sibling
- Previous death of an infant under the care of the same person

57. A child comes alone to the ED with abdominal pain. She does not want her mother called for permission and states that she is afraid of her mother. Is this a case of child abuse?

This is a difficult case. It may meet the criteria for emotional abuse, and you should attempt to report it. The diagnosis of abuse usually rests on the documentation of an injury. You may need a mental health consultation to document the nature and extent of the fear.

58. Does failure to thrive (FTT) always indicate abuse or neglect?

No. Some cases of FTT are based on the lack of proper child-rearing practices, others are due to an organic condition, and still others result from the combination of a child who is difficult to feed and a family without proper skills and resources. Cases that result from abuse, of course, must be reported.

59. What are some red flags that indicate that a patient with FTT may have an underlying medical cause?

Some of the red flags include cardiac findings, developmental delay, dysmorphic features, organomegaly, lymphadenopathy, recurrent infections, and other symptoms such as diarrhea, vomiting, and dehydration. Most children with FTT on a psychosocial basis have few signs or symptoms and are just not receiving adequate calories.

60. What forms of neglect are included in the definition of most state laws?
- Physical neglect
- Educational neglect
- Medical neglect
- Emotional neglect
- Abandonment

61. What are the two types of child abuse cases in the court system? What are the differences?

The two types are criminal and civil. Civil cases are brought in violation of specific child abuse laws. They require only proof that the injury occurred through nonaccidental means. The ultimate penalty is removal of the child from the family. The rules of evidence tend to be more lenient. In criminal cases, one must prove that a specific perpetrator committed a specific crime—a violation of the criminal code. The penalty is incarceration, and the rules of the courtroom are strictly enforced.

62. In testifying in a child abuse case, what is the role of the ED physician?

The physician must be fair, objective, and reasonable in the presentation of facts and medical data. There is no room for testimony that presents feelings, sentiments, or emotions. The role of the emergency physician is to offer and explain medical information.

63. What is the most important step in managing a child abuse case?

The most important step is to have a high degree of suspicion for every traumatic injury; to build a level of suspicion with objective findings and observations; and when the level of suspicion is high, to report all cases of suspected abuse. Failure to intervene can have serious consequences. Children returned to the primary caregiver without intervention after an event of maltreatment have an 11% to 50% chance of a second event.

64. **Does child abuse affect children only during their childhood?**
No. Many studies have proved that child abuse, and even the witnessing of abuse of others, may have long-term (lifelong) consequences. Abused children are at greater risk for posttraumatic stress disorder, attention-deficit/hyperactivity disorder, suicidal ideation, and substance abuse. Almost 70% of survivors of AHT have some degree of permanent neurological impairments, such as intellectual disability, cerebral palsy, static encephalopathy, cortical blindness, seizures, or behavioral problems.

BIBLIOGRAPHY

1. AAP Section on Radiology Diagnostic imaging of child abuse. *Pediatrics*. 2012;123(5):1430–1435.
2. Berger RP, Fromkin JB, Stutz H, et al. Abusive head trauma during a time of increased unemployment: a multicenter analysis. *Pediatrics*. 2011;128:637–643.
3. Chadwick DL, Bertocci G, Castillo E, et al. Annual risk of death rate resulting from short falls among young children: less than 1 in a million. *Pediatrics*. 2008;121:1213–1224.
4. Chaiyachati BH, Wood JN, Carter C, et al. Emergency department child abuse evaluations during COVID-19 a multicenter study. *Pediatrics*. 2022;150(1):e2022056284.
5. Christian CW. AAP Committee on Child Abuse and Neglect. Clinical report: The evaluation of suspected child physical abuse. *Pediatrics*. 2015;135(5):e1337–1354.
6. Deutsch SA. Abusive head trauma. *Ped Ann*. 2020;49:e347.
7. Farrell CA, Fleegler EW, Monuteaux MC, Wilson CR, et al. Community poverty and child abuse fatalities in the United States. *Pediatrics*. 2017;139(5):e20161616.
8. Fisher-Owens SA, Lukefahr JL, Tate AR. AAP Section on Oral Health, Committee on Child Abuse and Neglect. Clinical report: Oral and dental aspects of child abuse and neglect. *Pediatrics*. 2017;140(2):e20171487.
9. Kaiser SV, Kornblith AE, Richardson T, Pantell M, et al. Emergency visits and hospitalizations for child abuse during the COVID-19 pandemic. *Pediatrics*. 2021;147(4):e2020038489.
10. Lindberg DM, Stence NV, Grubenhoff JA, et al. Feasibility and accuracy of fact MRI versus CT for traumatic brain injury in young children. *Pediatrics*. 2019;144(4):e20190419.
11. Melville JD, Hertz SK, Steiner D, Lindberg DM. Use of imaging in children with witnessed physical abuse. *Pediatr Emerg Care*. 2019;35(4):245–248.
12. Mills R, Scott J, Alari R, et al. Child maltreatment and adolescent mental health problems in a large birth cohort. *Child Abuse Negl*. 2013;37(5):292–305.
13. Narang SK, Fingarson A, Lukefahr J, et al. AAP Council on Abuse and Neglect. Policy statement: Abusive head trauma in infants and children. *Pediatrics*. 2020;145(4):e20200203.
14. Paine WC, Fakeye O, Christian CW, Wood JN. Prevalence of abuse among young children with rib fractures. *Pediatr Emerg Care*. 2019;35(2):96–103.
15. Palusci VJ, Kay AJ, Batra E, Moon RY, et al. AAP clinical report: Identifying child abuse fatalities during infancy. *Pediatrics*. 2019;144(3):e20192076.
16. Sege RD, Amaya-Jackson L, et al. AAP Committee on Child Abuse and Neglect, Council on Foster Care, Adoption and Kinship Care. Clinical considerations related to the behavioral manifestations of child maltreatment. *Pediatrics*. 2017;139(4):e20170100.
17. Shenoi RP, Nassif A, Camp EA, Pereira FA. Previous emergency medical services use by victims of child homicide. *Pediatr Emerg Care*. 2019;35(9):589–595.
18. Shiau T, Levin AV. Retinal hemorrhages in children: the role of intracranial pressure. *Arch Pediatr Adolesc Med*. 2012;166:623–628.
19. Sowrey L, Lawson KA, Garcia-Fillon P. Duodenal injuries in the very young child: child abuse? *J Trauma Acute Care Surg*. 2013;74:136–142.
20. Sugar NF, Taylor JA, Feldman KW, et al. Bruises in infants and toddlers: those who don't cruise rarely bruise. *Arch Pediatr Adolesc Med*. 1999;153:399–403.
21. Wood JH, Connelly J, Callahan JH, Christian CW. Child abuse/assault. In: Shaw KN, Bachur RG, eds. *Fleisher & Ludwig's Textbook of Pediatric Emergency Medicine*. 8th ed. Wolters Kluwer; 2021:620–633.

CHAPTER 52

SEXUAL ASSAULT

Sara DiGirolamo and Jeannine Del Pizzo

1. **What is the approach to a child in the emergency department (ED) with concern for sexual assault?**

    When a child presents to the ED with concern for sexual assault, the fundamental job of the clinicians is the same as it would be for any chief complaint—evaluate for life-threatening emergencies and offer emergency medical care. For an acute sexual assault, emergency medical care also includes:
    - Ensuring there are no injuries that require emergent intervention
    - Testing and treatment for sexually transmitted infection (STI)
    - Pregnancy testing and emergency contraception (EC) when applicable
    - Consideration of the child's safety and well-being
    - A report to Child Protective Services (CPS)
    - Law enforcement notification
    - Behavioral health evaluation performed and/or behavior health resources offered

    In addition to providing medical care, the medical team partners with law enforcement to obtain forensic evidence. Forensic evidence, the evidence of an alleged perpetrator's DNA on a patient's body, is NOT medically necessary, and instead, its purpose is for potential legal proceedings. Until a decision is made by the medical team, patient, and their guardians whether forensic evidence is to be collected, instruct patients to leave their clothes on, avoid urinating or defecating if possible, and not to eat or drink. Gloves should also be worn during triage while obtaining vital signs to prevent the healthcare provider's DNA from contacting the patient's skin in the event evidence collection is recommended.

    Remember that the medical team is not the police. Our role is not to discover all information regarding an assault but rather to gather the data necessary to offer essential medical care. In this vein, the medical team should perform a minimal facts interview to ascertain information that will impact medical care, such as the nature, timing, body location of contact, identity of alleged perpetrator, and any symptoms the patient has (pain, bleeding, dysuria, etc.). Ideally, all necessary team members (clinician, social worker, sexual assault nurse examiner, etc.) should be present to limit the need for the victim to repeat the story. If possible, interview patients without parental or guardian presence, and document witnesses to the interview in the medical record. An in-depth history will be done later by law enforcement with an age-appropriate forensic interview.

2. **What should the exam for children with acute sexual assault include?**

    The exam should include a full head-to-toe evaluation looking for evidence of injuries on the body. Children who are sexually assaulted may have different injuries associated with the assault, such as bruising from being held, bite marks, oral injuries, and head injuries, among others. Obtain photographs of any injuries and document them in the medical record. Additionally, perform a detailed genital and perianal/anal exam, looking for signs of acute trauma and/or evidence of STIs. Photographs may be taken of the genitals and perianal area after consent is obtained from the guardian and/or child (depending on patient's age and your state's forensic consenting laws). It is most efficient to perform the physical exam, obtain photographs, STI testing, and evidence collection concurrently. By doing so the amount of time to perform the exam can be minimized, which further decreases trauma to the patient.

3. **Does every child with concern for sexual assault receive STI treatment?**

    After any sexual encounter, there is a risk for STIs, and this includes sexual assault cases. There are two kinds of STI treatments after a sexual assault: empiric treatment and postexposure prophylaxis (PEP). The purpose of empiric treatment is to treat the most common STIs: *Neisseria gonorrhoeae*, *Chlamydia trachomatis*, and *Trichomonas vaginalis*. It is not universally recommended that all children receive empiric treatment for these organisms after an acute sexual assault. In fact, the Centers for Disease Control (CDC) recommends that most prepubertal patients should NOT receive empiric treatment for these STIs after a sexual assault as there is an overall low incidence of STI in prepubertal children. Additionally, because follow-up is usually excellent in this age group, it is reasonable to test prepubertal children and treat only if positive.

    Considerations for empirically treating the prepubertal child after an assault are clear symptoms of an STI, oral, genital or anal injuries, evidence of ejaculation by an alternative light source, confirmed STI in a perpetrator, or if a child or parent requests treatment. Alternatively, in the adolescent population, there is a high rate of preexisting STIs (present before the assault) and adolescents have generally poor follow-up. If untreated, adolescent females are at risk for ascending infection causing pelvic inflammatory disease. Because of these reasons, empiric treatment for the above STIs is recommended in all pubertal patients.

4. **Does every child concerned for sexual assault receive human immunodeficiency virus (HIV) PEP?**
   The only infection that PEP is available for is HIV. The risk of acquiring HIV from a single encounter of sexual assault is unknown. For reference, the risk of acquiring HIV from consensual receptive vaginal intercourse is 0.1%, and from consensual receptive anal intercourse is 1% to 2%. HIV PEP with zidovudine alone has been shown to decrease the risk of acquiring HIV by 70% to 80% in mother-child horizontal transmission and health care workers exposed to needlestick injuries and, therefore, is highly effective. This risk reduction has been extrapolated to HIV exposure in victims of sexual assault. Most HIV PEP regimens now use two or more drugs, and this likely offers superior risk reduction to zidovudine alone. There are several considerations to take into account before deciding to start a child on an HIV PEP regimen. HIV PEP must be started within 72 hours of contact. HIV PEP is an involved course, and as mentioned above, usually involves two or more medications taken every day for 28 days. Most HIV PEP regimens have side effects ranging from mild (nausea, vomiting, diarrhea, fatigue, headaches) to severe (hepatitis, hyperglycemia, fever, rash, pancytopenia, and hepatotoxicity). It is worth noting that there is some evidence that newer HIV PEP medications that incorporate integrase inhibitors, such as dolutegravir and raltegravir, and newer nucleoside reverse transcriptase inhibitors (NRTIs), are better tolerated than prior regimens that included protease inhibitors and older NRTIs. The risks and benefits of starting HIV PEP must be carefully considered in each child. Consult with either a child abuse expert or an immunologist in cases that are not clear-cut.

5. **What are my responsibilities as a mandated reporter?**
   ED providers are mandated reporters. If there is reasonable concern that sexual abuse occurred, you are required to make a report to CPS. Make a report to CPS if a child discloses sexual contact with a perpetrator of any age. For consensual sexual contact, it is essential to know your state laws, as reporting laws may differ by jurisdiction. For example, in Pennsylvania (PA), it is a crime for any child <13 years old to have sexual intercourse, and therefore a report would be made to the police as well as CPS. In PA, for children 13 to 15 years old, if a sexual partner is 4 or more years older, even if it is consensual, it is a crime, so police would be notified in addition to CPS. It is not the responsibility of the provider to determine whether the assault actually took place, as that is left to the investigators, whether it is CPS or Law Enforcement performing the investigation. If it is determined that an assault is unlikely after an investigation, there are statutes that protect reporters from civil or criminal liability if the report was made in good faith.

6. **What are the indications for forensic evidence collection?**
   Forensic evidence collection is recommended within 72 hours for pubertal patients and within 24 hours for prepubertal patients. Studies have shown that the forensic evidence yield in prepubertal children collected diminishes with time. The yield is low enough after 24 hours from the assault that evidence collection has not been routinely recommended after this point. There are several possible explanations for this: child sexual assault is typically more coercive or manipulative rather than violent, decreasing the incidence of injury. Also, the pH in the prepubertal vagina is more alkaline and lacks estrogen, and the smaller volume of the vaginal cavity decreases the probability of deep penile penetration into the vaginal canal. Guidelines for pubertal patients are based on adult studies regarding the yield of forensic evidence. As the field of DNA technology has continued to advance, some experts advocate that evidence in both prepubertal children and pubertal children and adults should be collected past the routine cut-offs. Some centers have changed their guidelines to reflect these recommendations and will collect forensic evidence in prepubertal children for up to 72 hours and in some adults for up to 120 hours or greater, depending on the assault history and physical exam. As further studies occur using updated technology, these recommendations could be reassessed and changed.

7. **What are the general guidelines regarding obtaining consent for forensic evidence collection?**
   Although very important legally, forensic evidence is not considered medically necessary. Stabilize all medical emergencies before proceeding with forensic evidence collection. It is imperative to learn the consent requirements of your state and institution, as criminal laws regarding sexual assault can vary by jurisdiction. Sexual intercourse below a certain age is determined a crime, therefore that patient is presumed to lack capacity to provide valid consent. It is important to assess if the patient, parent, or legal guardian has the capacity to consent when provided appropriate medical information, communication supports, and technical assistance. The patient, parent, or legal guardian should be able to (1) understand the potential material benefits, risks, and alternatives; (2) make the health care decision on his or her own behalf; and (3) communicate the decision to another person. Lack of medical decision-making capacity can be caused by a variety of factors including stress, mind-altering substances, mental health problems, or intellectual disability. Consent for forensic evidence collection is its own consent process, separate from the hospital's medical treatment consent. The patient and family have the ability to withdraw consent at any time.

8. **Can an adolescent consent to forensic evidence collection?**
   Maintaining adolescent confidentiality, adolescents can consent to forensic evidence collection without the consent of their parent or legal guardian. A parent or legal guardian should not be able to overrule or withdraw a patient's ability to consent. Sexual assault patients may be victims of a drug-facilitated assault, whether voluntarily ingested or surreptitiously given by the assailant. If a known substance was ingested and it is anticipated that the patient should quickly regain capacity, forensic evidence collection may be briefly deferred to allow for the patient to consent. If the ingested substance is unknown or it is anticipated that the patient may be altered for a significant period, a parent or legal guardian can consent to forensic evidence collection.

9. **What are important considerations regarding consent for forensic evidence collection for young pediatric patients?**
   A parent or legal guardian must consent to forensic evidence collection for pediatric patients who are younger than the age of consent. A relative such as a grandparent, older sibling, or cousin typically cannot consent to forensic evidence collection. Children below the age of consent should be asked to assent to the examination and be allowed to maintain control over the conduct of the examination. The patient should be allowed to choose if a parent or other support person can be present in the examination room. If there is concern that a parent may be an alleged perpetrator and their refusal to consent may reflect a conflict of interest, contact the institution's Legal Department or Office of General Counsel. If a parent or legal guardian is unavailable or does not have the capacity to consent, the Legal Department or Office of General Counsel should also be contacted. Contact CPS for these instances and obtain the ability to provide medical consent through the local court system.

10. **What are key forensic evidence collection tips?**
    Upon arrival to the ED, advise victims not to undress, eat, or drink, and avoid urination and defecation if possible. However, if a younger patient is eager to eat or drink, which will allow them to cooperate better for the exam, you can open a forensic kit after family consents and obtain oral swabs. Ensure evidence is secured if needing to walk away from the patient's bedside. Perform STI screening, such as oral and rectal swabs for *N. gonorrhoea* and *C. trachomatis*, concurrently with forensic evidence collection to streamline the exam and minimize discomfort for the patient. Premoisten sterile swabs with sterile water or saline to better obtain DNA from the patient's body. When evidence is collected, two swabs are collected concurrently from each body site. Obtain all swabs together, moving in a rolling motion to evenly distribute DNA as swabs are typically sectioned into smaller pieces for testing at the crime lab. If a positive finding is discovered on one swab, a piece of the adjacent swab is tested. Obtain cervix swabs only with a speculum exam. Performing a vaginal exam on a prepubteral female is painful due to the thin un-estrogenized hymenal mucosa, and therefore, cervix swabs should not be obtained from a prepubertal patient unless under anesthesia. Internal vaginal swabs may also be deferred in prepubtertal patients depending on the hospital and jurisdictional evidence collection policies.

11. **What clothing is obtained as part of forensic evidence collection?**
    Obtain clothing that is worn during the sexual assault. Large items such as jackets and shoes are usually not collected unless the items show wet stains or biological material (blood, saliva, semen, etc.). Collect underwear and diapers even if they are not the original pair worn during or after the assault, as body secretions or debris may be present. If able, have the patient remove one article of clothing at a time while standing on a debris sterile sheet. Separate clothing and place in individual brown bags, labeled with patient identification sticker, date, time, and name of forensic examiner. Collect the debris sterile sheet and place this in the "debris collection" envelope of the forensic evidence kit. Store all evidence in paper bags as plastic bags promote the growth of mold and degrade evidence.

12. **What is the purpose of the alternate light source (ALS) exam?**
    Perform the ALS exam prior to obtaining forensic evidence swabs. While the patient is removing each article of clothing, use an ALS such as a blue light shining through an orange filter in a dark room, assessing the patient's skin, looking for any additional areas on the patient's body that produce a fluorescent light. This can indicate additional biological material on the patient's body not seen by the naked eye. Use two premoistened swabs with sterile saline or sterile water to swab the area and allow it to air-dry. When dry, place the swabs in a swab box, and into the "miscellaneous" envelope, noting from which body site the sample was collected. ALS technology provides additional data for the interpretation of findings further evaluated by a crime lab.

13. **What typical positioning is used during the anogenital physical exam?**
    Typical positioning during the genital exam includes the supine frog-leg position or modified lithotomic position (i.e., child is positioned on the lap of a parent or other support person) (Figs. 52.1 and 52.2). The prone knee-chest position is generally not preferred as it can feel like it is placing the patient in a compromising position but may be a position used for younger patients while being provided a book or tablet for distraction. If examining a pediatric patient on a stretcher, place a rolled towel underneath the patient's buttocks to prevent the patient from sinking into the stretcher and improve visualization for the GU exam and photo documentation. For the rectal exam, ask

Female Anatomy

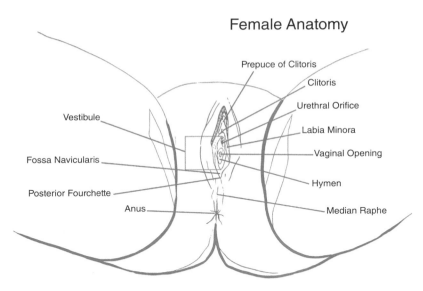

Prepuce of Clitoris

Clitoris

Urethral Orifice

Vestibule

Labia Minora

Vaginal Opening

Fossa Navicularis

Posterior Fourchette

Hymen

Anus

Median Raphe

Fig. 52.1 Normal female anatomy.

Normal Prepubertal Male Anatomy

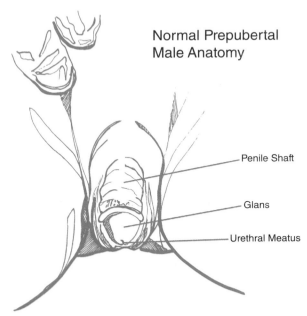

Penile Shaft

Glans

Urethral Meatus

Fig. 52.2 Normal prepubertal male anatomy.

the patient to "get into a cannon ball position" or supine-knee-chest position to allow for the best visualization. Use gynecological stretchers, if available, for ideal positioning of pubertal patients.

14. **Are there any tips to obtain good quality photo documentation?**
    To obtain photo documentation, use a colposcope, digital camera, or phone with secure access to the hospital's electronic medical record. For optimal focus on the colposcope, place the camera 11 inches from the GU region.

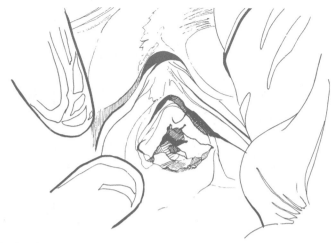

Fig. 52.3 Normal female anatomy close-up.

Use caution with the overhead light as it can produce too much light and overexposure of photos. For the female patient, perform labial traction and separation (Fig. 52.3). If difficult to visualize the hymen, ask the patient to cough or bear down to improve visualization of the introitus. A premoistened swab can be used to run the hymenal rim to improve visualization of the hymen for the pubertal patient. However, this is not recommended in the prepubertal patient as the hymen is not estrogenized and is very sensitive. If any blood is noted during the vaginal exam, use a swab to better identify the source of bleeding. For the male patient, take multiple photos displaying different angles of the penile shaft and scrotum. While obtaining photos of the rectum, place mild traction on the buttocks for improved visualization while the patient is in the supine-knee-chest position. While examining the body, obtain photos of any bruises, bite marks, or injuries, including oral injuries. When taking photos, perform a generalized photo of area of interest, then close-up photo of the region. Using a scale such as a small ruler can better identify the size of the site of injury.

15. **If the genital exam is normal, does that mean a sexual assault did not occur?**
    No. The majority of pediatric patients who are victims of sexual assault will have a normal anogenital exam. This is due to the rapid healing of the GU mucosa and the typical nonviolent nature of child sexual abuse. Studies show injuries are typically seen 20% to 25% of the time when a pediatric patient presents within 72 hours of assault. Factors such as timing of incident from exam, child age, and gender can affect the likelihood of injury. While debriefing, reassure the family of the normal exam. However, it is important to relay that the lack of injury does not mean the assault did not occur.

16. **What are common findings suggestive of sexual abuse?**
    Common areas of injury suggestive of abuse include acute lacerations or bruising of labia, penis, scrotum, perineum, posterior fourchette, vagina, or hymen (partial or complete laceration). Hymenal injuries most commonly occur from the 3 o'clock to 9 o'clock position of the hymen. Bruising, petechiae, or abrasions of the hymen are also concerning. Residual healing injuries to genital/anal tissues are suggestive of sexual abuse but may be difficult to diagnose unless the acute injury was noted first on a previous exam. The presence of an STI in a child past the perinatal period is highly suggestive of sexual abuse. Findings diagnostic of sexual abuse include pregnancy and semen identified in forensic specimens taken directly from a child's body.

17. **What are common conditions mistaken for sexual assault?**
    Diagnoses often mistaken for sexual abuse include normal variants such as vestibular bands, hymenal skin tags or clefts, median raphe, and failure of midline fusion. Accidental trauma to the genital area includes straddle injuries, impalement to anogenital structures, zipper injuries, suction drain injuries, or toilet seat injuries. Additional conditions include urethral prolapse, rectal prolapse, folliculitis of mons pubis, molluscum contagiosum, venous congestion or venous pooling in the perianal area, or lichen sclerosis. Vulvar ulcers such as aphthous ulcers or those seen in Bechet disease or Stevens-Johnson syndrome can be mistaken for sexual assault. Erythema, inflammation, and fissuring of the perianal or vulvar tissues such as seen in vulvovaginitis can be due to other bacteria, fungus, viruses, parasites, or other infections that are not sexually transmitted. Anal dilatation in

children with predisposing conditions such as constipation or encopresis, or children who are under sedation or anesthesia, or with impaired neuromuscular tone can also be commonly mistaken as abuse.

18. **What is Emergency Contraception (EC)?**
There are four methods of EC available in the United States: ulipristal, levonorgestrel, combined oral contraceptives, and copper intrauterine device. Of these, two methods are Food and Drug Administration approved: ulipristal and levonorgestrel. The most commonly available EC is levonorgestrel, also known as Plan B, which is available over the counter and can be taken as a one-time dose. Although labeled for use up to 72 hours after sexual contact, Plan B still has some effectiveness if taken up to 96 hours later but is most effective if taken as soon as possible after sexual contact. Depending on the timing of a female's cycle, Plan B can delay ovulation or inhibit it altogether. However, it has not been shown to prevent implantation of a fertilized embryo and therefore is not an abortifacient. Common side effects include nausea, vomiting, headaches, irregular bleeding, delayed menstrual cycle, breast tenderness, dizziness, and fatigue. Ulipristal is more effective 72 to 96 hours after sexual intercourse and for those patients with higher BMI >26. Offer EC to all pubertal females after an acute sexual assault.

19. **What are important documentation tips to know as a Pediatric Emergency Medicine provider while caring for sexual assault patients?**
Recommended documentation templates for the care of sexual assault patients are typically standardized by each state, whether that is performed on paper or electronically. While documenting the history of the present illness as reported by the patient or family member, the medical record should reflect the exact details of the history obtained. If a more thorough forensic interview is to occur after the ED visit, perform the minimal facts interview and limit documentation of the details of the assault to avoid further trauma for the patient retelling their story and reduce discrepancies in the record. Quote the patient's responses regarding timing, type of sexual contact, and symptoms, which will direct the medical evaluation and treatment plan. At the end of the ED visit, document all forensic swabs and clothing on the evidence receipt form that accompanies the forensic evidence kit. Capturing the appearance and description of injuries through assessments, documentation, and imaging provides vital evidence to corroborate or refute a history of injury. Therefore, careful review of documentation is critical.

20. **What type of medical follow-up care do sexual assault patients receive?**
Discharge sexual assault patients with a specific plan of care that includes follow-up with their primary care provider (PCP) or child abuse specialist, child advocacy center, and mental health services. Follow-up with the PCP or child abuse specialist is recommended within 1 to 2 weeks to assess healing and symptoms. For patients receiving HIV PEP medication, follow-up is indicated to monitor the side effects of medication and adherence to the regimen. It is recommended to repeat complete blood count and LFTs in 2 to 3 weeks. Serologic tests for syphilis are recommended 4 to 6 weeks and 12 weeks after the ED visit and fourth-generation HIV testing should be repeated at 6 weeks and 12 weeks after the ED visit. Also, perform a repeat pregnancy test 2 to 3 weeks after the ED visit. Repeat human papillomavirus and Hepatitis B vaccine administration can be performed following the CDC Vaccine Schedule, according to the patient's age, if initiated during the ED visit.

21. **What services do Child Advocacy Centers (CAC) provide?**
CAC are county-based community agencies that provide support for pediatric victims of child abuse in a developmentally appropriate manner. Following an ED visit, CACs are able to provide a thorough pediatric forensic interview. The interview is typically recorded and viewed in a separate room by detectives, CPS, and the district attorney's office to best minimize trauma to the pediatric victim. Following the forensic interview, CACs can provide mental health services or refer patients to local Victim Service Centers or community mental health partners for behavioral health support. Victims of sexual assault are at risk for short- and long-term psychological disturbances including depression, anxiety, or suicidality; therefore, referral to mental health services is vital to the healing process. CACs also provide support to patients and families during the investigation and court proceeding process. Some CACs also provide medical services on-site.

KEY POINTS: SEXUAL ASSAULT

1. When evaluating a victim of sexual assault, first ensure there are no injuries that require emergent intervention.
2. Forensic evidence is very important legally but is not medically necessary.
3. Forensic evidence collection in prepubertal children has been routinely recommended within 24 hours since the assault, however, collection can be considered beyond that period depending on local and jurisdictional evidence collection policies.
4. If forensic evidence is to be collected, instruct patients to leave clothes on, avoid defecating or urinating if possible, and not to eat or drink until supplies and personnel are available.

5. Have all necessary team members take a history together to limit the need for the victim to repeat the story.
6. Empiric treatment for STI is not recommended after sexual assault evaluation in most prepubertal patients. It is recommended for pubertal patients.
7. ED providers are mandated reporters—know your state laws for reporting.
8. An STI in a child (past prenatal period) is highly suggestive of sexual abuse.
9. Lack of injury does not mean an assault did not occur.

BIBLIOGRAPHY

1. ACOG Practice Bulletin No. 112: Emergency contraception. *Obstet Gynecol.* 2010;115(5):1100–1109.
2. Adams J. Understanding medical findings in child sexual abuse: an update for 2018. *Acad Forensic Pathol.* 2018;8(4):924–937.
3. Banvard-Fox C, Linger M, Paulson D, et al. Sexual assault in adolescents. *Primary Care.* 2020;47(2):331–349.
4. *Centers for Disease Control and Prevention.* 2022 Immunization schedules. <https://www.cdc.gov/vaccines/>; 2022 Accessed 07.06.22.
5. *Centers for Disease Control and Prevention.* HIV risk and prevention. <https://www.cdc.gov/hiv/risk/index.html> Accessed 12.06.22.
6. *Centers for Disease Control and Prevention.* Sexually transmitted infections treatment guidelines. <https://www.cdc.gov/std/treatment-guidelines/sexual-assault.htm>; 2021 Accessed 12.06.22.
7. *Centers for Disease Control and Prevention.* Updated guidelines for antiretroviral postexposure prophylaxis after sexual, injection drug use, or other nonoccupational exposure to HIV—United States. <https://stacks.cdc.gov/view/cdc/38856>; 2016 Accessed 12.06.22.
8. Hornor G, Benzinger E, Doughty K, Hollar J, Wolf K. Pediatric forensic analysis: the benefits of DNA collection beyond 24 hours. *J Forensic Nurs.* 2022;8(4):E29–E37.
9. Kaplan R, Adams J, Starling S, Giardino A. *Medical Response to Child Sexual Abuse—A Resource for Professionals Working With Children and Families.* STM Learning Inc; 2011:10.
10. Mackenzie B, Jenny C. The use of alternate light sources in the clinical evaluation of child abuse and sexual assault. *Pediatr Emerg Care.* 2014;30(3):207–210.
11. Mayer KH, Mimiaga MJ, Gelman M, Grasso C. Raltegravir, tenofovir DF, and emtricitabine for postexposure prophylaxis to prevent the sexual transmission of HIV: safety, tolerability, and adherence. *J Acquir Immune Defic Syndr.* 2012;59(4):354–359.
12. Molnar J, O'Connell MS, Mollen C, Scribano P. Sexual assault: child and adolescent. In: Shaw KN, Bachur RG, eds. *Fleisher & Ludwig's Textbook of Pediatric Emergency Medicine.* Wolters Kluwer Health; 2021:1448–1459.
13. Robinson E, Ketterer T, Molnar J, et al. Emergency department visits for behavioral health concerns after sexual assault: a retrospective mixed methods study. *Pediatric Emergency Care.* 2021;37(12):1251–1254.
14. Scafide K, Ekroos R, Mallinson R, et al. Improving the forensic documentation of injuries through alternate light: a researcher-practitioner partnership. *J Forensic Nurs.* 2023;19(1):30–40.
15. Thackeray J, Hornor G, Benzinger E, Scribano P. Forensic evidence collection and DNA identification in acute child sexual assault. *Pediatrics.* 2011;128(2):227–232.
16. Trotman G, Young-Anderson C, Deye K. Acute sexual assault in the pediatric and adolescent population. *J Pediatr Adolesc Gynecol.* 2016;29(6):518–526.
17. Workowski K, Bachmann L, Chan P, et al. Sexually transmitted infections treatment guidelines. *MMWR Recomm Rep.* 2021;70(4):1–187.

CHAPTER 53

DENTAL INJURIES

Amy D. Thompson and Laura Santry

1. **What are the priorities in evaluating a child with dental trauma?**
   As with all trauma patients, it is important to manage life-threatening injuries first. Dental injuries are rarely life-threatening. However, airway obstruction is possible with facial trauma due to an aspirated tooth or blood in the oral cavity and pharynx. When evaluating a child with a dental injury, carefully examine the patient's airway, head, cervical spine, orbits, and jaw. Consider the possibility of child abuse in your assessment.

2. **How common are pediatric dental injuries?**
   Pediatric dental injuries occur in up to 50% of all children and adolescents. The incidence of injuries to primary teeth is equal in males and females, and most injuries are caused by falls. Injuries to the permanent dentition occur more often in males. Trauma to permanent dentition typically occurs on playgrounds, during fights, sporting events, or in motor vehicle accidents.

3. **What are some risk factors for dental injuries in children?**
   Risk factors for dental injury include participation in sports, exposure to violence, need for intubation, severe overjet of the maxillary incisors, and chronic health conditions including attention-deficit hyperactivity disorder, epilepsy, and cerebral palsy.

4. **What are the components of the tooth?**
   A tooth can be considered in two parts: the crown and the root. Components of the crown include dentin, a softer, microtubular structure, and pulp, which provides the tooth's neurovascular supply (Fig. 53.1). Enamel is the hard mineralized substance that covers and protects the crown. The root of the tooth, which anchors it to the alveolar bone, consists of cementum, the periodontal ligament, and the alveolar bone.

5. **How do I make the distinction between primary and permanent teeth?**
   - *Primary (deciduous) teeth* begin to erupt at about 6 months of age and are complete by 3 years. A full complement of primary teeth consists of 10 mandibular and 10 maxillary teeth, including 4 central incisors, 4 lateral incisors, 4 canines, and 8 molars. Usually, mandibular teeth erupt before their maxillary counterparts (Fig. 53.2).
   - *Permanent teeth* typically begin to erupt at 6 years of age and are complete by 16 years of age. A full complement of permanent teeth consists of 16 mandibular teeth and 16 maxillary teeth, including 4 central incisors, 4 lateral incisors, 4 canines, 8 bicuspids (premolars), and 12 molars (see Fig. 53.2).
   - If in doubt, parents usually can distinguish the child's primary from permanent teeth. If a parent is unavailable, two other hints are helpful:
   - Primary teeth are often much smaller than permanent teeth.
   - The occlusive or chewing surface of the permanent tooth is ridged, whereas the occlusive surface of the primary teeth is smooth.

5. **How do I accurately describe which tooth is injured?**
   There are two ways to describe an injured tooth. The first way is to divide the mouth into quadrants: right maxillary, right mandibular, left maxillary, and left mandibular. Then, describe the type of tooth and the quadrant in which it is located. For example, the terms *right maxillary central incisor* and *left mandibular canine* denote both the type of tooth and the quadrant of the mouth in which it is found (see Fig. 53.2). The second way is the lettering (primary teeth) and numbering (permanent teeth) system. Teeth are assigned starting from the right-most maxillary tooth and then proceeding to the left-most maxillary tooth (A through J for primary; 1 through 16 for permanent). The mandibular teeth are assigned starting from the left-most tooth and then proceeding to the right-most tooth (K through T for primary; 17 through 32 for permanent) (Fig. 53.3).

6. **How do I perform an extraoral examination on a patient with dental trauma?**
   Palpate the facial skeleton evaluating for swelling, crepitus, depression, and asymmetry.
   Palpate the temporomandibular joint and test range of motion looking for mandibular deviation, trismus, or malocclusion. Examine any lip or intraoral wounds for tooth fragments or foreign bodies. Inspect for teeth displacement by assessing lip competency. Examine for any evidence of numbness of the lips, nose, and cheeks.

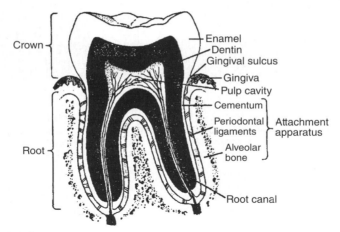

Fig. 53.1 Anatomy of a tooth.

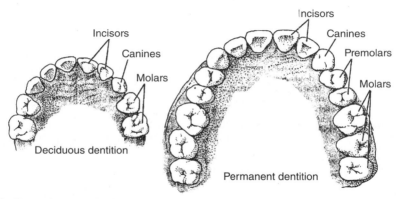

Fig. 53.2 Deciduous and permanent dentition of the upper jaw.

7. **How are broken or fractured teeth classified?**
   There are multiple methods for describing fractures, including the Ellis Classification. The system that the American Academy of Pediatric Dentistry uses describes four types of fractures: infraction, crown, crown-root, and root fractures.
   - An **infraction** is an incomplete fracture, or crack, only of the enamel without loss of tooth structure. These injuries are not sensitive to palpation.
   - A **crown fracture** is a complete fracture through the crown portion of the tooth and can be categorized either as:
     - An **uncomplicated** fracture involving either the enamel alone or extending through the enamel involving the yellow dentin. Fractures that involve the dentin can be painful and are often sensitive to heat, cold, and air.
     - A **complicated** fracture involving the enamel, dentin, *and pulp*. Pulp will appear as a red dot with bleeding from the tooth itself. Pain can be severe as the neurovascular bundle of the tooth is exposed.
   - A **crown-root fracture** is a fracture of enamel, dentin, and cementum. It too can be either an uncomplicated or complicated fracture depending on whether pulp is involved.
   - A **root fracture** is a fracture of the root of the tooth involving the dentin, pulp, and cementum.

8. **How are fractured teeth treated?**
   Treatment depends on the classification of the tooth fracture:
   - **Infractions** may require etching and bonding to prevent discoloration. Nonurgent dental follow-up is recommended.

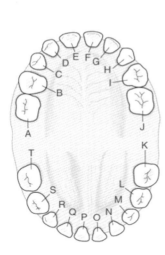

Primary teeth

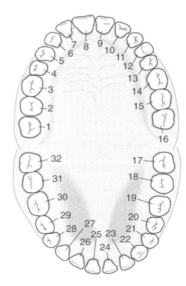

Secondary teeth

Fig. 53.3 Lettering and numbering system of deciduous and permanent dentition.

- **Uncomplicated crown fractures of the enamel** require the filing of sharp tooth edges to prevent oral soft tissue injury. The tooth fragment can be bonded to the tooth if it is available. Nonurgent dental follow-up is recommended.
- **Uncomplicated crown fractures of the enamel-dentin** require prompt treatment. In the ED setting, a temporary protective composite coating should be applied to the exposed dentin and dental follow-up should occur within 48 hours.
- **Complicated crown fractures** require dental follow-up within 24 hours. In the ED setting, a temporary calcium hydroxide pulp cap should be applied over the exposed pulp.

9. How are root fractures diagnosed and treated?
   Root fractures present with bleeding from the gingival sulcus, tooth mobility, or crown displacement. An intraoral dental radiograph is required for diagnosis. The closer the fracture is to the apex of the root, the better the prognosis. Treatment is based on the location of the fracture and may require reduction, splinting, or extraction.

10. When should I suspect an alveolar ridge fracture?
    Malocclusion, pain, and segment mobility (the movement of multiple continuous teeth with palpation) are common findings for an alveolar fracture. Identification of subtle fractures may be possible by palpating the gingiva and looking for any evidence of crepitus or step-offs. These fractures often occur with luxation injuries of adjacent teeth.

KEY POINTS: TOOTH FRACTURES

1. Crown tooth fractures most commonly occur in the anterior dentition and are classified as uncomplicated or complicated.
2. Uncomplicated crown fractures of the enamel-dentin and complicated crown fractures require urgent dental referral.
3. Suspect alveolar ridge fractures in the case of multiple continuous teeth that move with palpation. Suspect root fractures in the case of mobile teeth with gingival bleeding.

11. How are concussion and subluxation injuries diagnosed and treated?
    - **Concussion** is defined as a traumatic injury to the tooth and supporting structures without displacement or mobility. Signs and symptoms include exaggerated tooth sensitivity during percussion, chewing, occlusion, or

mobility testing. Treatment includes a soft diet and analgesics for 7 to 10 days with dental follow-up to monitor tooth viability.
- **Subluxation** is defined as trauma to the tooth with minor mobility but no displacement. Signs and symptoms include tooth sensitivity to percussion, minor mobility on tooth examination, and blood in the gingival sulcus. Treatment is the same as for tooth concussion, but dental follow-up is more important—not only to monitor tooth viability but also to rule out a root fracture. Subluxation injuries in permanent teeth may be splinted if there is excessive mobility or tenderness.

12. **What is a luxation injury?**
Luxation injuries cause physical displacement of the tooth within the alveolar socket, tearing of the periodontal ligament, and possible injury to the alveolar bone.
- **Intrusion** describes impaction of the tooth into the alveolar socket.
- **Extrusion** describes vertically dislodgement of the tooth from the alveolar socket.
- **Lateral luxation** describes displacement of the tooth in any lateral direction.

13. **Which injuries in primary and permanent dentition are most common?**
Crown fractures are the most common traumatic injuries in permanent dentition, whereas luxation injuries are the most reported in primary teeth.

14. **How are extrusion and lateral luxation injuries in *primary* teeth treated?**
Treatment decisions are based on the degree of displacement and mobility. If there is no malocclusion, the tooth should be allowed to spontaneously reposition itself. In the case of severe lateral luxation, the tooth can also be gently repositioned and splinted. If the tooth is excessively mobile or extruded more than 3 mm, it should be extracted, and an immediate dental referral is required. If there is a risk for aspiration, urgently remove the tooth in the ED.

15. **How are extrusion and lateral luxation injuries in *permanent* teeth treated?**
These injuries require emergent dental referral. Ideally, the tooth should be repositioned and splinted within 2 hours. These injuries may ultimately require root canal treatment.

16. **How is an intrusion injury to a *primary* tooth treated?**
Allow the tooth to spontaneously reposition itself. In most cases, this occurs within 6 months. Patients should be seen by their dentist within 48 hours. Past guidelines recommended that if the traumatized primary tooth root was directed toward the permanent tooth germ, it should be immediately extracted. However, observation is now supported by newer evidence that the intruded primary teeth spontaneously erupt and extraction could further damage the tooth germ.

17. **How is an intrusion injury to a *permanent* tooth treated?**
Patients with intruded permanent teeth can be managed conservatively in the ED and instructed to see their dentist within 48 hours. In adolescents and patients with mature roots, management is based on the depth of intrusion. If the tooth is intruded less than 3 mm, spontaneous re-eruption is allowed. If the tooth is intruded more than 3 mm, surgical repositioning is required. In younger patients with an immature root, the tooth usually is allowed to re-erupt spontaneously.

18. **What is an avulsion injury?**
An avulsion injury is the complete displacement of the tooth (crown and root) from the alveolar socket. This injury is a dental emergency and a permanent tooth must be reimplanted promptly to increase the chance of tooth salvage.

19. **What storage medium is best for an avulsed tooth prior to reimplantation?**
If replantation at the accident site is not possible, it is imperative to store the tooth in an appropriate solution to keep the periodontal ligament alive and to ensure successful reimplantation. Appropriate fluids, in descending order of preference, are Hank's Balanced Salt Solution (HBSS) (commercially marketed as Save-a-Tooth) or cold milk, saliva, or saline. Tap water is not recommended because its low osmolality will cause cell rupture within minutes. It is not advised to have the child keep the tooth in his/her mouth as it can be aspirated or swallowed.

20. **What is the procedure for reimplanting an avulsed permanent tooth?**
1. Hold the crown of the tooth, not the root, and remove debris with gentle rinsing using sterile saline or storage medium. To avoid injury to the periodontal ligament, do not handle or scrub the root of the tooth.
2. Insert the root of the tooth into the alveolar socket. The concave part of the tooth should face the tongue.
3. Splint the tooth for 10 to 14 days.

4. If the alveolar socket is filled with blood, it may be necessary to irrigate the socket with saline prior to successful tooth reimplantation.
5. Occasionally, it is necessary to perform a local nerve block to accomplish the procedure.
6. Check tetanus status and prescribe a soft diet, analgesics, and antibiotics.

21. **Why is it so important to reimplant a permanent tooth within 30 minutes?**
There is a 90% likelihood of tooth survival if a permanent tooth is reimplanted within 30 minutes. The survival rate declines rapidly with time, by approximately 1% for each minute beyond 30 minutes. A tooth reimplanted after 60 minutes of extraoral dry time has a poor long-term prognosis because the periodontal ligament becomes necrotic and ankylosis-related root resorption occurs.

22. **Why not reimplant an avulsed primary tooth?**
An avulsed primary tooth should never be reimplanted because of a risk of ankylosis—a bony fusion of the tooth with the alveolar bone that may result in facial deformities. In addition, reimplantation of a primary tooth may interfere with the eruption of the underlying permanent tooth. Temporary prosthetic devices can be made if a cosmetic effect is desired after a primary tooth is avulsed.

KEY POINTS: TOOTH AVULSIONS

1. Never reimplant avulsed primary teeth because of the risk of ankylosis and resultant facial deformities.
2. Fluids suitable to store avulsed permanent teeth, in descending order, are HBSS or cold milk, saliva, or saline.
3. The prognosis for avulsed permanent teeth is highly time-dependent. Complete the reimplantation as soon as possible.

23. **When should a radiograph be obtained in patients with dental injury?**
If the patient has a fractured or avulsed tooth and the entire missing segment cannot be found, obtain a chest radiograph. Patients requiring lobectomies from aspirated teeth have been reported. Intraoral soft tissue radiographs may also be necessary if there is concern that tooth fragments may have become embedded in lacerations.

24. **What is the maximum recommended dose for common injectable local anesthetics used for dental anesthesia?**
While the manufacturer's recommended dose (MRD) for lidocaine is 7 mg/kg, the American Academy of Pediatric Dentistry in conjunction with the American Academy of Pediatrics recommends a more conservative maximum dose of 4.4 mg/kg. The maximum dose for bupivacaine is 1.3 mg/kg. The duration of lidocaine is 90 to 200 minutes, whereas the duration of bupivacaine is 180 to 600 minutes.

25. **When should prophylactic antibiotic therapy be prescribed for patients with dental injuries?**
Antibiotics are recommended following reimplantation of avulsed permanent teeth. For children under 12 years of age, amoxicillin twice daily for 7 days is recommended. Clindamycin can be substituted in the case of severe penicillin allergy. For older children, doxycycline is recommended. Dental trauma that occurs with concomitant oral wounds may also require antibiotics. In addition, antibiotics may be recommended for immunocompromised patients and those at risk for developing bacteremia. Antibiotics are not indicated for isolated luxation injuries, primary tooth avulsion, or tooth fractures.

26. **What dental anomalies can be seen in permanent teeth after trauma to primary dentition?**
Dental trauma to a primary tooth can damage the underlying permanent teeth either by direct impact or through periapical infection. Traumatic avulsion, extrusion, and intrusive injuries have the highest risk. Frequent consequences in permanent dentition include white or yellow spots, enamel hypoplasia, malposition, and early or delayed eruption. Children less than 3 years of age at the time of the injury are at highest risk for developing anomalies.

27. **What discharge instructions should be provided after dental trauma?**
   - Avoid contact sports.
   - Take appropriate analgesics (e.g., acetaminophen, ibuprofen).
   - Apply cold compresses as needed.
   - Eat a soft diet.
   - Use chlorhexidine mouth rinse.
   - Use a soft toothbrush if able to brush teeth.
   - For certain injuries, restrict the use of straws/pacifiers.

28. **What is recommended to prevent sports-related dental injuries?**
    The incidence of dental injuries can be significantly reduced through mandatory protective equipment policies. A properly fitted mouthguard is recommended in all collision and contact sports. The National Federation of State High School Associations currently mandates mouthguards only for football, ice hockey, lacrosse, field hockey, and wrestlers wearing braces. However, basketball, baseball, and softball also have a high incidence of dental injuries.
    Multiple types of mouthguards are available on the market including custom-fitted, mouth-formed, or boil-and-bite and stock. Better-fitted mouthguards, primarily those that are custom-fitted, will generally be more comfortable and provide better protection against dental injuries.

29. **What dental injuries raise suspicion for child abuse or neglect?**
    Facial and intraoral trauma has been described in up to 40% to 60% of toddlers and infants who have been abused. Any suspicion of child abuse or neglect should always be reported. Findings that raise suspicion for abuse or neglect include:
    - Lacerations of the oral frena in nonambulatory children
    - Posterior pharyngeal injuries
    - Gray and discolored teeth
    - Scarring or bruising at the corners of the mouth
    - A discrepant injury history or multiple injuries in different stages of healing

30. **Summarize the timing for dental consultation following dental trauma.**
    Immediate dental consult:
    - Avulsed permanent tooth
    - Extrusion or lateral luxation injury of a permanent tooth
    - Malocclusion or significant tooth mobility in a primary tooth with extrusion or lateral luxation injury
    - Root fracture with crown displacement
    Alveolar ridge fractureUrgent dental consult (within 48 hours):
    - Uncomplicated crown fracture of enamel-dentin
    - Complicated tooth fracture (pulp exposed)
    - Subluxation injury
    - Intrusion injury
    - Extrusion or lateral luxation injury of a primary tooth other than listed above
    Nonurgent dental consult (within 1 week):
    - Uncomplicated crown fractures of the enamel
    - Infraction injury
    - Concussion injury

KEY POINTS: PEDIATRIC DENTAL TRAUMA

1. In the evaluation of children with dental injuries, it is important to understand normal dental development, as proper identification of primary versus permanent dentition affects diagnosis and treatment.
2. Primary teeth may be distinguished from permanent teeth because they are usually found in children younger than 6 years of age, are smaller in size, and have a smooth, not ridged, occlusive surface.
3. In the ED, it is important to promptly reimplant an avulsed permanent tooth.
4. It is possible to prevent many sports-related dental injuries with the use of properly fitted mouthguards.

Acknowledgments
The authors wish to thank Dr. Steven Chan, Dr. Evaline A. Alessandrini, and Dr. Linda L. Brown for their contributions to this chapter in the previous editions.

BIBLIOGRAPHY

1. Adnan S, Lone MM, Khan FR, et al. Which is the most recommended medium for the storage and transport of avulsed teeth? A systematic review. *Dent Traumatol.* 2018;34(2):59–70.
2. American Academy of Pediatric Dentistry. *Use of local anesthesia for pediatric dental patients. The Reference Manual of Pediatric Dentistry.* American Academy of Pediatric Dentistry; 2021:332–337.
3. American Academy of Pediatric Dentistry. *Use of antibiotic therapy for pediatric dental patients. The Reference Manual of Pediatric Dentistry.* American Academy of Pediatric Dentistry; 2021:461–464.
4. American Academy of Pediatric Dentistry. *Antibiotic prophylaxis for dental patients at risk for infection. The Reference Manual of Pediatric Dentistry.* American Academy of Pediatric Dentistry; 2021:465–470.
5. American Academy of Pediatric Dentistry. *Policy on prevention of sports-related orofacial injuries. The Reference Manual of Pediatric Dentistry.* American Academy of Pediatric Dentistry; 2021:110–115.

6. Bardellini E, Amadori F, Pasini S, Majorana A. Dental anomalies in permanent teeth after trauma in primary dentition. *J Clin Pediatr Dent.* 2017;41(1):5–9.
7. Bourguignon C, Cohenca N, Lauridsen E, et al. IADT guidelines for the management of traumatic dental injuries: 1. Fractures and luxations. *Dent Traumatol.* 2020;36(4):314–330.
8. Casey RP, Bensadigh BM, Lake MT, Thaller SR. Dentoalveolar trauma in the pediatric population. *J Craniofac Surg.* 2010;21(4):1305–1309.
9. Day PF, Flores MT, O'Connell AC, et al. IADT guidelines for the management of traumatic dental injuries: 3. Injuries in the primary dentition. *Dent Traumatol.* 2020;36(4):343–359.
10. Fida Z, Chase II, Padwa BL. Dental trauma. In: Bachur RG, Shaw KN, eds. *Textbook of Pediatric Emergency Medicine.* 8th ed. Wolters Kluwer/Lippincott Williams & Wilkins; 2021:1104–1111.
11. Fisher-Owens SA, Lukefahr JL, Tate AR, et al. Oral and dental aspects of child abuse and neglect. *Pediatrics.* 2017;140(2):e20171487.
12. Fouad AF, Abbott PV, Tsilingaridis G, et al. IADT guidelines for the management of traumatic dental injuries: 2. Avulsion of permanent teeth. *Dent Traumatol.* 2020;36(4):331–342.
13. Glendor U. Epidemiology of traumatic dental injuries—a 12 year review of the literature. *Dent Traumatol.* 2008;24(6):603–611.
14. Hall E, Hickey P, Nguyen-Tran T, Louie J. Dental trauma in a pediatric emergency referral center. *Pediatr Emerg Care.* 2016;32(12):823–826.
15. Keels MA. Management of dental trauma in a primary care setting. *Pediatrics.* 2014;133(2):e466–e476.
16. Klein BL, Larson BJ. Reimplanting an avulsed permanent tooth. In: King C, Henretig FM, eds. *Textbook of Pediatric Emergency Medicine Procedures.* 2nd ed. Wolters Kluwer/Lippincott Williams & Wilkins; 2008:669–673.
17. Levin L, Day PF, Hicks L, et al. IADT guidelines for the management of traumatic dental injuries: general introduction. *Dent Traumatol.* 2020;36(4):309–313.
18. Li JL. Emergency department management of dental trauma: recommendations for improved outcomes in pediatric patients. *Pediatr Emerg Med Pract.* 2018;15(8):1–23.
19. Patidar D, Sogi S, Patidar DC, Malhotra A. Traumatic dental injuries in pediatric patients: a retrospective analysis. *Int J Clin Pediatr Dent.* 2021;14(4):506–511.

WEBSITES

American Dental Association: Oral Health Topics:
http://www.ada.org/en/member-center/oral-health-topics
International Association of Dental Trauma:
http://www.iadt-dentaltrauma.org
American Academy of Pediatric Dentistry:
http://www.aapd.org/research/oral-health-policies--recommendations/

CHAPTER 54

EXTREMITY INJURIES

John M. Loiselle and Maria Carmen G. Diaz

1. How does the pediatric musculoskeletal system differ in its response to stress as compared to adults?
   - The pediatric skeleton is less densely calcified than the adult version. It is composed of a higher percentage of cartilage. Pediatric bones are lighter and more porous than adult bones, with Haversian canals making up a greater percentage.
   - The pediatric musculoskeletal system is an actively growing structure. Long bones contain growth plates or physes that are the primary site of this growth. The ends of the bone contain a chondro-osseous segment termed the *epiphysis* or secondary site of ossification.
   - The bones in a child are surrounded by a thick and very active periosteum. This structure provides additional support as well as a high capacity for remodeling injured bone.
   - The relative strengths of the different musculoskeletal components differ from child to adult. In the child, the ligaments and periosteum are stronger than the bone and less likely to give way under stress. The physis is the weak link. As a result, fractures tend to be relatively more common than sprains or ligamentous injuries in children than in adults.
   - The degree of ossification, the thickness of the periosteum, and the width of the growth plate vary with age. Therefore, the age of the child and the corresponding anatomy dictate the response of the musculoskeletal system to trauma.

2. What unique categories of fractures are commonly seen in pediatrics as a result of these differences?
   - Physeal or Salter-Harris fractures
   - Plastic deformation fractures
   - Avulsion fractures

3. Describe the Salter-Harris classification of fractures.
   - **Salter I:** A fracture within the growth plate. The fracture line itself is not visible on radiographs, but a widening of the physis or displacement of the epiphysis may be suggestive of such a fracture.
   - **Salter II:** A fracture that extends through the growth plate and metaphysis.
   - **Salter III:** An intraarticular fracture that extends through the growth plate and the epiphysis.
   - **Salter IV:** An intraarticular fracture that involves the metaphysis, growth plate, and epiphysis.
   - **Salter V:** A compression fracture of the growth plate. This injury is unlikely to be detected initially by radiographs and often becomes evident only as the result of eventual growth arrest in the affected limb.

4. Why is the Salter-Harris classification important?
   The Salter-Harris classification of fractures categorizes fractures that involve the growth plate. The classification has implications for both prognosis and treatment. Fractures categorized within the higher numbers of the classification are more likely to affect joint congruity and disrupt the blood supply to the growth centers of the bone, leading to greater potential for future growth disturbance.

5. At what age are physeal injuries most likely to occur?
   Eighty percent occur between 10 and 16 years of age, with a median age of 13 years. Hypertrophy of the physis during the growth spurt and increased participation in physical activity and sports at this age are responsible for the increased incidence.

6. What are plastic fractures?
   Plastic fractures result from the pliability of the bones in childhood. Pediatric bones respond to compressive and transverse forces through plastic deformation. With a small amount of force, the bone is capable of bending slightly and then returning to its natural state. If excessive force is applied, the bone eventually exceeds its capacity for full elastic recoil and deforms. Depending on the degree of force and how it is applied, one of the three plastic fractures of childhood may result.

7. Name three types of plastic fractures in childhood.
   - Buckle or torus fracture
   - Greenstick fracture
   - Bowing or bending fracture

8. Why is it important to reduce a forearm bowing fracture?
   These fractures do not include injury to the periosteum and therefore do not undergo vigorous stimulation to remodel. This may result in permanent angulation of the bone, which can have deleterious effects on the normal range of motion and function of the involved forearm.

9. In what order do the growth centers in the elbow ossify? Why is this clinically important?
   The mnemonic **CRITOE** is a useful reminder of the sequence in which these ossified growth centers appear. An ossified fragment that is present out of its expected order suggests a fracture rather than a normal ossification center (Table 54.1).

10. What is a FOOSH? What is its significance to pediatric extremity injuries?
    A **FOOSH** stands for **F**all **O**n an **O**ut-**S**tretched **H**and. This is the most common mechanism of forearm, elbow, and wrist injuries in children.

11. Describe the initial approach to the trauma victim with a significantly deformed extremity fracture.
    The initial approach to any trauma patient should focus on potential life-threatening injuries. The primary survey consists of the evaluation and stabilization of the airway, breathing, and circulation. The physician should not be distracted by the more obvious extremity injuries, which are rarely life-threatening. Extremity fractures are more appropriately addressed as part of the secondary survey.

12. Describe pain management for pediatric extremity injuries.
    Several studies demonstrate inadequate attention to analgesia for pediatric extremity injuries. Provide oral or parenteral analgesics in weight-based dosages early in the visit. Intranasal fentanyl is fast acting and can be administered for severe pain. Intravenous administration of morphine (0.05-0.1 mg/kg/dose, max 5 mg) mg as per Lexicomp is recommended for displaced fractures. The superiority of oral opiates over nonsteroidal anti-inflammatory drugs (NSAIDs) has not been proven. Early immobilization of the injured extremity through application of a splint results in significant reduction in pain scores.

13. What motor and sensory nerve functions should be assessed when evaluating an upper extremity injury?
    These data are mentioned in Table 54.2.

Table 54.1 Ossification Centers and Age of Calcification in the Pediatric Elbow

OSSIFICATION CENTER	APPEARANCE (YEARS)
C = Capitellum	1
R = Radial head	3
I = Internal (medial) epicondyle	5
T = Trochlea	7
O = Olecranon	9
E = External (lateral) epicondyle	11

Table 54.2 Motor and Sensory Functions of Upper Extremity Nerves

NERVE	MOTOR FUNCTION	SENSORY FUNCTION
Radial	Wrist extension Thumb extension "thumbs up sign"	Web space between thumb and index finger on dorsum of hand
Ulnar	Fingers spread Crossing index and middle finger	Little finger and ulnar side of the ring finger
Median	Tip of index finger to tip of thumb "OK sign"	Thumb, index, middle, and radial sides of ring fingers
Anterior Interosseous	Tip of index finger to tip of thumb "OK sign"	No sensory component

14. **What factors determine the need for fracture reduction?**

   Pediatric bones have a high capacity to remodel. As a general rule, remodeling should not be relied upon to correct all deformities. Immobilize fractures as close to anatomic position as possible. The decision to actively reduce a particular fracture or to rely on remodeling depends on several factors:
   - **Patient's age:** The older the child, the less time for growth and remodeling.
   - **Location of the fracture:** Fractures farther from the physis have less capacity to remodel.
   - **Bone involved:** Different bones are subjected to different muscular stresses that in part determine their growth and healing capacity.
   - **Type of fracture:** In general, the greater the disruption of periosteum, the greater the stimulation for repair and remodeling.
   - **Degree and direction of disruption:** Rotational deformities are particularly poor at remodeling.

15. **Which pediatric extremity injuries require emergent orthopedic consultation?**
   - Femur fracture
   - Complete fractures of the tibia or fibula
   - Open fracture
   - Fractures associated with neurovascular compromise
   - Dislocation of a large joint, with the possible exception of the shoulder
   - Fractures with significant displacement
   - Fractures involving a large joint
   - Displaced supracondylar fractures

16. **List the key information that should be communicated when an orthopedic consultation is requested.**
   - Age and gender of the patient
   - Mechanism of injury
   - Bone or bones involved in the injury
   - Type of fracture
   - Neurovascular status of the extremity
   - Presence and amount of displacement
   - Presence and degree of angulation
   - Presence or absence of an open fracture

17. **What is the most commonly injured nerve in acute shoulder dislocation?**

   The axillary nerve, which innervates the upper arm, must be carefully examined for acute shoulder dislocation. Shoulder dislocation is most likely to occur when the arm is abducted and externally rotated. Anterior dislocations are far more common and recurrent.

18. **What is little league shoulder and how does it present?**

   Little league shoulder, also known as proximal humeral epiphysiolysis, is an overuse injury most often seen in high-performance pitchers between 11 and 16 years of age. It may also be seen in tennis players, swimmers, and gymnasts. The chief complaint is gradual pain localized to the proximal humerus during the act of throwing or serving. The physical exam may be negative, or there may be tenderness to palpation of the proximal humerus. Radiographs may reveal a widening of the proximal humeral physis. Treatment is almost always nonsurgical and includes a 3-month rest period and physical therapy.

19. **What radiologic findings on a lateral elbow film suggest the presence of an occult fracture?**

   A visible posterior fat pad or outward displacement of the anterior fat pad away from the humerus is evidence of an elbow effusion. Assume a fracture to be present when an elbow effusion is seen in the setting of elbow trauma.

   A malaligned anterior humeral line (one that passes anterior to the capitellum rather than through the middle or posterior third) suggests the presence of a supracondylar fracture with dorsal displacement of the capitellum and distal humerus.

   Malalignment of the radiocapitellar line, as determined by a line through the center of the radius that does not pass through the center of the capitellum on either the anteroposterior or lateral radiograph, is evidence of a dislocated radius.

20. **What are the three classifications of supracondylar fractures?**

   The three Gartland classifications of supracondylar fractures are:
   - **Type I:** Nondisplaced fracture
   - **Type II:** Mild displacement with intact posterior cortex
   - **Type III:** Displaced fracture with no anterior and posterior cortical contact

   All type III fractures and most type II supracondylar fractures (Fig. 54.1) require percutaneous pinning to obtain appropriate reduction and to reduce complications.

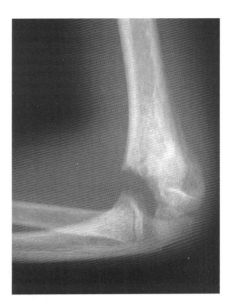

Fig. 54.1 Supracondylar fracture.

21. What are two long-term complications that can result from supracondylar fractures?
    1. **Volkmann contracture:** Deformation that results from ischemia of the muscles and other soft tissues. It occurs most commonly in the forearm as the result of a compartment syndrome. The predisposing injury in children is frequently a supracondylar fracture.
    2. **Gunstock deformity or cubitus varus deformity:** A deformity that occurs when a supracondylar fracture heals with poor alignment. This results in medial displacement of the distal humerus. It is the most common complication of supracondylar fractures. Cubitus varus is most often a cosmetic rather than a functional deformity.

22. What is the most common nerve injury resulting from a supracondylar fracture and how do you clinically assess for it?
    Median, radial, and ulnar nerve injuries can all occur as a complication of a supracondylar fracture. The anterior interosseous branch of the median nerve is the most common nerve injury; typically occurring in extension-type supracondylar fractures. This nerve may be injured in up to 50% of patients with type III supracondylar fractures. A nerve palsy of the anterior interosseous nerve results in isolated motor loss and is often missed due to a lack of sensory changes. The injury results in an inability to tightly approximate the tips of the index finger and thumb while maintaining flexion of the distal interphalangeal joint of the index finger and the interphalangeal joint of the thumb forming the "OK" sign. Alternatively, the patient is unable to extend the interphalangeal joint of the thumb against resistance.

23. Explain the term *nursemaid's elbow*.
    The term refers to the most common mechanism for obtaining a radial head subluxation (or annular ligament displacement) injury. A "nursemaid" or caretaker may abruptly lift a young child by the wrist while crossing a street or attempting to prevent a stumbling child from falling. Traction is applied to the forearm with the elbow extended and the forearm in pronation. A nursemaid's elbow can occur without a history of this classic mechanism. The result is a tear or displacement of the annular ligament that becomes interposed between the capitellum and the radial head.

24. What is the typical clinical presentation for a nursemaid's elbow?
    Children typically do not appear to be in pain but refuse to use the affected arm. The arm is held in pronation and slight flexion at the side of the body. The examiner detects no swelling, point tenderness, bruising, or warmth over the joint, but resistance to supination, flexion, and pronation is noticeable. The child may hold the wrist on the affected side to support the extremity, often leading the parents and examiner to believe that the wrist is involved. Mild dependent edema of the hand may appear as swelling and further confuse the picture.

25. **Name the classic radiographic findings for a radial head subluxation (nursemaid's elbow).**
    There are no diagnostic radiographic findings for a radial head subluxation. Radiographs appear *normal*. They should be obtained only when the diagnosis is in question after the history and physical examination. In this setting, radiography is performed to rule out alternative causes of elbow pain.

26. **Describe two accepted maneuvers for reducing a radial head subluxation.**
    In both procedures, the child is seated in the parent's lap, facing the examiner. The examiner grasps the elbow and provides stabilization with the nondominant hand. With the dominant hand, the examiner holds the wrist or hand of the child's affected side and either (1) extends the elbow and hyperpronates the forearm or (2) supinates the forearm and then flexes the elbow in one smooth motion so that the child's hand comes up to the ipsilateral shoulder. A palpable "pop" may be appreciated at the elbow as the reduction occurs. The hyperpronation maneuver has a higher success rate and is perceived to be less painful.

27. **What is little league elbow?**
    Little league elbow, or medial epicondylar apophysitis, results from repetitive stress to the medial epicondyle in the skeletally immature elbow. It is most commonly seen in children between the ages of 8 and 12 years who are baseball pitchers, gymnasts, or tennis players. An excessive number of pitches thrown, and a sidearm pitching style have both been implicated as etiologies. The athlete presents with gradual onset of pain in the medial elbow and proximal forearm while throwing. Examination reveals localized tenderness at the medial epicondyle. Radiographs may be normal or reveal medial epicondylar apophyseal widening. Treatment is complete rest from throwing activities, ice, nonsteroidal anti-inflammatory agents, and physical therapy. After the 4- to 6-week rest period, asymptomatic athletes may partake in a 4- to 8-week progressive throwing program.

28. **What is the difference between Galeazzi and Monteggia fractures?**
    Both injuries involve a combination of forearm fracture and dislocation. The Galeazzi fracture is a fracture of the radius with dislocation of the distal radioulnar joint. The Monteggia fracture is an ulnar fracture with radial head dislocation (Fig. 54.2). Failure of a line drawn through the center of the radius to intersect with the capitellum

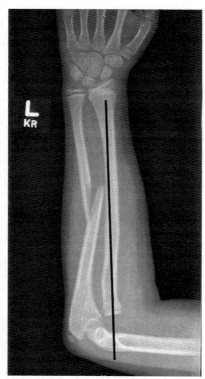

Fig. 54.2 Monteggia fracture with radiocapitellar line.

Table 54.3 Differences Between Mallet Finger and Jersey Finger

	MALLET FINGER	JERSEY FINGER
Injury	Extensor digitorum tendon disruption	Flexor digitorum tendon disruption
Physical exam	Forced flexion of an extended distal interphalangeal joint	Forced extension of a flexed distal interphalangeal joint
Mechanisms	Finger struck on the tip by a ball	Football player grabs another player's jersey
	Forcefully tucking in a bedspread	Lifting a latch on a car door
	Pushing off a sock with an extended finger	

From Bielak KM, Kafka J, Terrell T. Treatment of hand and wrist injuries. *Prim Care Clin Office Pract.* 2013;40:431–451.

(the radiocapitellar line) is diagnostic of a dislocation of the radial head. The dislocations associated with these fractures are at risk of being overlooked once the fracture has been identified. Failure to diagnose and reduce these injuries in a timely manner can result in permanent disability.

29. **What is the acute management and recommended follow-up of a distal radius buckle fracture?**
Buckle fractures of the distal radius are stable injuries with a high potential for complete remodeling. These are common injuries accounting for 40% of distal forearm fractures in young children. Immobilization in a removable brace for 2–3 weeks has been shown to provide more rapid functional recovery, greater convenience and is preferred by patients and parents. This management can be monitored in a primary care setting.

30. **What is the mechanism of injury in a "boxer's fracture"?**
Fractures of the fourth or fifth metacarpal ("boxer's fractures") are sustained when a person strikes an object with a closed fist. Destructive infections of the hand and metacarpophalangeal joint can occur when one person strikes another in the teeth and mouth flora are introduced into the resulting lacerations.

31. **Describe the mechanism of injury in a gamekeeper's thumb.**
Gamekeeper's thumb, also known as skier's thumb, is a sprain of the ulnar collateral ligament of the metacarpophalangeal joint of the thumb. The injury is the result of forced abduction and extension of the thumb that occurs when falling on an outstretched hand or colliding with an object. These patients exhibit point tenderness over the ulnar collateral ligament and have no radiographic findings. Treatment includes immobilization and compression with a thumb spica splint. If the patient has an open physis, this mechanism of injury will produce a Salter-Harris Type III fracture of the proximal phalanx.

32. **How does a mallet finger deformity differ in children and adults?**
The adult mallet finger is the result of disruption of the extensor tendon. In young children, the presence of the relatively weaker growth plate of the distal phalanx often leads to a Salter I fracture with displacement of the epiphysis. In older children or teenagers, the injury may result in an avulsion or Salter III fracture through the epiphysis. Such injuries may cause difficulty in reducing the finger although the majority can be managed nonoperatively.

33. **What is the difference between a mallet finger and a jersey finger?**
The difference is mentioned in Table 54.3.

34. **How do you evaluate distal nerve function in an uncooperative or preverbal child following extremity or digit injury?**
Placing the fingers in a bowl of warm water for several minutes results in wrinkling of the skin on the finger pads if distal nerve function is intact.

35. **How do pelvic avulsion fractures occur?**
Pelvic avulsion fractures result from sudden muscular contractions and are usually associated with vigorous running or jumping. These are most commonly seen in skeletally immature athletes and in sports that require rapid acceleration or deceleration, or quick changes of direction.

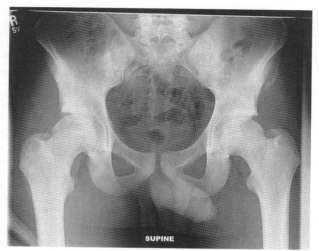

Fig. 54.3 Pelvic avulsion fracture, left side.

Table 54.4 Pelvic Avulsion Fracture Locations and Involved Muscle

LOCATION	INVOLVED MUSCLE
Ischial tuberosity	Hamstrings and adductors
Anterior superior iliac spine	Sartorius
Anterior inferior iliac spine	Rectus femoris

36. **What are the most common locations of pelvic avulsion fractures and what muscle attachment contributes to the fracture?**
An image of a pelvic avulsion fracture (left side) can be found in Fig. 54.3.
Table 54.4 details the muscle attachment that contributes to the pelvic avulsion fracture.

37. **What is the typical mechanism for an injury to the anterior cruciate ligament (ACL) in children?**
As in adults, injury to the ACL results from a sudden deceleration accompanied by hyperextension and a rotatory force on a planted foot. This is often accompanied by a popping sensation and the acute onset of hemarthrosis. Whereas adults and older adolescents will probably tear the ligament itself, younger children may avulse a bony segment of the tibia at the ACL insertion site. Plain radiography followed by magnetic resonance imaging is used to delineate the specifics of the injury. Management of the ACL injury is complicated by the open physes in skeletally immature children, requiring careful consideration of operative versus nonoperative treatment plans by the orthopedist.

38. **What is the most common type of patellar dislocation and the most common mechanism of injury?**
Lateral dislocations are the most common type of patellar dislocation. It usually occurs when an internal rotatory force is applied to a flexed knee with the foot planted. This may happen in sports that require cutting or pivoting such as gymnastics, football, or wrestling.

39. **How do you reduce a laterally dislocated patella?**
A laterally dislocated patella almost always reduces spontaneously when the leg is placed in extension; it remains dislocated only when the patient maintains the leg in flexion. Flexion of the hips to relax the quadriceps muscles may aid in the reduction. Occasionally a small amount of pressure applied on the medial side of the patella is necessary. Sedation and/or analgesia are often needed before movement of the extremity. After reduction, immobilize the joint and obtain radiographs to rule out associated fractures. Whether prereduction radiographs are useful or simply prolong the patient's discomfort remains controversial.

40. Name the two types of apophysitis syndromes that occur surrounding the patellar tendon.
    - Osgood-Schlatter disease: An apophysitis at the anterior tibial tubercle due to traction by the inferior aspect of the patellar tendon.
    - Sinding-Larsen-Johansson: An apophysitis of the inferior pole of the patella due to traction by the superior aspect of the patellar tendon. Sinding-Larsen-Johansson is differentiated from "Jumper's Knee" in that Jumpers Knee is not an apophysitis but rather an inflammation within the proximal patellar tendon itself.

41. What is the most common overuse injury in the young athlete?
    Osgood-Schlatter disease, an apophysitis at the anterior tibial tubercle, commonly affects adolescents during periods of rapid growth. Symptoms include tenderness and prominence at the tibial tubercle, with pain worsened by high-impact sports, kneeling, or squatting. Plain radiographs may demonstrate enlargement or fragmentation at the anterior tibial tubercle due to the traction force at the insertion of the patellar tendon. However, radiographs are not necessary in typical cases. Management includes ice, NSAIDs, and stretching regimens to increase the flexibility of the quadriceps and hamstrings. It is most important to avoid activities that place stress on the tibial tubercle. Activity can be resumed when the patient is pain-free. The problem usually (90% of cases) resolves with conservative management in 12 to 24 months.

42. What injuries may be associated with proximal tibial physeal fractures?
    - Ligamentous injuries may be seen with Salter-Harris III and IV fractures of the proximal tibia.
    - Injuries that posteriorly displace the proximal tibial metaphysis may stretch and tear the popliteal artery.
    - Tibial tubercle avulsion fractures may be associated with bleeding of the anterior tibial recurrent artery into the anterior compartment thus leading to compartment syndrome.

43. List the most common locations for stress fractures in pediatric athletes.
    - Tibia 51%
    - Fibula 20%
    - Pars interarticularis 15%
    - Femur 3%
    - Metatarsal 2%
    - Tarsal navicular 2%

44. What is a toddler's fracture?
    A toddler's fracture is described most commonly as a hairline, nondisplaced spiral, or oblique fracture of the distal third of the tibia. It occurs, as its name suggests, in ambulatory children up to approximately 4 years of age. It often results from relatively minor force, such as a fall from a step or the end of a sliding board. Others have expanded the definition to include any subtle or occult injury such as a distal buckle fracture of the tibia.

45. What name is associated with a Salter III fracture of the distal tibia? How is this fracture related to the age and growth of a child?
    A Salter III fracture of the distal tibia is called a Tillaux fracture (Fig. 54.4). It classically occurs in teenagers shortly before growth plate closure. The medial segment of the distal tibial physis fuses last, and the medial aspect of the distal epiphysis remains anchored to the fibula by the anterior tibiofibular ligament. External rotation of the foot with sufficient force produces an avulsion fracture through the unfused medial segment of the growth plate and down through the epiphysis.

46. What is a triplane ankle fracture and what imaging modality may help determine treatment?
    Triplane ankle fractures are complex traumatic Salter-Harris IV fractures of the distal tibia. The triplane configuration represents fractures of the epiphysis in the sagittal plane, posterior metaphysis in the coronal plane, and the physis in the transverse plane. Computed tomography (CT) helps determine fracture pattern, degree of displacement, and treatment.

47. What is the low-risk ankle rule?
    The low-risk ankle rule is a clinical prediction rule that was validated in children between 3 and 16 years of age and identifies which ankle injuries in children are low risk and thus may not need imaging. In a prospective study of 2151 children, this rule had 100% sensitivity, 53.1% specificity, and reduced imaging by 22%. Low-risk ankle injuries include lateral ankle sprains, isolated nondisplaced distal fibular Salter-Harris I, Salter-Harris II, and avulsion fractures.
    Ankle injuries in children are considered low risk and do not need radiographs if:
    - There is tenderness and swelling isolated to the distal fibula or adjacent lateral ligaments distal to the tibial anterior joint line.
    - Injury is acute (<72 hours old).
    - Child not at risk for pathologic fractures.

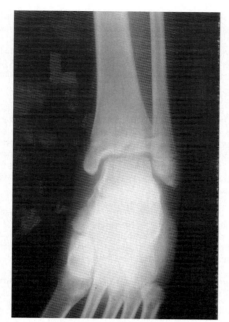

Fig. 54.4 Salter III fracture of the distal tibia, commonly called a Tillaux fracture.

- No congenital anomaly of the feet or ankles.
- Child can reliably express pain/tenderness.
- No gross deformity, neurovascular compromise, or distracting injury.

48. **What are the limitations of the Ottawa Ankle Rules in children?**
    The Ottawa Ankle Rules are criteria developed for predicting ankle fractures based on examination features in adults with the goal of reducing unnecessary radiographs. They allow, however, for "insignificant fractures" (such as small avulsion fractures) to be undiagnosed. They are not universally applicable to the pediatric population due to the questionable significance of Salter I and avulsion fractures on children's future growth and development. A 2003 meta-analysis of 15,581 adults and children from 27 studies demonstrated an overall sensitivity and specificity for the Ottawa Ankle Rules of 97.6% and 31.5%, respectively. In a 2009 pooled analysis of 12 studies representing 3,130 children with 671 fractures, the authors reported a sensitivity of 98.5% and a negative likelihood ratio of 0.11. This data estimates a missed fracture rate of 1.2% in children.

49. **What is the recommended management for Sever's disease?**
    Sever's disease, an apophysitis resulting from repetitive stresses on the calcaneal ossification center by the Achilles tendon, is often seen in young runners. The athlete will complain of heel pain and often has had a recent growth spurt and increase in activity level. Management includes rest, NSAIDs, Achilles tendon stretching, and the use of heel cups in cleats or sneakers. It usually resolves in 2 to 4 months' time without the need for surgery.

50. **How do you differentiate an avulsion fracture at the proximal fifth metatarsal from the normal secondary site of ossification?**
    Avulsion injuries of the proximal fifth metatarsal occur during the inversion of the ankle. Stress is transmitted through the peroneus brevis ligament, which inserts on the proximal fifth metatarsal. The resulting fracture line is transverse to the foot, whereas the secondary site of ossification (os vesalianum) occurs in a longitudinal orientation. A comparison view of the normal foot may be helpful. Palpating for tenderness over the area is a simpler means of making the distinction.

51. **What types of toe fractures warrant orthopedic consultation?**
    - Orthopedics should be consulted for open fractures of the proximal phalanges.
    - Salter-Harris III or IV intraarticular fractures of the proximal phalanx of the great toe require urgent orthopedic consultation if there is more than 25% of the joint surface involved and there is displacement of more than 2 to 3 mm of the joint surface.

52. **What extremity fractures are associated with abuse?**

    Up to 10% of all extremity injuries in children are inflicted. Almost any extremity injury may be the result of abuse. Certain classic extremity fractures are more specific for abuse:
    - Metaphyseal chip fractures/corner fractures/bucket handle fractures
    - Multiple fractures in different stages of healing
    - Fractures inconsistent with the history or developmental abilities of the child
    - Femur fractures in children under a year of age or in preambulatory children
    - Spiral long bone fractures in preambulatory children
    - Fractures in association with other injuries suggestive of abuse

KEY POINTS: UNIQUE CHARACTERISTICS OF THE PEDIATRIC MUSCULOSKELETAL SYSTEM

1. Less densely calcified
2. Thick periosteum
3. Presence of the growth plate
4. Relatively strong ligaments

KEY POINTS: PEDIATRIC FRACTURES

1. Because of its increased pliability, the pediatric bone can go through several stages of deformity prior to fracture.
2. Salter-Harris fractures are those involving the growth plate.
3. The relative strength of the ligaments may predispose to avulsion fractures over ligamentous injuries.
4. Normal ossification centers in the pediatric skeleton are often mistaken for fractures.

KEY POINTS: FINDINGS IN RADIAL HEAD SUBLUXATION

1. History of forearm traction in pronation
2. Refusal to use arm
3. Lack of elbow swelling or bruising
4. Negative radiographs (if obtained)

KEY POINTS: ELBOW TRAUMA

1. The most common mechanism of pediatric elbow injury is hyperextension associated with a fall on an outstretched hand.
2. The presence of a posterior fat pad or elevated anterior fat pad on x-ray is evidence of a supracondylar fracture.
3. Most type II and all type III Gartland fractures typically require surgical pinning for adequate reduction.
4. Secondary ossification centers in the elbow appear in a predictable order.

BIBLIOGRAPHY

1. Antevy PM, Saladino RA. Management of finger injuries. In: King C, Henretig FM, eds. *Textbook of Pediatric Emergency Procedures.* 2nd ed. Williams & Wilkins; 2008:939–953.
2. Bednar ED, Kay J, Memon M, Simunovic N, et al. Diagnosis and management of little league shoulder: a systematic review. *Orthop J Sports Med.* 2021;9(7):23259671211017563.
3. Bekkens R, Washburn FJ, Eygendaal D, et al. Effectiveness of reduction maneuvers in the treatment of nursemaid's elbow: a systematic review and meta-analysis. *Am J Emerg Med.* 2017;35(1):159–163.
4. Boutis K, Grootendorst P, Willan A, Plint AC, et al. Effect of the low risk ankle rule on the frequency of radiography in children with ankle injuries. *CMAJ.* 2013;185(15):E731–738.
5. Boutis K. The emergency evaluation and management of pediatric extremity fractures. *Emerg Med Clin N Am.* 2020;38:31–59.
6. Diaz MCG, Werk LN, Crutchfield JH, et al. A provider-focused intervention to promote optimal care of pediatric patients with suspected elbow fracture. *Pediatr Emerg Care.* 2021;37(12):e1663–e1669.
7. Dowling S, Spooner CH, Liang Y, et al. Accuracy of Ottawa ankle rules to exclude fractures of the ankle and midfoot in children: a meta-analysis. *Acad Emerg Med.* 2009;16:277.
8. Duthon VB. Acute traumatic patellar dislocation. *Orthop Traumatol Surg Res.* 2015;101(1 Suppl):S59–67.

9. Eismann EA, Stephan ZA, Mehlman CT, Denning J, et al. Pediatric triplane ankle fractures: impact of radiographs and computed tomography on fracture classification and treatment planning. *J Bone Joint Surg Am.* 2015;97(12):995–1002.

10. Fares MY, Salhab HA, Khachfe HH, Fares J, Haidar R, Musharrafieh U. Sever's disease of the pediatric population: clinical, pathologic, and therapeutic considerations. *Clin Med Res.* 2021;19(3):132–137.

11. Frank JS, Gambacorta PL. Anterior cruciate ligament injuries in the skeletally immature athlete: diagnosis and management. *J Am Acad Orthop Surg.* 2013;21(2):78–87.

12. Frick SL, Mehlman CT. The community orthopaedic surgeon taking trauma call: pediatric supracondylar humeral fracture pearls and pitfalls. *J Orthop Trauma.* 2017;31:S11–S15.

13. Johnson FC, Okada PJ. Reduction of common joint dislocations and subluxations. In: King C, Henretig FM, eds. *Textbook of Pediatric Emergency Procedures.* 2nd ed. Williams & Wilkins; 2008:962–990.

14. Joffe MD, Loiselle JM. Musculoskeletal emergencies. In: Shaw KN, Bachur RG, eds. *Fleisher & Ludwig's Textbook of Pediatric Emergency Medicine.* 8th ed. Wolters Kluwer; 2021:1358–1381.

15. Kim HHR, Menashe SJ, Ngo A, et al. Uniquely pediatric upper extremity injuries. *Clin Imaging.* 2021;80:249–261.

16. Ladenhauf HN, Seitlinger G, Green DW. Osgood-Schlatter disease: a 2020 update of a common knee condition in children. *Curr Opin Pediatr.* 2020;32(1):107–112.

17. Lin JS, Samora JB. Outcomes of splinting in pediatric mallet finger. *J Hand Surg.* 2018;43(11):1041.e1–1041.e9.

18. Liu D, Lin Y. Current evidence for acute pain management of musculoskeletal injuries and postoperative pain in pediatric and adolescent athletes. *Clin J Sport Med.* 2019;29(5):430–438.

19. McIntosh AL, Crawford H. Ch 30, Fractures, dislocations, and other injuries of the foot. In: Waters PM, Skaggs DL, Flynn JM, eds. *Rockwood and Wilkins' Fractures in Children.* 9th ed. Lippincott Williams & Wilkins; 2020:1212. Available from: http://ovidsp.ovid.com. Accessed 30.05.22.

20. Sawark JF, LaBella CR. Overuse injuries *Pediatric Orthopaedics and Sports Injuries: A Quick Reference Guide.* 3rd ed. American Academy of Pediatrics: Itaska; 2021:IL311–342.

21. Rathjen KE, Kim HKW, Alman BA. The injured immature skeleton. In: Waters PM, Skaggs DL, Flynn JM, eds. *Rockwood and Wilkins' Fractures in Children.* 9th ed. Lippincott Williams & Wilkins; 2020:13–39.

22. Shea KG, Frick SL. Chapter 29. Ankle fractures. In: Waters PM, Skaggs DL, Flynn JM, eds. *Rockwood and Wilkins' Fractures in Children.* 9th ed. Lippincott Williams & Wilkins; 2020:1125. Available from: http://ovidsp.ovid.com. Accessed 30.05.22.

23. Shore BJ, Edmonds EW. Ch. 26. Proximal tibial physeal fractures. In: Waters PM, Skaggs DL, Flynn JM, eds. *Rockwood and Wilkins Fractures in Children.* 9th ed. Lippincott Williams & Wilkins; 2001:993. Available from: http://ovidsp.ovid.com. Accessed 30.05.22.

24. Shore BJ, Gillespie BT, Miller PE, et al. Recovery of motor nerve injuries associated with displaced, extension-type pediatric supracondylar humerus fractures. *J Ped Orthop.* 2019;39(9):e652–e656.

25. Thompson RW, Hannon M, Lee LK. Musculoskeletal trauma. In: Shaw KN, Bachur RG, eds. *Fleisher & Ludwig's Textbook of Pediatric Emergency Medicine.* 8th ed. Wolters Kluwer; 2021:1170–1213.

26. Wang Y, Doyle M, Smit K, Varshney T, Carsen S. The toddler's fracture. *Pediatr Emerg Care.* 2022;38(1):36–39.

CHAPTER 55

EYE INJURIES

Martha W. (Molly) Stevens

1. **What is the leading cause of vision loss in children?**
   Eye injuries are the leading cause. It is estimated that there are 8 to 15/100,000 children with eye injuries annually. Boys are four times more likely to have an eye injury than girls. Many eye injuries are related to sports, and many are preventable with the use of proper eye protection.

2. **Which sports are associated with a high risk for eye injuries?**
   - Paintball and use of an air rifle or BB gun
   - Basketball
   - Baseball/softball
   - Lacrosse
   - Ice, field, and street hockey
   - Squash and racquetball
   - Fencing
   - Boxing, wrestling, and full-contact martial arts

3. **What are the recommendations for the use of protective eyewear in athletes?**
   Appropriately fitted protective eyewear has been shown to decrease the incidence of injury by 90%. Almost 42,000 sports-related eye injuries occur each year in the United States, and more than one-third involve children. The American Academy of Pediatrics and the American Academy of Ophthalmology recommend eye protection for all athletes and mandate it in functionally one-eyed patients and in patients whose ophthalmologist recommends eye protection after surgery or trauma. *Functionally one-eyed* is defined as the best corrected visual acuity of less than 20/40 in the weaker eye.

4. **Name two injuries that are ophthalmologic emergencies.**
   Injuries that lead to incremental vision loss without early recognition and prompt initiation of treatment are ophthalmologic emergencies. Two such injuries include chemical burns and globe rupture. Both warrant emergent (same-day) ophthalmologic consultation after emergent initiation of treatment/stabilization in the emergency department (ED).

KEY POINTS: EVALUATION OF AN EYE INJURY

1. The mechanism of injury and timing of injury are critical points of information.
2. It is imperative to test visual acuity.
3. Investigate the possibility of a foreign body; metallic foreign bodies, if not removed, can stain the cornea.

5. **List the important aspects of the history of all patients with eye injuries.**
   - Change in visual acuity
   - Change in eye appearance (unilateral change pupil size/shape, en- or exophthalmos)
   - Discomfort or pain (including photophobia)
   - History of trauma, including details of the mechanism (blunt/sharp, significant impact, soil or chemical contamination, foreign-body risk)
   - Corrective lenses (contacts currently in place?)
   - Medications
   - Eye surgeries
   - History of ocular problems
   - Systemic diseases (sickle cell, connective tissue, or rheumatologic disease; hypertension; diabetes; human immunodeficiency virus infection)
   - Tetanus immunization history

6. **What should be included in the routine physical examination for all pediatric patients with eye injuries (except when temporarily deferred in absolute emergencies)?**
   - Visual acuity
   - Extraocular muscles

- Pupillary reactions
- External examination (including lids and bulbar/palpebral conjunctivae)
- Direct ophthalmoscopy/red reflex
- Other tests as indicated: visual field testing, slit-lamp examination, intraocular pressure (palpation or tonometer). The last two tests often are performed by an ophthalmologist for pediatric patients.

7. **What are the common pitfalls in evaluating children with eye injuries?**
   - Failure to treat life-threatening injuries before the more obvious (but less serious) eye injury
   - Failure to examine and assess visual acuity in both eyes
   - Failure to consider globe injury (in the setting of other facial injuries or more superficial eye injury)

8. **How do you test visual acuity in infants?**
   Check pupillary reaction to light and fixation reflex. Infants should be able to fix on a high-contrast object held in their central vision, such as the caretaker's or examiner's face or a bright toy. By 2 to 3 months of age, they should be able to fix on and start to follow an object or light, and by about 6 months, to fix and follow all visual fields. Central, steady, maintained fixation is estimated to be equivalent to 20/40 vision, unsteady fixation equivalent to 20/100, and eccentric wandering gaze equivalent to less than 20/400.

9. **How do you test visual acuity in preschool and school-aged children?**
   - 2½ to 3½ years old: Picture chart (Allen object recognition)
   - 3½ and older: Picture chart, tumbling E chart, or Sheridan-Gardner visual acuity test
   - School-aged: Snellen chart (letters in rows of diminishing size)

10. **What pearls should be kept in mind for visual acuity testing in children?**
    - Have the child identify the objects on the chart up close before testing at a distance.
    - Test one eye at a time, "bad" eye first.
    - Use a card or the child's palm to cover the other eye; children "peek" between fingers.
    - Always test with corrective glasses if available.

11. **For patients without their glasses or contact lenses, how can you differentiate between decreased acuity and baseline refractive error?**
    Pinhole testing—with a premade device, a card with a hole punched with an 18-gauge needle, or multiple pinholes in a rigid eye shield—corrects refractive errors to about 20/30.

12. **How do you record decreased acuity in patients unable to visualize a chart?**
    - Ability to count fingers from a specified number of feet
    - Ability to perceive hand motion
    - Light perception (with or without directionality, eyelids open or closed)

KEY POINTS: PEDIATRIC EYE INJURY EXAMINATION

1. Examine the child in a position of comfort (parent lap, sitting on a chair, etc.).
2. Pain control (consider topical anesthetic drops *early*, if globe rupture is not suspected).
3. Check visual acuity in both eyes.
4. For a young child, it is best to inspect the peripheral eye first: observe eyelids, degree of swelling, ecchymosis, laceration, eye movement, and the anterior surface of the eye all without upsetting the patient.
5. If a ruptured globe is suspected, stop the examination.

13. **What should you consider if you find an irregularly shaped pupil (e.g., "teardrop pupil")?**
    - Ocular rupture, corneal or other globe perforation
    - Iris injury or scarring from prior iritis
    - Prior ocular surgery

14. **What are the causes and expected course of subconjunctival hemorrhage?**
    Subconjunctival hemorrhage, the localized rupture of small subconjunctival vessels, may be spontaneous or may be due to direct trauma or increased intrathoracic pressure (e.g., coughing, nose-blowing, vomiting). It usually is benign and resolves in up to 2 to 3 weeks without treatment or sequelae. Very large hemorrhages or those that fully encircle the iris raise concern for an underlying injury, such as globe perforation or a bleeding diathesis.

15. **What is the most common pediatric eye injury?**
   Corneal or conjunctival abrasion is the most common pediatric eye injury.

16. **Which eye injuries are seen when a child is hit by an airbag in a car crash?**
   Pediatric eye injuries from airbag deployment are caused by blunt force trauma and chemical burns. Injuries can be monocular or binocular and include eyelid and corneoscleral abrasions and lacerations, lens dislocation, iris detachment, hyphemas and vitreous hemorrhages, globe rupture, retinal injuries, and alkaline burns (from the alkaline combustion byproduct of sodium azide). Wearing glasses at the time of the crash protects against chemical injury but increases the risk of penetrating trauma to the eyes. Using seatbelts in combination decreases injuries due to airbags. It is recommended that children are not allowed to sit in the front seat of an automobile until age 13.

17. **How does a child with corneal abrasion typically present?**
   The common presentation is a red eye with tearing, intense pain, resistance to eye-opening, and, less frequently, lid swelling or photophobia. The child often does not know what caused the injury and may complain of a foreign-body sensation.

18. **How is a corneal abrasion diagnosed?**
   - Larger abrasions can be seen with tangential light (surface irregularity or dry-appearing area).
   - Fluorescein staining and cobalt blue light (or Wood lamp) best delineate abrasions.
   - Use a topical anesthetic to greatly facilitate the examination and aid in the diagnosis (pain will be fully alleviated with an ocular surface problem—superficial foreign body, abrasion, or superficial ulcer). Persistent pain after a topical anesthetic suggests injury of deeper structures.
   - Check thoroughly for a retained foreign body when evaluating corneal or conjunctival abrasions, particularly for vertical linear abrasions.
      Pediatric pearl: Consider the application of a topical anesthetic *before* your first examination attempt in suspected corneal or conjunctival abrasions (when presentation is not concerning for globe rupture). In young children, this is most easily accomplished by letting the child keep the eye shut, having the child lie in a supine position, and pooling drops of the topical anesthetic medially at the corner of the eye. Gentle traction caudally on the cheek will crack apart the lids, and the drops will run onto the eye surface. Let the child sit up, and in a few seconds, he or she will usually spontaneously open the eye and your examination can proceed without a fight!

19. **Which corneal abrasions are most worrisome and why?**
   Corneal abrasions over the visual axis, abrasions in patients with a history of ocular herpes, and corneal abrasions in contact lens wearers are concerning. Those who wear contact lenses and develop a corneal abrasion are predisposed to fungal and bacterial infections and corneal ulceration.

20. **Describe the management of a corneal or conjunctival abrasion.**
   Most abrasions heal quickly without sequelae. Antibiotic ophthalmic ointment or artificial tears provide lubrication and some pain relief. Patching is rarely appropriate for children. If asymptomatic in 24 hours after a small superficial lesion, follow-up is not required. Large abrasions and those involving the visual axis are treated with antibiotic ointment; consider follow-up with ophthalmology in 24 hours for these lesions. Instruct patients to return or see an ophthalmologist for pain or foreign-body sensation that persists for more than 2 to 3 days, or if pain and redness worsen at any time. Instruct those who wear contact lenses to discontinue their use until the patient is seen by an ophthalmologist.

21. **Describe the management of the child with "something in my eye."**
   - Most patients with an external foreign body (conjunctival or superficial corneal) report just that.
   - If there is no suspicion of a perforated globe or deep corneoscleral laceration, instill a topical anesthetic, which will relieve pain fully and allow thorough examination.
   - Thoroughly examine the bulbar conjunctival surface, cornea, palpebral conjunctivae, and superior and inferior fornices.
   - Perform a full conjunctival surface evaluation: Evert (flip-up) the upper lid, while the child is looking down, to visualize the inner lid surface. Exert outward traction on the lower lid with an upward gaze to visualize the lower bulbar and palpebral conjunctivae.
   - Vertical linear abrasions should trigger a search for a foreign body adherent to the inner lid.
   - The foreign body usually can be loosened and removed with saline irrigation or a moistened sterile swab or gauze. If the foreign body is still adherent, consider removal under slit-lamp magnification or ophthalmology referral. Be sure to complete a full eye examination after removal of the foreign body; treat associated abrasions.
   - Seek emergent/urgent ophthalmology consultation for a corneal or scleral laceration or an embedded foreign body that you cannot remove.

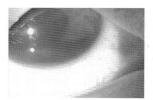

Fig. 55.1 Hyphema. Note the layering of blood in the right eye.

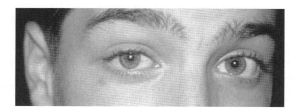

Fig. 55.2 Iritis.

22. **What is a hyphema?**

    A hyphema is bleeding into the chamber between the cornea and iris or lens after blunt or sharp trauma. It may range from microscopic bleeding to a full-chamber or "eight-ball" hyphema.

23. **How are hyphemas diagnosed and treated?**

    Suspect a hyphema (Fig. 55.1) in any child with a tearing, painful eye and injected bulbar conjunctiva immediately after blunt or lacerating eye trauma. It is often diagnosed by careful physical examination. Very small and microscopic hyphemas require microscopic slit-lamp examination to visualize, but these are not usually clinically significant. All hyphemas require urgent ophthalmologic consultation for evaluation, management, and follow-up. With treatment, 66% to 97% of isolated hyphemas will fully resorb without complication.

    Children with large or complex hyphemas are occasionally admitted to the hospital for management, particularly if the patient is young or has sickle cell hemoglobinopathy (including trait) or hemophilia, or if inadequate follow-up is a concern. Most children with hyphemas are managed at home with frequent outpatient follow-up after the initial visit. Consider cycloplegics, analgesics, elevation of the head of the bed to 45 degrees, and control of nausea and vomiting. Antifibrinolytic agents and corticosteroids may also be indicated but should be prescribed only after consultation with ophthalmology. Restricted activity or bed rest is essential.

24. **What is the major potential vision-threatening sequela of hyphemas? Who is at risk?**

    Rebleeding, with the development of intraocular pressure elevation or corneal staining, is the most serious sequela. Rebleeding is most likely within 3 to 5 days of the initial injury. Patients with sickle cell disease or trait are at particularly high risk of ocular complications; a screening test or hemoglobin electrophoresis is recommended for patients at risk for undiagnosed hemoglobinopathy.

25. **Why are patients with sickle cell hemoglobinopathies at high risk for complications secondary to a hyphema?**

    Sickle cell patients have a high risk for complications from increased intraocular pressure (acute glaucoma) even with small amounts of anterior chamber blood. Erythrocytes with sickle cell hemoglobin will sickle in the relatively hypoxic and academic aqueous humor and cause mechanical obstruction, leading to increased pressure and optic neuropathy or corneal staining.

26. **When and how does traumatic iritis present?**

    Traumatic iritis (Fig. 55.2), which may accompany other ocular injuries or be the sole manifestation of blunt eye trauma, is most often characterized by a delayed presentation, typically 24 to 72 hours after injury. Physical examination reveals a painful, red eye (perilimbal conjunctival injection), tearing, and pain with pupillary constriction (on accommodation or concentric constriction to light). The affected eye also may have slight miosis and a decreased or sluggish pupillary response. The pain is secondary to inflammation in the anterior chamber. Slit-lamp evaluation is diagnostic when it reveals white blood cells and a protein "flare" in the aqueous humor.

27. **How is traumatic iritis treated?**
In children, request an ophthalmology consultation for a full evaluation, initial management, or follow-up. Management includes mydriatics for pain control, topical steroids, and close outpatient follow-up.

28. **What is an orbital "blow-out" fracture?**
An orbital blow-out fracture involves the bony orbital walls caused by blunt trauma to the face. The presentation may include periorbital ecchymosis, facial asymmetry, lid swelling or ptosis, proptosis or enophthalmos, ophthalmoplegia, localized anesthesia of the face, and, in rare cases, orbital emphysema. The patient may have entrapment or restriction of an extraocular muscle and restriction of extraocular movement on examination or the complaint of diplopia. The inferior rectus is most commonly involved, with limitation in upward gaze; the most common fracture sites are the inferior and medial walls (rarely lateral). Superior wall fractures have the potential to communicate with the intracranial space. Computed tomography (CT) or magnetic resonance imaging typically delineates the fracture. Plain films are not helpful. A full ocular examination is needed to rule out other eye injuries, including retinal trauma.

29. **What are important historical questions regarding orbital fractures?**
    - Is there epistaxis or cerebrospinal fluid (CSF) rhinorrhea/otorrhea? CSF rhinorrhea is seen with an orbital fracture.
    - Does the patient have vision changes such as blurry vision or double vision? Blurry vision can be seen with hyphema, retinal detachment, and vitreous hemorrhage.
    - Is there diplopia with lateral or upward gaze? Diplopia is concerning for lens dislocation.
    - Does the patient have pain with eye movement? Pain is indicative of extraocular muscle entrapment.
    - Is photosensitivity present? Photophobia is concerning for iritis.
    - Does the patient complain of flashes of light? Flashes of light are seen in retinal detachment.

30. **What is the major pitfall when diagnosing an orbital wall fracture?**
Failure to consider and appropriately rule out other eye injuries. The incidence of concomitant globe injury with orbital fractures has been reported in up to 20% of cases.

31. **What are the indications for obtaining a CT scan of the orbits when a patient has a blow to the face and presents with pain, periorbital swelling, and ecchymosis?**
    - Evidence of or concern for fracture on examination
    - Limitation of extraocular motility, diplopia
    - Decreased visual acuity
    - Severe pain
    - Inadequate examination of the eye (soft tissue swelling prevents eye examination)
    - Altered mental status

32. **How are orbital fractures managed?**
Address any life-threatening injuries before focusing on the eye injury. If globe rupture is suspected, stop the examination, keep the patient calm (crying can increase intraocular pressure), apply an eye shield, and consult ophthalmology. Therapeutic interventions for orbital fracture include sleeping with the head of the bed elevated, nasal decongestants, and ice packs. Pain control is very important. Caution for patients with this injury is to avoid blowing their nose. Prophylactic antibiotics and corticosteroids have little benefit. Some fractures may require surgical intervention. Usually, there is no intervention unless there is suspicion of muscle entrapment after swelling resolves, a few days after the injury.

KEY POINTS: REASONS TO SUSPECT GLOBE PERFORATION OR RUPTURE

1. History of hammering/grinding metal (for a child, standing nearby).
2. Significant eye trauma causing decreased vision.
3. Physical examination findings of a severe lid swelling, large or circumferential subconjunctival hemorrhage, large hyphema; posttraumatic corneal or conjunctival edema; enophthalmos; extruded vitreous, iris, or choroid; irregularly shaped pupil.
4. The more difficult it is to examine the patient after trauma (because of pain, edema, hyphema, or intraocular hemorrhage), the greater the concern for globe rupture.

KEY POINTS: ED MANAGEMENT OF GLOBE RUPTURE/LACERATION

1. Stop your examination.
2. Place a rigid shield (span bone to bone) over the affected eye.
3. Keep the patient at rest, with the head elevated.
4. Avoid agitation of the child; treat pain and nausea/vomiting if present.
5. Ensure that the patient consumes nothing by mouth.
6. Seek emergent ophthalmologic consult.
7. Consider intravenous (IV) antibiotics.

33. **What physical examination findings are consistent with a ruptured or perforated globe?**
    - Significantly decreased visual acuity and severe pain
    - Irregularly shaped or characteristic teardrop pupil, pointing toward perforation
    - Mucoid, fleshy, or pigmented-appearing mass on the ocular surface (extrusion through the perforation or rupture by vitreous or aqueous humor, choroid, or iris; do not mistake this for a foreign body!)
    - Large, overlying subconjunctival hemorrhage (often fully around the iris) or hyphema
    - An unusually shallow anterior chamber

34. **What aspects of the history place patients at high risk for globe perforation or rupture?**
    - Hammering/grinding metal (for children, ask about standing nearby these activities)
      - Significant eye trauma causing decreased vision
      - The patient continues to complain of foreign body in the eye
    Note: It is sometimes difficult to see a globe rupture, especially if the cause was a rapidly penetrating foreign body (from hammering). The more difficult it is to examine the patient after trauma (because of pain, edema, hyphema, or intraocular hemorrhage), the greater the likelihood of globe rupture.

35. **What are the initial treatments/stabilization for globe rupture?**
    - Stop the examination; place a rigid eye shield.
    - Have the patient rest in bed with the head elevated.
    - Keep the patient calm; treat pain, agitation, and nausea/vomiting as needed (to avoid increased pressure to the globe, which can cause further extrusion of vitreous or aqueous humor).
    - Consider administration of tetanus and IV antibiotic prophylaxis (delay if IV placement will cause excessive agitation).
    - Order imaging studies as indicated (concern for fracture, retained foreign body, intraorbital hematoma).

36. **What are the important considerations in evaluating lacerations of the eyelids?**
    - Evaluate for full-thickness laceration and underlying orbital/globe injury.
    - Check the inner (conjunctival) surface (superficial-appearing lacerations may be full thickness).
    - Assess the integrity of the levator muscle (both lids raise equally with upward gaze).
    - Lacerations of the medial third of the upper or lower lid potentially involve the lacrimal canaliculi (see Fig. 55.3)
    - Adipose tissue exposed/extruding in an upper lid laceration indicates full-thickness lid laceration (upper lid has no adipose; this is orbital fat).
    - Full-thickness lacerations, lacerations through the lid margin or tarsal plate, and lacerations involving lacrimal canaliculi require ophthalmologic consultation for multilayer repair.
    - Consider consultation for lacerations with ptosis or significant avulsions or if you are unable to rule out other ocular/globe injuries.

37. **Describe the emergency initial management of chemical burns to the eye.**
    - Recommend that parents put the child under running water immediately, to clean the eyes prior to transport to the ED.
    - Upon ED arrival, *irrigate immediatelyirrigate immediately* (begin in triage if possible) and copiously with normal saline or lactated Ringer solution, at least 1 to 2 L via IV tubing set.
    - Consider a similar, perhaps less severe, injury to the other eye.
    - Use topical anesthetic early and every 20 minutes; retract lids (with gauze or retractors) to ensure thorough irrigation; remove particulate matter from fornices.
    - Monitor the pH of the conjunctival fossa after irrigation and recheck 10 to 20 minutes later. Continue irrigation until a pH of 7.4 to 7.6 is maintained on rechecks.
    - Arrange emergent (same-day) ophthalmologic consultation for patients with evidence of a significant burn (such as persistent pain, corneal lesions, or decreased acuity).

38. **Which are more severe—alkali or acid burns?**
Alkali burns are potentially more severe. Alkaline substances penetrate more deeply than acids, which coagulate with surface proteins. Common alkaline agents include lye, lime, ammonia, and aluminum-containing or magnesium hydroxide containing fireworks (flares and sparklers). Automobile airbag deployment is a reported cause of alkali eye burns (combustion byproduct of sodium azides). Acidic solutions coagulate proteins in the superficial layers of the eye, forming a protective barrier against further penetration. The severity of the injury is also related to the volume and duration of exposure.

KEY POINTS: ED MANAGEMENT OF ABSOLUTE EMERGENCIES IN PEDIATRIC EYE INJURIES

1. Initiate copious irrigation immediately in chemical injury (at home, in triage).
2. For suspected globe rupture, stop the examination, place a rigid eye shield, avoid agitation of the child, and place an emergent ophthalmologic consult. Do not use topical anesthetic or other drops.

39. **An emergency physician attempts to repair a forehead laceration of a young child using cyanoacrylate glue. Some of the glue drips down the child's face and the child's eyelashes become stuck together. The child's parent is quite concerned. Which eye injuries are likely?**
Usually none. The eyelashes may be stuck together by the glue, but the eye is very rarely injured in this scenario. Parents may be concerned, as the child cannot open his/her eyes. Avoid forceful attempts to pry open the eyelids. Instead, place petroleum jelly on the eyelashes and wait patiently (30-60 minutes) or massage gently with a cotton swab until the glue dissolves. Avoid the use of acetone to dissolve the glue, as this could cause an eye injury. Ophthalmologic consultation is rarely needed.

KEY POINTS: EYE INJURIES THAT WARRANT EMERGENT/SAME-DAY OPHTHALMOLOGIC CONSULTATION

1. Ruptured globe
2. Orbital hematoma
3. Severe chemical burns
4. Hyphema
5. Retinal/vitreous detachment
6. Retinal hemorrhage
7. Intraocular foreign bodies
8. Contact lens abrasions
9. Complicated eyelid lacerations
10. Decreased visual acuity
11. Limitation of extraocular muscles

BIBLIOGRAPHY

1. Almahmoud T, Barss P. Vehicle occupant restraint systems impact on eye injuries: a review. *Surv Ophthalmol.* 2014;59(3):334–344. https://doi.org/10.1016/j.survophthal.2013.08.005. Epub 2013 Dec 19. PMID: 24359757.
2. Blende MS. Irrigation of conjunctivae. In: King C, Henretig FM, eds.*Textbook of Pediatric Emergency Procedures.* 2nd ed. Williams & Wilkins; 2008:555–558.
3. Boese EA, Karr DJ, Chiang MF, Kopplin LJ. Visual acuity recovery following traumatic hyphema in a pediatric population. *J AAPOS.* 2018;22(2):115–118.
4. Matsa E, Shi J, Wheeler KK, McCarthy T, et al. Trends in US ED visits for pediatric acute ocular injury. *JAMA Ophthal.* 2018;136(8):895–903.
5. Roskind CG, Levin AV. Chapter 122 Ocular trauma. In: Shaw KN, Bachur RG, eds. *Fleisher & Ludwig's Textbook of Pediatric Emergency Medicine.* 7th ed. Wolters Kluwer; 2016.
6. Miller KN, Collins CL, Chounthirath T, Smith GA. Pediatric sports, recreation related eye injuries treated in US emergency departments. *Pediatrics.* 2018;141(2): e20173083.

7. Mir T, Iftikhar M, Seidel N, Trang M, Goldberg MF, Woreta FA. Clinical characteristics and outcomes of hyphema in patients with sickle cell trait: 10-year experience at the Wilmer Eye Institute. *Clin Ophthalmol.* 2020;14:4165–4172. https://doi.org/10.2147/OPTH.S281875. PMID: 33293789.
8. Neuman MI, Bachur RG. Orbital fractures. *UpToDate.* <http://www.uptodate.com>; 2022.
9. SooHoo JR, Davies BW, Braverman RS, et al. Pediatric traumatic hyphema: a review of 138 consecutive cases. *J AAPOS.* 2013;17(6):565–567.
10. Turner A, Rabiu M. Patching for corneal abrasion. *Cochrane Database Syst Rev.* 2006(2): CD004764.

HEAD TRAUMA

Caroline G. Kahane and Sara A. Schutzman

CHAPTER 56

1. **How common is head trauma in children?**
   Pediatric head trauma accounts for more than 800,000 emergency department (ED) visits and 25,000 hospitalizations per year. Hospitalizations have decreased since the last surveillance report.

2. **What is the most common cause of head trauma in children?**
   Younger children are more likely to suffer from head injuries related to falls or abuse. Older children are more commonly injured from accidents—motor vehicles, pedestrians, or bicycles.

3. **What kinds of head injuries commonly present to the ED?**
   Head injuries occur to the scalp, skull, and intracranial contents. Although most injuries are minor, there is a wide spectrum ranging from simple contusion to lethal brain injury. Lacerations and contusions are common scalp injuries. Injuries to the cranial vault include skull fractures, traumatic brain injuries (TBIs), concussions, cerebral contusions, bleeding (epidural, subdural, subarachnoid, and intracerebral), and acute brain swelling. Most head injuries result from blunt head trauma, but penetrating injuries rarely occur and are caused by bullets, teeth (e.g., dog bites), or other sharp objects (e.g., dart, pellet, pencil).

4. **How common are head injuries related to non-accidental trauma?**
   Although most head trauma is accidental, the incidence of abusive head trauma for children younger than 1 year is 17 per 100,000 person-years. Abusive head trauma is the most common cause of traumatic death in children, and nearly 25% of patients aged 2 years and younger who present with abusive head trauma die from the injury. Because these children are preverbal and abusive caretakers are rarely forthcoming, the clinician must have a heightened sense of awareness to diagnose non-accidental trauma.

5. **Name the ways in which children <2 years differ from older children with regard to head trauma.**
   Children younger than 2 years of age differ in several ways, making it prudent to have a low threshold for head imaging:
   - Clinical assessment is more difficult.
   - TBI is frequently asymptomatic (i.e., patients may have scalp swelling but no symptoms of brain injury).
   - Skull fractures and TBI may result from relatively minor trauma.
   - Inflicted injury occurs more frequently.
   - Young children are more sensitive to the effects of ionizing radiation due to a longer lifetime to manifest cancer and providers must therefore be judicious in computed tomography (CT) utilization.

6. **How is head trauma severity defined?**
   There is no standard definition for minor head trauma, which accounts for more than 90% of injuries evaluated. The American Academy of Pediatrics defines children with minor head injury as those who have normal mental status at the initial examination, a normal neurologic examination, and no physical evidence of skull fracture (i.e., no palpable skull defect and no signs of basilar skull fracture (BSF) such as hemotympanum, cerebrospinal fluid (CSF) oto- or rhinorrhea, or periocular or posterior auricular hematomas). Moderate head trauma is typically defined as a Glasgow Coma Scale (GCS) score of 9 to 12, and severe head trauma, as a GCS score of 3 to 8.

7. **What are TBIs?**
   TBIs represent any insult to the brain. These injuries include concussion, post-traumatic seizures, contusions, hemorrhages, hematomas, cerebral edema, diffuse axonal injuries, penetrating trauma, and retained foreign bodies.

8. **How do we define clinically important traumatic brain injuries (ciTBIs)?**
   Researchers have focused more recently on patients deemed to have injuries that were of significant clinical importance (i.e., not just a tiny abnormality noted on CT requiring no intervention). One large study published by the Pediatric Emergency Care Applied Research Network (PECARN) defined clinically important injuries as those resulting in death, neurosurgery, intubation for more than 24 hours, or hospital admission for two or more nights. A large Canadian study (CATCH, Osmond and colleagues) defined clinically important injuries as those requiring neurologic intervention, neurosurgery, monitoring of intracranial pressure (ICP), intubation, or resulting in death.

9. **What is the incidence of ciTBI?**
   Approximately 3% to 7% of children with minor head injuries who present for evaluation have a TBI noted on CT. Of note, however, rates of clinically important TBI range from 0.02% to 4.4%.

10. **What imaging modality is recommended to diagnose ciTBI?**
    CT identifies essentially all significant TBIs requiring intervention. Injuries such as diffuse axonal injury may not be evident on CT and will require magnetic resonance imaging.

11. **Which children are at high risk for ciTBI and should undergo CT?**
    Evidence indicates that children with a GCS score <15, abnormal neurologic examination, or evidence of skull fracture are at high risk for TBI and should undergo CT. Additional criteria for infants include irritability, bulging fontanel, or suspected abuse.

12. **If CT identifies major complications, why not image all children with head injuries?**
    Although a very useful imaging modality, CT carries disadvantages, most importantly exposure to ionizing radiation. Children are at higher risk of radiation-induced cancer since they have a longer lifetime to manifest cancer and have increased radiation sensitivity of developing tissues. The greatest lifetime risk occurs in the youngest patients and decreases as age increases. The estimated rate of lethal malignancies from CT is between 1 in 1500 and 1 in 5000 pediatric cranial CT scans, with a higher risk in younger patients. Therefore CT should be used selectively.

13. **Which children are at low risk for significant head injury and do not need an emergent head CT?**
    PECARN published a decision rule identifying children at low risk for ciTBI, for whom imaging is not indicated. For children older than 2 years with no altered mental status, loss of consciousness (LOC), vomiting, severe headache, signs of BSF, or significant mechanism (e.g., fall >5 feet) the likelihood of having a clinically important injury was <0.05% and thus imaging can be avoided. For children younger than 2 years, the low-risk predictors were having normal mental status, no non-frontal scalp hematoma, no LOC, no palpable skull fracture, no significant mechanism (e.g., fall >3 feet), and acting normally per parents.

14. **Which patients have an intermediate risk for TBI and is there a role for observation?**
    Not all patients in this group require imaging; however, imaging should be considered more strongly if symptoms are more intense, worsening, of longer duration, or if more than one symptom is present. For children with mild symptoms, careful observation in the ED or at home may be an alternative approach, with reevaluation and CT for persistent or worsening symptoms.

15. **What are additional factors to consider for children younger than 2 years old?**
    The PECARN study identified low-risk predictors for children <2 years with ciTBI, as above. It is important to note that these predictors should not be used to determine risk for any infant for whom there is a concern for non-accidental trauma. Additionally, because there are no long-term studies of infants and children with TBI on CT who do not meet the criteria for clinically important TBI, the long-term implications of these findings, especially in the youngest patients, are unknown.
    Infants with isolated non-frontal hematomas (i.e., no other PECARN risk factors) are not considered low risk. However, this large, heterogeneous group can be further risk stratified by using the Infant Scalp Score (ISS). This validated score (ranging from 0 to 8) uses patient age, hematoma size, and location to determine the risk of TBI. In one large study, no infants with a scalp score <4 had TBI, and no infant with a score <5 had a clinically important TBI.

RISK POINTS	PATIENT AGE (MONTHS)	HEMATOMA SIZE	HEMATOMA LOCATION
0	>12	None	Frontal
1	6-11	Small (<1 cm)	Occipital
2	3-5	Medium (1-3 cm)	Temporal/parietal
3	0-2	Large (>3 cm)	

16. **Describe the different types of skull fractures.**
    Skull fractures are described in terms of location and characteristics. They may involve the frontal, parietal, occipital, and temporal bones of the skull (calvarium). The skull base consists of portions of the temporal and occipital bones, along with the maxillary, sphenoid, and palatine bones. Fractures in this area are referred to as BSFs.

Fractures may be linear, depressed (if the inner table of the skull is displaced by more than the thickness of the entire bone), or diastatic (traumatic separation of the cranial bones at one or more suture sites). Compound fractures communicate with lacerations, and comminuted fractures are those with several fragments.

17. **Name the most important complications of BSFs.**
    - **TBI:** 10% to 50% of patients with BSF have an associated TBI.
    - **CSF leak:** An associated dural tear may lead to CSF leak through the nose or ear and occurs in approximately 10% to 30% of children with BSFs.
    - **Meningitis:** Meningitis occurs in 0.7% to 5% of children with BSF (due to CSF leak and exposure to microorganisms); the rate is <1% for children with GCS score >13 and no TBI.
    - **Cranial nerve impairment:** This occurs in up to 23% of cases, with cranial nerves VI, VII, and VIII most commonly injured. The impairment may be transient or permanent.
    - **Hearing loss:** This occurs in up to half of patients with BSF; it can be conductive (from hemotympanum or otic canal disruption) or sensorineural.

18. **Define primary and secondary brain injury.**
    Primary brain injury is the neural damage sustained at the time of trauma. Secondary brain injury is neuronal damage sustained after the initial traumatic event to cells not initially injured, and results from numerous causes including hypoxia, hypoperfusion, and metabolic derangements. Because many causes of secondary brain injury are potentially preventable, the clinician's main goal is to monitor for and attempt to prevent these complications in order to limit further neuronal damage.

19. **How does increased ICP occur, and how can this lead to secondary injury?**
    After infancy (when the cranial sutures fuse), the cranial vault becomes stiff and poorly compliant. The normal intracranial contents include brain, blood, and CSF. Because intracranial volume is fixed, any increase in the volume of one of the components (e.g., cerebral edema, expanding epidural hematoma) must be accompanied by a proportional decrease of the other components; otherwise, ICP will increase. Increased ICP is associated with a significant risk of brain tissue herniation, ischemia, and death.

    Cerebral perfusion pressure (CPP) is the difference between the mean arterial pressure (MAP) and the intracranial pressure (ICP) (CPP = MAP − ICP). Therefore significant decreases in mean arterial pressure or significant increases in ICP can lead to inadequate CPP, with resultant cerebral ischemia and secondary brain injury.

KEY POINTS: INTRACRANIAL INJURY

1. Most head injuries are minor; about 5% of children with minor head injuries have TBI, and ~1% have clinically important intracranial injuries.
2. The goal is to identify children with ciTBI to avoid further neuronal injury while limiting unnecessary neuroimaging.
3. Altered mental status, focal neurological examination, and skull fractures are predictors for increased risk of TBI.
4. Children older than 2 years with a nonsevere injury mechanism, no LOC, no vomiting, no severe headache, no signs of BSF, and who have normal mental status have an extremely low likelihood of a *clinically important* TBI.
5. Children younger than 2 years with a nonsevere injury mechanism, no LOC, no scalp hematoma (except frontal), no palpable skull fracture, and who have normal mental status and are acting normally per parents have an extremely low likelihood of a *clinically important* ICP.

20. **What is the cerebral herniation syndrome?**
    The cranial cavity is separated by dural folds and bony prominences into the anterior, middle, and posterior fossa. Cerebral herniation occurs when increased ICP causes the brain parenchyma to shift into an anatomic area that it does not normally occupy.

    Uncal herniation is the most common form, in which the uncus (inferomedial-most structure of the temporal lobe) slides through the tentorial notch, passing from the middle to the posterior fossa. Initial symptoms include headache and decreased level of consciousness, followed by ipsilateral pupillary dilatation and contralateral hemiplegia. Altered respiration, bradycardia, and systemic hypertension may ensue with decerebrate posturing or flaccid paresis. If the process continues unchecked, ultimately brain stem failure with respiratory arrest, cardiovascular collapse, and death will occur.

21. **Outline the ED treatment for increased ICP.**
    - Manage the ABCs (airway, breathing, and circulation). This is essential to avoid hypoxia and hypercarbia, and to maintain adequate CPP. Carbon dioxide is one of the main determinants of cerebrovascular tone. While low

levels produce vasoconstriction and decreased blood flow, thus lowering ICP, levels too low can lead to cerebral ischemic injury. Therefore maintaining a $PaCO_2$ of 35 to 40 mm Hg is recommended. Consider temporary, mild, therapeutic hyperventilation ($PaCO_2$ 30-35 mm Hg) in patients with intracranial hypertension and signs of impending herniation.
- Avoid secondary brain injury from other metabolic causes, including hypoglycemia, hyperthermia, and seizures.
- Ensure appropriate positioning with an elevation of the head of the bed 30 degrees and maintain the midline position of the neck. This promotes venous drainage and can decrease ICP.
- Obtain emergent head CT to identify mass lesions that require surgical evacuation.
- Consider osmotic agents: Mannitol and 3% hypertonic saline can lower ICP.
- Secure an airway in all patients with GCS <9, inability to protect the airway or maintain adequate SpO_2 despite supplemental oxygen, or clinical signs of cerebral herniation.
- Use sedation: Conscious patients who are paralyzed for intubation require sedation.

22. Which children need to be admitted following acute head trauma?

Children with TBI or depressed or BSFs usually require hospital admission. Consult a neurosurgeon regarding their management and disposition. Also, consider hospital admission for patients with persistent neurologic deficits (despite normal CT scan), significant extracranial injuries, unremitting vomiting, or caretakers who are unreliable or unable to return if necessary. Strongly consider admission for any child with suspected non-accidental trauma.

Children with an isolated nondepressed, linear skull fracture with a normal neurologic examination and no other injuries identified by neuroimaging may be discharged from the ED as long as clear discharge instructions are provided and proper follow-up can be ensured.

23. What is a concussion?

An international multidisciplinary conference defined a *concussion* as a complex pathophysiologic process affecting the brain, induced by traumatic biomechanical forces. It typically results in the rapid onset of short-lived impairment of neurologic function that resolves spontaneously and reflects a functional disturbance rather than a structural injury. Therefore concussions are associated with grossly normal neuroimaging, if obtained. Concussions result in a graded set of clinical symptoms that may or may not involve LOC. Resolution of the clinical and cognitive features often follows a sequential course; however, in certain cases, symptoms may be prolonged.

A simpler, perhaps more useful working definition is a trauma-induced alteration in mental status that may or may not involve LOC. From a practical standpoint, concussion is often used to refer to a head injury when the Glasgow Coma Scale (GCS) is 14 to 15, the patient has some symptoms (e.g., headache, dizziness, vomiting, amnesia, or confusion), there is no evidence of a fracture, there are no focal neurologic deficits and neuroimaging (if obtained) is normal.

24. What are the major symptoms associated with concussion?

Signs and symptoms of concussion can be classified into five categories, including somatic, vestibular, oculomotor, cognitive, emotional, and sleep. Headache is the most frequently reported symptom (seen in 86%-96% of patients with a concussion), followed by dizziness (65%-75%), difficulty concentrating (48%-61%), and confusion (40%-46%). A postconcussion symptom checklist, such as the Acute Concussion Evaluation ED tool, can be useful in assessing a patient after a concussion.

25. What should families be advised regarding a child's return to activities and follow-up after a concussion?

Children with concussions should have a brief period of physical and cognitive rest (24-48 hours, although the optimal duration has not been determined). They should then follow a gradual and progressive return to activities, individualized to avoid symptom exacerbation, and also avoiding activities that could result in a second head injury. While recent evidence suggests that return to physical activity within 1 week may improve recovery, the current evidence evaluating the effect of rest and treatment following a sports-related concussion is sparse.

The timing for return to school and exercise vary from patient to patient, depending on their individual clinical course, and cannot reliably be predicted in the ED. Therefore ED clinicians should not be managing these decisions beyond the immediate postdischarge period and should discuss outpatient follow-up for symptom management and return to/liberalization of physical and cognitive activity decisions. Primary care follow-up is appropriate for most concussion patients, however, additional evaluation and guidance from concussion specialists may be appropriate for certain higher-risk patients (e.g., patients with a history of multiple prior concussions or prolonged recovery from previous concussions) as well as those with a prolonged or more difficult course.

26. Why are discharge instructions important for children with head trauma?

Even well-appearing children with head trauma who have no evidence of complications (either clinically or radiographically) have a small chance of subsequent deterioration. Therefore it is mandatory that competent caretakers are available to observe the child at home and they should be educated about signs and symptoms concerning complications of head trauma. Children who develop a change in mental status, seizure, worsening pattern of vomiting, severely worsening headache, or a new unsteady gait should be brought back to the ED immediately for further evaluation.

BIBLIOGRAPHY

1. Chen C, Shi J, Stanley RM, Sribnick EA, et al. US trends of ED visits for pediatric traumatic brain injuries: implications for clinical trials. *Int J Environ Res Public Health*. 2017;14(4):414.
2. Goodman TR, Mustafa A, Rowe E. Pediatric radiation exposure: where we were, and where we are now. *Pediatr Radiol*. 2019;49(4):469–478.
3. Gelineau-Morel RN, Zinkus TP, Le Pichon JB. Pediatric head trauma: a review and update. *Pediatr Rev*. 2019;40(9):468–481.
4. Halstead ME, Walter KD, Moffatt K, Council on Sports Medicine and Fitness Sport-related concussion in children and adolescents. *Pediatrics*. 2018;142(6):e20183074. https://doi.org/10.1542/peds.2018-3074.
5. Ide K, Uematsu S, Tetsuhara K, et al. External validation of the PECARN trauma prediction rules in Japan. *Acad Emerg Med*. 2017;24(3):308–314.
6. Kochanek PM, Tasker RC, Bell MJ, Adelson PD, et al. Management of pediatric severe traumatic brain injury: 2019 consensus and guidelines-based algorithm for first and second tier therapies. *Pediatr Crit Care Med*. 2019;20(3):269–279.
7. Kuppermann N, Holmes JF, Dayan PS, et al. Identification of children at very low risk of clinically-important brain injuries after head trauma: a prospective cohort study. *Lancet*. 2009;374:1160.
8. Mannix R, Bazarian JJ. Managing pediatric concussion in the emergency department. *Ann Emerg Med*. 2020;75(6):762–766. https://doi.org/10.1016/j.annemergmed.2019.12.025.
9. McLendon LA, Kralik SF, Grayson PA, Golomb MR. The controversial second impact syndrome: a review of the literature. *Pediatr Neurol*. 2016;62:9–17. https://doi.org/10.1016/j.pediatrneurol.2016.03.009.
10. Narang SK, Fingarson A, Lukefahr J, Council on Child Abuse and Neglect Abusive head trauma in infants and children. *Pediatrics*. 2020;145(4):e20200203.
11. Osmond MH, Klassen TP, Wells GA, et al. CATCH: a clinical decision rule for the use of computed tomography in children with minor head injury. *CMAJ*. 2010;182:341.
12. Peterson AB, Xu L, Daugherty J, Breiding MJ. *Surveillance Report of Traumatic Brain Injury-related Emergency Department Visits, Hospitalizations, and Deaths: United States, 2014*. Centers for Disease Control and Prevention, National Center for Injury Prevention and Control; 2019.
13. Powell EC, Atabaki SM, Wootton-Gorges S, Wisner D, et al. Isolated linear skull fractures in children with blunt head trauma. *Pediatrics*. 2015;135(4):e851–857.
14. Schonfeld D, Fritz B, Nigrovic L. Effect of the duration of emergency department observation on computed tomography use in children with minor blunt head trauma. *Ann Emerg Med*. 2013;62(6):597–603.
15. Schutzman SA, Barnes P, Duhaime AC, et al. Evaluation and management of children younger than two years of age with apparently minor head trauma: proposed guidelines. *Pediatrics*. 2001;107:983–993.
16. Tunik MG, Powell EC, Mahajan P, et al. Clinical presentations and outcomes of children with basilar skull fractures after blunt head trauma. *Ann Emerg Med*. 2016;68(4):431–440. e1.
17. Zemek R, Barrowman N, Freedman SB, et al. Clinical risk score for persistent postconcussion symptoms among children with acute concussion in the ED. *JAMA*. 2016;315:1014–1025.

CHAPTER 57

MINOR TRAUMA

Sabina B. Singh and Magdy W. Attia

1. **What are the most important principles of wound care management?**
   - Hemostasis
   - Infection prevention
   - Cosmesis
   - Pain/anxiety control

2. **How commonly are lacerations cared for in pediatric emergency departments (EDs)?**
   Lacerations represent up to 40% of all injuries presenting to pediatric EDs. Blunt trauma accounts for the majority, while the rest are related to animal bites.

3. **How does the location of injury affect assessment?**
   - **Injuries over a joint or adjacent to tendons** should be checked for crepitus or "sucking" sound, which may signify disruption of the joint capsule. Loss of motor function may indicate tendon injury.
   - **Lacerations close to the neurovascular bundle** may cause nerve damage. Assess capillary refill and pulses and conduct a careful neurologic examination of motor and sensory functions.
   - Wounds in proximity to **areas of high bacterial concentration**, such as the perineum, axilla (particularly in adolescents), and exposed parts (hands and feet) are at a higher risk for infection.

4. **What is the ideal time frame for the repair of wounds?**
   Ideally, wounds should be repaired within 6 hours of injury. Clean wounds can be closed within 12 to 24 hours after injury. Delayed closure can be considered 3 to 5 days after the original injury for wounds with high potential for infection (heavily contaminated wounds, bite wounds, puncture wounds) and wounds in areas of low cosmetic concern in immunocompromised patients.

5. **Which wounds are allowed to heal by secondary intention?**
   Allow infected wounds and small puncture wounds in areas of low cosmetic concern to close by secondary intention. Close follow-up in 2 to 3 days following the initial evaluation is recommended to check for the signs of infection. Give patients with high-risk wounds (i.e., animal bites, punctures) strict return precautions for the development of fever, purulent drainage, significant swelling, and/or pain out of proportion to the injury.

6. **How should the emergency physician approach sedation and pain control?**
   Discuss options, risks, and benefits with parents and older children. Parents often can predict the level of cooperation expected from their children. Distraction techniques with the help of a trained child life specialist, local anesthetics, and midazolam (intranasal or oral) reduce the anxiety associated with procedures and improve tolerance.

7. **When should consultation be obtained for wound care?**
   Consider consultation with a surgical or orthopedic specialist for the following types of wounds:
   - Associated with fracture or violation of a joint cavity
   - Injury to a tendon, nerve, or large vessel
   - Wounds requiring complex repair located in areas of high cosmetic concern

8. **When are radiographic studies indicated as part of wound management?**
   Obtain radiographs for wounds associated with fractures or joint disruption or if a foreign body is suspected. Plain radiographs identify fragments of metal and glass if they are larger than 0.5 cm. Wood is identified in only 15% of cases. Ultrasonography has 90% sensitivity and specificity for nonopaque foreign bodies if the location is not near a bony or gaseous structure. Ultrasound can also aid in foreign body removal, but this is technically challenging. Consider computed tomography or magnetic resonance imaging (MRI) if a surgical approach is planned for the removal of a foreign body near vital structures. If the retained object is metallic, it may limit the use of MRI.

9. **How can you decrease the chances of missing a retained foreign body in a wound?**
   A detailed history of the mechanism and circumstances surrounding the injury is important. Good exploration with visualization of the base of the wound significantly reduces the risk. In one study, wounds less than 0.5 cm deep had a low risk of an embedded foreign body. Glass fragments can penetrate deeply and have the potential of not being visualized. Persistent or extreme pain, pain on passive movement, and a mass with discoloration at the site of a wound are highly suggestive of a retained foreign body.

10. **Should a retained foreign body be removed?**
In general, foreign bodies should be removed; however, limit removal attempts to a reasonable amount of time. Consider the following factors prior to attempted removal:
- **Location:** Intra-articular, intravascular, or in close proximity to vital structures or has the potential to migrate toward vital structures (e.g., lung, spleen). Consult a surgical specialist in these cases.
- **Material:** Risk of toxicity (e.g., lead, venom from spines).
- **Tissue response:** Production of inflammatory response (e.g., organic matter, silica that causes large granuloma formation), persistent pain, infection, or cosmetic disfigurement.
   Explore foreign bodies associated with penetrating injuries to the abdomen, neck, or chest and arrange for removal in the operating room. Small, deeply embedded foreign bodies may be difficult to locate without ultrasound guidance. They can be left in place with close follow-up or removed electively.

11. **Should hair be removed from a wound site before repair?**
The presence of hair usually does not interfere with the repair of the wound. Petroleum jelly can be used to keep hair away from the wound site during repair. If hair removal is needed, use clippers because they have a lower rate of infection than razors. *Do not remove eyebrow hair during wound repair, because regrowth can be slow or absent.*

12. **Outline the steps in preparing a child for wound closure.**
- Follow standard precautions.
- Prepare the child and the family. An honest and caring explanation of the various steps is important to reduce anxiety.
- Use distraction techniques to decrease anxiety. A child life specialist can be extremely helpful in providing an easy-to-understand explanation of the steps and in distracting during the repair.
- Determine whether sedation or anxiolysis is required.
- Cleanse and irrigate the wound.
- Use local anesthesia topical application (preferred) or by injection.
- Use sterile draping and technique.

13. **How is irrigation and cleansing of the wound best achieved?**
Irrigation is best achieved with normal saline, sterile water, or tap water under pressure using a 20- or 30-mL syringe on a 19- or 22-gauge plastic intravascular catheter and 50 to 100 mL of fluid for irrigation per centimeter of laceration. Although studies have shown no difference in outcome between irrigation with sterile water and tap water, sterile water is used most commonly for irrigation. Splash shields decrease the splattering of irrigation fluid. Avoid excessive pressure during irrigation, because it can distort the anatomy and damage the tissues. Remove road rash (tar), dirt, and foreign material gently with irrigation and mild scrubbing to prevent tattooing. Limit scrubbing because it can damage tissues, leading to poor cosmetic outcomes. Several studies have shown that the use of povidone-iodine affects fibroblasts and hence wound defenses. Irrigation is best done after analgesia is obtained.

14. **What agents are used for local anesthesia?**
Topical anesthetics such as LET (**l**etlidocaine 4%, **e**pinephrine 1:1000, **t**etracaine 0.5%) are the mainstay in achieving local anesthesia in smaller and superficial wounds. LET is applied to the wound locally in the form of a gel for 15 to 20 minutes and produces anesthesia with 97% efficacy. Avoid topical agents containing epinephrine in areas of end-blood supply, such as the fingers, ears, nose, toes, and penis. Occasionally, deeper and larger wounds require infiltration with another agent, such as lidocaine 1% with or without epinephrine. Bupivacaine, which has a longer duration of action, is an alternative in lidocaine-allergic patients.

15 **What is the maximum dose of lidocaine in local anesthetic medications?**
The dose of lidocaine with epinephrine should not exceed 7 mg/kg body weight; the dose of lidocaine alone should not exceed 4 mg/kg.

KEY POINTS: TIPS TO REDUCE PAIN OF ANESTHETIC INFILTRATION

1. Prior application of LET gel.
2. Rubbing the skin near the site of injection (stimulates other nerve endings and thereby decreases the perception of pain).
3. Buffering lidocaine with 8.4% sodium bicarbonate (ratio of 9:1).
4. Warming the buffered lidocaine to 40°C.
5. Using a 27- or 30-gauge needle to slow the rate of injection and 3-cc syringe. Larger syringe will generate higher pressure and may cause more discomfort during injection.
6. Injecting from inside the wound through devitalized tissue.

16 **What is the best method of obtaining hemostasis during wound repair?**
A tourniquet, such as a rubber band or blood pressure cuff, and a local anesthetic with epinephrine can decrease the amount of bleeding during wound repair. Inflate the blood pressure cuff to just above systolic blood pressure. Use a tourniquet for only 20 to 30 minutes at a time. Release it periodically for 2 to 3 minutes to allow reperfusion. Prolonged continuous use can lead to nerve and vascular damage, with subsequent thrombosis and gangrene.

17 **What are the key points for proper wound approximation?**
- Some prefer to place the first suture at the midpoint.
- Slight eversion of the wound edges prevents tethering of the scar line.
- Remove any clots from the wound to help prevent infection and allow for better approximation.
- Reach the floor of the wound to obliterate any potential cavity to decrease the chance of infection and fibrosis.
- Minimize tension on the scar line by doing a layered closure if needed.
- Shift the knot lateral to the laceration so as not to impede approximation.

18 **What are the appropriate types of sutures and techniques for the closure of various wounds?**
For skin closure, use fast-absorbing gut or synthetic nonabsorbable monofilament nylon (Ethilon or Dermalon) whenever possible. Fine absorbable synthetic sutures (e.g., coated Vicryl or Dexon) are used for deeper layers or nail bed repairs. Suture size depends on the site and size of the wound. Use smaller needles (e.g., PS or P1) for wounds that require fine cosmetic outcomes. Table 57.1 lists suggested suture types for various locations.

KEY POINTS: ACHIEVING IDEAL WOUND APPROXIMATION

1. Plan ahead.
2. Consider placing the first suture at the midpoint for good alignment.
3. Ensure slight eversion of the wound edges.
4. Remove clots from gaping wounds.
5. Keep wound tension to a minimum.
6. In layered closures, close each layer individually.

19. **How do alternative wound care techniques compare?**
See Table 57.2 for a comparison of alternative wound care techniques.

20. **When can tissue adhesives be used?**
Tissue adhesives are nearly painless, do not require local anesthesia or removal, and have cosmetic results similar to those of sutures. Use tissue adhesives for wounds with straight edges that are less than 5 to 6 cm long and no wider than 2 to 4 mm. During application, ensure a good approximation of the wound and take care to prevent the adhesive from dripping into the wound cavity. The presence of adhesive in the wound acts like a foreign body and can produce intense inflammation and poor approximation. Instruct parents to avoid the use

Table 57.1 Suggested Suture Types for Various Locations

WOUND SITE	SUTURE TYPE	RECOMMENDED TECHNIQUE	REMOVAL (DAYS)
Scalp	Staples	Simple interrupted	7
Face	6-0 FA or SNA for skin 5-0 AS for deeper layers	Simple interrupted or continuous for skin; interrupted for deeper layers	3-5
Extremity	3-0 or 4-0 SNA 4-0 or 5-0 AS	Simple interrupted mattress or continuous for skin; interrupted for deeper layers	7-10
Hands or feet	5-0 SNA 4-0 AS	Simple interrupted or continuous for skin; interrupted for deeper layers	7-10
Joints	3-0 or 4-0 SNA 4-0 AS	Simple interrupted mattress or continuous for skin; interrupted for deeper layers	10-14

AS, Absorbable synthetic; FA, fast-absorbing gut; SNA, synthetic nonabsorbable.

Table 57.2 Comparison of Alternative Wound Care Techniques

TYPE OF CLOSURE	WOUND TYPE	EASE OF APPLICATION	COSMETIC RESULT	PAIN	COST	NEED FOR REMOVAL
Suture	Any	Poor	Excellent	High	High	Yes
Staple	Scalp*	Good	Poor	High	Medium	Yes[†]
Surgical glue	Small	Good	Good	None	Medium	None
Steri-Strips	Small[†]	Good	Fair	None	Low	Yes

*Should be avoided in areas of cosmetic concern or in patients needing computed tomography or magnetic resonance imaging. Requires special removal forceps.
[†]Small, straight lacerations that are not located over joints, hair-bearing areas, or moist areas.
Data from Farion K, Osmond MH, Hartling L, et al. Tissue adhesives for traumatic lacerations in children and adults. *Cochrane Database Syst Rev.* 2002;(3):CD003326.

of ointments or cream at the site of the wound because they lead to premature peeling of the adhesive. Tissue adhesive (cyanoacrylate) polymerizes on the surface of the approximate wound edges, forming a strong bond to maintain the achieved approximation. Routine follow-up is not necessary, and no removal is needed because the glue will slough off after 7 to 10 days. Take special care to avoid dripping the glue on the eyes/eyelashes if the wound is in close proximity.

21. **When should tissue adhesives be avoided?**

    Do not use tissue adhesives alone for deep wounds. Do not use glue to repair wounds from animal bites or other wounds at high risk for infection. Also, do not use tissue adhesives for wounds on the hands (the glue is likely to wear off and hands are at high risk of infection) or for those subject to great tension (located over a joint). It may be best to avoid the use of tissue adhesives in hair-bearing areas.

22. **What are the complications of tissue adhesives?**

    Occasionally, skinfolds are inadvertently glued together, the glove of the operator may become glued to the patient's skin, or adhesive drips into the patient's eyelashes. If these complications occur, massage petroleum jelly or eye ointment into the site to help dissolve the glue. Refrain from clipping the eyelashes, because their regrowth is uncertain. The strength of the wound after repair with an adhesive is 10% to 15% less than that of wounds closed by sutures. Dehiscence occurs in 1% to 5% of all wounds closed by adhesives. If the wound dehisces, allow it to heal by secondary intention unless the result will be cosmetically unacceptable.

23. **What are some important considerations in the evaluation of puncture wounds?**

    Puncture wounds account for 3% to 5% of all injuries. The most common site is the forefoot (50%). The rate of complications is directly proportional to the depth of penetration. Infection occurs in 6% to 10% of all puncture wounds, with staphylococci, streptococci, and anaerobes being the most common organisms. Injuries penetrating through a foam or rubber insole of a sneaker are often contaminated by *Pseudomonas aeruginosa.* The most common offending object in puncture wounds is a nail (>90%). It is essential to examine the wound well for the possibility of damage to deeper structures and for retained foreign bodies. Puncture wounds have a greater incidence of infectious complications, such as cellulitis, soft tissue abscess, pyarthrosis, osteomyelitis (0.4%-0.6% of wounds), and foreign body granuloma.

24. **A 10-year-old boy presents with persistent pain in his right forefoot after sustaining a puncture wound from a nail 10 days ago. Some redness and swelling are seen at the site. What are your major concerns and management course?**

    Osteomyelitis is a major concern with a puncture wound when persistent pain is accompanied by local signs of infection, even without systemic involvement. Obtain a complete blood count and erythrocyte sedimentation rate, along with imaging studies. MRI is more sensitive in detecting a periosteal reaction or bony destruction than radiography in the first week. Treat osteomyelitis with intravenous (IV) antistaphylococcal and possibly antipseudomonal antibiotics. If no improvement is noted in 48 hours, surgical débridement may be necessary.

25. **What is coring of a puncture wound?**

    Coring removes a 2-mm circular rim of the puncture track. Prepare the area with povidone-iodine, local anesthetic, or regional nerve block, followed by irrigation and packing with iodoform gauze. Instruct the patient to avoid weight-bearing for 5 days. Consider coring in wounds that are grossly contaminated or have a foreign body in an area of low cosmetic concern and high risk for infection, such as the foot.

26. **How are forehead lacerations generally repaired?**
Superficial transverse lacerations of the forehead are easy to repair. They can be repaired using tissue adhesive if superficial with minimal tension or with interrupted or continuous cuticular sutures using 6-0 absorbable suture materials (fast-absorbing gut), which has the same cosmetic result as nonabsorbable sutures. The absorbable suture material has the added advantage of not requiring suture removal. Repair deeper transverse lacerations involving the deep fascia, frontalis muscle, or periosteum in layers. If the deeper tissue planes are not closed, the function of the frontalis muscle (eyebrow elevation) may be compromised. Vertical forehead lacerations tend to have wider scars because they traverse the tension lines if proper tension and coaptation are not achieved. Forehead lacerations are rarely associated with skull fractures, but it is advised to rule out facial, neck, and intracranial injuries.

27. **How are lacerations of the eyelid repaired?**
Lacerations of the eyelid are mostly simple transverse wounds of the upper eyelid just inferior to the eyebrow. Repair does not require special skills. Consider ophthalmology referral for complicated lacerations potentially involving the levator palpebrae muscle or medial canthal ligament or those close to the lacrimal duct (medial third of the lower eyelid). Evaluation of associated injuries to the globe is imperative.

28. **How are lacerations of the external ear treated?**
To avoid necrosis and auricular deformity, minimize débridement and cover the perichondrium with the lacerated, thin but vascular skin. Simple closure with the least possible tension is usually advised. Include the perichondrium in the sutures to ensure that the suture material does not tear through the friable cartilage and to restore nutrient and oxygen supply. If ear trauma has led to an auricular hematoma, drain this promptly to avoid necrosis of the cartilage, which leads to a deformed auricle or cauliflower ear. After the repair of ear lacerations or evacuation of an auricular hematoma, apply a pressure dressing. Follow-up in 24 hours is recommended to evaluate vascular integrity.

29. **What is the recommended technique for the repair of lip lacerations?**
Proper repair of lip lacerations is important because they are highly visible. The vermilion border is a relatively pale line that identifies the junction of the dry oral mucosa and facial skin. It is an important landmark for proper repair. Avoid the use of epinephrine with local anesthesia, because it causes swelling that distorts the border. A mental nerve block provides good anesthesia while preserving the landmarks. Lacerations involving the vermilion border must be aligned precisely. Warn parents that although the lip is still anesthetized, the child might bite off the sutures. They should distract the child from doing so. After local anesthesia has worn off, the site typically is sore enough that the child does not attempt to manipulate the area.

30. **Describe the proper approach to lacerations of the tongue and buccal mucosa.**
    - Small isolated lacerations of the buccal mucosa, usually due to teeth impaction after falls, require no suturing. Lacerations greater than 2 to 3 cm in length or with flaps are best closed with simple interrupted stitches using absorbable material.
    - Tongue lacerations often bleed excessively at the time of injury, but the bleeding usually ceases quickly as the lingual muscle contracts. Most tongue lacerations can be left alone with good results. Repair large lacerations involving the free edge, large flaps, and bleeding lacerations. Full-thickness repair with interrupted 4-0 absorbable sutures is recommended.
    - Local or regional anesthesia is often sufficient.
    - Pay attention to potential airway problems during the repair.
    - Hold the mouth open with a padded tongue depressor. The tongue can be maintained in the protruded position by a gentle pull using a towel clip or by placing a suture through the tip.
    - As in lip lacerations, children may chew off the stitches; warn parents of this possibility. They should attempt to distract the child, at least until the local anesthesia has worn off.

31. **How are fingertip avulsions repaired?**
Most fingertip avulsions are contused lacerations or partial avulsions. Sharp injuries are more common in older children and less likely to be associated with fractures. Evaluate for associated nail bed injury and obtain radiographs for possible fracture of the phalanx. In general, this type of injury is managed conservatively, as tissue regeneration is excellent in preadolescent children. For complete amputation reattachment, skin flap and grafting are options used by the hand specialist. Consider antibiotic coverage if the bone is exposed or fractured in the fingertip injury.

32. **Describe the approach to nail bed injuries.**
Trauma in the distal fingers is often associated with nail and nail bed (matrix) injuries. Nail avulsion may be partial or complete and may be associated with nail bed laceration and/or underlying fracture of the distal phalanx. Injury to the fingertip often is associated with subungual hematoma. Unrepaired nail bed lacerations may permanently

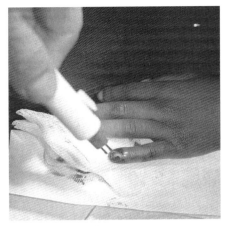

Fig. 57.1 Trephination of a subungual hematoma by cauterization.

disfigure new nail growth from the cicatrix nail bed. If the nail is partially avulsed but is firmly attached to its bed, exploring the nail bed is not warranted. A good outcome is expected because the nail holds the underlying lacerated nail bed tissues in place.

When the nail is completely avulsed or attached loosely, perform a digital block and then lift the nail to assess the nail bed for a laceration. A recent case report describes the successful use of ultrasound to identify nail bed injury. If the nail bed is lacerated, repair it by using 6-0 or smaller absorbable material. After its soft proximal portion is cleansed and trimmed, replace the nail between the nail bed and nail fold (eponychium) and then anchor it in place with a few stitches. This technique splints the nail fold away from the nail bed and prevents obliteration of the space between the two. Preserving this space allows the new nail to grow undisturbed.

The preferred method of local anesthesia for nail bed repair is digital block or sedation for a young child. The use of a finger tourniquet during repair allows a bloodless field. Apply a finger splint after repair, especially in patients with an associated fracture.

33. **How should a subungual hematoma be managed?**
A subungual hematoma is a collection of blood between the nail plate and the nail bed. It is commonly seen with blunt and crushed fingertip injuries and presents with throbbing pain and discoloration of the nail. It may be associated with nail bed injury or fracture of the distal phalanx. Drain a subungual hematoma involving 50% or more of the nail. Drainage of the hematoma relieves pain and prevents deformity of the nail bed. Local anesthesia is not required for a simple trephination by cauterization of the nail (Fig. 57.1). Postdrainage care includes elevation of the hand and warm soaks for a few days. Discuss the possibility of nail deformity in the future with the family.

When the injury is more involved, the digital block is advised. If the hematoma is large and extends to the tip of the nail, separation of the nail from the nail bed allows drainage. In the presence of a distal phalangeal fracture, be careful not to transform a closed fracture into an open fracture by communicating a subungual hematoma to the exterior surface of the nail. If this possibility exists, antibiotic coverage and close follow-up are appropriate.

34. **What should you consider in the management of an animal bite?**
- Vaccine (tetanus and rabies) status of the patient
- Vaccine (rabies) status of animal
- Ability to observe animal
- Necessity of animal bite report (varies per state)
- Antibiotic prophylaxis
- Wound closure: balancing cosmesis versus the risk of infection

35. **When is rabies prophylaxis indicated?**
The rabies virus is shed in the saliva of infected animals for 10 to 14 days before they become symptomatic. Postexposure guidelines are summarized in Table 57.3. Bites from animals such as squirrels, hamsters, guinea pigs, gerbils, chipmunks, rats, mice, rabbits, hares, and other rodents rarely require rabies prophylaxis.

Table 57.3 Guidelines for Rabies Prophylaxis		
TYPE OF ANIMAL	**AVAILABILITY OF ANIMALS FOR OBSERVATION**	**POSTEXPOSURE PROPHYLAXIS**
Dog or cat	Healthy or can be observed for 10 days	Only if the animal develops signs of rabies
	Suspected to be rabid or unknown	RIG + HDCV
Livestock, ferrets, rodents	Consider individually	As per the advice of public health official
Skunks, raccoons, bats, foxes, woodchucks, and other carnivores	Consider rabid unless a geographic area is known to be free of rabies	RIG + HDCV

HDCV, Human diploid cell vaccine; RIG, rabies immunoglobulin.

36. **What is the regimen for postexposure rabies prophylaxis?**
Active immunization with rabies human diploid cell vaccine (HDCV) is given as soon as possible after the exposure, starting on the day of injury and on days 3, 7, and 14. Immunocompromised patients should receive a fifth dose on day 28. Administer the vaccines as a 1.0-mL intramuscular injection in the deltoid. In small infants, use the gluteal area. Give rabies immunoglobulin (RIG) along with the first dose of rabies vaccine, but at a different site. The dose of RIG is 20 IU/kg body weight. Infiltrate as much as possible of the total dose of RIG at the wound site and inject the remainder intramuscularly. Give RIG as soon as possible, and within 7 days after exposure. For patients previously immunized with rabies vaccine give only two doses of HDCV, on days 0 and 3.

37. **A 15-year-old male presents with a hand laceration after punching a classmate in the mouth. In addition to achieving hemostasis and cosmesis, what additional intervention is necessary?**
This wound is likely to have devitalized tissue and is at high risk for developing infection. This is especially concerning if the wound is over a metacarpophalangeal joint. Manage lacerations caused by a fist punch to the mouth as a human bite. Antibiotic prophylaxis is recommended.

38. **What are the signs of wound infection?**
Signs of wound infection include marked or worsening pain or tenderness at the wound site beyond that which would be expected from the initial trauma. Local erythema, warmth, swelling, and discharge, such as pus or serosanguineous fluid, also are signs of infection. In severe infections, fever, phlebitis (streaking), regional lymphadenopathy, and other systemic manifestations may be seen.

39. **For which wounds should prophylactic antibiotics be considered?**
   • Human and animal bites
   • Crush injuries
   • Extensive wounds
   • Exposed cartilage
   • Open fractures
   • Joint cavity violated
   • Hand and foot wounds
   • Moist areas (axilla, perineum)
   • Contaminated wounds
   • Immunocompromised host

40. **Which antibiotics are recommended as prophylaxis for animal bites?**
Prescribe amoxicillin-clavulanic acid (oral) or ampicillin-sulbactam (IV) for animal/human bites to provide additional coverage against anaerobes. For patients with penicillin allergies, prescribe extended-spectrum cephalosporin or trimethoprim-sulfamethoxazole AND clindamycin.

41. **For all other high-risk wounds requiring prophylaxis, which antibiotics are recommended?**
Use a first-generation cephalosporin to cover staphylococci and streptococci or use clindamycin or trimethoprim-sulfamethoxazole if methicillin-resistant *Staphylococcus aureus* is a concern.

42. **What are the key elements of post-repair wound care?**
    - Apply antibiotic ointment to keep the wound area moisturized and to reduce infection by preventing scab formation.
    - Elevate the affected area to decrease edema.
    - Immobilize wounds over joints with a splint or apply a bulky dressing.
    - Provide discharge instructions regarding wound care, signs of infection, and follow-up.
    - Instruct the patient to avoid bathing for 24 to 48 hours; after that time, the wound should be washed with mild soap and water and gently dried.
    - Arrange for the wound recheck in 24 to 48 hours to assess healing and signs of infection.
    - Remove sutures in a timely manner to prevent scars from suture tracks.
    - Instruct the patient to use sunscreen for 6 to 12 months after injury to prevent hyperpigmentation of the scar.

43. **When does a wound regain its strength?**
    A wound regains 5% of its strength in 2 weeks, 30% in 1 to 2 months, and full strength in 6 to 8 months. The scar achieves its final appearance in 6 to 12 months.

44. **What are the indications for tetanus prophylaxis?**
    Tetanus is a potential risk in all wounds. There were an average of 30 cases of tetanus per year from 2001 to 2018 in the United States, of which 10% to 20% were fatal. Wounds at a higher risk for tetanus are those contaminated by soil or feces and those with devitalized tissue (e.g., puncture, crush, missile, or avulsion wounds). Burns and frostbite are also prone to tetanus. Prophylaxis depends on the type of wound and the patient's immunization status (Table 57.4).

45. **A young boy is brought to the ED after being stuck by a needle on the playground. The needle has crusted blood along the metallic edge. What are your concerns? What is the best course of management?**
    A needlestick injury raises concerns about exposure to tetanus and blood-borne pathogens, such as hepatitis B virus (HBV), hepatitis C virus (HCV), and human immunodeficiency virus (HIV). Give tetanus prophylaxis after considering the potential for contamination and the immunization status of the child. HBV can survive on fomites for several days, and prompt postexposure prophylaxis reduces the risk of transmission. Table 57.5 summarizes the recommendations for hepatitis prophylaxis. The risk of infection with HIV causes great anxiety to the family.

Table 57.4 Guidelines for Tetanus Prophylaxis

HISTORY OF TETANUS TOXOID DOSES	TIME SINCE LAST DOSE	CLEAN WOUND		ALL OTHER WOUNDS	
		DTaP/ Tdap/Td*	TIG	DTaP/ Tdap/Td	TIG
>3 vaccines	<5 years	No	No	No	No
	5-10 years	No	No	Yes	No
	>10 years	Yes	No	Yes	No
<3 vaccines or unknown		Yes	No	Yes	Yes

DTaP, Diphtheria, tetanus, acellular pertussis toxoid for children younger than 7 years; Td, tetanus toxoid, reduced diphtheria; Tdap, tetanus toxoid, reduced diphtheria toxoid, acellular pertussis vaccine; TIG, tetanus immunoglobulin.
*Tdap is preferred to Td for >7 years who have never received Tdap.

Table 57.5 Hepatitis Prophylaxis After a Needlestick Exposure

NUMBER OF DOSES OF HBV VACCINE ALREADY RECEIVED	IMMUNOPROPHYLAXIS
>3	None
1-3	Additional dose of HBV vaccine; complete the rest of the schedule with or without HBIG
None	Begin vaccination series + HBIG

HBIG, Hepatitis B immunoglobulin; HBV, hepatitis B virus.

However, the risk of transmission of HIV from a discarded needle is less than 0.3%. Testing the syringe is neither practical nor reliable. Testing the patient for HIV is controversial, but if testing is elected, it should be done at the time of injury and at 6 weeks, 12 weeks, and 6 months after exposure. Consult a specialist in HIV before using prophylaxis. Start antiretroviral therapy if the syringe had fresh blood.

The risk of transmission of HCV from a discarded needle is low. Testing is done if there is known exposure or high risk of HCV. Assess for anti-HCV antibodies by enzyme immunoassay at the time of injury and 3 to 6 months after exposure. There is no prophylaxis for HCV.

46. **What is the best course of management for a fishhook embedded in soft tissue?**
Fishhooks have a straight shank and a curved belly that has an eyelet with a barb pointed away from the tip. Do not attempt removal in the ED if the fishhook is buried near vital structures. If the fishhook is not in a dangerous location, consider using a digital block or local infiltration. Wear protective eyewear to avoid injury during the removal. Remove lures and additional hooks first with a hemostat and wire cutter.

There are several methods of removal. The push-through method is most effective when the barb is close to the skin. After providing local anesthesia, push the barb forward (antegrade) through the skin. Then clip it with a wire cutter and pull the rest of the barb back through the original wound.

With the string technique, loop a long piece of string around the hook at the point of entry and around the clinician's finger. While the clinician applies pressure downward over the straight part of the fishhook to disengage the barb, pull the hook away rapidly. Local anesthetics are rarely needed with this technique.

47. **What is the best way to remove a ring that is stuck on a child's finger?**
If vascular compromise is present, remove the constricting ring as soon as possible. The risk of gangrene is present in any obstruction that persists beyond 10 to 12 hours. A ring cutter is useful. It is easiest to cut the thinnest part of the ring, which is usually on the palmar surface of the hand. Once cut, separate the ends manually. The string-pull method is best used for broad or metallic bands. One end of a suture is slipped under the band. After the application of lubricant, grasp the string with a hemostat and pull in a circular motion until it slides off.

BIBLIOGRAPHY

1. Al-Mubarak L, Al-Haddab M. Cutaneous wound closure materials: an overview and update. *J Cutan Aesthet Surg.* 2013;6(4):178–188. https://doi.org/10.4103/0974-2077.123395.
2. American Academy of Pediatrics. Hepatitis C. Red Book: 2021–2024 Report of the Committee on Infectious Diseases, Red Book Online, American Academy of Pediatrics. <https://www.aap.org>; Accessed June 2023.
3. Centers for Disease Control and Prevention: Vaccines and Immunizations. Chapter 16: Tetanus. Manual for the surveillance of vaccine-preventable diseases. <http://www.cdc.gov/vaccines/pubs/surv-manual/chpt16-tetanus.html>; Accessed June 2023.
4. Cho C. *Fleisher & Ludwig's Textbook of Pediatric Emergency Medicine.* In: Shaw KN, Bachur RG, eds. *Minor trauma.* 8th ed. Wolters Kluwer; 2021:1153–1169.
5. Ernst AA, Gershoff L, Miller P, et al. Warmed versus room temperature saline for laceration irrigation—a randomized clinical trial. *South Med J.* 2003;96:436–439.
6. Gungor F, et al. The value of point-of-care ultrasound for detecting nail bed injury in. *Am J Emerg Med.* 2016;34(9):1850–1854. https://doi.org/10.1016/j.ajem.2016.06.067.
7. Gursky B, Kestler LP, Lewis M. Psychosocial intervention on procedure related distress. *J Dev Behav Pediatr.* 2010;31:217–222.
8. Karounis H, Gouin S, Eisman H, et al. A randomized, controlled trial comparing long-term cosmetic outcomes of traumatic pediatric lacerations repaired with absorbable plain gut versus nonabsorbable nylon sutures. *Acad Emerg Med.* 2004;11:730–735.
9. Moran B, et al. Photographic assessment of postsurgical facial scars epidermally sutured with rapidly absorbable polyglactin 910 or nylon: a randomized clinical trial. *J Am Acad Dermatol.* 2020;83(5):1395–1399.
10. Resende MMC, et al. Tap water versus sterile saline solution in the colonisation of skin wounds. *Int Wound J.* 2016;13(4):526–530.
11. Cristal NS, et al. Child life reduces distress and pain and improves family satisfaction in the pediatric emergency department. *Clin Pediatr.* 2018;57(13):1567–1575.
12. Silva JB, Becker AS, Leal BLM, et al. Subungual hematoma: nail bed repair or nail trephination? A systematic review. *Eur J Plast Surg.* 2022. https://doi.org/10.1007/s00238-022-02003-7.
13. Volk A, Zebda M, Abdelgawad AA. Plantar and pedal puncture wounds in children: a case series study from a single level I trauma center. *Pediatr Emerg Care.* 2017;33(11):724–729. https://doi.org/10.1097/PEC.0000000000000615.
14. Zempsky WT, Parrotti D, Grem C, Nichols J. Randomized controlled comparison of cosmetic outcomes of simple facial lacerations closed with Steri-Strip skin closure or dermabond tissue adhesive. *Pediatr Emerg Care.* 2004;20(8):519–524.

CHAPTER 58

MULTIPLE TRAUMA

Laurie H. Johnson and Anne Runkle

1. **Why is trauma such an important topic in pediatric emergency medicine?**
   Injury is the leading cause of death and disability in children older than 1 year. Although injury death rates in the U.S. population have continued to decline, trauma is still the number one killer of children. Trauma is responsible for about 10,000 deaths per year in children aged 19 years and younger. Significant differences in outcome are observed for specific mechanisms of injury based on age, injury severity, and mortality risk. The sequelae from these injuries can often have a substantial impact on the mental and physical functioning of children as they mature.

2. **What factors interfere with the detection of injuries in the pediatric patient?**
   - Lack of cooperation of the child due to any of the following: preverbal or nonverbal, fearful, in pain, or with altered mental status due to injury or ingested substances
   - Lack of trauma team activation
   - Occult injuries, which are not initially apparent
   - Nonaccidental trauma/physical abuse, where injury is not disclosed by the parent or caretaker

3. **What are the leading causes of traumatic death in children?**
   - Gunshot wounds. In 2017, firearm injuries overtook motor vehicle collisions as the leading cause of death for children and adolescents (0-24 years of age).
   - Motor vehicle traffic–related crashes are the second leading cause of death from injuries in children, both as passengers and as pedestrians struck.
   - Drowning is the third leading cause of pediatric injury death nationally.
   - Deaths from burns and smoke inhalation have declined but remain fourth.
   - Falls are the most common mechanism of nonfatal injury; severity of the injury is minor except in falls greater than 10 to 20 feet.

4. **What injury patterns are expected with specific mechanisms (such as motor vehicle crashes, bicycle crashes, and falls)?**
   In addition to the details of the mechanism (speed of a vehicle, height of a fall, protective equipment worn), the age and size of the pediatric patient are factors in predictable patterns of injury.

5. **Discuss the importance of sports-related injuries.**
   Sports-related injuries are common but do not often lead to death. Neck injuries sustained due to falls in equestrian sports and football injuries are an important cause of severe injury and death despite a low incidence. Blunt trauma from sports can lead to serious head, intra-abdominal solid organ, and eye injury. In terms of visits for emergency care, sports injuries are responsible for large numbers of musculoskeletal injuries, fractures, and joint injuries.

6. **Describe the prehospital care capability for children with potentially serious injuries.**
   Emergency medical technicians have vast experience in advanced life support for adults, but skills such as endotracheal intubation and intravenous (IV) access can be challenging in younger patients. A systematic review suggests endotracheal intubation results in equivalent or less favorable outcomes than bag-valve-mask ventilation or placement of a supraglottic airway. Rates of success with IV access have been fair in infants, good in preschoolers, and excellent in adolescents. Even with programs conducted to improve these rates (such as procedures in the operating room [OR] and field courses), in settings with less experienced providers and short transit distances, the best procedure is safe extrication/preparation and immediate transfer to the hospital. Advances in prehospital management of pediatric trauma include increased use of intraosseous (IO) access and the ability to administer intranasal medications to treat pain from injuries.

7. **Describe the initial approach to children with potentially serious injuries (ABCDEs).**
   The ABCDEs are used during the initial assessment (called the primary survey) to define underlying injuries and to reverse potential life-threatening problems. The team must assess and stabilize each step in order (e.g., control of the airway always precedes control of circulation). While there has been a modification of this sequence in combat and disaster settings to prioritize massive hemorrhage control prior to airway and breathing assessment, current trauma guidelines have not changed this sequence for the civilian population.
   - **A**irway management: Assess and secure the airway while maintaining cervical spine control.
   - **B**reathing: Ensure adequate oxygenation and maximize oxygen delivery.

- Circulation: Establish vascular access, control hemorrhage, and restore circulatory volume.
- Disability: Assess potentially critical injury to the central nervous system.
- Exposure: Visualize every part of the patient to assess for injury and control body temperature (especially important in young infants and children).

8. **What factors raise suspicion for cervical spine injury in a patient with blunt trauma?**
   The multicenter observational Pediatric Emergency Care Applied Research Network study on cervical spine injury in children less than 18 years identified seven factors associated with cervical spine injury with 92% sensitivity (confidence interval [CI] 85.7%-98.1%) and 50.3% specificity (CI 48.7%-51.8%). These factors were the following: (1) diving, (2) axial load, (3) neck pain, (4) inability to move neck, (5) altered mental status, (6) intubation, (7) respiratory distress.

9. **How can one appropriately clear the cervical spine in a pediatric trauma patient?**
   There is currently no validated prediction rule for pediatric cervical spine injury, unlike in adults where the National Emergency X-Radiography Utilization Study (NEXUS) and Canadian Cervical Spine rules are both validated tools to clinically clear the cervical spine without imaging. In pediatric patients over the age of 8 years, NEXUS has been retrospectively validated. In the alert patient with no distracting injury and no midline cervical pain with palpation, the cervical spine can be cleared clinically by assessing midline tenderness and active range of motion. Maintain proper immobilization and obtain plain film images if any of the following are present: cervical spine tenderness to palpation, altered mental status or neurologic deficits (presence or history of numbness, tingling sensation, decreased sensory or motor function), or distracting injury (such as an extremity fracture or abdominal pain). Initial imaging is center dependent and often consists of anteroposterior and lateral films of the cervical spine. Cervical spine computed tomography (CT) scan may be the initial imaging of choice in polytrauma patients or those with altered mental status.

10. **What is the reason for the use of hypertonic saline in the trauma patient with severe traumatic brain injury (TBI)? What are the other emergency department (ED) interventions for severe TBI?**
    Studies performed on pediatric and adult trauma patients in the intensive care unit setting have demonstrated the safety and efficacy of hypertonic saline for acutely decreasing intracranial pressure compared to traditional therapies. The proposed mechanism for the use of hypertonic solutions is that increased serum osmolality decreases intracranial pressure via the osmotic pressure gradient. Early administration of hypertonic saline may therefore be helpful in supporting blood pressure as well as decreasing intracranial pressure. Other ED treatments to improve outcomes in severe TBI are maintaining normothermia, normocapnia ($PaCO_2$ 35-45 mm Hg), avoiding hypoxia, and elevating the head of the bed (reverse Trendelenburg in patients with suspected concomitant spinal injuries).

KEY POINTS: INITIAL MANAGEMENT OF POTENTIALLY SERIOUS INJURIES

1. Assess the airway first.
2. Once the airway is secure, stabilize breathing.
3. Confirm or establish stable circulation.
4. Maintain cervical spine immobilization and control.

11. **Describe the secondary survey.**
    The secondary survey is a detailed head-to-toe physical examination that follows the initial ABCDE survey and resuscitation. Survey the head, neck, and face first for evidence of blood or occult injury while maintaining control of the cervical spine. This includes assessment of maxillary and mandibular stability, eyes, ears, and oropharynx. Careful assessment of the bony thorax, lungs, and cardiovascular system is next, followed by the assessment of the abdomen, pelvis, and external genitourinary tract. Log roll the child in a neutral position to assess the back, posterior chest, and spine. Lastly, assess the extremities carefully for obvious and occult injury, along with neurovascular status. Evaluation of the central nervous system may be conducted during each part of the examination or performed at the end.

12. **What components of the neurologic examination should be conducted during the secondary survey?**
    Evaluate pupillary size, symmetry, and reactivity. Report the child's level of consciousness using the Glasgow Coma Scale (GCS), but in preverbal children (usually children <2 years), the verbal response score should be modified as follows:
    Coos, babbles: +5
    Irritable cries: +4
    Cries in response to pain: +3
    Moans in response to pain: +2
    No response: +1

13. **What initial radiographic and laboratory studies are important in trauma?**
In unstable or high-risk patients, the most important studies to be obtained in the first 5 to 10 minutes include a complete blood count, type, and cross-match for packed red blood cells (pRBCs), and coagulation studies (prothrombin time, partial thromboplastin time). Obtain portable radiographs of the chest and pelvis. Portable lateral cervical spine films and Focused Assessment of Sonography for Trauma (FAST) examination using point-of-care ultrasound may also be performed. Due to its low sensitivity in pediatric patients, a negative FAST examination does not rule out significant intra-abdominal hemorrhage or injury. After stabilization, severely injured patients may undergo further CT imaging or be transported directly to the OR.

   In patients with mild-to-moderate trauma, screening blood studies and radiographs, although standard in the past, are no longer routine and are usually of low utility. It is always appropriate to reassess the patient and obtain studies as needed.

14. **Should one remove a penetrating foreign body?**
No, leave any foreign body in place. This is especially important in foreign bodies to the neck, chest, abdomen, or back, or a foreign body that has the possibility of neurovascular compromise in any other location. These objects should be stabilized and only be removed by a surgeon in a controlled environment.

15. **List the major signs of intra-abdominal bleeding.**
   - Abdominal tenderness
   - Abdominal distention that does not improve after nasogastric decompression
   - Shock
   - Bloody nasogastric aspirate, blood on rectal examination, or grossly bloody urine
   - Positive FAST examination

16. **Describe the presentation and treatment of tension pneumothorax.**
Tension pneumothorax results from penetrating chest trauma or acute barotrauma after blunt injury. Air is trapped behind a one-way flap-valve defect in the lung, collapsing the lung and displacing the mediastinum contralaterally. The child presents with moderate-to-severe respiratory distress and may have contralateral tracheal deviation. Systemic perfusion is often compromised significantly by obstructed venous return. Treatment requires needle decompression followed by chest tube placement. While adult guidelines recommend the fourth or fifth intercostal space anterior to the midaxillary line as the location for needle decompression, the second intercostal space in the midclavicular site is still recommended for prepubertal pediatric patients. After needle decompression, a chest tube must be placed. The size of the chest tube (including whether pigtail catheter chest tubes are used for traumatic pneumothorax without hemothorax) depends on the age of the child and hospital guidelines.

17. **Define open pneumothorax. How is this injury managed?**
Open pneumothorax, or a "sucking chest wound," which may occur after a penetrating chest wound, allows free bidirectional flow of air between the affected hemithorax and surrounding atmosphere. Sucking chest wounds are extremely rare in children. Management centers on positive-pressure ventilation and covering the wound with an occlusive dressing taped securely on three sides to allow for air to escape with exhalation and avoid air-trapping during inhalation.

18. **What findings are associated with mild blood volume loss?**
Mild blood volume loss (<30% blood loss) is associated with mild tachycardia, mild tachypnea, decreased urine output, normal pulse pressure, prolonged capillary refill, and normal blood pressure (usually). Hypotension is a late finding, associated with ongoing hemorrhage, and indicates that the child is near decompensation.

19. **Which physical examination findings indicate shock in injured children?**
Shock may be difficult to recognize because the signs are subtle and mimic those of fright or pain. Tachycardia and tachypnea are early signs. The child will be anxious or confused. Urine output is decreased and capillary refill is prolonged. Hypotension may not be evident until the child has lost 25% to 40% of blood volume and is thus a late finding.

20. **When is a blood transfusion indicated for an injured child?**
A blood transfusion is necessary for children when signs of shock from hemorrhage persist despite one bolus of crystalloid (20 mL/kg). In cases of massive hemorrhage with signs of shock, initial resuscitation with blood transfusion before crystalloid may be appropriate. Administer blood as a bolus of pRBCs in aliquots of 10 mL/kg. Warming the blood to body temperature is recommended to increase the speed of transfusion and prevent hypothermia. Give type-specific, cross-matched blood. O-negative blood may be imperative if shock is present, and type-specific blood is not available. If the massive transfusion protocol is activated, or transfusion of more than 40 mL/kg of pRBCs is anticipated, 1:1:1 transfusion may be indicated.

21. **What is the 1:1:1 rule for transfusion? What else is helpful with severe hemorrhage?**

    The 1:1:1 rule is applied when there is severe hemorrhage, and the massive transfusion protocol is activated. This rule dictates that pRBCs, plasma, and platelets are transfused in a predefined equal ratio. This has shown improved outcomes (prevention of coagulopathy) in adult studies over previous transfusion strategies, which emphasized pRBC transfusion over plasma and platelets.

    Another recent advance in the treatment of severe hemorrhage in pediatrics is the addition of tranexamic acid (TXA) as an adjunctive therapy. TXA is an antifibrinolytic medication, which is administered for uncontrolled hemorrhage in the adult population and has been used in elective pediatric surgery cases. TXA was successful in reducing inpatient mortality in combat victims but has not yet been found to be successful in reducing mortality due to pediatric trauma. TXA is more frequently used as an adjunct to the massive transfusion protocol.

KEY POINTS: ABNORMAL VITAL SIGNS IN THE INJURED CHILD

1. Tachycardia in an injured patient may be due to pain, anxiety or agitation, or blood loss.
2. Carefully evaluate the tachycardic trauma patient for the possibility of compensated shock.
3. An older child in compensated shock may be deceivingly responsive and alert.
4. Treat shock in the trauma patient with a rapidly infused 20 mL/kg bolus (maximum of 1 L) of crystalloid fluids (normal saline, lactated Ringer solution, or other isotonic fluid).
5. If the patient is refractory to treatment with crystalloid, rapidly infuse pRBCs, plasma, and platelets in a balanced ratio and closely follow coagulation studies while emergently seeking operative or other definitive intervention.

---

22. **Which visceral injuries are more common in children than adults?**

    Duodenal hematoma and blunt pancreatic injury may occur when a handlebar strikes the child in the right upper quadrant, due to undeveloped abdominal muscular tone. Small bowel perforations at or near the ligament of Treitz and mesenteric small bowel avulsion injuries are more common in children. The shallowness of the pelvis leads to more frequent occurrences of bladder rupture. Because of the proximity of the peritoneum to the perineum, intraperitoneal injuries occur more commonly after straddle injuries in children.

23. **What are the indications for endotracheal intubation of the injured child?**
    - Inability to oxygenate or ventilate with a bag-valve-mask device
    - Need for prolonged airway control
    - Prevention of aspiration in a comatose child
    - Severe TBI (GCS score of 8 or less)

24. **What is the most appropriate way to intubate the trachea of a seriously injured child?**

    Rapid sequence intubation should be performed to maximize the chances of successful intubation. Always precede tracheal intubation with adequate preoxygenation.

    The patient's neck must remain in the neutral position and *should not be hyperextended* during the procedure. This goal is best accomplished with the jaw-thrust spinal stabilization maneuver. Place two fingers on each side of the lower jaw and lift the jaw upward and outward. The head-tilt/chin-lift maneuver may cause manipulation of the neck, which can convert an incomplete spinal cord injury to a complete one. Ideally, one team member should stabilize the neck (bimanually) after removing the front of the cervical spine collar while another performs the endotracheal intubation. The Sellick maneuver (cricoid pressure) is not routinely recommended for tracheal intubation. Have a rigid suction device immediately available. A hyperangulated video laryngoscope blade may also be useful. Discuss a backup plan with the trauma team in the event that intubation is unsuccessful and oxygenation and ventilation are compromised; supraglottic airway devices may be contraindicated in extensive facial trauma, and rescue with a surgical airway may be necessary.

25. **What can lead to gastric distention in an injured child? Why is gastric distention important, and how should it be managed?**

    Gastric distention can occur when the child swallows air at the time of injury, or when crying after the injury occurs. It also may be due to ventilation with a bag-valve-mask device or a leak around an endotracheal tube. Gastric distention is dangerous because it can compromise ventilation. It limits diaphragmatic motion, reduces lung volume, and increases the risk of vomiting and aspiration.

    Place a nasogastric tube as soon as the airway is controlled and decompress the stomach. Consider decompression before intubation to decrease the probability of emesis and improve preintubation preoxygenation. Use an orogastric tube instead of nasogastric decompression if the child has significant facial trauma or a maxillofacial or basal skull fracture.

26. **List the current child passenger safety recommendations.**
    - All infants and toddlers should be in a rear-facing car safety seat for as long as possible (until the maximum height/weight limit has been reached for the specific car safety seat as listed by the manufacturer).
    - Children should be secured in a forward-facing car safety seat with a harness until at least 4 years of age or when the maximum height/weight limit for the car seat has been reached.
    - Children who have outgrown the forward-facing limit of a car seat should use a belt-positioning booster seat until they reach a height of 4 feet 9 inches (typically between 8 and 12 years of age).
    - Children younger than 13 years should be properly restrained with a lap-and-shoulder seat belt in the rear seat of the vehicle.

27. **How might airbags and pediatric restraint devices in vehicles influence motor vehicle crash-related injuries?**
    Children younger than 12 years seated in the front seat of the car are at risk for injuries from airbag deployment, such as facial burns, lacerations, contusions, abrasions, and eye injuries. More devastating injuries such as spinal cord transection and blunt head and neck trauma have also been reported in children who were restrained in the front seat. Children restrained in the rear seat are one-half to two-thirds as likely to be injured as those restrained in the front seat. Unrestrained and improperly restrained children are at risk of being ejected during a motor vehicle collision. Age-appropriate restraint devices have been shown to decrease rates of mortality and significant injury in children 6 years old and younger.

28. **Can the IO route be used to establish vascular access in an injured child?**
    Yes. The IO route is expeditious and may be lifesaving if an IV line cannot be established quickly. It can be used to deliver crystalloid fluids, blood, or medications. Placement sites include the proximal tibia, proximal humerus, and distal femur. Placement of an IO line is contraindicated in a fractured long bone, an extremity with a vascular injury, an area with an overlying skin infection or burn, or an extremity where an IO line was recently attempted or placed. Patients with underlying bone fragility syndromes (such as osteogenesis imperfecta) are not good candidates for IO placement.

29. **What are the indications for ED thoracotomy in pediatric trauma?**
    Thoracotomy is performed in the ED as an attempt to resuscitate patients who go into cardiac arrest due to trauma. Thoracotomy allows direct access to the chest, and the performance of potentially life-saving procedures including release of cardiac tamponade, cross-clamping the aorta for control of severe hemorrhage, and direct control of cardiac or pulmonary injuries. In adults, survival after ED thoracotomy is approximately 10%. In pediatrics, survival is lower. A recent study has shown overall survival of 3.4%, with higher rates of survival in adolescents (4.8%) than in children <15 years (0%). Survival rates were highest for arrest due to penetrating thoracic trauma. Survival rates were lowest in blunt trauma and children with severe TBI. Partially because of these very low survival rates, as well as the paucity of data, there are no current pediatric-specific recommendations for ED thoracotomy. Center-specific guidelines may be adapted from adult guidelines from the Western Trauma Association and the Eastern Association for the Surgery of Trauma, which both recommend ED thoracotomy for penetrating thoracic trauma, but have differing recommendations for blunt trauma and extrathoracic trauma.

30. **What are the possible causes of shock in a patient with severe TBI without signs of external bleeding?**
    The child most likely has a serious injury of the chest, abdomen, or pelvis with internal bleeding. Isolated head trauma rarely results in shock, although a significant scalp laceration can produce excessive blood loss. Femur fractures from high-impact injuries in adolescents may lead to shock. Consider neurogenic shock after a thorough evaluation for possible causes of hemorrhagic shock.

31. **How does the anatomy of young children result in different injury patterns than in adolescents and young adults?**
    Because of their smaller size, children sustain injuries to multiple organ systems more commonly than adults exposed to the same mechanism. The immature skeletons of children result in less frequent bone injuries and more frequent soft tissue injuries and internal organ damage. Bone injury may be more subtle because children have open growth plates at the epiphyses. Owing to a flexible and less muscular chest wall, rib fractures and flail chest are less common, but forces are more easily transmitted to internal organs. Likewise, the solid organs in the abdomen are disproportionately larger and more exposed than in adults. Children have larger heads relative to their bodies and are more likely to land on their heads when they fall. The large head also contributes to cervical spine injuries at a higher level (C2-C3) in children than in adults. Because children have more skin surface area in relation to their overall size than adults, they can lose heat quickly after injury, resulting in hypothermia.

32. **What are the key aspects of the medical history in seriously injured children?**
In managing a critically injured child, it is not appropriate to divert attention to a long, detailed history. Instead, the American College of Surgeons recommends an AMPLE history:
   - **A:** Allergies
   - **M:** Medications
   - **P:** Past illnesses
   - **L:** Last meal
   - **E:** Events surrounding the injury

33. **What are the criteria for admission to a pediatric trauma center?**
   - GCS score of 12 or less
   - Decompensated shock (low systolic blood pressure for age)
   - Shock unresponsive to fluid resuscitation
   - Abnormal respiratory rate (adjusted for age)

34. **When a trauma patient requires transfer to a trauma center, what are the responsibilities of the transferring physician?**
   - Identification of the patient requiring transfer
   - Initiation of the transfer process via phone contact with the receiving physician
   - Maximal stabilization using the capabilities of the local institution
   - Determination of the best mode of transport
   - Assurance that the level of care allows the patient to remain stable and not deteriorate
   - Transfer of all relevant records, results, and radiographs to the receiving facility

35. **When should prehospital care providers withhold/terminate resuscitation for injured children?**
Withholding of prehospital resuscitative efforts in pediatric trauma patients is not a common occurrence. Termination of resuscitation should be considered only if injuries are not survivable (i.e., decapitation), evidence of rigor mortis or dependent lividity, or prolonged resuscitation (>30 minutes) without return of spontaneous circulation with the nearest treatment facility greater than 30 minutes away.

BIBLIOGRAPHY

1. American College of Surgeons Committee on Trauma *Advanced Trauma Life Support ATLS: Student Course Manual. Committee on Trauma.* 10th ed. American College of Surgeons; 2018.
2. American College of Surgeons Committee on Trauma American College of Emergency Physicians Pediatric Emergency Medicine Committee National Association of EMS Physicians American Academy of Pediatrics Committee on Pediatric Emergency Medicine Fallat ME. Withholding or termination of resuscitation in pediatric out-of-hospital traumatic cardiopulmonary arrest. *Pediatrics.* 2014;133(4):e1104–e1116. https://doi.org/10.1542/peds.2014-0176 PMID: 24685948.
3. Arbogast KB, Kallan MJ, Durbin DR. Front versus rear seat injury risk for child passengers: evaluation of newer model year vehicles. *Traffic Inj Prev.* 2009;10(3):297–301.
4. Burlew CC, Moore EE, Moore FA, et al. Western Trauma Association critical decisions in trauma: resuscitative thoracotomy. *J Trauma Acute Care Surg.* 2012;73(6):1359–1363.
5. Calder BW, Vogel AM, Zhang J, et al. Focused assessment with sonography for trauma in children after blunt abdominal trauma: a multi-institutional analysis. *J Trauma Acute Care Surg.* 2017;83(2):218–224.
6. *Centers for Disease Control and Prevention, National Center for Health Statistics.* National vital statistics system, mortality 1999-2020 on CDC WONDER online database. <https://wonder.cdc.gov>Released 2021. Accessed 17.05.22
7. *Centers for Disease Control and Prevention, National Center for Injury Prevention and Control.* Web-based Injury Statistics Query and Reporting System (WISQARS). <https://www.cdc.gov/injury/wisqars/LeadingCauses.html> Accessed 17.05.22
8. Diab YA, Wong EC, Luban NL. Massive transfusion in children and neonates. *Br J Haematol.* 2013;161(1):15–26.
9. Dieckmann RA, Brownstein D, Gausche-Hill M, et al. *Pediatric Education for Prehospital Professionals (PEPP).* In: Dieckmann RA, ed. *Trauma.* 4th ed. Jones & Bartlett; 2020.
10. Durbin DR, Hoffman BD, AAP Council on Injury, Violence, and Poison Prevention Child passenger safety. *Pediatrics.* 2018;142(5):e20182460.
11. Egloff AM, Kadom N, Vezina G, Bulas D. Pediatric cervical spine trauma imaging: a practical approach. *Pediatr Radiol.* 2009;39(5):447–456.
12. Fox JC, Boysen M, Gharahbaghian L, et al. Test characteristics of focused assessment of sonography for trauma for clinically significant abdominal free fluid in pediatric blunt abdominal trauma. *Acad Emerg Med.* 2011;18(5):477–482.
13. Gausche M, Lewis RJ, Stratton SJ, et al. Effect of out-of-hospital pediatric endotracheal intubation on survival and neurological outcome: a controlled clinical trial. *JAMA.* 2000;283(6):783–790.
14. Hamele M, Aden JK, Borgan MA. Tranexamic acid in pediatric combat trauma requiring massive transfusions and mortality. *J Trauma Acute Care Surg.* 2020;89(2S Suppl 2):S242–S245.
15. Holcomb JB, Tilley BC, Baraniuk S. Transfusion of plasma, platelets, and red blood cells in a 1:1:1 vs a 1:1:2 ratio and mortality in patients with severe trauma: the PROPPR randomized clinical trial. *JAMA.* 2015;313(5):471–482.
16. Kochanek PM, R.C. RC, Carney N, Totten AM, et al. Guidelines for the Management of Pediatric Severe Traumatic Brain Injury, 3rd Edition: update of the Brain Trauma Foundation guidelines. *Pediatr Crit Care Med.* 2019;20(3S Suppl 1):S1–S82. Erratum in: Pediatr Crit Care Med. 2019;20(4):404. PMID: 30829890. 10.1097/PCC.0000000000001735.

17. Kornelsen E, Kupperman N, Nishijima D, et al. Effectiveness and safety of tranexamic acid in pediatric trauma: a systematic review and meta-analysis. *Am J Emerg Med.* 2022;55:103–110.
18. Leonard JC, Browne LR, Ahmad FA, et al. Cervical spine injury risk factors in children with blunt trauma. *Pediatrics.* 2019;144(1):e20183221.
19. Lee LK, Douglas K, Hemenway D. Crossing lines—a change in the leading cause of death among US children. *N Engl J Med.* 2022;386(16):1485–1487.
20. Moore HB, Moore EE, Bensard DD. Pediatric emergency department thoracotomy: a 40-year review. *J Pediatr Surg.* 2016;51(2):315–318.
21. Saldino R, Gaines B. *Fleisher & Ludwig's Textbook of Pediatric Emergency Medicine.* In: Shaw KN, Bachur RG, eds. *Abdominal trauma.* 8th ed. Wolters Kluwer; 2021:1084–1094.
22. Seamon MJ, Haut ER, Van Arendonk K, et al. An evidence-based approach to patient selection for emergency department thoracotomy: a practice management guideline from the Eastern Association for the Surgery of Trauma. *J Trauma Acute Care Surg.* 2015;79(1):159–173.
23. Weihing VK, Crowe EH, Want HE, Ugalde IT. Prehospital airway management in the pediatric patient: a systematic review. *Acad Emerg Med.* 2021 https://doi.org/10.1111/acem.14410.
24. Woodward GA, Keilman A. *Fleisher & Ludwig's Textbook of Pediatric Emergency Medicine.* In: Shaw KN, Bachur RG, eds. *Neck trauma.* 8th ed. Wolters Kluwer; 2021:1214–1253.

CHAPTER 59

NECK AND CERVICAL SPINE TRAUMA

Nadine Smith and Howard Kadish

1. **What are the differences in neck anatomy comparing children and adults?**

   Compared to adults, children have a larger head, larger mandible, and a shorter neck in proportion to the rest of their body. These differences protect the child's anterior neck at the time of injury; therefore the head and face absorb the major force of impact. However, a child's smaller neck area with a larger number of vital organs and structures puts them at risk for increased severity of injury after a direct penetrating or blunt injury, especially if hyperextended at the time of injury.

   Infants and children also have a smaller larynx in regards to both size and dimensions compared to adults. In children, the arytenoids are larger, the epiglottis has an omega shape, and the larynx has a funnel shape, which is the narrowest in the subglottic region. In adults, the narrowest point of the trachea is located at the level of C7, whereas in children, it is at the cricoid cartilage ring at the level of C4. These anatomic differences, along with the ring-like cricoid cartilage, result in a narrowed laryngeal inlet in children. Adolescents and adults can tolerate up to 50% narrowing of the airway without obvious respiratory distress, whereas infants and children experience significant respiratory compromise with this degree of restriction.

   Children, specifically under the age of 8 years, have more elastic cervical spines. The increased elasticity places them at high risk for translational mobility and movement during flexion/extension. Also, they can tolerate significant stretching without tearing, which can cause pseudosubluxation. In addition, their relatively large heads, hypermobile spines, and weak neck muscles (specifically the underdeveloped paraspinous muscles) make them particularly susceptible to upper cervical fractures. Higher fulcrum location in the necks of children also contributes to an increased incidence of upper cervical fractures, specifically those fractures located from the occiput to C2. In infants, the fulcrum is present at C2-C3. By the age of 5 to 6 years, the fulcrum shifts to C3-C4. It is not until the age of 8 years that the fulcrum is similar to those of adults, being located at C5-C6.

2. **Describe the three anatomic zones of the neck.**

   Zone I is the area between the thoracic inlet and the cricoid. Zone II extends from the cricoid to the angle of the mandible. Zone II is the most common site for penetrating trauma. Zone III includes the area above the angle of the mandible. Awareness of these landmarks and the anatomy present within each are valuable when evaluating and managing neck injuries.

3. **Name the major signs and symptoms of a laryngotracheal injury.**
   - Airway obstruction
   - Aphonia (loss of voice)
   - Cough
   - Crepitus
   - Drooling
   - Dysphagia (difficulty swallowing)
   - Dysphonia (change in voice)
   - Hoarseness
   - Hemoptysis
   - Neck deformity
   - Neck pain/tenderness
   - Odynophagia (painful swallowing)
   - Pneumomediastinum
   - Pneumothorax
   - Retractions
   - Stridor
   - Subcutaneous emphysema

4. **Describe the initial management for patients with penetrating neck injury.**

   The goals of management follow trauma guidelines with strict attention to airway, breathing, and circulation (ABCs). After the airway is assessed and breathing stabilized, control any hemorrhage and maintain good cervical spine precautions. Stabilize all penetrating objects in the neck, but keep them in place until they can be removed surgically. Obtain routine trauma laboratory studies, including type and crossmatch of blood for packed red blood cells. Minimal radiographic evaluation includes cervical spine films and chest radiographs.

5. How should the airway and breathing be managed in a child with a neck injury?
Most importantly, give all patients supplemental oxygen and treat them as if they have a cervical spine injury until proven otherwise.

Elective endotracheal intubation is not recommended unless backup measures, such as a surgical airway or fiberoptic intubation equipment, are available. If endotracheal intubation is to be completed, take special care to avoid hyperextension by using inline neck immobilization. If intubation is necessary, always intubate with two providers in order to ensure cervical spine safety.

Attempted placement of an endotracheal tube through an already injured airway may cause a small mucosal laceration to progress to complete transection. In cases of laryngotracheal separation, the transected ends of the trachea may separate by as much as 8 cm. Successful passage of an endotracheal tube across this distance is difficult and may delay or preclude airway control. Trauma to the airway may also produce a blind path and an inability to pass an endotracheal tube successfully. In the unstable airway, blind nasotracheal intubation is not recommended. If orotracheal intubation needs to be performed emergently, ensure that backup measures, such as surgical and anesthesia consultation, fiberoptic bronchoscopy, cricothyrotomy, and tracheostomy, are available in case of complications.

6. What are the major indications for surgical evaluation in patients with neck trauma?
   - Active bleeding/hemorrhagic shock
   - Airway obstruction
   - Cord paralysis
   - Decreased level of consciousness
   - Displaced fracture
   - Dysphagia
   - Dysphonia or hoarseness
   - Expanding or massive hematoma
   - Exposed cartilage
   - Foreign bodies
   - Hematemesis
   - Hemoptysis
   - Hemothorax
   - High-velocity wounds (gun, rifle, or explosion wounds)
   - Neurological deficits
   - Pneumothorax
   - Progressive respiratory distress
   - Unstable vital signs

7. How common are cervical spine injuries in children?
Cervical spine injuries are rare, occurring in only 1% to 2% of pediatric patients with injuries due to blunt trauma. Motor vehicle accidents account for most cervical spine injuries; however, falls, sports, firearms, nonaccidental trauma, and obstetric complications can also account for such injuries. Because a cervical spine injury can result in permanent disability or death, carefully evaluate patients with suspicious mechanisms of injury.

8. Which preexisting conditions put children at higher risk for cervical spine trauma?
   - Achondroplasia
   - Acute soft tissue or bony infection/infiltration
   - Cervical stenosis
   - Chiari malformation
   - Down syndrome
   - Klippel-Feil syndrome (congenital fusion of the cervical spine)
   - Morquio syndrome (odontoid hypoplasia)
   - Rheumatic disease

9. Which methods are helpful in immobilizing a patient with suspected cervical spine injury?
Soft cervical collars offer no stability to a potentially unstable cervical spine. Even hard collars (C-Breeze, XTW, Philadelphia, the Stifneck, Miami J, and Aspen) allow a significant amount of motion. Place patients with a suspected cervical spine fracture in a rigid cervical collar and immobilize them on a hard spine board. Sizing of the collar will depend on both the age of the patient and the type of collar used. Generally, apply the longest collar that does not hyperextend the neck. It should also not interfere with airway management but should provide support for the chin and jaw. Even with adequate immobilization, the patient may be able to flex or extend the neck approximately 20% to 60% depending on the type of collar used. Contraindications to the placement of a cervical collar include cervical swelling or the need for surgical intervention of the airway.

10. **Name symptoms or signs of cervical spine injury.**
    - Abnormal motor examination (paresis, paralysis, flaccidity, ataxia, spasticity, loss or decreased rectal tone)
    - Abnormal sensory examination
    - Altered mental status
    - Clonus without rigidity
    - Decreased bladder function
    - Diaphragmatic breathing without retractions
    - Hypothermia or hyperthermia
    - Fecal retention
    - Limitation of motion
    - Neck muscle spasm
    - Neck pain
    - Priapism
    - Spinal shock (hypotension with bradycardia, blood pressure variability with flushing and sweating)
    - Torticollis

11. **What type of cervical spine radiographs should I order for a child with a suspected neck injury?**
    Ideally, obtain three views—lateral, anteroposterior (AP), and odontoid (open mouth view). An adequate lateral view of the cervical spine should include the base of the skull and C1-T1. This has a sensitivity of 79% for the detection of fractures. With the addition of an AP view (visualization of C3-C7) and an odontoid view (visualization of C1-C2), sensitivity increases to 95%. However, the odontoid view is difficult to obtain and may not be useful in children less than 8 years of age. Be sure the initial three views adequately demonstrate all cervical vertebrae, including the relationship of C7 to T1. If C7-T1 is not visualized, obtain a swimmer's view.
    Pediatric cervical spine films can also be difficult to interpret due to the large amount of cartilage and variability of the retropharyngeal space related to the child's crying or respiratory patterns. Therefore if a patient is still symptomatic, consider further imaging tests such as cervical spine computed tomography (CT) or magnetic resonance imaging (MRI) of the cervical spine.

12. **What about flexion-extension views? Are they helpful?**
    The clinical value of flexion-extension views is questionable, and their use in the acute evaluation of neck injuries is controversial. Do not obtain these routinely. They should not be used in an acute trauma evaluation or in a patient with preexisting neck pain at rest. For alert patients with neck pain, normal plain films (three views), and no neurological deficits, flexion-extension views are sometimes ordered. These x-rays are obtained while the patient independently flexes and extends the neck, only until the child feels pain or discomfort.

13. **What is the best way to read cervical spine radiographs?**
    Use a systematic approach, such as the ABCS method:
    - **A: A**lignment. Assess the following four lines: anterior vertebral line, posterior vertebral line, spinolaminar line, and spinous process line. The spinal cord lies between the posterior vertebral line and the spinolaminar line. Also assess for lordotic curves, malalignment, subluxation, or distraction.
    - **B: B**ones. Evaluate for fractures in all parts of the vertebrae.
    - **C: C**artilage. Cartilage is radiolucent on cervical spine radiographs. Compression or widening of the intervertebral space may indicate a cartilage disruption.
    - **S: S**oft tissues. Because a child's spinal column contains a significant amount of cartilage, prevertebral soft tissue swelling may be the only clue to a cartilage or ligament injury. The prevertebral space at C2 or C3 should be less than half the width of the adjacent vertebral body. Abnormal swelling of the prevertebral space may be due to blood or edema.

14. **When should a CT or MRI of the cervical spine be ordered for a suspected cervical spine injury?**
    CT identifies fractures but is not ideal for evaluation of the spinal cord or ligaments. It is useful in the secondary evaluation of a possible cervical spine fracture when plain radiographs are difficult to obtain/interpret, are noted to be abnormal, or if there is a high suspicion of injury despite normal radiographs. CT is often also used for younger children who are unable to obtain an odontoid view and have a high suspicion of a C1-C2 traumatic injury. Given the low incidence of pediatric cervical spine injuries and the increased radiation exposure with CT, do not use CT as a primary radiographic evaluation in patients with a possible cervical spine fracture. The National Institute for Health Care Excellence advises a CT scan of the cervical spine for these risk factors: Glasgow Coma Scale <13 on arrival, if intubated, focal neurological signs, paresthesia of the upper/lower limbs, a strong suspicion of injury despite negative radiographs or inadequate radiographs.
    MRI is not ideal for identifying bony fractures. If a cervical spine injury is diagnosed, obtain an MRI to evaluate the ligaments and spinal cord for potential injuries, such as disk herniation, spinal cord edema, hemorrhage, compression, or transection. MRI is also valuable in the obtunded, intubated, or uncooperative patient, as well as the child with persistent or delayed neurological symptoms.

15. **What is the National Emergency X-Radiography Utilization Study (NEXUS)?**
   The NEXUS was a multicenter, prospective, observational study of emergency department (ED) patients with blunt trauma for whom cervical spine imaging was ordered. The results of the study suggested which patients would benefit from imaging and which would not. According to the NEXUS, patients must meet *all five* of the following criteria to be considered low risk and therefore would not need cervical spine imaging:
   1. No midline cervical tenderness
   2. No evidence of intoxication
   3. No altered level in mental status
   4. No focal neurological deficit
   5. No distracting or painful injury
       If a patient does not meet all five of these criteria, evaluate for a possible cervical spine injury with radiographic imaging. Do not use this rule in children younger than 9 years of age as the original study included only a small population of children under this age (and no children under the age of 2 years). Therefore these criteria may not have the same validity in comparison to older children and adults. A recent systematic review showed weak support (low sensitivity, reliability, clinical acceptability) for applying NEXUS criteria to determine the need for cervical spine imaging in children.

16. **What is pseudosubluxation of C2 on C3? How do you differentiate it from the anterior subluxation of C2 on C3?**
   Pseudosubluxation is a normal variant seen in approximately 25% of patients up to 16 years of age. It is due to ligamentous laxity and horizontal positioning of facet joints. Anterior subluxation of C2 on C3 is usually caused by a hyperflexion injury following a hyperextension injury with a possible associated spinal cord injury. Swischuk's "posterior cervical line" (Fig. 59.1) is helpful in distinguishing pseudosubluxation from true anterior subluxation on a lateral cervical film. A line is drawn from the cortex of the spinous process of C1 to the cortex of the spinous process of C3. If the line is located more than 1.5 to 2.0 mm anterior to the cortex of the spinous process of C2, suspect a fracture of C2.

17. **What is a Jefferson fracture?**
   A Jefferson fracture (Fig. 59.2) is a burst fracture of C1. C1 becomes compressed between the occipital condyles of the skull on the lateral masses of C2 secondary to an axial load, such as with a diving injury. Patients may

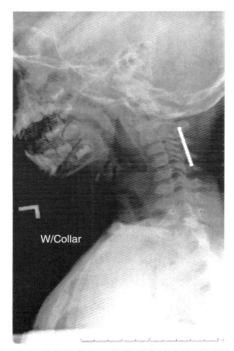

W/Collar

Fig. 59.1 Posterior cervical line. (From Easter JS, Barkin R, Rosen CL, Ban K. Cervical spine injuries in children, part II: management and special considerations. *J Emerg Med.* 2011;41(3):252–217.)

present with severe neck pain, especially with rotation. Although patients rarely have neurological symptoms because the fracture bursts outward and does not impair the spinal cord, a Jefferson fracture is unstable and needs to be immobilized immediately. The odontoid view may show the lateral masses offset or overriding the vertebral body of C2. Radiographic criteria include a lateral offset of the lateral masses of C1 greater than 1 mm from the vertebral body of C2.

This fracture can be confused with a pseudo-Jefferson fracture, which is a normal variant due to the child's growth. Children's lateral masses of C1 grow faster than the vertebral body of C2; often the lateral masses override C2 either unilaterally or bilaterally. A pseudo-Jefferson fracture can be present in up to 90% of children under the age of 2 years but usually normalizes by the age of 4 years. If in doubt, CT of the cervical spine at C1 and C2 is helpful in making the diagnosis.

18. **What is a hangman's fracture?**
A hangman's fracture (Fig. 59.3) results from severe hyperextension of the neck. During hyperextension, there is compression of the posterior elements of C2, which can cause a fracture of the pars interarticularis of C2. This type of fracture can also have ligamentous damage secondary to hyperflexion after the hyperextension. Ligamentous damage can lead to anterior subluxation of C2 on C3 and thus damage the cervical spinal cord. Use Swischuk's "posterior cervical line" in distinguishing pseudosubluxation from a subtle hangman's fracture on a lateral cervical film. Patients with this injury usually present after a motor vehicle crash, and they may have neck pain but often no neurological findings. Immobilize the cervical spine of these patients.

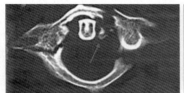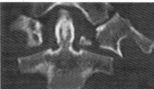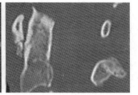

Fig. 59.2 Jefferson fracture (*arrow*) with offset of lateral masses. (From Lekic N, Sheu J, Ennis H, Lebwohl N, Al-Maaieh M. Why you should wear your seatbelt on an airplane: burst fracture of the atlas (Jefferson fracture) due to in-flight turbulence. *J Orthop.* 2019;17:78–82.)

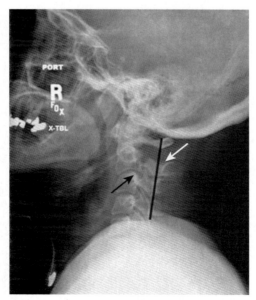

Fig. 59.3 Hangman's fracture: fracture of the pars interarticularis of C2. Anteriolisthesis of C2 on C3 (*black arrow*). Posterior displacement of C2 (*white arrow*). Spinolaminar line (*black line*). (From Giauque AP, Bittle MM, Braman JP. Type I hangman's fracture. *Curr Probl Diagn Radiol.* 2012;41(4):116–117.)

19. **Why is it recommended that patients with Down syndrome receive cervical spine screening radiographs prior to sports participation?**
Approximately 15% of patients with Down syndrome have atlantoaxial subluxation (AAS) secondary to atlantoaxial instability (AAI), and many with this condition will be asymptomatic. AAI occurs because of transverse ligament laxity (the most common reason in patients with Down syndrome) or when a fractured den allows movement between C1 and C2. If AAI progresses to AAS, it will be demonstrated on the lateral cervical spine radiograph with a widening of the predental space. A normal predental space should be less than 3 mm in adults and less than 4 to 5 mm in children. Neurological symptoms such as abnormal gait, loss of sphincter control, and/or paralysis may be seen if the predental space is 7 to 10 mm. In addition to Down syndrome, AAI has been associated with minor trauma in patients with connective tissue disorders, arthritis, and pharyngitis.

20. **What is SCIWORA?**
SCIWORA (i.e., **S**pinal **C**ord **I**njury **W**ith**O**ut **R**adiographic **A**bnormality) describes an acute spinal cord injury with sensory and/or motor deficits but no radiographic evidence of vertebral fracture or bony misalignment on plain radiographs or computed tomography (CT). It is usually seen in children younger than 8 years because of the increased amount of cartilage and elastic nature of the younger child's vertebral column. The child with a spine injury may present with an abnormal neurological examination caused by a vascular or ligamentous injury and no evidence of a fracture on plain radiography or CT. Neurosurgical consultation is recommended for this type of injury, as is MRI to further evaluate the cervical spine and spinal cord. MRI is the gold standard for spinal cord injuries and has made it possible to identify injuries missed by plain radiography and CT scans. Children diagnosed with SCIWORA who have normal MRI findings have better outcomes than those with cervical cord abnormalities noted on MRI.

21. **Describe the initial appropriate treatment of a child with a spinal cord injury.**
First, focus on the ABCs of trauma management. Children with spinal cord injury may present with hypotension, bradycardia, and warm or flushed peripheral extremities (spinal shock) because of the loss of sympathetic input. They need fluid resuscitation and inotropic support. A common mistake is to treat patients with spinal shock as if they have hypovolemic shock and to overload them with fluids. (Remember that patients with hypovolemic shock present with tachycardia.) If the child is not improving after aggressive fluid resuscitation, consider spinal shock and use inotropic support to stabilize their blood pressure.

22. **Why is the administration of steroids in pediatric spinal cord injuries controversial and no longer recommended?**
Experts in emergency medicine and neurosurgery questioned the potential benefit of steroids for a traumatic cervical spine injury. Children younger than 13 years of age were excluded from the studies, and some experts feel the potential risks of steroids are greater than the potential neurological benefits. The administration of high-dose steroids is not recommended in most types of pediatric spinal cord injury. Give steroids only after consultation with a neurosurgeon or trauma surgeon.

23. **How do you differentiate benign torticollis from atlantoaxial rotary subluxation?**
Benign torticollis is due to a muscular spasm of the sternocleidomastoid muscle (SCM). On examination the patient's head will be tilted toward the affected SCM and the chin will be rotated away. If there is a history of trauma prior to the development of pain, plain radiographs may help differentiate benign torticollis from other serious causes. Treatment generally includes soft collar placement, rest, and analgesia.
Atlantoaxial rotary subluxation is due to a rotational displacement of C1 on C2 and can occur after minor trauma, upper respiratory tract infections, pharyngeal surgery, or with certain congenital cervical malformations. These patients look similar to those with benign torticollis; however, the spasm of the SCM is on the same side toward which the chin points. With this condition, odontoid views can be helpful. They may demonstrate asymmetry of the lateral masses of C1 in relation to the odontoid. Specifically, one of the lateral masses of C1 is medially offset and will appear rotated forward, wider, and closer to the midline. The other lateral mass is laterally offset and will appear more narrow and farther from the midline. Reconstructive CT views can help evaluate the location of C1 upon C2, but if there are neurological changes on examination, MRI is the preferred test of choice to evaluate for cord compression. Treatment includes management of the underlying cause and neck immobilization. Treatment for mild rotary subluxation includes soft collar and analgesia, although more severe cases require neurosurgical consultation and may require further immobilization, traction, and possibly fusion of the cervical spine.

24. **What are the main differences between anterior cord syndrome, central cord syndrome, Brown-Séquard syndrome, and complete cord syndrome?**
Anterior cord syndrome is due to hyperflexion injuries and anterior cord compression. Compression of the anterior cord involves injury to the spinothalamic tract, which is responsible for motor function and the body's response to pain, light touch, and temperature sensation. Injury of the anterior cord results in paralysis and loss of pain, light touch, and temperature sensation below the level of vertebral injury. Proprioceptive functions and vibratory sense remain intact.
Central cord syndrome is usually seen in older patients with degenerative spinal disease; however, it can be seen in children with hyperextension injuries. Injury of the central cord results in weakness that is greater in the

upper extremities in comparison to the lower extremities. Patients can also have a transient burning sensation in their hands.

Brown-Séquard syndrome is caused by hemisection of the spinal cord, most often secondary to penetrating trauma. Injury to this area results in contralateral loss of pain and temperature sensation with ipsilateral loss of motor function, light touch sensation, and proprioception below the level of vertebral injury.

Complete cord syndrome is due to complete transection of the spinal cord, most often from penetrating or blunt trauma. It results in a complete loss of all neurological function below the level of injury. This type of injury is most often responsible for neurogenic shock.

25. **How should a spine board be modified when immobilizing an injured young child?**
The standard backboard may be hazardous to a young child with a neck injury. A young child's head is disproportionately large compared to that of an adult. On a standard hard spine board, the young child's neck is forced into a relative kyphotic position. It is therefore important to take steps to allow neutral positioning of the cervical spine of an injured young child. Use a special board with an occipital recess or modify a standard spine board with a mattress pad under the trunk to achieve neutral positioning of the cervical spine. Remove the patient from the spinal board as soon as you are able to do so, to avoid complications such as pressure sores, pain, or respiratory compromise.

KEY POINTS: NECK AND CERVICAL SPINE TRAUMA

1. Pediatric anatomy differs significantly from adults. Consider this when diagnosing and managing children with cervical spine injuries.
2. Cervical spine injuries occur in only 1% to 2% of pediatric patients.
3. Obtain radiographs for any pediatric trauma patient with an altered mental status, abnormal neurological examination, point tenderness of the cervical spine, or pain with rotation. Use CT and MRI as adjuncts and not for first-line imaging.
4. One view is no view—at a minimum, for patients with suspected cervical spine injuries, order lateral, anteroposterior, and odontoid radiographs.
5. The administration of high-dose steroids is not recommended for most types of spinal cord injuries. Consult a neurosurgeon or trauma surgeon before giving steroids.
6. When in doubt, immobilize, obtain imaging studies, and consult a neurosurgeon or trauma surgeon.

BIBLIOGRAPHY

1. Abujamra L, Joseph MM. Penetrating neck injuries in children: a retrospective review. *Pediatr Emerg Care.* 2003;19(5):308–313.
2. Atesok K, Tanaka N, O'Brien A, Robinson Y, et al. Posttraumatic spinal cord injury without radiographic abnormality. *Adv Orthop.* 2018;2018:7060654.
3. Babcock L, Olsen C, Jaffe D, et al. Cervical spine injuries in children associated with sports and recreational activities. *Pediatr Emerg Care.* 2018;34(10):677–686.
4. Bauer JM, Dhaliwal VK, Browd SR, Krengel WF. Repeat pediatric Trisomy 21 radiographic exam: Does atlantoaxial instability develop over time? *J Pediatr Orthop.* 2021;41(8):e646–e650.
5. Caruso MC, Daugherty MC, Moody SM, Falcone RA, et al. Lessons learned from administration of high-dose methylprednisolone sodium succinate for acute pediatric spinal cord injuries. *J Neurosurg Pediatr.* 2017;20(6):567–574.
6. Cheng J, Cooper M, Tracy E. Clinical considerations for blunt laryngotracheal trauma in children. *J Pediatr Surg.* 2017;52(5):874–880.
7. Copley PC, Tilliridou V, Kirby A, Jones J, et al. Management of cervical spine trauma in children. *Eur J Trauma Emerg Surg.* 2019;45(5):777–789.
8. Ekhator C, Nwankwo I, Nicol A. Implementation of National Emergency X-Radiography Utilization Study (NEXUS) criteria in pediatrics: a systematic review. *Cureus.* 2022;14(10):e30065.
9. Hurlbert RJ, Hadley MN, Walters BC. Pharmacolgical therapy for spinal cord injury. *Neurosurgery.* 2013;72(S2):93–105.
10. Kalanjiyam GP, Kanna RM, Rajasekaran S. Pediatric spinal injuries—current concepts. *J Clin Orthop Trauma.* 2023;38:102122. https://doi.org/10.1016/j.jcot.2023.102122.
11. Khan SN, Erickson G, Sena MJ, et al. Use of flexion and extension radiographs of the cervical spine to rule out acute instability in patients with negative computed tomography scans. *J Orthop Trauma.* 2011;25(1):51–56.
12. Leonard JR, Jaffe DM, Kupperman N, et al. Cervical spine injury patterns in children. *Pediatrics.* 2014;133:e1179–e1188.
13. Low GM, Inaba K, Chouliaras K, et al. The use of anatomic zones of the neck in the assessment of penetrating neck injury. *Am Surg.* 2014;80(10):970–974.
14. Mahajan P, Jaffe DM, Olsen CS, Leonard JR, et al. Spinal cord injury without radiologic abnormality in children imaged with magnetic resonance imaging. *J Trauma Acute Care Surg.* 2013;75(5):843–847.
15. Shin JI, Lee NJ, Cho SK. Pediatric cervical spine and spinal cord injury: a national database study. *Spine.* 2016;41:283–292.
16. Slaar A, Fockens M, Wang J, et al. Triage tools for detecting cervical spine injury in pediatric trauma patients. *Cochrane Database Syst Rev.* 2017;12CD011686.
17. Stone ME, Farber BA, Olorunfemi O, Kalata S, et al. Penetrating neck trauma in children: an uncommon entity described using the National Trauma Data Bank. *J Trauma Acute Care Surg.* 2016;80(4):604–609.
18. Wagner R, Jagoda A. Spinal cord syndromes. *Emerg Med Clin North Am.* 1997;15(3):699–711.
19. Woodward GA, Keilman A. Neck trauma. In: Shaw KN, Bachur RG, eds. *Fleisher & Ludwig's Textbook of Pediatric Emergency Medicine.* 8th ed. Wolters Kluwer; 2021:1214–1253.

PELVIC TRAUMA AND GENITOURINARY INJURY

Hannah Carron and Timothy Brenkert

1. **Why are children more likely to sustain renal injuries than adults?**
   - Children have weaker abdominal musculature, less-ossified thoracic cage, and less-developed perirenal fat and fascia to protect the kidneys.
   - Kidneys are disproportionately larger in relation to body size.
   - Kidneys retain fetal lobulations that allow for easier parenchymal disruption.

2. **Describe the most common mechanisms for renal injury in pediatric patients.**
   More than 90% of pediatric renal injury is secondary to blunt trauma, with <10% of cases involving a penetrating mechanism. Trauma that involves either a direct blow to the flank or rapid deceleration is an important predictor for potential kidney trauma. Thus accidents involving motor vehicles or bicycles, falls from heights, or direct blows in sports are often responsible for renal injury.

3. **Describe the potential complications, both immediate and delayed, of renal injury.**
   Contusion and minor cortical lacerations typically heal without sequelae. More severe injuries may be associated with secondary or delayed hemorrhage, perinephric abscess formation, or extravasation of urine. Later complications include impaired renal function, urinomas, or development of arteriovenous fistulas. Chronic hypertension following renal trauma has been shown to occur for up to 32 years after injury. Regular, long-term monitoring of blood pressure is recommended for these patients.

4. **What is the cardinal laboratory marker of renal injury?**
   Hematuria is the most important laboratory evidence of renal injury, and yet it has been reported to be absent in up to 36% of renal pedicle injuries and in 29% of patients with penetrating injuries. In addition, the degree of hematuria does not correlate well with the level of injury. In stable patients sustaining blunt trauma, imaging is recommended for those with >50 red blood cells per high-power field (RBCs/hpf) on urinalysis. Imaging is also indicated in trauma patients with gross hematuria, microscopic hematuria with shock, >5 RBCs/hpf in the setting of penetrating trauma, or those with clinical findings indicative of renal trauma.

5. **How are renal injuries classified?**
   The Organ Injury Scaling Committee of the American Association for the Surgery of Trauma developed a scaling system to facilitate clinical research, to risk-stratify patients for quality measures, and for billing and coding purposes. These were revised in 2018 to the following:
   - Grade I: Subcapsular hematoma or parenchymal contusion without laceration
   - Grade II: Perirenal hematoma confined to Gerota fascia, or lacerations <1 cm in depth without urinary extravasation
   - Grade III: Vascular injury with bleeding confined to Gerota fascia or parenchymal lacerations >1 cm in depth without urinary extravasation or collecting system rupture
   - Grade IV: Vascular injury with bleeding beyond Gerota fascia and into retroperitoneum or peritoneum, vessel thrombosis with renal infarction and absence of active bleeding, or lacerations of renal pelvis or parenchyma that extend into the collecting system with urinary extravasation
   - Grade V: Shattered kidney, organ devascularization with active bleeding, avulsion of the hilum, or laceration of the main renal artery or vein

6. **Which imaging modality is considered the diagnostic test of choice for the evaluation of renal injuries?**
   CT is considered the diagnostic test of choice for the detection of renal injury in pediatric trauma patients. It not only delineates the degree of renal parenchymal injury with high accuracy but also assesses other intra-abdominal, retroperitoneal, and pelvic injuries simultaneously. However, this test is relatively expensive, subjects the child to radiation, and requires a hemodynamically stable patient who can tolerate transport to the radiology suite. Currently, there remains a lack of evidence with regards to the diagnostic accuracy of ultrasound for renal trauma in the pediatric population. While the use of Focused Assessment with Sonography for Trauma (FAST) evaluation addresses many of the issues with CT use, the operator dependence and varied sensitivity of this test do not allow it to replace CT as the preferred initial imaging modality for renal injuries.

7. **How common are bladder injuries in pediatric patients?**
   Up to 18% of children with pelvic fractures have a concomitant bladder injury. As compared to adults, the bladder's location in children is more exposed above the protective pelvic ring, increasing the risk of potential injury. Although symptoms may be nonspecific, maintain a high suspicion in patients with abdominal distention, urinary retention, suprapubic tenderness, or gross hematuria, particularly if a pelvic fracture is present.

8. **In what clinical scenario should you suspect a ureteral injury?**
   Ureteral lesions occur in <1% of pediatric abdominal trauma. Penetrating trauma and iatrogenic injuries during surgical procedures are the most common cause, though a sudden hyperextension of the pediatric spine in high-energy deceleration trauma can also result in ureteral injury as the ureter is disrupted from the renal pelvis. The physical examination may be unremarkable, but an enlarging flank mass in the absence of other signs of retroperitoneal bleeding may indicate underlying urinary extravasation. Hematuria is an unreliable marker, as the urinalysis can be normal in >40% of these patients. If the presentation is delayed, symptoms can include fever, chills, lethargy, pyuria or bacteriuria, or flank pain or mass.

9. **What are the hallmark signs of urethral injury?**
   - Blood at the urethral meatus
   - Perineal/penile hematoma
   - Pain with voiding, or inability to void

10. **What are the indications for urethrography in pediatric trauma patients?**
    Retrograde urethrography is the radiological method of choice for the diagnosis of urethral injuries. It should be performed in any child with penetrating trauma and suspected genitourinary injuries; perineal trauma with hematuria; inability to void or to advance a urinary catheter; vaginal laceration or bleeding; swelling, hematoma, or ecchymosis of the perineum; blood at the urethral meatus; and high-riding or boggy prostate.

14. **Describe the most common mechanisms causing blunt perineal injury in children.**
    Pediatric perineal injury is uncommon; it occurs in <1% of all pediatric injuries. Eighty percent of cases are secondary to straddle injuries, in which a child straddles a long horizontal object during a fall, such as playground equipment, a bicycle bar, or the edge of a bathtub. Other perineal injuries occur after motor vehicle collisions, usually in the setting of other multisystem trauma. Sexual assault is another mechanism for perineal injury; its incidence is highest in children 0 to 4 years old and is responsible for 17% of injuries in this population.

15. **Describe the management considerations of a pediatric patient with straddle injury.**
    In straddle injuries, soft tissues become compressed between the object and the pelvic bones, leading to hematomas and edema. Swelling may lead to urethral obstruction. The practitioner should consider early placement of a Foley catheter to avoid this complication. Given the highly vascular nature of genital tissue, minor abrasions and lacerations not only can lead to profuse bleeding but can also often heal rapidly with conservative management. Surgical consultation may be needed for vaginal bleeding, anorectal involvement, or inability to maintain hemostasis of an external laceration. The evaluation of a child with genital trauma is frequently limited secondary to fear, anxiety, and pain. In a cooperative child, the genitalia can be gently irrigated and inspected to determine if the injury is superficial or extensive. Superficial injuries can be managed at home with analgesics

and sitz baths. Extensive wounds need surgical consultation. These patients sometimes require a more thorough examination under sedation or anesthesia.

16. **When should a vulvar hematoma be drained?**
    Vulvar hematomas are more common in children than adults due to underdeveloped protective fat pads in the highly vascularized labia majora, and the increased risk of straddle injury especially involving bicycles. Drainage should be avoided; bleeding is often from multiple venous sites (making isolation of vascular injury difficult), and opening the area places the patient at risk for infection. Most hematomas will resolve with conservative management including ice, pain control, and bed rest to allow for tamponade. If swelling from a large hematoma obstructs the urethra, a Foley catheter may be placed. Drainage is indicated only in cases of quickly expanding hematomas causing a drop in hemoglobin and/or clinical instability, or if there is tissue necrosis.

17. **When is surgical evaluation needed prior to the repair of a scrotal laceration?**
    Laceration of the scrotal skin can occur with any scrotal trauma. Blunt trauma may occur in the setting of falls, kicks, straddle injuries, or motor vehicle collisions. Penetrating trauma may occur from falls with impalement, animal or human bites, or gunshot wounds. The scrotum is highly vascularized and has inherent elasticity, making most scrotal wounds relatively superficial. Lacerations involving only the skin layer can be repaired with absorbable suture. Lidocaine with epinephrine usually provides appropriate analgesia, given locally or regionally through a penile block. Lacerations involving the dartos layer warrant surgical evaluation given the high rate of associated testicular rupture, in which the tunica albuginea is breached, leading to extravasation of testicular contents into the scrotal sac. This is a surgical emergency; there is a higher chance of testicular salvage if exploration is done within 24 hours after the injury.

18. **Describe the management of zipper entrapment of the penis or foreskin.**
    Numerous methods to release zipper entrapment of the foreskin have been utilized; most use bone or wire cutters. The tool is used to split the median bar of the zipper fastener, thus allowing the two sides of the zipper to release the entrapped tissue (Fig. 60.1). Alternatively, a simple, noninvasive method to free the foreskin involves the use of mineral oil. Liberally apply mineral oil to the involved tissue and allow the penis/foreskin to soak for 15 to 20 minutes. The trapped skin may then be easily released. One report notes that the head of a small flat-head screwdriver may be inserted between the faceplates of the fastener opposite the median bar from the site of entrapped tissue. With a rotating motion, the faceplates can be separated from one another, releasing the injured tissue. Warm soaks may be used after the procedure to control edema. Some children may require sedation or local anesthetics to assist with pain control.

19. **When can depilatory agents be used to manage hair-thread tourniquet syndrome?**
    Hair-thread tourniquet syndrome occurs when a hair or thread becomes tightly wound around a finger, toe, or genitalia (such as penis, clitoris, or labia). This most commonly happens after a parent's hair falls onto an infant during bathing or diapering. There is constricted lymphatic and venous drainage, with subsequent pain, swelling,

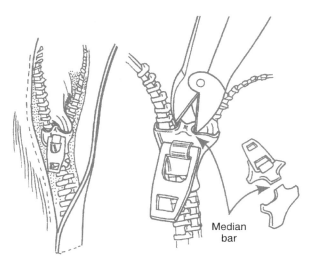

Median
bar

Fig. 60.1 Standard zipper fasteners contain a median bar; bone or wire cutters can be used to split this median bar and release entrapped tissue.

discoloration, and irritability. In more severe cases, the thread can become embedded in the soft tissue and cause tissue ischemia or necrosis. In pediatrics, the use of depilatory agents is especially helpful given the decreased need for sedation and analgesia. To use depilatory agents, the area must have minimal skin breakdown, cannot be near a mucosal surface (i.e., not involve the clitoris or labia), and should be constricted by a known hair. If contraindicated or unsuccessful, the provider can attempt mechanical removal using fine forceps, a blunt probe, and a scalpel. Topical lidocaine may be helpful.

20. **What are the potential complications of burns to the perineum and/or genitalia, and how can they be prevented?**
Burns to the perineum and genitalia usually occur in the setting of other burns. Accidental scald burns are most common, in which children spill hot food or beverage onto their lap. These burns will demonstrate a splash pattern with irregular borders and depth. If this is inconsistent, consider child abuse. Major sequelae from perineal burns include genitourinary and sexual dysfunction and infection. In the acute setting, have a low threshold for urinary catheter placement to avoid obstruction secondary to edema and stricture formation. Surgical consultation can help optimize successful and minimally traumatic placement. Careful cleaning and debridement are also important to prevent infection, given the polymicrobial nature of the area.

KEY POINTS: MANAGEMENT CONSIDERATIONS FOR PERINEAL INJURY

1. This highly vascularized area leads to profuse bleeding and likely heals with conservative management.
2. Swelling and/or hematoma can lead to compressive urethral obstruction requiring urinary catheter placement.
3. Management will likely require anxiolytic and/or sedative medications to assist in thorough evaluation and interventions.
4. Always consider abuse with injuries in the perineal region.

---

21. **How does pediatric pelvic trauma differ from that of adults?**
Pediatric bones are more pliable with thicker periosteum compared to adult bones. Also, pediatric ligaments and tendons are relatively stronger than their adjacent bones and apophyses. These differences make pelvic avulsion fractures and isolated pelvic ring fractures more common in children; complete pelvic ring fractures require significantly higher force.

22. **How do children with pelvic fractures typically present?**
Pediatric pelvic fractures have a reported incidence of 0.3% to 4% of pediatric injuries. Given the pliability of their bones relative to adults, pelvic fractures in pediatric patients are usually (83.3%) the result of high-energy blunt trauma such as motor vehicle collisions and are associated with multisystem injury. Patients with significant pelvic fractures may present with unstable vital signs (62.8% of cases) as brisk bleeding collects in the pelvis or in massive retroperitoneal hematomas and in isolated ring fractures. However, vital signs are often close to normal. Examination findings suggestive of pelvic ring fractures include pain and instability elicited by pelvic rocking at the anterior iliac spines, and pain and crepitus with firm pressure over the pubis.

23. **What are the indications for CT scan to assess for pelvic fracture in pediatric trauma patients?**
Plain radiographs have limited sensitivity for detecting pediatric pelvic fractures; however, they are often done before a CT scan in a patient with blunt trauma in accordance with Advanced Trauma Life Support guidelines. CT imaging is much more specific and is helpful to better characterize pelvic fractures (to more clearly view the posterior pelvic ring, for example). Indications for obtaining CT of the abdomen and pelvis include the following:
- Radiograph showing pelvic ring injury
- Concern for unstable pelvis on examination
- Concern for intra-abdominal injury on examination, radiograph, or ultrasound

24. **Is a pelvic fracture predictive of a genitourinary injury in pediatric patients?**
A review of the literature has found that associated genitourinary injury is seen in 11% to 12% of pediatric pelvic fractures. This incidence increases to 40% to 50% with multiple fractures to the pelvic ring. The presence of multiple pelvic fractures is also the best predictor of intra-abdominal injury in these patients.

BIBLIOGRAPHY

1. Casey JT, Bjurlin MA, Cheng EY. Pediatric genital injury: an analysis of the National Electronic Injury Surveillance System. *Urology.* 2013;82(5):1125–1130.
2. Coccolini F, Moore EE, Kluger Y, et al. Kidney and uro-trauma: WSES-AAST guidelines. *World J Emerg Surg.* 2019:14–54.
3. Dangle PP, Fuller TW, Gaines B, et al. Evolving mechanisms of injury and management of pediatric blunt renal trauma: 20 years of experience. *Urology.* 2016;90:159–163.

4. Fein J, Zderic SA. Management of zipper injuries. In: Henretig FM, King C, eds. *Textbook of Pediatric Emergency Procedures.* Williams & Wilkins; 2008:980.
5. Fernandez-Ibieta M. Renal trauma in pediatrics: a current review. *Urology.* 2018;113:171–178.
6. Gänsslen A, Heidari N, Weinberg AM. Fractures of the pelvis in children: a review of the literature. *Eur J Orthop Surg Traumatol.* 2013;23:847–861.
7. Kozar RA, Crandall M, Shanmuganathan K, et al. Organ injury scaling 2018 update: spleen, liver, and kidney. *J Trauma Acute Care Surg.* 2018;85(6):1119–11122.
8. Kwok MY, Yen K, Atabaki S, et al. Sensitivity of plain pelvis radiography in children with blunt torso trauma. *Ann Emerg Med.* 2015;65:63.
9. O'Brien K, Fei F, Quint E, Dendrinos M. Non-obstetric traumatic vulvar hematomas in premenarchal and postmenarchal girls. *J Pediatr Adolesc Gynecol.* 2022;35(5):546–551.
10. O'Gorman A, Ratnapalan S. Hair tourniquet management. *Pediatr Emerg Care.* 2011;27:203.
11. Raveenthiran V. Releasing of zipper-entrapped foreskin: a novel nonsurgical technique. *Pediatr Emerg Care.* 2007;23(7):463–464.
12. Singer G, Arneitz C, Tschauner S, et al. Trauma in pediatric urology. *Semin Pediatr Surg.* 2021;30(4):151085.
13. Starnes M, Demetriades D, Hadjizacharia P, et al. Complications following renal trauma. *Arch Surg.* 2010;145(4):377–381.
14. Kovell R, Tasian GE, Belfer RA. Genitourinary trauma. In: Shaw KN, Bachur RG, Shaw KN, Bachur RG, eds. *Fleisher & Ludwig's Textbook of Pediatric Emergency Medicine.* 8th ed. Wolters Kluwer; 2021:1131–1142.

CHAPTER 61

THORACIC TRAUMA

Howard Kadish

1. **How common are thoracic injuries, and why are they important?**
   Among injured children, thoracic trauma is relatively uncommon. About 4% to 6% of pediatric trauma victims have a thoracic injury. Blunt mechanisms account for 85% of these injuries. Recognition of thoracic injuries is important because the mortality rate is high (15%-26%) for children with such trauma.

2. **What are the most common injuries in blunt and penetrating thoracic trauma?**
   - **Blunt thoracic trauma:** Lung contusions are most common, followed by pneumothorax or hemothorax, and then rib fractures.
   - **Penetrating thoracic trauma:** Pneumothorax and/or hemothorax are the predominant diagnoses, followed by diaphragmatic lacerations, cardiac injuries, and vascular injuries.

3. **How does thoracic trauma differ in children and adults?**
   Pediatric thoracic trauma differs from adult thoracic trauma in the mechanism of injury, type of injury, and other organ systems involved. Falls are the most common mechanism of injury in infants and children. Older children are often injured as pedestrians or unrestrained passengers in motor vehicle accidents. Adolescents are more likely to be occupants in motor vehicle–related accidents and to experience penetrating injuries secondary to violence.

   Overall, lung contusions are the most common pediatric thoracic injury, with intrapleural injury second. Only 30% of children, compared with 50% to 75% of adults, sustain rib fractures because of increased compliance in the pediatric thoracic cage due to increased cartilage content and greater elasticity of the bones. Thus a child may have an internal injury (lung contusion) without external evidence of trauma (rib fracture, laceration, bruising).

   The pediatric trachea has a smaller internal diameter than the adult trachea; therefore a small amount of obstruction secondary to blood, secretions, or edema can cause significant respiratory distress and hypoxia. The younger pediatric patient is also more sensitive to hypoxia and may develop reflex bradycardia or asystole.

   In evaluating pediatric patients with thoracic trauma, consider head, neck, and intra-abdominal injuries because approximately 80% of cases of thoracic trauma in children are part of a multisystem injury. Thoracic trauma is routinely associated with abdominal trauma in children because the chest and abdominal cavities lie in close proximity.

4. **How do I evaluate a patient with thoracic trauma?**
   The ABCDEs (airway, breathing, circulation, disability, exposure) of trauma management apply to patients with suspected thoracic injury. Indications for endotracheal intubation in pediatric patients with thoracic trauma include depressed neurologic status, inadequate oxygenation or ventilation, compromised circulatory status, and an unstable airway (including burns). If a patient has an abnormal examination but appears to be oxygenating and ventilating well and is not in shock, chest radiography is indicated. If breathing is inadequate after endotracheal intubation, with asymmetry of breath sounds, intervention is required prior to chest radiography. Consider pericardial tamponade, tension pneumothorax, or hemothorax in poorly perfused patients with signs of shock in whom other sources of blood loss have been excluded and volume resuscitation has not improved clinical status. Once the patient is stabilized and immediate life-threatening injuries, such as airway obstruction, tension pneumothorax, hemothorax, and pericardial tamponade, are treated, chest radiography and thoracic computed tomography (CT) provide valuable information about other potentially life-threatening and/or operative injuries.

5. **Which thoracic injuries require operative intervention?**
   - Tracheal/bronchial rupture
   - Laceration of lung parenchyma, internal mammary artery, or intercostal artery
   - Esophageal disruption
   - Diaphragmatic hernia
   - Pericardial tamponade
   - Great vessel laceration

6. **Describe signs and symptoms/findings related to each operative thoracic injury.**
   See Table 61.1 for the signs and symptoms of thoracic injuries.

7. **What signs and symptoms are associated with pulmonary contusion?**
   Most pulmonary contusions result from blunt trauma, generally a motor vehicle crash or a child hit by a car. Patients with moderate-to-severe pulmonary contusions may be tachypneic, with abnormal breath sounds and

Table 61.1 Signs and Symptoms/Findings of Thoracic Injuries

INJURY	SIGNS AND SYMPTOMS/FINDINGS
Tracheal/bronchial rupture	Active chest tube air leak
Lung parenchyma	Chest tube bleeding >2-3 mL/kg/hr
Internal mammary or intercostal artery laceration	Hypotension unresponsive to transfusions
Esophageal disruption	Abnormal esophagogram (leak) or esophagoscopic result
	Gastric contents in the chest tube
Diaphragmatic hernia	Abnormal gas pattern in hemithorax
	Displaced nasogastric tube in hemithorax
Pericardial tamponade	Distant heart sounds Poor perfusion Positive pericardiocentesis
Great vessel laceration	Widened mediastinum
	Tracheal or nasogastric tube deviation
	Blurred aortic knob
	Abnormal aortogram (gold standard)

an oxygen requirement secondary to shunting within the lung. In one study of patients with mild pulmonary contusions, a finding of tachypnea, tenderness, or abnormal breath sounds was 100% sensitive for all positive radiographs. However, the clinical features of pulmonary contusion may be subtle, especially just after the injury. Even the initial chest radiograph can appear normal or show only minimal abnormality. Carefully observe the patient's respiratory status after thoracic trauma.

8. **How should rib fractures be characterized?**
   Rib fractures may be characterized as upper zone (ribs 1-4), midzone (ribs 5-8), and lower zone (ribs 9-12). The location of the rib fracture determines the likelihood of serious associated injuries. The upper zone ribs are protected by the scapula, humerus, and clavicle; therefore a significant amount of force is required to fracture these ribs. When evaluating a patient with an upper zone rib fracture, it is important to consider other serious injuries such as a pulmonary contusion, injury to intrathoracic vessels, or cervical spine injury. Consider liver and spleen injuries with lower zone rib fractures. Children with rib fractures will likely splint and hypoventilate secondary to pain. Adequate pain control is, therefore, very important in the management of children with rib fractures. Otherwise, most isolated rib fractures will heal without complications in about 6 weeks. Rib fractures in children under 2 years of age are highly suggestive of child abuse.

9. **Describe flail chest and discuss the respective management.**
   Flail chest refers to paradoxical movement of a segment of the chest wall secondary to associated rib fractures, typically from a crush-type injury. If in distress, intubate the patient's trachea to improve lung expansion and ventilation. If the patient is stable, pain control and pulmonary care are prudent, as patients can develop atelectasis from hypoventilation. Flail chest is uncommon in children due to the increased compliance of the chest wall in comparison to adults but should be treated aggressively if identified.

10. **What signs and symptoms are associated with a pneumothorax?**
    Patients may be asymptomatic, report pleuritic chest pain, have tachypnea, or be in severe respiratory distress. Physical examination may be normal or reveal diminished or absent breath sounds, crepitus, or hyperresonance to percussion on the side of the pneumothorax.

11. **How do I diagnose and treat patients with pneumothorax?**
    In asymptomatic or mildly symptomatic patients, a chest radiograph is helpful in diagnosing and determining the type of treatment. If the pneumothorax is small and the patient is asymptomatic, hospital observation and administration of 100% oxygen may be all that is necessary. A small pneumothorax is classically described as smaller than 15%, although it is common to underestimate the size of a pneumothorax on plain films and to find a much more extensive lesion on a CT scan. If the patient is in respiratory or cardiovascular distress, the diagnosis is made clinically. Place a chest tube or a pigtail catheter when this is noted. Use a pigtail catheter only with a

pure pneumothorax (no blood). Chest tube or pigtail placement is also indicated in patients undergoing positive-pressure ventilation or requiring air transport. An asymptomatic patient may rapidly become symptomatic if a small, simple pneumothorax progresses to a tension pneumothorax.

12. **Should thoracic CT replace chest radiography in the initial management of blunt trauma in the pediatric patient?**
No. Even though CT has been shown to be more sensitive than chest radiography in diagnosing thoracic injuries, thoracic trauma makes up less than 20% of all pediatric traumas. Performing thoracic CT on all pediatric patients in trauma would increase costs and patient radiation dose, with little clinical improvement. Obtain a thoracic CT only in patients with suspected thoracic injury from clinical examination or chest radiograph.

13. **What is the role of bedside thoracic ultrasound in the initial management of blunt trauma in the pediatric patient?**
Thoracic ultrasound can also be used in the evaluation of thoracic trauma and is sensitive in identifying pleural air or fluid or a hemopericardium. It can be done quickly in the emergency department (ED) and avoid radiation. One disadvantage of bedside ultrasound is that it is operator dependent. CT remains the gold standard for the evaluation of underlying lung parenchyma injury.

14. **Should I be concerned about sternal and scapular fractures?**
Sternal and scapular fractures occur infrequently among children and usually are associated with significant mechanisms such as motor vehicle crashes. Sternal fractures may be associated with a pulmonary contusion, vertebral spine injury, and rib fractures. Blunt cardiac injury occurs uncommonly. Those with scapular fractures are more likely than those without scapular fractures to have serious associated injuries. Besides the usual intracranial, intrathoracic, and intra-abdominal injuries, consider axillary artery, brachial plexus, and great vessel injuries in these patients.

15. **How do I treat a patient with a tension pneumothorax?**
Initial treatment consists of needle decompression performed while the team is preparing for pigtail catheter or tube thoracostomy placement. A placement site at the fifth intercostal space in the anterior or midaxillary line or the traditional second or third intercostal space in the midclavicular line is appropriate. With a tension pneumothorax, an immediate release of air should be noted. If this sign is positive, needle decompression is only a temporizing measure and must be followed by tube thoracotomy. Tube thoracotomy or insertion of a pigtail catheter is usually done in the midaxillary line at the level of the fifth intercostal space (nipple level). Obtain chest radiography only after insertion of the chest tube/pigtail catheter. Do not use a radiograph to diagnose tension pneumothorax in symptomatic patients. One of the advantages of bedside thoracic ultrasound is that it can be done quickly in the ED while prepping the patient for a chest tube. If significant air leak continues after chest tube placement, consider a tracheobronchial rupture.

16. **How can I tell if a patient has a tracheobronchial injury?**
Injury to the tracheobronchial tree in children is rare (incidence <1%). The mortality rate for these injuries is very high, and many patients with a tracheobronchial injury will die at the scene. This injury is most commonly caused by acceleration or deceleration forces. The mechanism of injury (fall, crush, and direct blow) provides an important clue. Clinical signs include cyanosis, hemoptysis, tachypnea, and subcutaneous emphysema (cervical, mediastinal, or both). A continued air leak after the insertion of a thoracostomy tube should alert the physician to the possibility of a bronchial tear. In the absence of pneumothorax, suspect tracheal rupture if pneumomediastinum or cervical emphysema is present. Immediately consult a surgeon when this injury is suspected.

17. **How is a tracheobronchial injury treated?**
Treatment includes initial airway stabilization followed by bronchoscopic evaluation of the airway. According to numerous reports in the literature, a partial tracheal tear may become complete after endotracheal intubation. Therefore if the airway is stable, perform orotracheal intubation in the operating room under bronchoscopic guidance. If the airway is unstable and emergent endotracheal intubation is needed, prepare for backup measures, such as cricothyroidotomy, tracheostomy, or fiberoptic bronchoscopy.

18. **How can I tell if a patient has an esophageal injury?**
Esophageal injury is very rare in children but presents a diagnostic challenge when it does occur. The most common cause of esophageal perforation in children is iatrogenic, followed by penetrating trauma (gunshot or stab wound). Patients with an esophageal rupture in the cervical region may report neck stiffness or neck pain. They may regurgitate bloody material and have cervical subcutaneous emphysema or odynophagia. In the thoracic region, patients may present with abdominal spasms and guarding, chest pain, subcutaneous emphysema, tachycardia, or dyspnea. A lateral neck radiograph may show retroesophageal emphysema. A chest radiograph may show pneumothorax, pneumomediastinum, or an air-fluid level in the mediastinum. Esophagography, esophagoscopy, or both can make the diagnosis of esophageal perforation.

19. **How are esophageal injuries treated?**
Treat patients who have suspected esophageal perforation with adequate volume resuscitation, placement of a nasogastric tube, and antibiotics covering gram-positive, gram-negative, and anaerobic organisms. Once the diagnosis is made, prompt surgical correction is mandatory. If the diagnosis is made within 24 hours, the mortality rate is approximately 5%. Diagnosis delayed for more than 24 hours after injury is associated with a mortality rate of 70%.

20. **In the setting of thoracic trauma, what are some signs or symptoms concerning blunt cardiac injury?**
    * Arrhythmia or heart failure
    * Ecchymosis, abrasions, or deformity of the chest wall
    * Focal tenderness over the sternum or scapula
    * Muffled heart tones or a new murmur
    * Abnormal upper or lower extremity pulses

21. **How is the diagnosis of a traumatic rupture of the aorta (TRA) made?**
Consider a CT scan with contrast when an aortic injury is suspected clinically or by chest radiograph. Thoracic CT is only 55% to 65% accurate but helps to diagnose associated injuries. The gold standard for diagnosing TRA is aortography. In one study, transesophageal echocardiography was shown to be highly sensitive and specific for detecting injury to the thoracic aorta. If the patient is stable and TRA is a concern, obtain an aortography study. Evaluate for life-threatening intracranial, thoracic, or intra-abdominal injuries and stabilize the patient before aortography. If the patient is unstable, transesophageal echocardiography can be performed in the operating room while other life-threatening injuries are treated. Early diagnosis is imperative for patients with TRA. Morbidity and mortality rates increase threefold if operative intervention is delayed more than 12 hours.

22. **How do patients with pericardial tamponade present?**
Pericardial tamponade initially may be difficult to diagnose because associated injuries obscure the clinical signs and symptoms. Patients may present with distant heart sounds, low blood pressure, poor perfusion, narrow pulse pressure, or electromechanical dissociation. Pulsus paradoxus, with blood pressure falling more than 10 mm Hg during inspiration, occurs in less than half of patients with pericardial tamponade. Do not rely on this to make the diagnosis. Chest radiography may show an enlarged heart, and an electrocardiogram (ECG) may show low-voltage QRS waves. Neither of these tests is diagnostic for pericardial tamponade. In stable patients, an echocardiogram can demonstrate fluid within the pericardial sac. Do not delay treatment (pericardiocentesis) for unstable patients.

23. **What is the evaluation for a _stable_ patient at risk for a blunt cardiac injury?**
Obtain a plain chest radiograph. In cases of blunt cardiac injury, the radiograph may demonstrate cardiomegaly or noncardiac injuries (rib or sternal fractures).
    Obtain an ECG in any child with chest wall tenderness, chest pain, chest wall ecchymosis, abnormal heart sounds, or abnormal upper or lower extremity pulses. Biomarkers are not routinely obtained. The patient may be discharged to home in 4 to 6 hours if stable and if the chest radiograph and ECG are normal.

24. **What is the evaluation for an _unstable_ patient at risk for blunt cardiac injury?**
Besides a chest radiograph and ECG, performing a bedside ultrasound is helpful in identifying hemopericardium. If there is a persistent concern for cardiogenic shock, then a formal transthoracic echocardiogram looking for wall motion or valvular abnormalities is indicated. Troponin may be obtained and used as an adjunct in patients who are either clinically symptomatic or who have abnormal findings on chest radiograph or ECG.

25. **What conditions lead to sudden circulatory arrest after a nonpenetrating blow to the chest (commotio cordis)?**
    1. The blow strikes the chest in the area of the heart with force.
    2. The object has sufficient mass (baseball, hockey puck, lacrosse ball, knee).
    3. The blow strikes the chest during the ventricular vulnerable period (T wave).
    4. The ventricles have a large enough mass (>3.5 kg).

26. **We know that sudden cardiac arrest can be managed in the field with bystander cardiopulmonary resuscitation (CPR) and early defibrillation. How can physicians advocate for appropriate preparation for these events in the community?**
    * Working with local athletic associations (i.e., little league, football organizations) to ensure that coaches are CPR certified and that automated external defibrillators exist at each site.
    * Pediatricians can counsel families to ensure that protective equipment is worn by athletes, though commercially available chest wall protectors have not been proven to prevent cardiac arrest.

KEY POINTS: THORACIC TRAUMA

1. The most common injuries in blunt thoracic trauma are lung contusions, pneumothorax or hemothorax, and rib fractures.
2. Thoracic CT should be part of the initial evaluation for pediatric patients with trauma if a lung contusion, pneumothorax, or a hemothorax is suspected or the cause of the patient's respiratory distress is unknown. Thoracic ultrasound can be used at the bedside to diagnose a pneumothorax or hemothorax.
3. Myocardial contusion is the most common, and ventricular rupture is the most lethal of blunt cardiac injuries.
4. Patients with a TRA may present with hypotension, paraplegia, anuria, or absent/diminished femoral pulses.
5. Radiographic findings of a TRA may include a widened mediastinum, blurred aortic knob, pleural cap, or tracheal or nasogastric tube deviation.
6. Suspect commotio cordis and ventricular fibrillation in any patient who has become unconscious immediately after a blow to the chest.

BIBLIOGRAPHY

1. Arbuthnot M, Onwubiko C, Osborne M, Mooney DP. Does the incidence of thoraic aortic injury warrant the routine use of chest CT in children? *J Trauma Acute Care Surg.* 2019;86(1):97–100.
2. Chalfin AV, Mooney DP. Pediatrric sternal fracutres: a single center retrospective review. *J Pediatric Surg.* 2020;55:1224.
3. Eisenberg M, Collins J. Thoracic trauma. In: Shaw KN, Bachur RG, eds. *Fleisher & Ludwig's Textbook of Pediatric Emergency Medicine.* 8th ed. Wolters Kluwer; 2021:1274–1289.
4. Farrokhian AR. Commotio cordis and contusio cordis: possible cause of trauma-related cardiac death. *Arch Trauma Res.* 2016;5(4):e41482.
5. Frishman WH, Alpert JS. Commotio cordis and the triumph of out-of-hospital cardiopulmonary resuscitation. *Am J Med.* 2023;136(5):401–402.
6. Holmes JF, Sokolove PE, Brant WE, Kuppermann N. A clinical decision rule for identifying children with thoracic injuries after blunt torso trauma. *Ann Emerg Med.* 2002;39:492.
7. Link MS. Pathophysicology, prevention and treatment of commotio cordis. *Curr Cardiol Rep.* 2014;16:495.
8. Maron BJ, Link MS. Don't forget commotio cordis. *Am J Cardiol.* 2021;156:134.
9. Moore MA, Wallace EC, Weston SJ. The imaging of paediatric thoracic trauma. *Pediatr Radiol.* 2009;39:485.
10. Patel RP, Hernanz-Schulman M, Hilmes MA, et al. Pediatric chest CT after trauma: impact on surgical and clinical management. *Pediatr Radiol.* 2010;40:246.
11. Pearson EG, Fitzgerald CA, Santore MT. Pediatric thoracic trauma: current trends. *Semin Pediatr Surg.* 2017;26(1):36–42.
12. Weinstein J, Maron BJ, Song C, et al. Failure of commercially available chest wall protectors to prevent sudden cardiac death induced by chest wall blows in an experimental model of commotio cordis. *Pediatrics.* 2006;117(4):e6565-e6562.

BITES AND STINGS

Kate M. Cronan

CHAPTER 62

1. **Which age group has the highest risk for dog attacks?**
   Dog bites account for the majority (80%-90%) of mammalian bites. The highest number of dog bites occurs in boys from 5 to 14 years. In this group, the injury happens in or near home and is often due to large-breed or mixed-breed dogs. Children in this age group tend to get head, neck, and upper extremity injuries. They are at particular risk of serious injury due to dog bites.

2. **What are some of the statistics for dog bites?**
   Each year, there are approximately 4.5 million dog bites in the United States. More than 885,000 people seek medical care for these bites. Often the dog has been provoked and has not been known to have bitten anyone previously. In 85% to 95% of cases, the dog's owner can be identified. Many dog owners are unaware of the risk of injury to a young child. Pit bulls are responsible for the highest percentage of reported bites across all studies (22.5%). The incidence of dog bites increased dramatically during the COVID-19 pandemic, as families and dogs were quarantined at home for extended periods of time.

3. **A 2-year-old child was attacked by a large dog, and she has multiple significant facial lacerations. Besides the obvious wounds, what other injuries should you consider?**
   When a small child is attacked by a large dog, a fracture of the skull or facial bones must be considered. The dog's powerful jaws exert a strong force and can encircle the child's head. This can cause considerable damage to a child, and fractures are common. Consider radiographs of the skull or a computed tomography scan of facial bones and skull.

4. **What is the rate of wound infection after common animal bites?**
   - Cat bites: as high as 50%
   - Dog bites: 20%
   - Human bites: 10%

5. **What are the common microbiologic organisms involved with dog, cat, and human bites?**
   - **Dog bites**: *Staphylococcus aureus*, streptococci, *Pasteurella canis*
   - **Cat bites**: *Pasteurella multocida*, *S. aureus*, streptococci
   - **Human bites**: *Streptococcus viridans*, *S. aureus*, anaerobes, Bacteroides, and Peptostreptococcus species
     Note: Methicillin-resistant *S. aureus* is a potential bite wound pathogen.

6. **Which bites should be treated with prophylactic antibiotics?**
   - All dog bites involving hands and feet
   - All human bites
   - All cat bites
   - Puncture wounds
   - Bites that penetrate a joint
   - Bites for which treatment has been delayed for more than 24 hours
   - Bites in immunosuppressed and asplenic patients
     Amoxicillin-clavulanate is the antibiotic of choice for prophylaxis and empirical therapy for children who are not allergic to penicillin.

7. **In penicillin-allergic patients who present with a human bite or a high-risk animal bite, what antibiotic regimen is recommended?**
   Prophylaxis and treatment for penicillin-allergic children are challenging problems. Erythromycin and tetracycline activity against *S. aureus* and anaerobes is unreliable. Tetracycline is effective against *Pasteurella* spp. but consider the risk of dental staining in children younger than 8 years. Therefore combination treatment with oral or parenteral trimethoprim-sulfamethoxazole (effective against *S. aureus*, *Eikenella corrodens*, and *Pasteurella* spp.) and clindamycin (effective against anaerobes, streptococci, and *S. aureus*) is used for preventing or treating bite wound infections. Ceftriaxone may be used if the patient can tolerate cephalosporins. Metronidazole provides excellent anaerobic coverage and may be used as an alternative to clindamycin.

8. True or false: Wounds due to some animal bites should be closed with cyanoacrylate tissue adhesive.
   False. Avoid the use of tissue adhesive in treating animal bites because of the risk of infection.

KEY POINTS: DOG BITES

1. Frequently involve young children who may have unintentionally provoked the dog
2. Could involve fractures of the facial bones and skull if a small child is attacked by a large dog
3. Must be carefully irrigated with saline to prevent infection
4. Often require closure with sutures for cosmetic reasons
5. Should not be closed if at high risk for infection

---

9. Which organisms cause rat bite fever?
   Rat bite fever is an infectious disease that is most commonly caused by *Streptobacillus moniliformis*. Transmission to humans can happen via rat and other rodent bites and scratches. It can also be transmitted by handling infected animals or ingesting food or water contaminated by excreta.

10. What are the symptoms of rat-bite fever?
    Patients with *S. moniliformis* infection present with fever, chills, myalgia, headache, and vomiting. Within a few days of the onset of fever, a rash develops and is typically found on the extremities including the palms and soles. The bite area heals quickly and is followed by migratory polyarthritis in approximately 50% of patients. Complications of infection such as pneumonia, endocarditis, myocarditis, and meningitis may occur.

11. Describe the bite of fire ants. How is this treated?
    Fire ants are nonwinged *Hymenoptera* found in the Southeastern and South Central and Northern United States. They are aggressive insects. They bite with their jaws, then pivot around and sting at multiple sites in a circular pattern. The sting causes painful reactions. A wheal forms quickly on the skin and the reaction varies from 1 mm up to 10 cm. During the next 4 hours a vesicle appears, and later looks cloudy. After 24 hours, the area becomes red and painful and this can last for a few days, up to 10 days. Treatment consists of local wound care, antihistamines, and steroids for severe cases.

12. True or false: Stings from fire ants *(Solenopsis invicta)* can cause severe systemic reactions.
    True. Local reactions can consist of a wheal, a pustule, or a large local reaction. Systemic reactions may range from urticaria to life-threatening anaphylaxis.

13. What is the best multipurpose insect repellent?
    DEET (*N,N*-diethyl-m-toluamide) is the best multipurpose insect repellent and is the active ingredient in most commercial insect repellents. It is available in various forms, including sprays, gels, liquids, and sticks, and in concentrations of 4% to 100%. DEET can be applied to skin or clothes. It should not be applied under clothes. It does not work against stinging insects but is quite effective against mosquitoes, biting flies, chiggers, fleas, and ticks. It is important to note that the application of DEET may reduce the efficacy of sunscreen. Protection with DEET is shortened by swimming, washing, rainfall, sweating, and wiping.

14. Are there precautions to take when using DEET?
    Yes. Avoid DEET completely for children younger than 2 months of age. Oral ingestion of large quantities of DEET may cause seizures, coma, or death. For those concerned about the possible toxicity of DEET, citronella, a plant-derived insect repellent, is a good alternative.

15. What is the role of permethrin in helping to avoid insect bites?
    Permethrin is not an insect repellent. It causes toxicity to the nervous system of insects. It is available as a spray and should be applied to clothing or bedding. Do not apply this to the skin for the purpose of preventing insect bites.

16. Describe papular urticaria.
    Papular urticaria is a skin condition that causes intensely pruritic wheals and papules. These lesions are from arthropod bites in specifically sensitized children. A number of arthropods have been identified as culprits: dog lice, mosquitoes, bedbugs, fleas, mites, and chiggers. The wheals represent an immediate hypersensitivity reaction to insect bites. The wheals then evolve into papules, which represent a delayed hypersensitivity reaction.

The lesions usually appear on exposed areas. The differential diagnosis includes varicella, scabies, pediculosis, urticaria, and insect bites without papular urticaria.

17. **How is papular urticaria treated?**
Use a multipurpose insecticide for the entire home. Household pets should be included in the treatment. When the cause of the lesions is removed, clinical symptoms usually improve significantly, but supportive treatment is necessary. Oral antihistamines and topical steroid creams help to control the itching.

18. **Which tick-borne infectious diseases occur in the United States?**
    - **Bacterial:** Lyme disease, tularemia, relapsing fever
    - **Rickettsial:** Rocky Mountain spotted fever, ehrlichiosis
    - **Viral:** Colorado tick fever
    - **Protozoal:** Babesiosis

KEY POINTS: MAMMALIAN BITES AT HIGH RISK FOR INFECTION

1. Puncture wounds
2. Minor wounds on the hands or feet
3. Wounds with care delayed more than 12 hours
4. Cat and human bites
5. Wounds in immunocompromised children

19. **Explain the *Hymenoptera* sting.**
A sting consists of an injection of venom via a tapered shaft that projects from the venom sac located in the abdomen of females of the *Hymenoptera* species. Stings usually occur in warm weather.

20. **Which group of the order *Hymenoptera* is considered aggressive—apids or vespids?**
Vespids are aggressive. The yellow jacket is the most aggressive in this family. Yellow jackets are thought to be the principal cause of allergic reactions to insect stings in the United States.
    Apids include honeybees and bumblebees; vespids include yellow jackets, hornets, and wasps. Apids tend to be docile and sting only when provoked. Bees, wasps, and hornets are responsible for many of the anaphylactic reactions to venomous insects in the United States. The bumblebee is large, slow-moving, and very noisy. Honeybees may cause problems among beekeepers.

21. **How are reactions to bee stings categorized?**
    - **Small local reaction**: It is the most common reaction. It presents as a painful pruritic lesion smaller than 5 cm at the site of the sting and lasts briefly (several hours).
    - **Large local reaction**: After a sting, it manifests with swelling and erythema in the area of the sting. It is usually larger than 5 cm in diameter, often is very painful and itchy, and lasts for longer than 24 hours, sometimes up to 1 week.
    - **Systemic reactions**: They occur in approximately 0.5% of *Hymenoptera* stings, begin within minutes to hours after the sting, and can be mild or severe.
    - **Mild systemic reactions**: They most commonly consist of dermal signs and symptoms: generalized urticaria, pruritus, flushing, and angioedema. Gastrointestinal symptoms, such as abdominal pain, nausea, and diarrhea, may also occur.
    - **Severe systemic reactions**: They include life-threatening signs, such as upper airway edema with hoarseness and stridor; shock, manifested by pallor and fainting; and bronchospasm, characterized by coughing, dyspnea, and wheezing.
    - **Unusual reactions**: Such reactions to bee stings include vasculitis, nephrosis, encephalitis, and serum sickness. Symptoms usually occur several days to several weeks after the sting and tend to last for a long time.

22. **Describe the best way to remove a stinger after a bee sting.**
The aim should be to remove the stinger as soon as possible to avoid further deposition of venom. During a sting, the apparatus of a bee becomes lodged in the skin along with the venom sac. Venom is released in the first few seconds. If possible, flick the stinger off the skin as soon as possible. If you have a credit or other card use it to swipe it sideways. Grasping and pulling the stinger may squeeze the remaining venom from the venom sac into the sting site.

23. **What is the treatment for anaphylaxis due to an insect sting?**
The treatment is the same as for anaphylaxis from other causes. First, pay attention to airway, breathing, and circulation. Give intramuscular epinephrine in a 1:1000 dilution immediately; repeat the dose every 30 minutes as

needed. Intravenous (IV) epinephrine is rarely indicated except in the case of profound shock. Antihistamines, such as diphenhydramine or hydroxyzine, given parenterally, may reduce urticaria and pruritus. In some cases, steroids, such as methylprednisolone, should be administered early in the treatment plan. Depending on the severity of the reaction, other treatment modalities may be indicated (vasopressors, supplemental oxygen, IV fluids, bronchodilators). After recovery, be sure to provide an emergency kit for the self-administration of epinephrine. Provide detailed instructions about the technique and appropriate use to the patient and family.

24. **Why does the Southwestern desert scorpion,** *Centruroides exilicauda*, **have significance?**
C. exilicauda is the only scorpion species of medical importance in the United States. Also called the Arizona bark scorpion, it is found mainly in Arizona, Texas, and California. Arizona bark scorpions are yellow or brown and are usually 5 cm in length. Their appearance resembles that of a shrimp. The stinger is contained in its long mobile tail. They tend to reside in brush areas and trees and sting mostly at night. Children are usually stung on their extremities.

25. **Describe how the venom of the Arizona bark scorpion works.**
The venom of Arizona bark scorpions contains four neurotoxins. It overstimulates the parasympathetic and sympathetic nervous systems and results in agitation, tachycardia or bradycardia, hypertension, dysrhythmias, and increased secretions. Cranial nerve dysfunction may cause rapid dysconjugate eye movements and contractions of muscles of the face and tongue. Peripheral motor neuron involvement presents as muscle contractions and frequent jerking movements of the extremities. Respiratory distress may result from low pharyngeal tone and uncoordinated contraction of respiratory muscles.

26. **How are scorpion envenomations treated?**
Treatment of scorpion envenomation is usually supportive. Provide local wound care and tetanus prophylaxis. To reduce swelling, cryotherapy at the location of the sting has been advocated. Admit children with systemic signs and symptoms to the hospital. Give analgesics and benzodiazepines for pain and agitation. Many authorities prefer a continuous infusion of midazolam. Scorpion antivenom, Anascorp, is the first US Food and Drug Administration–approved antivenom that is available in the United States. It is used for severe envenomation.

27. **Name the four kinds of sharks in the United States that are responsible for most shark bites.**
They are gray reef, great white, blue, and mako sharks. Bites from these sharks can cause extensive injury, including fractures, amputations, and penetration of internal organs.

28. **Which two spiders in the United States cause significant envenomations?**
The black widow spider *(Latrodectus mactans)* and the brown recluse spider *(Loxosceles reclusa)* are the only two spiders known to cause significant envenomations.

29. **Describe the brown recluse spider and the black widow spider.**
Brown recluse spider bites occur much more frequently than black widow spider bites. Brown recluse spiders are nonaggressive and usually bite only when threatened. They have a brown or yellow violin-shaped marking on the dorsal thorax. They are found most commonly in the Southern and Midwestern states. They prefer dark, warm, protected areas, such as closets and garages. Most bites occur in bedrooms while people are sleeping or dressing.
Black widow spiders inhabit all states except Alaska and are found mostly in the South, Ohio Valley, Southwest, and West Coast. They are found in attics, barns, trash piles, and other dimly lit areas. In the warmer months, the bites are more frequent. The black widow spider is jet black, with an hourglass-shaped red mark on the underside of the abdomen.

30. **What are the symptoms of the bite of a brown recluse spider?**
In many cases, the bite of the brown recluse spider may not be noticed. Some children may feel stinging. Increased pain and pruritus may develop within several hours. Discomfort can occur from mild local irritation to large necrotic skin lesions and systemic reactions. A central vesicle with surrounding erythema is often discovered at the site of the bite. Within 24 hours, subcutaneous discoloration can spread up to 10 to 15 cm. This is followed by pustular drainage leaving an ulcerated area that does not last. Systemic signs and symptoms occur in approximately 40% of envenomations, including fever, nausea, vomiting, headache, and arthralgias.

31. **Describe how the bite of a brown recluse spider is treated.**
Most bites can be treated with minimal intervention. Treatment consists of local wound care; extensive dermal injuries may require skin grafting. Nonsteroidal anti-inflammatory drugs in children older than 6 months, and tetanus immunization are the mainstays of therapy. If substantial intravascular hemolysis occurs, it is crucial to maintain high urinary flow rates with alkalinization of the urine via sodium bicarbonate infusion.

32. **What is latrodectism?**

Latrodectism refers to systemic symptoms due to the spread of the neurotoxin from black widow spider bites. There are three phases of latrodectism:

- The **exacerbation** phase, from less than 6 and up to 24 hours after the bite. It is characterized by muscle spasms at the site of the bite or elsewhere.
- The **dissipation** phase, from 1 to 3 days after the bite and is a time when symptoms subside.
- The **residual** phase occurs weeks to months after the bite and may consist of persistent tremors, weakness, and fatigue.

33. **How is the bite of a black widow spider treated?**

Treatment consists of analgesia, including oral opioids for milder cases and IV morphine for more severe cases. Benzodiazepines can relieve anxiety and relax the muscles. After the bite is confirmed and testing shows no hypersensitivity, children who weigh less than 40 kg should get 2.5 mL of latrodectus antivenin. This is usually effective in 30 minutes. If necessary, it may be repeated once within 2 hours if the child has shown symptoms.

34. **Are iguanas good pets for young children?**

Despite iguanas being popular pets, they are not good for young children. They can inflict injury by scratching, biting, and tail-whipping. They frequently carry unusual subtypes of fecal salmonella. The Centers for Disease Control and Prevention recommend that children under the age of 5 years and those who are immunocompromised should not have iguanas and other salmonella-carrying pets, such as turtles, in the home.

35. **What are the poisonous snakes indigenous to the United States?**

Snakes in the Crotalidae family (pit vipers) and Elapidae family (coral snakes) are poisonous. Rattlesnakes, copperheads, and water moccasins are pit vipers and account for 99% of poisonous snakebites. The coral snake accounts for less than 1% of poisonous snakebites.

36. **Describe how pit vipers can be distinguished from nonpoisonous snakes.**

Pit vipers have two pits, one on either side of their head. Their pupils are elliptical and vertically oriented. The head is triangular, and they have two curved fangs that are widely spaced. The scales caudal to the anal plate continue in a single row.

Nonpoisonous snakes have oval heads with round pupils, teeth, and a snout. The anal plate has a double row of subcaudal plates.

37. **How does a patient with a snake bite present?**

It is understandable that most patients will be anxious and have tachycardia, dry mouth, and hyperventilation (leading to carpopedal spasm, paresthesia, and lightheadedness). Depending on the species, many bites (10%-80%) have no venom (dry bites). Common symptoms of bites with venom include pain, swelling, and tenderness that spreads up the affected limb. There can be bleeding from the bite wounds. Nausea, vomiting, and syncope may develop. With bites from pit vipers, blistering may develop within hours and tissue necrosis is possible. Hypovolemia, hypotension, and coagulation abnormalities are common.

38. **What are the possible complications of Crotalid bites?**

Complications of Crotalid bites can be coagulopathy, tissue necrosis, rhabdomyolysis, compartment syndrome, dysrhythmia, shock, multisystem failure, and death.

39. **How can you get information about the treatment of snakebites and how to obtain antivenom?**

Contact the local poison center. Also, try a local zoo or aquarium. Many have antivenom available for bites by snakes in their collections.

40. **What is tularemia?**

Tularemia is an infection caused by *Francisella tularensis*, a gram-negative pleomorphic coccobacillus. Human infections can occur after contact with wild-infected animals. Sources of this organism include many species of wild mammals, some domestic animals (e.g., sheep, cattle, cats), and the blood-sucking arthropods that bite these animals (e.g., ticks and mosquitoes). In the United States, rabbits and ticks are major sources of infection.

41. **How does tularemia present?**

There are a number of tularemic syndromes. Most patients present with a sudden onset of fever, chills, myalgia, and headache. This usually happens 3 to 5 days after a person has been exposed. The most common type is ulceroglandular syndrome. This presents with a painful maculopapular lesion at the bite site and painful, acutely inflamed lymph nodes. Other less common syndromes are the glandular, oropharyngeal, oculoglandular typhoidal, intestinal, and pneumonic presentations.

42. **How is tularemia treated?**
Treatment should be started promptly for patients with suspected or confirmed tularemia. The first choice for treatment is gentamicin for 10 days. Ciprofloxacin is an alternative for mild disease. Treatment usually lasts for 10 days.

43. **Which type of jellyfish sting is highly toxic?**
Stings from *lion's mane* (*Cyanea capillata*) are highly toxic. This type of jellyfish is found along both coasts of the United States. Contact with the tentacles of lion's mane causes severe burning. Prolonged exposure results in muscle cramps, and respiratory failure may ensue.

44. **What is the treatment for toxic jellyfish stings?**
Treatment of toxic jellyfish stings relies on relieving pain, alleviating the effects of the venom, and giving supportive therapy. To avoid further nematocysts discharging, first remove the tentacles. Then apply vinegar (acetic acid) for 30 minutes. This may inactivate the remaining nematocysts. In many species, vinegar may cause pain and exacerbation of nematocyst discharge. Hot water immersion (104°F to 113°F) as tolerated and topical lidocaine are beneficial in improving pain symptoms. If these are not available, consider removing the nematocysts and washing the area with saltwater. Use gloved hands or instruments to remove the residual tentacles. No antivenin is available. Antihistamines, steroids, and analgesics may be indicated. In some cases, cardiac and respiratory support may be required.

45. **Describe the best way to remove a tick embedded in the skin.**
Ticks should be removed as soon as possible. There is no need to put petroleum jelly or other substances on the tick.
    Using fine-tipped forceps or tweezers, grasp the tick with the forceps as close to the skin's surface as possible. Pull up steadily and do not twist or jerk the tick as you pull back.
    Do not squeeze or crush the tick. This could regurgitate material into the wound during removal.
    Clean any residual parts that are found on the skin, then remove them with forceps. After removal, cleanse the bite wound and your hands with rubbing alcohol or soap and water.

46. **How important is the duration of attachment of ticks to the skin?**
Duration of attachment to the host plays a major role in the transmission of pathogens. *Borrelia burgdorferi* from an infected tick has a higher likelihood of transmission after 24 hours, and this increases after 72 hours of attachment.

47. **How can one avoid Lyme disease?**
The most effective precautions are as follows:
    - Wear long sleeves and keep them buttoned. Wear long pants that are tucked in when tics are nearby.
    - Apply DEET to the skin and clothes. Permethrin can be applied to clothes along with DEET.
    - Parents should check their children after they have spent time in risky areas. If a tick is found on the skin, they should wash the area. This can be effective before attachment occurs.
    - Replace brush with wood chips.

48. **How soon after an exposure should immunoprophylaxis for rabies begin?**
After the wound care is completed, passive and active immunoprophylaxis are required. Begin prophylaxis as soon as possible after exposure. This should happen ideally within 24 hours. A delay of several days or more may not compromise effectiveness. Begin prophylaxis, if indicated, regardless of the time of exposure.

49. **Should rabies prophylaxis be given after a bite from a bat?**
Consider rabies prophylaxis when direct contact between a human and a bat has occurred. Also, think about rabies prophylaxis for a child who has been in a room with a bat and may be unable to rule out any physical contact. These patients might include (1) a sleeping child who awakens to find a bat in the room, (2) a young child, (3) an unattended child, (4) a mentally disabled person, or (5) an intoxicated person.
    Rabies prophylaxis is not necessary if the person is aware of the bat at all times while in an enclosed space and is certain that there was no bite, scratch, or mucous membrane exposure. If the bat is captured and can be tested for rabies, rabies prophylaxis can await the results of prompt testing. If uncertainty about the need for prophylaxis still exists, consult the local public health authority.

50. **When there is a concern for rabies exposure, what is the best way to prevent the rabies virus from entering neural tissue?**
Immediate and thorough care of all lesions is crucial. Otherwise, the virus may remain close to the area of the bite. Wounds should be flushed thoroughly and then cleaned with soap and water. Tetanus prophylaxis and bacterial control should be considered as needed.

51. **Which animals are rarely found to be infected with rabies in the United States?**
    Squirrels, hamsters, guinea pigs, chipmunks, mice, rats, gerbils, rabbits, hares, and pikas are almost never found to be infected with rabies. They do not transmit rabies to humans. Therefore those bitten by these animals rarely need prophylaxis.

52. **What are the recommendations for rabies prophylaxis?**
    Give human rabies vaccine 2.5 International Units of rabies antigen (1 mL) intramuscularly in the deltoid area or the anterolateral aspect of the thigh. It is not recommended to inject into the gluteal area. Give this on the day of exposure and then on days 3, 7, and 14.
    In addition, on the day of exposure give rabies immunoglobulin (RIG) 20 international units/kg by local infiltration around the wound, with the remaining immunoglobulin administered intramuscularly in an anatomical site distant from where the vaccine was placed. For children with small muscle mass, it may be necessary to administer RIG at multiple sites.

53. **How are bedbug bites detected?**
    Bedbug bites are not obvious initially. This is because they are painless and may look like flea or mosquito bites. Usually, the bites become pruritic and are then noted. Bites usually occur on the face, neck, hands, legs, and arms. The bite marks may be in a straight line or in random locations. Often the bites become very itchy and some children have trouble sleeping due to scratching the bites.

54. **How are bedbug bites treated?**
    Bedbug bites do not always need treatment. The lesions may resolve on their own. However bothersome pruritus may occur. In some cases, it may improve with a topical corticosteroid or an oral antihistamine. Of note, antihistamines can suppress the symptoms and signs of bites and may reduce the patient's ability to detect an ongoing infestation.

55. **What infection can result from a mouse bite?**
    Rickettsialpox is a rare infection that can be seen after a mouse bite. Most cases are seen in urban settings, associated with mouse infestations. The child will likely present with a classic triad of fever, eschar, and rash. Seven to 10 days after the painless bite, a papular skin lesion appears at the bite location. It becomes vesicular with a surrounding area of erythema and ruptures to form the eschar that is almost always present at the time of diagnosis. About 3 to 7 days after this initial lesion appears, patients develop systemic symptoms such as fever, chills, malaise, myalgia, and headache. These symptoms may last 6 to 10 days. A few days after the onset of systemic symptoms, a generalized papular rash can be noted on the face, trunk, and extremities. This can be mildly pruritic. Laboratory findings commonly include leukopenia and thrombocytopenia.
    Rickettsialpox is usually a self-limited disease, and constitutional symptoms resolve in 7 to 10 days. The prognosis is excellent, and there are no known fatalities. Treatment with doxycycline decreases the course of illness.

BIBLIOGRAPHY

1. *American Academy of Pediatrics*, Committee on Infectious Diseases. Red Book: Report of the Committee on Infectious Diseases, 32nd ed. American Academy of Pediatrics; 2021: 180, 606–607, 621.
2. Amine L, Eldos Y. Envenomation, scorpion. In: Hoffman RJ, Wang VJ, eds. *Fleisher & Ludwig's 5-Minute Pediatric Emergency Medicine Consult.* 2nd ed. Wolters Kluwer; 2019:256–257.
3. Bula-Rudas FJ, Olcott JL. Human and animal bites. *Pediatr Rev..* 2018;39(10):490–500.
4. *Centers for Disease Control and Prevention (CDC), National Center for Emerging and Zoonotic Infectious Diseases.* <https://www.cdc.gov/ncezid/dw-index.html>; Last accessed 2021.
5. Freeman T. Bee, yellow jacket, wasp and other Hymenoptera stings: reaction types and acute management. In: Golden DB, ed. *UpToDate;* 2022.
6. Hadvani T, Vallejo JG, Dutta A. Rat bite fever: variability in clinical presentation and management in children. *Pediatr Infect Dis J..* 2021;40(11):e439–e442.
7. Hananiya A, Douglas L, Fagan M. Rickettsialpox in a pediatric patient. *Pediatr Emerg Care..* 2017;33(4):260–262.
8. Kamath S, Kenner-Bell B. Infestations, bites, and insect repellents. *Pediatr Ann..* 2020;49:e124–e131.
9. Koutroulis I, Agarwal D. Environmental emergencies, radiological emergencies, bites and stings *Fleisher & Ludwig's Textbook of Pediatric Emergency Medicine.* 8th ed. Wolters Kluwer; 2021:706–723.
10. Warrell DA. Venomous bites, stings and poisoning. *Infect Dis Clin North Am..* 2019;33(1):17–38.

CHAPTER 63

DROWNING

Brian L. Park and William B. Prince

1. **What is drowning?**
   The World Health Organization defines drowning as "the process of experiencing respiratory impairment from submersion or immersion in liquid." While drowning is one of the leading causes of injury death in young children and adolescents (third most common worldwide), it does not imply death or any morbidity associated with the event. Drowning outcomes are classified as "death," "morbidity," or "no morbidity." Terminologies such as "near," "wet," "dry," "secondary," "silent," "passive," and "active" are no longer used.

2. **What is the pathophysiology of drowning?**
   A conscious, drowning person will attempt to keep water from entering the airway by spitting or swallowing the water, which is followed by breath-holding. Typically, after no longer than a minute (10-20 seconds in children), increased respiratory drive will overcome breath-holding, resulting in aspiration of water which then leads to reflexive coughing and laryngospasm. Aspirated water causes surfactant washout and disruption of the alveolar-capillary membrane, leading to decreased lung compliance, atelectasis, bronchospasm, and pulmonary edema. Prolonged hypoxemia can precipitate a cardiac arrest (most commonly asystole). Eventual brain hypoxia is the main physiologic mechanism leading to morbidity and mortality in drowning patients.

3. **What does drowning look like?**
   Drowning is often a silent and quick process. "Instinctive Drowning Response" described by Pia in 1974 is a reaction to keep the mouth above the water by a person who is close to drowning. The body will be upright, the head tilted back, and the arms extended to the side. There may be repeated submersion of the head as the person struggles to keep buoyant. Yelling or waving for help is unlikely during this period. A person can struggle for about 20 to 60 seconds before the final submersion occurs and the person drowns.

4. **What are the risk factors for drowning?**
   Children 0 to 4 years of age have the highest rate of drowning. This typically occurs in bathtubs or buckets for infants and in swimming pools for preschool-aged children. Adolescents (15-19 years of age) have the second highest rate of drowning, and most commonly occurs in natural water settings (e.g., rivers, lakes, beaches). These drownings are often associated with alcohol use. Other risk factors include male sex, rural setting, Black race, low socioeconomic status (barrier to swimming lessons), epilepsy (7.5- to 10-fold increase compared to children without epilepsy), autism spectrum disorder, and cardiac abnormalities (e.g., long QT syndrome, myocarditis, arrhythmias).

5. **Is hypothermia protective?**
   Therapeutic hypothermia, the medical intervention of cooling a drowning victim with the intention to improve neurologic outcome (targeted temperature management), should be distinguished from patients who present with hypothermia (<34°C) after a drowning event. Therapeutic hypothermia was thought to reduce the degree of brain injury after cardiac arrests by reducing cerebral metabolic rate; however, this is now controversial with recent randomized controlled trials demonstrating no improvement in neurologic outcomes or survival over normothermia in both adult and pediatric cardiac arrests. Additionally, while there are few case reports of good neurologic outcomes in hypothermic children with prolonged cardiac arrest after drowning in icy cold water, most children who present with hypothermia after drowning-related cardiac arrests have an extremely poor prognosis as it may reflect prolonged submersion.

6. **What is a cold water drowning?**
   There is no strict temperature definition for cold water drowning/immersion. "Cold shock," a physiologic response to a sudden decrease in skin temperature, occurs at ~25°C and peaks between 15°C and 10°C. Resulting gasp reflex and subsequent hyperventilation significantly decrease breath-holding time. Cold water also increases the risk of supraventricular tachyarrhythmias, which is thought to be caused by an "autonomic conflict" between "cold shock response" and "diving response." Both processes increase the risk of drowning. Additionally, a large case-control study found no association between water temperature and drowning outcomes.

7. **Is there a clinical difference between saltwater and freshwater drowning?**
   There is no clinical difference. While a recent large multicenter retrospective study demonstrated that freshwater was independently associated with increased mortality compared to saltwater, freshwater drownings were associated with more psychiatric comorbidities, apparent suicide attempts, drug/alcohol intoxication, and cardiac

arrests. Old animal models demonstrated electrolyte and hemodynamic changes based on the salinity of the aspirated water; however, numerous studies since then have failed to show similar associations in humans. One explanation is that humans generally do not aspirate large volumes of water during a drowning. Any significant electrolyte or acid-base disturbances are attributable to hypoxia. Underlying pathophysiology and management of a drowning victim are the same regardless of the salinity of the aspirated fluid.

8. **What are the key tenants in resuscitation of an unresponsive drowning patient?**
   The key to resuscitating an unresponsive drowning patient is to prevent or reverse cerebral hypoxia as soon as possible via high-quality cardiopulmonary resuscitation (CPR). Thus the most crucial interventions occur in the prehospital setting. For those with apnea or hypopnea, early rescue breaths whether by bag-valve-mask or even mouth-to-mouth by a bystander are vital. In instances in which a drowning person is far from shore, in-water respiratory-only resuscitation for up to 1 minute by trained personnel is recommended. In some cases, spontaneous respiration may return only after a few rescue breaths. Positive pressure ventilation and supplemental oxygen should be initiated as soon as it is available to support ventilation and oxygenation. Intubation is indicated for those who continue to have inadequate ventilation, depressed neurologic status, and/or hemodynamic instability despite noninvasive positive pressure ventilation.
   Any drowning person who is pulseless, severely bradycardic, or hypotensive should be managed per Pediatric Advanced Life Support/Advanced Cardiovascular Life Support with high-quality CPR. It is important to note that drowning cardiac arrests are usually due to hypoxia from respiratory failure thus compression-only CPR is not recommended. Additionally, chest compressions should be prioritized over automated external defibrillator placement as most common rhythms in drowning cardiac arrests are non-shockable (asystole and pulseless electrical activity).
   Hypothermia, as discussed above, is a controversial topic. Severe hypothermia ($<32°C$) should be addressed (e.g., removing wet clothes) as it can depress myocardial function and cause arrhythmias. Hyperthermia, on the other hand, is detrimental and should be avoided.

9. **Is the Heimlich maneuver/subdiaphragmatic thrusts helpful?**
   No. While drowning involves some aspiration of water into the airway, there is no evidence that it causes airway obstruction or that the Heimlich maneuver is effective in expelling water from the airway. Review of the literature by the International Liaison Committee on Resuscitation showed that chest compressions create greater mean peak airway pressure than the Heimlich maneuver. In addition to its lack of efficacy, the Heimlich maneuver can cause harm including aspiration of stomach contents, injuries to visceral organs, and, most importantly, delay in ventilation and chest compressions.

10. **Should prophylactic antibiotics be given to the drowning patient?**
    No. While aspiration of water increases the risk of developing pneumonia, studies do not support the use of prophylactic or empiric antibiotics. Decision to administer antibiotics should be based on symptoms and available laboratory evaluation (e.g., sputum or endotracheal aspirate cultures, blood cultures). Diagnosis of pneumonia can be challenging in drowning patients as aspiration can produce radiographic findings similar to that of pneumonia and the stress of drowning can cause leukocytosis and fever.

11. **Should corticosteroids be given to the drowning patient?**
    No. Prophylactic intravenous steroids were previously given as it was thought to facilitate surfactant production and improve post-drowning pulmonary inflammation. Review of the current literature, while limited to retrospective reviews and case series, does not show any mortality or morbidity benefit. Thus routine administration of corticosteroids is not recommended in the management of a drowning patient.

12. **Which tests are helpful in managing the drowning patient?**
    Drowning patients can present in a variety of ways, therefore, tests should reflect the severity of their presentation and characteristics of the event. At a minimum, serial monitoring of vital signs and oxygenation by pulse oximetry, repeated pulmonary examination, and neurologic assessment should be performed in all drowning patients. For the alert patient with mild to no respiratory distress, oximetry monitoring may be all that is needed and is a more reliable treatment guide than chest radiography. Several studies have recommended against using an abnormal radiograph as the sole criterion for hospital admission. Blood gas, chest radiography, complete blood count, electrolytes, and urine toxicology can be reserved for the unresponsive patient who is at great risk for complications and poor outcomes. Additionally, a glucose level is a useful prognostic factor. While not specific for drowning patients, close glycemic control (80-110 mg/dL) was associated with better outcomes for critically ill patients in the intensive care unit.

13. **Can some drowning patients be sent home from the emergency department (ED)?**
    Most well-appearing drowning patients who are alert and in minimal to no respiratory distress are unlikely to clinically worsen after 6 hours postsubmersion. Thus these patients should be observed in the ED for a minimum of 4 to 6 hours (after the drowning event) with a focus on neurologic and pulmonary status, including

cardiorespiratory monitoring with pulse oximetry. Some initially asymptomatic, alert patients may develop mild respiratory distress (tachypnea, mild hypoxemia) and cough at the scene or within a few hours of the submersion. In many cases, their symptoms respond to a brief period of low-flow oxygen and they can be discharged to home if they are asymptomatic at 6 hours.

14. **What is the most common cause of death and disability in hospitalized drowning victims?**
Cerebral edema secondary to irreversible hypoxic-ischemic injury is the biggest contributor to morbidity and mortality in a drowning patient. This can develop rapidly over several hours after a drowning-associated cardiac arrest, and the resulting increased intracranial pressure worsens cerebral ischemia. Many children who survive a drowning-associated cardiac arrest have poor neurological outcomes. Additionally, drowning can result in other end-organ dysfunction leading to acute respiratory distress, acute kidney injury, arrhythmias, thrombocytopenia, and/or hemolysis.

15. **Do all survivors of drowning in the wilderness need emergency evacuation?**
Not all survivors of a drowning event require an emergency evacuation. A large retrospective study of 42,000 lifeguard rescues found that patients who were asymptomatic or with a mild cough without abnormal lung sounds had 0% mortality after a drowning event. However, patients with hypotension have an increased risk of mortality (>19%) and should be emergently evacuated. If a child is asymptomatic with a normal pulmonary examination, release from the scene with another individual (e.g., parent or guardian) to monitor them for the next 4 to 6 hours may be appropriate.

16. **Does every drowning patient need evaluation for cervical spine injury?**
No. Routine cervical spine imaging is not indicated for most patients. Cervical spine injury is very rare (<0.5%) in drowning patients and is almost never seen in preadolescent children. It is typically associated with diving, surfing, or accidents involving motor vehicles, boats, or other personal watercraft. In two large studies with over 2000 patients, all cases of cervical spine injury had a history consistent with high-speed mechanism or clinical signs of serious injury on physical examination. A careful history and examination of the neck are sufficient screening for cervical spine injury for most patients.

17. **What are the predictors of the outcome of drowning?**
The key predictor is the patient's mental status after the drowning. Patients who are alert on arrival to the ED or at hospital admission will likely survive with normal neurologic status. For patients arriving at the ED unresponsive or with mental status changes, neurologic outcome is difficult to predict. Factors associated with poor outcomes including persistent vegetative state or death include duration of submersion >5 minutes, absent pupillary reflexes, hyperglycemia after resuscitation (glucose level > 250 mg/dL), acidosis (pH < 7.10), hypothermia, and CPR >25 minutes without return of spontaneous circulation. Early Glasgow Coma Scale assessments are poor predictors of neurologic outcomes. Since no single factor or combination of factors at the time the patient arrives in the ED has achieved greater than 96% accuracy in predicting poor outcomes, some recommend resuscitation attempts for all drowning victims on arrival to the ED.

   Neurologic examination and progression of symptoms during the first 24 to 72 hours are currently the best prognosticators of neurologic outcomes. Children who regain consciousness and neurologic function within 48 to 72 hours, even after prolonged resuscitation, are unlikely to have serious neurologic sequelae. Survivors with good outcomes typically have spontaneous purposeful movements and normal brainstem function within 24 hours, while most of those who remain comatose at 24 hours will die or survive with severe neurologic sequelae.

18. **How does one recognize child abuse as the etiology of drowning?**
Drowning as child abuse or homicide is most often recognized in the young child whose submersion occurred in the bathtub. Drowning may be the primary injury as well as a secondary injury when the abuser attempts to revive the child or to conceal other physical injuries by placing the child in the tub. The key to recognition of intentional trauma is usually in history. A caregiver's explanation for the injury that is not compatible with the child's developmental age, or a changing or vague history, should prompt consideration of child abuse. The physical examination must include a careful search for signs of physical abuse and signs of multiple trauma. A critical part of any childhood drowning, regardless of the concern for abuse, is evaluation by social services.

19. **How can pediatric drowning be prevented?**
The most effective way to prevent drowning is to create "layers of protection" with multiple preventative strategies (think "Swiss cheese" model of medical error prevention). The five best evidenced-based interventions are the following: four-sided pool fencing, lifejackets, swim lessons, adequate supervision, and lifeguards. It has been shown that four-sided pool fencing (at least 4 feet tall and with self-closing and latching gates) can prevent >50% of childhood drownings. Any personal flotation devices (PFDs) should be U.S. Coast Guard-approved as not all PFDs are effective and may create a false sense of security. Formal swim lessons can decrease rates of drowning in children as young as 1 to 4 years. Supervision must be constant and attentive as drowning is often a silent process. For beginner swimmers, children should be within arm's reach (touch supervision).

KEY POINTS: DROWNING

1. Major risk factors for drowning include age (young children and adolescents), male sex, rural settings, Black race low socioeconomic status, epilepsy, autism spectrum disorder, and cardiac abnormalities.
2. Multilayered protection (e.g., four-sided pool enclosure, close one-on-one supervision, swimming lessons, lifejacket) is the best way to prevent and reduce the burden of drowning.
3. Thorough history and physical examination can best identify child abuse in drowning.
4. Patients who experienced a drowning, but are asymptomatic after 4 to 6 hours of observation, can be safely discharged to home if the social situation permits.
5. Social work involvement is important in the evaluation of any drowning patient for possible abuse, homicide, suicide, or risk-taking behaviors, especially alcohol use.

KEY POINTS: POOR PROGNOSTIC SIGNS AFTER DROWNING

1. Duration of submersion longer than 5 minutes
2. Depressed neurologic status
3. Hyperglycemia
4. Hypothermia
5. No spontaneous circulation after 25 minutes of CPR

BIBLIOGRAPHY

1. Colls Garrido C, Riquelme Gallego B, Sánchez García JC, Cortés Martín J, Montiel Troya M, Rodríguez Blanque R. The effect of therapeutic hypothermia after cardiac arrest on the neurological outcome and survival: a systematic review of RCTs published between 2016 and 2020. *Int J Environ Res Public Health.* 2021;18(22):11817. https://doi.org/10.3390/ijerph182211817.
2. Denny SA, Quan L, Gilchrist J, et al. Prevention of drowning. *Pediatrics.* 2019;143(5): https://doi.org/10.1542/peds.2019-0850. e20190850.
3. Dyson K, Morgans A, Bray J, Matthews B, Smith K. Drowning related out-of-hospital cardiac arrests: characteristics and outcomes. *Resuscitation.* 2013;84(8):1114–1118.
4. McIntosh SE, Freer L, Grissom CK, et al. Wilderness Medical Society clinical practice guidelines for the prevention and treatment of frostbite: 2019 update. *Wilderness Environ Med.* 2019;30(4 Suppl):S19–S32. https://doi.org/10.1016/j.wem.2019.05.002.
5. Quan L, Mack CD, Schiff MA. Association of water temperature and submersion duration and drowning outcome. *Resuscitation.* 2014;85(6):790–794. https://doi.org/10.1016/j.resuscitation.2014.02.024.
6. Reizine F, Delbove A, Dos Santos A, et al. Clinical spectrum and risk factors for mortality among seawater and freshwater critically ill drowning patients: a French multicenter study. *Crit Care.* 2021;25(1):372. https://doi.org/10.1186/s13054-021-03792-2.
7. Shattock MJ, Tipton MJ. 'Autonomic conflict': a different way to die during cold water immersion? *J Physiol.* 2012;590(14):3219–3230. https://doi.org/10.1113/jphysiol.2012.229864.
8. Szpilman D, Bierens JJ, Handley AJ, Orlowski JP. Drowning. *N Eng J Med.* 2012;366(22):2102–2110. https://doi.org/10.1056/NEJMra1013317.

CHAPTER 64

ELECTRICAL AND LIGHTNING INJURIES

Sarah N. Weihmiller

ELECTRICAL INJURY

1. **How common are electrical injuries?**
   - About 30,000 incidents a year
   - Approximately 1000 deaths per year (50-300 due to lightning)
   - Up to 40% of serious electrical injuries are fatal
   - About 20% of all electrical injuries occur in children

2. **What age group is at greatest risk for electrical injury?**
   Younger children are at high risk of household electrical injuries, while adolescents are at the risk of high-voltage injury due to power lines. Incidence decreases after the teenage years and rises again during working adulthood.

3. **What is current, and what is the difference between alternating current (AC) and direct current (DC?)**
   - Current is the volume of electrons that flows across a gradient.
   - **AC current**: Flow changes direction rapidly in a cyclic fashion and causes intense muscle contractions. An example is household current of 110V flows at 60 cycles/second.
   - **DC current**: Flow is in one direction and can cause significant trauma by throwing the patient from the source. Examples include batteries, lightning, and high-tension power lines.
   - AC is approximately three to five times more damaging than DC current of equal voltage.

4. **What are the mechanisms of electrical injury?**
   - Direct effect of current on organ systems—arrhythmias, apnea, rhabdomyolysis
   - Blunt mechanical injury—muscle contraction, falls
   - Conversion of electrical injury to thermal injury—burns

5. **What is the "let go" current?**
   The maximum current a person can actively grasp *and still release* an electrical source before locking on due to tetany.

6. **What influences the extent of electrical injury?**
   - Voltage
   - Tissue resistance
   - Pathway of current
   - Duration of contact
   - Type of current, AC versus DC

7. **What is considered a low-voltage injury versus a high-voltage injury?**
   - 60 to 1000V = low voltage
   - >1000V = high voltage

8. **Which tissues have the highest resistance to electricity? Which tissues have the least resistance?**
   - Highest resistance to electricity: bone (most resistant), fat, skin
   - Lowest resistance (conducts electricity readily): nerves (least resistant), blood vessels, muscle, and mucosa

9. **What is the difference in electrical injury between wet and dry skin?**
   Dry skin has higher resistance and greater superficial tissue damage but less damage to deeper structures. Wet skin has lower resistance and less superficial tissue damage, however, causes more extensive injury to internal organs.

10. **What systems are affected by electrical injury? List some examples of injury for each.**
    Cutaneous:
    - Superficial burns
    - Deep burns may require skin grafting or amputation

Pulmonary:
- Respiratory failure due to cardiac arrest or paralysis of respiratory muscles
- Pneumothorax due to falls
- Later-pneumonitis, pneumonia, pulmonary effusions

Cardiovascular: Rare, a result of both high- and low-voltage injury
- Cardiac arrest due to ventricular fibrillation or asystole
- Arrythmias
- Myocardial injury and myocardial infarction

Musculoskeletal:
- Rhabdomyolysis
- Compartment syndrome
- Fractures/dislocations due to trauma or severe muscle contractions

Renal:
- Myoglobinuria resulting in acute kidney failure

Vascular:
- Thrombosis
- Vasospasm

Neurological: Common
- Loss of consciousness, altered mental status
- Numbness, weakness, paresthesias, difficulty concentrating (may be delayed)
- Spinal cord injury—more common in high-voltage injuries

11. **What are some key components of the history of electrical injury patients?**
- Electrical source: High versus low voltage
- Type of current: AC versus DC
- Duration of contact
- Environment: Indoors versus outdoors, raining, potential for trauma due to a fall.

12. **Describe the ED management of a patient who presents to the ED with high-voltage electrical injury.**
Initially, it is most important to focus on the airway, breathing, circulation, disability, and exposure (ABCDEs) according to Pediatric Advanced Life Support and Advanced Trauma Life Support protocols. All patients should be *fully examined*, from head to toe in a gown. Consider early intubation for patients with face and neck burns. Be certain that backup airway devices are available, along with a surgical airway setup. Maintain cervical spine immobilization as there is a risk of neck trauma when a patient is thrown after a high-voltage electrical injury. Place the patient on continuous cardiac monitoring. Administer intravenous (IV) isotonic fluids to maintain a urine output of 1 to 1.5 mL/kg/hour. Perform a thorough neurovascular examination. Manage pain with opioids as needed.

Take a thorough history. Clean any burns and cover them with sterile dressings. Give tetanus prophylaxis if indicated. Perform frequent neurovascular checks and assess for compartment syndrome.

13. **Should significant patients with electrical injury be considered trauma patients?**
Yes. Patients who experience significant electrical injury may have been thrown from the scene, suffering significant internal trauma. It is important to maintain c-spine immobilization in these patients. Perform a full trauma evaluation. If transfer to another medical facility is indicated, a trauma center should take precedence over a burn center.

14. **Should every patient with an electrical injury have an electrocardiography (EKG)?**
All patients with electrical injury should have an EKG. However, there are no specific guidelines for pediatric patients. If the EKG is normal, the injury was low voltage, and there was no loss of consciousness or cardiac arrest, then a repeat EKG or cardiac monitoring is not indicated.

15. **What labs and imaging should be considered for a patient with an electrical injury?**
- **Labs**: For high-voltage exposure, lightning strikes, significant burns, or trauma, obtain a *complete blood count* (CBC), *chemistry panel* (including glucose, BUN, creatinine), *urinalysis*, *creatinine kinase* (CK), and *urine myoglobin*. Consider *CK-MB and LDH* for markers of tissue damage; however, this is controversial. *Troponin* has not been shown to be a reliable indicator of cardiac injury. Perform a *pregnancy test* in reproductive-aged females. For those with abdominal trauma, consider *coagulation studies*, *liver enzymes*, and *pancreatic enzymes*.
- **Imaging**: Perform a *chest x-ray* on any patient with cardiac/respiratory arrest or chest pain. Patients with loss of consciousness, trauma, or altered mental status should have a *head CT*. Consider a *c-spine CT* if there is a concern for a neck injury. Perform *E-fast* for trauma patients.

16. **What is the recommended disposition of patients who present with low-voltage electrical injury?**
    Patients with no loss of consciousness, normal EKG, no trauma, and no major burns can be considered for discharge with close primary care follow-up.

17. **Are minor surface burns reassuring?**
    No. The extent of surface burns may not accurately reveal the extent of burns to visceral and deep tissue. This is especially true with wet or lacerated skin, which allows more current to pass to deeper structures.

18. **Should the Parkland formula be used to determine fluid needs in patients with electrical burns?**
    No. IV fluid requirements in electrical burns can be very high and may be underestimated with the Parkland formula. The Lund-Browder chart can be used for a more accurate estimate of burn percentage. Fluids should be given to maintain urine output of 1 to 1.5 mL/kg/hour.

19. **What are the indications for hospital admission in patients with electrical injury?**
    • Neurological instability, loss of consciousness
    • Cardiac history or cardiac symptoms/chest pain, abnormal EKG
    • Significant burns (transfer to a burn center)
    • High-voltage and lightning exposures

20. **What is concerning about a child biting an electrical cord?**
    These children can suffer from a burn to the oral commissure. The danger is a possible (up to 24%) life-threatening hemorrhage of the labial artery that can occur 2 to 21 days after the injury.

21. **Can a child who bites an electrical cord be discharged home?**
    Patients with superficial oral commissure burns and who are tolerating fluids can be discharged with local wound care and instructions to manage bleeding if it occurs. They need follow-up with an oral or plastic surgeon within 1 week. Admit patients with more extensive burns and have them seen urgently by an oral or plastic surgeon.

KEY POINTS: ELECTRICAL INJURIES

• Obtain an EKG for all patients with electrical injury.
• Manage those with high-voltage electrical injury like trauma patients.
• Superficial burn severity is not representative of deeper injury.
• An asymptomatic patient with low-voltage exposure and no loss of consciousness may safely be discharged home.
• Children with oral commissure burns are at risk for severe bleeding 2 to 21 days after injury and need follow-up with an oral or plastic surgeon.

---

22. **Are taser injuries concerning?**
    Taser is a brand name for a conducted electrical weapon (CEW). These weapons vary but typically use two barbed projectiles to conduct rapid, high-voltage (50,000 V) electricity to a subject. While there have been case fatalities after CEW use, the consensus is that they cause minimal harm. These patients, if asymptomatic, do not require labs, EKG, or admission.

23. **What usually causes damage in Taser injuries?**
    Trauma from the Taser barbs. To remove an imbedded barb, grab it with a forceps and pull straight out with a quick motion. Follow with standard wound care.

LIGHTENING INJURY

24. **What is the mortality rate of lightning injuries?**
    The mortality rate is around 17.5%. The most common cause of death is cardiac arrest due to asystole.

25. **What voltage level occurs with lightning strike injuries?**
    • Millions of volts over a very short period (milliseconds)

26. **What is "reverse triage" for lightning injury victims?**
Unlike with standard mass casualty triage, the priority is to resuscitate those who appear dead. Victims with cardiac arrest due to lightning generally do well with aggressive cardiopulmonary resuscitation. As a result of autonomic dysfunction, these patients may present with a blown pupil, which should not be used as an indicator of neurological status.

27. **Can lightning strikes occur when there is no rain or thunder?**
Yes. Lightning can travel horizontally as far as 10 miles and strike when it is sunny out, preceding a storm. Approximately 10% of lightning strikes occur when there is no rain.

28. **What are Lichtenberg figures?**
These are feather-like skin manifestations that are pathognomonic of lightning injury. They are transient and do not cause skin damage.

29. **What is keraunoparalysis?**
Temporary paralysis that occurs with lightning strikes is likely due to vasospasm and usually resolves within hours.

30. **List four ways lightning injuries differ from high-voltage electrical injuries.**
   - Energy level: Lightning injuries have a higher voltage.
   - Time of exposure: Lightning injuries are very brief/instantaneous versus longer exposure to high-voltage injuries.
   - Cardiac: Lightning injuries cause asystole versus high-voltage injuries that cause ventricular fibrillation.
   - Burns: Lightning burns are more superficial, causing little to no damage. High-voltage burns are deeper and more likely to result in the need for fasciotomy.

31. **What is the initial management of a patient struck by lightning?**
These patients should be managed like other patients with multiple injuries. Focusing on ABCDE is the first priority. Airway management is essential because hypoxic cardiac arrest is the major cause of death. Hemorrhage control and fracture management are likely unnecessary since blunt trauma is unusual. Full-thickness burns are also rare. It is important to obtain an EKG and look for QT prolongation, T-wave inversion, and ST alterations. Order diagnostic studies including CBC, basic metabolic panel, creatine phosphokinase, creatine kinase-MB, coagulation panel, troponin, and urinalysis. Monitor sodium levels carefully as hyponatremia can increase their risk for cerebral edema.

32. **Which two additional systems need to be thoroughly evaluated in lightning injuries?**
   a. Ocular: Ocular damage can occur in up to 50% of patients injured by lightening. Cataracts may develop hours, days, or months after lightning exposure.
   b. Auditory: Tympanic membrane rupture occurs in 60% to 80% of patients with lightning injuries. Patients usually heal well with complete restoration of their hearing. Any otorrhea or hemotympanum should prompt an emergent CT scan for skull fracture.

33. **Do all patients with lightning strikes need to be admitted?**
All patients with lightning should be admitted for observation due to possible delayed cerebral edema. After 24 hours, patients who are stable may be considered for discharge with adequate follow-up and anticipatory guidance on common delayed sequelae such as cataracts, neurological dysfunction, visceral injury, and depression.

KEY POINTS: LIGHTNING INJURIES

- Lightning injury can occur when it is sunny out, preceding a storm.
- The most common cause of death from lightning is cardiac arrest due to asystole.
- With lightning strikes, perform reverse triage and treat those who appear dead first.
- Blown pupils should not be used as an indicator of neurological status.
- All patients with lightning injuries should be admitted to the hospital.

Acknowledgment

The author wishes to thank Dr. Amanda Pratt for her contributions to this chapter in the previous edition.

BIBLIOGRAPHY

1. Gardner AR, Hauda WE, Bozeman WP. Conducted electrical weapon (TASER) use against minors: a shocking analysis. *Pediatr Emerg Care.* 2012;28(9):873–877.
2. Gatewood MO, Zane RD. Lightning injuries. *Emerg Med Clin N Am.* 2004;22:369–403.
3. Gentes J, Schleche C. Electrical injuries in the emergency department: an evidence-based review. *Emerg Med Pract.* 2018;20(11):1–19.
4. Glastein MM, Ayalon I, Miller E, Scolnik D. Pediatric electrical burn Injuries. Experience of a large tertiary care hospital and a review of electrical injury. *Pediatr Emerg Care.* 2013;29(6):737–740.
5. Roberts S, Meltzer JA. An evidence-based approach to electrical injuries in children. *Pediatr Emerg Med Pract.* 2013;10(8):1–20. EBMedicine.net.
6. Schissler K, Pruden C. Pediatric electrical injuries in the emergency department: an evidence based review. *Pediatr Emerg Med Pract.* 2021;18(12):1–24. EBMedicine.net.
7. Spies C, Trohman RG. Narrative review: electrocution and life-threatening electrical injuries. *Ann Intern Med.* 2006;145:531–537.
8. Van Ruler R, Eikendal T, Kooij FO, Tan ECTH. A shocking injury: a clinical review of lightning injuries highlighting pitfalls and a treatment protocol. *Injury.* 2022;53(10):3070–3077.
9. Yilmaz AA, et al. Evaluation of children presenting to the emergency room after electrical injury. *Turk J Med Sci.* 2015;45:325–328.

CHAPTER 65

HYPOTHERMIA AND HYPERTHERMIA

Brenda J. Bender

HYPOTHERMIA

1. **How do you define hypothermia?**
   There are three stages of hypothermia:
   - Mild: Core temperature 32°C to 35°C
   - Moderate: Core temperature 28°C to 32°C
   - Severe: Core temperature below 28°C

2. **Why are children more prone to hypothermia than adults?**
   Children are more prone to hypothermia because their bodies have larger surface-to-mass ratios. In addition, infants cannot shiver and increase heat production, young children have limited glycogen stores to support heat production, and children may not recognize and avoid cold exposure.

3. **Why is hypothermia often overlooked in pediatric patients?**
   Some clinical thermometers only measure as low as 34°C. In addition, clinicians may think of hypothermia only with severe environmental exposure. In fact, it may occur after prolonged exposure in less cold conditions, after any immersion in cold or warm water, with any major illness or trauma, after resuscitation or transport, and with other causes such as drug ingestion or child abuse.

4. **How can physicians not recognize a "cold patient"?**
   Only in the early stages of hypothermia do patients appear cold. In severe hypothermia, signs such as shivering, pallor, cyanosis, and agitation are replaced by flushing, edema, and muscular rigidity, so that the coldest patients are the most likely to have their hypothermia overlooked.

5. **What is the effect of hypothermia on the brain?**
   For every fall in body temperature of 1°C, there is a 6% decline in cerebral blood flow.
   At 29°C to 31°C, there will be confusion or delirium and muscle rigidity. At 25°C to 29°C, a patient will be comatose, have absent deep tendon reflexes, and have fixed and dilated pupils.

6. **What are some risk factors for hypothermia?**
   - Trauma
   - Severe illness
   - Immersion or submersion
   - Central nervous system (CNS) illness or injury
   - Hypothalamic dysfunction
   - Endocrine disease
   - Metabolic impairment
   - Rescue/resuscitation/transport
   - Intoxication, especially with alcohol, barbiturates, or phenothiazines
   - Bums and weeping dermatoses
   - Child abuse (e.g., cold water immersion)

7. **What are the key pathologic changes in hypothermia?**
   The key changes seen in hypothermia are as follows:
   - Hypovolemia due to vascular leak
   - Respiratory depression occurs late
   - Circulatory collapse due to decreased cardiac output, myocardial contractility, and systemic vascular resistance
   - Arrhythmias due to increased myocardial irritability
     - Ventricular fibrillation is often seen with severe hypothermia (<28°C)

8. **Is there an electrocardiogram (ECG) clue to hypothermia?**
   The J (Osborne) wave is pathognomonic but is not always seen. It is the convex upward deflections at the junction of QRS and ST segments.

9. **How should temperatures be taken to detect hypothermia?**

   A low-reading thermometer must be used. Oral, axillary, and skin scanning thermometers are unreliable, and tympanic temperatures have not been studied. Rectal temperatures must be taken deep in the rectum for at least several minutes, and may still be subject to damping, artifact, and time lags. In critical patients or those with marked hypothermia, flexible temperature probes in the bladder, esophagus, or nasopharynx best reflect core temperatures and provide the vital ability to track temperature over time.

10. **What is clinically seen in each stage of hypothermia?**

    - Mild hypothermia: The body attempts to combat heat loss by shivering, increasing metabolism, and vasoconstriction.
    - Moderate hypothermia: Compensatory mechanisms begin to fail. Mental status, respiration, and circulation may diminish.
    - Severe hypothermia: Failed thermoregulation, metabolic shutdown, and paradoxical vasodilatation accompanied by hypovolemia, decreased perfusion, and stupor or coma.

11. **What treatment does every hypothermic patient need to receive?**

    Every patient needs oxygen to correct hypoxia and hypercarbia. Patients often have electrolyte abnormalities and it is important to correct hypoglycemia and hypokalemia. All patients need fluid replacement, initially with warmed intravenous (IV) saline or Ringer's lactate.

12. **How should you rewarm a patient?**

    Patients can receive passive or active rewarming. Active rewarming includes external and core rewarming. Core rewarming is more rapid. Patients with temperatures at or above 32°C can be warmed using passive rewarming or simple external rewarming techniques such as warm blankets. Patients with core temperatures below 32°C due to acute causes should receive external or core rewarming. Those with temperatures less than 32°C due to chronic causes need core rewarming.

13. **What are methods of active rewarming?**

    - External rewarming includes forced-air warming.
    - Core rewarming includes warmed IV fluids (to about 43°C) in a blood-warming coil and heated, humidified oxygen, warmed irrigation of the bladder, stomach, or, most effectively, left pleural cavity, and finally to rewarming using heart-lung pumps or extracorporeal membrane oxygenation (ECMO).

14. **What are the risks of rewarming a patient?**

    Risks of rewarming include afterdrop, arrhythmias, hypotension, pulmonary edema, coagulopathy, shock, acute kidney injury, and CNS dysfunction. There are fewer risks in core rewarming than in external rewarming.

15. **What is afterdrop?**

    Afterdrop is when core temperature drops. This is seen when you do early rewarming of the skin and extremities. This leads to peripheral vasodilation and therefore shunting of cold, acidemic blood to the core, dropping the core temperature.

16. **What common treatments are not routinely recommended for hypothermia?**

    Prophylactic antibiotics or corticosteroids are not beneficial in hypothermia. Acidosis is physiologic in the hypothermic state, and the use of bicarbonate has provoked dangerous alkalosis after rewarming. Insulin for hyperglycemia is contraindicated; the condition will usually resolve with rewarming, and the insulin will begin to work only at that time.

17. **What is the ideal rewarming rate?**

    There is no established goal rate of rewarming, but 1°C/hour is adequate. If patients fail to rewarm at a rate of at least 0.5°C/hour, then you should progress to a more aggressive method.

18. **How long should the resuscitation of a hypothermic patient last?**

    All patients should receive treatments as per the Pediatric Advanced Life Support algorithm until the core temperature is 34°C to 35°C. This is because of the neuroprotective effects of hypothermia. There have been many cases documented of complete recovery of patients with hypothermia and cardiac arrest despite prolonged resuscitation.

19. **What is frostbite?**

    Frostbite is injury and destruction of skin and its underlying tissue after prolonged exposure to cold. This most commonly involves toes, fingers, ears, and nose.

20. **How do you treat frostbite?**
    There are three phases of treatment:
    - First, the pre-thaw period—get out of the cold and remove cold clothing. Apply soft padding to affected areas. Do not rub or apply pressure to the injured digits as this can cause further tissue damage.
    - Second, the rewarming period—immerse affected areas in water from 40°C to 42°C for 15 to 30 minutes.
    - Finally, the post-thaw period—apply loose sterile dressings to wounds, separate digits with cotton, and splint extremities.
        Patients need analgesia because rewarming is very painful. Consider tetanus prophylaxsis.

21. **Are there exceptions to the rule that "no one is dead until he is warm and dead"?**
    Yes. This does not apply when there are injuries that are incompatible with life, if a patient cannot be rescued from a cold environment in the first place, or if maximal available rewarming methods are ineffective and transport is not an option. Standard time limits may be employed if there is no return of spontaneous circulation within 30 minutes of warming from 32°C to 35°C.

22. **Is there an association between hypothermia and the mortality rate in severe acute respiratory syndrome coronavirus 2 (SARS-CoV-2) infection?**
    Patients with SARS-CoV-2 have a higher mortality rate if they also have hypothermia.

KEY POINTS: HYPOTHERMIA IN CHILDREN

1. Children are particularly prone to hypothermia, especially with serious illness or injury.
2. Hypothermia often goes undetected by clinicians lacking a high degree of suspicion.
3. Severe hypothermia mimics death.
4. The number one cause of hypothermia is environmental.

KEY POINTS: TREATMENT OF HYPOTHERMIA

1. Patient with mild hypothermia should receive passive rewarming.
2. Patients with moderate or severe hypothermia should receive active rewarming—either external or core rewarming.
3. Watch out for risks, especially afterdrop.

KEY POINTS: TREATMENT OF FROSTBITE

1. Rapidly rewarm frostbitten parts in a bath of water at 40°C to 42°C.
2. Give narcotic analgesics.
3. Give tetanus prophylaxsis.

HYPERTHERMIA/HEAT-RELATED ILLNESS

23. **What is in the spectrum of heat-related illness?**
    Heat-related illness includes heat cramps, heat exhaustion, and heat stroke.

24. **What is the difference between heat exhaustion and heat stroke?**
    Heat exhaustion and heat stroke are on a continuum of heat-related illnesses that occur when the body's heat loss mechanisms are overwhelmed or insufficient to respond to environmental demands. Heat exhaustion is the less severe of the two conditions and is believed to represent reversible heat overload without end-organ tissue damage. Heat stroke is characteristically associated with irreversible tissue damage. Heat stroke is life-threatening and is distinguished by the presence of neurologic dysfunction, anhidrosis, and a temperature >41°C (see Question 45).

25. **How does high humidity affect heat loss?**
    In addition to high ambient temperature, humidity plays an important role in heat-related illness. Evaporation of sweat is the primary and most important method for cooling the body. High humidity limits sweat evaporation, and there is less and less cooling as humidity rises. Eventually, when it is very humid, perspiration is not at all effective to cool the person.

26. **Who is at increased risk for heat-related illness?**

People at increased risk include those involved in extreme activities in a hot, humid atmosphere, people with an underlying illness or obesity, those with decreased fluid intake, and those who are drinking alcohol or using certain drugs such as cocaine, salicylates, amphetamines, phenothiazines, antihistamines, and anticholinergics.

Heat stroke typically occurs in extremes of age after excessive exertion in hot weather such as heat waves. Young children who rely on others for liquid intake are at higher risk. Neonates are perhaps at the greatest risk because they have poorly developed thermoregulatory mechanisms and depend on others to remove them from a hot environment and provide adequate hydration.

27. **Why are children at increased risk for hyperthermia compared to adults?**

Children are at higher risk due to their greater body surface area. Children produce more metabolic heat per kilogram of body weight and have a higher set point. They are less efficient at thermoregulation: they have a slower speed of acclimatization. In addition, children have a lower sweating rate. Finally, children may be less cognizant of the need to stay hydrated when exercising or playing in warm weather, and they may be dependent on others to help them rehydrate.

28. **Which diseases increase the risk for heat-related illness?**

- Diabetes insipidus, diabetes mellitus (associated with excessive fluid loss)
- Skin diseases (no sweat glands)
- Cystic fibrosis (salt losses in sweat)
- Mental retardation (inadequate drinking)
- Spina bifida (sweat gland dysfunction, suboptimal sweating)
- Hypothyroidism
- Cardiovascular disease (excessive sweating in some cyanotic heart diseases)
- Anorexia nervosa (abnormal hypothalamic function)
- Obesity
- Sickle cell trait (see Question 29)

29. **How can having sickle cell trait impact a patient with heat-related illness?**

Although sickle cell trait is often thought of as a benign condition, deaths from *exertional heat stroke* have been reported in adolescent athletes with sickle cell trait. Patients with sickle cell trait can have increased sickling with hypoxemia, acidosis, hyperthermia, and red blood cell dehydration. Patients with sickle cell trait are at increased risk for rhabdomyolysis or sudden death during exercise, even if not in an extremely warm environment. This danger is especially likely when the exercise is intense, done by unconditioned people, and done at high altitudes. These factors are all made worse if the individual is hyperthermic or dehydrated, but this is not always the case with exertional heat stroke (see Question 49).

The exact pathophysiology is not known, but rhabdomyolysis in these patients is most likely related to the sickling of the red blood cells in the exercising muscle. Recent research has shown that the skeletal muscle capillary structure in patients with sickle cell trait may differ when compared to control subjects. The biopsies from muscles of patients with sickle cell trait demonstrate a higher proportion of larger microvessels and a decrease in capillary density and degree of vascular tortuosity. These changes affect muscle perfusion and contribute to exercise-related acidosis and rhabdomyolysis.

30. **How is heat produced?**

Heat is produced as a byproduct of basal metabolism, through muscle activity (shivering), or through the effects of thyroxine and sympathetic stimulation on cellular processes.

31. **How is heat lost?**

Heat is lost through *conduction* to objects and air, *convection* through air or liquid that surrounds tissues, *evaporation*, and *radiation* of infrared energy.

32. **What is acclimatization?**

Acclimatization is the natural physiologic adjustment to heat exposure that usually occurs over 7 to 14 days. This adjustment allows for improved sweating and cardiac performance.

33. **What happens to the body's salt production in the heat?**

Initially, with heat exposure a child will lose a lot of salt, up to 15 to 20 g/day. Over time, aldosterone production increases, causing more NaCl reabsorption in the sweat gland ducts, and salt production normalizes to 3 to 5 g/day.

34. **What is the cause of heat cramps?**

Heat cramps are caused by electrolyte depletion. It occurs when a teenager loses excessive salt from heavy sweating after strenuous physical activity, leading to electrolyte depletion.

35. What are the symptoms of heat cramps?

    Symptoms of heat cramps include sudden onset of intermittent, brief severe cramps or spasms, usually in large muscles such as the hamstrings or gastrocnemius, or in the abdomen. Pain usually occurs after exercise, when the child is relaxing or showering.

36. Are there any abnormal laboratory values with heat cramps?

    • Blood levels of sodium and chloride are often decreased.
    • There is no urinary sodium.

37. Who most often suffers from heat cramps?

    Heat cramps are most often seen in highly conditioned persons who are acclimatized. They usually have good water replacement but inadequate salt replacement.

38. How are heat cramps treated?

    A patient suffering from heat cramps should rest in a cool place, drink fluids, and increase salt intake.

39. What causes heat exhaustion?

    Heat exhaustion is caused by dehydration and excessive sweating with inadequate water and salt intake. The two types of heat exhaustion are water depletion and salt depletion.

40. What causes water depletion heat exhaustion, and what are the symptoms?

    Water depletion heat exhaustion occurs in the unacclimatized person who exerts himself in the heat and has poor water replacement. Symptoms typically include high body temperature (38°C-39°C), intense thirst, headache, vomiting, hypotension, lethargy or agitation, tachycardia, myalgias, muscle cramps, and dizziness. If unattended, heat exhaustion may progress to heat stroke.

41. Which laboratory abnormalities may be present with water depletion heat exhaustion?

    • Hypernatremia
    • Hyperchloremia
    • Elevated hematocrit
    • Elevated urine specific gravity

42. What causes salt depletion heat exhaustion and what are the symptoms?

    Salt depletion heat exhaustion is seen in an unacclimatized person who exerts himself in hot weather and has poor salt replacement. It is also seen in patients with cystic fibrosis. Symptoms include a temperature of 39°C to 40°C, weakness, fatigue, frontal headache, nausea, vomiting, diarrhea, muscle cramps, tachycardia, and orthostatic hypotension.

43. Which laboratory abnormalities may be found with salt depletion heat exhaustion?

    • Hyponatremia
    • Elevated hematocrit
    • Severely decreased urinary sodium

44. How is heat exhaustion treated?

    Treat a patient with heat exhaustion with rest in a cool location and rehydration, either orally or IV. Increase salt and fluid intake. Give salty fluids and avoid hypotonic fluids, like water. Correct serum sodium slowly to avoid iatrogenic cerebral edema. Advise the patient to avoid alcohol and caffeine. If the patient is not able to orally hydrate, give isotonic saline IV. In severe salt depletion from heat exhaustion, with seizures, consider giving IV hypertonic saline.

45. What is heat stroke?

    Heat stroke is a life-threatening emergency. This condition has a greater than 50% mortality rate. It is the third most common cause of exercise-related death among U.S. high school athletes (after head injury and cardiac disorders). Heat stroke is characterized by a body temperature higher than 40°C, flushed appearance, red and hot skin, change in mental status with severe CNS dysfunction, and anhidrosis. Often, sweating stops before the onset of heat stroke. The patient may have circulatory collapse, rhabdomyolysis, renal failure, lightheadedness, muscle cramps, nausea, vomiting, tachycardia, tachypnea, and CNS dysfunction.

46. What are the CNS manifestations of heat stroke?

    CNS dysfunction can be manifested in many ways, including a sense of impending doom, headache, dizziness, weakness, confusion, euphoria, gait disturbance, combativeness, seizures, posturing, and coma. The early clinical symptoms are sometimes overlooked because they often are perceived to be the normal result of exertion. Often the severity of the problem is realized only when the victim collapses suddenly.

Table 65.1 Serious Complications of Heat Stroke

Acidosis	Rhabdomyolysis
Electrolyte imbalance	Disseminated intravascular coagulation
Adynamic ileus	Renal failure
Arrhythmias	Hepatic damage
Shivering	Permanent neurologic sequelae
Seizures	Death

47. **What cardiac findings are present in heat stroke?**
   Initially, there is a rapid and full pulse and an elevated pulse pressure. As heat stroke progresses, peripheral vascular resistance decreases and vasodilation occurs to increase cardiac output. If hyperpyrexia is not corrected, the patient may become cyanotic with a thin rapid pulse from decreased cardiac output.

48. **List the possible serious complications of heat stroke.**
   See Table 65.1.

49. **What are the two types of heat stroke and how do they differ?**
   Classic heat stroke usually involves a child with poor water intake in a very warm climate. It has a slow onset and there is no hypoglycemia or rhabdomyolysis. *Exertional heat stroke* typically affects a child who has been involved in prolonged activity, usually during the initial phases of training. Exertional heat stroke is less common and is usually seen in younger individuals. It is not associated with a markedly elevated core temperature or anhidrosis. In many cases, the ambient temperature is not as high as that seen in cases of classic heat stroke. Exertional heat stroke has a rapid onset, and there is often lactic acidosis, hypoglycemia, hypocalcemia, and rhabdomyolysis.

50. **Which laboratory abnormalities are seen in heat stroke?**
   - Sodium and chloride can be normal or elevated.
   - Glucose can be normal or decreased.
   - Calcium is usually decreased.
   - Serum creatinine kinase (CK) is typically elevated.

51. **What are the priorities for treating heat stroke?**
   The two priorities of treating heat stroke are eliminating hyperpyrexia and supporting the cardiovascular system. First, bring the patient into a cool location and remove all clothing. Actively cool the child by *evaporative cooling*. This is done by spraying the patient with lukewarm water and positioning fans to blow air across the body and applying ice packs to the neck, groin, and axilla. In extreme cases consider iced peritoneal lavage. Active cooling can be discontinued when the rectal temperature falls to 38.5°C. Consider sedation and paralysis of the patient.
   Use 5% dextrose in 0.5 normal saline for maintenance fluid and bolus with normal saline or lactated Ringer's solution (20 mL/kg) as needed for resuscitation. Use other fluids as needed to correct electrolyte abnormalities. Monitor the child's temperature using a rectal probe, heart rate, ECG, blood pressure, pulses, perfusion, urine output, and CNS function. Consider ECMO in extreme situations.

52. **What medication should you use for cardiovascular support for patients with heat stroke?**
   Use dobutamine at 5 to 20 mcg/kg/minute as needed to support the cardiovascular system. Dobutamine is a β-receptor agonist that increases myocardial contractility and maintains peripheral vasodilation.

53. **What medication should you use to stop shivering?**
   Use IV benzodiazepines, such as lorazepam, to prevent or stop shivering. You do not want the patient to be shivering because this increases endogenous heat production.

54. **Which medications should be avoided in managing patients with heat stroke?**
   Avoid alpha-agonists, such as epinephrine and norepinephrine, because they cause peripheral vasoconstriction leading to poor heat dissipation. Do not use atropine and other anticholinergic drugs because they inhibit sweating. Antipyretics, such as acetaminophen and ibuprofen, are not useful to lower core temperature. Likewise, dantrolene, which is used to treat malignant hyperthermia, has no role in managing heat stroke. There are no specific medications available for this condition.

55. **How do you treat myoglobinuria related to heat stroke?**
    Treat myoglobinuria with diuresis. Maintain urine output at more than 1 mL/kg/hour, and if needed use furosemide at 1 mg/kg. Some recommend giving mannitol at 0.25 to 1 g/kg.

56. **Which laboratory values need to be assessed in heat stroke?**
    Check the following:
    - Complete blood count
    - Prothrombin time/partial thromboplastin time
    - Electrolytes, blood urea nitrogen, creatinine, calcium, phosphorus
    - CK
    - Urinalysis (including myoglobin)
    - Arterial blood gas
       Even after the patient is stabilized and cooled, there is still a high risk of multiorgan failure, metabolic abnormalities, and coagulopathies.

57. **What is the prognosis for a patient with heat stroke?**
    Severe heat stroke has a mortality rate of at least 10%. Up to one-third will have permanent moderate or severe neurologic impairment. Patients with higher initial temperatures, hypotension, and a lower Glasgow Coma Scale (GCS) are more likely to die. The outcome is directly related to how quickly cooling is initiated and the duration of hyperthermia. A patient is most likely to survive if that person can maintain cardiac output.

58. **What happens to an infant left in a car on a hot day?**
    Every year, dozens of infants die in the United States when they are left unattended in unventilated automobiles in the sun. Temperatures can reach 60°C within 15 minutes when a car is left in the sun at 30°C to 40°C. The average temperature increase in a closed vehicle is 3.20°F for every 5-minute interval, with 80% of the temperature rise happening during the first 30 minutes.
       Unfortunately, keeping the vehicle windows slightly open DOES NOT decrease the rate of temperature rise or decrease the maximum temperature reached in the vehicle.

59. **How can heat-related illnesses be avoided?**
    Encourage children to wear loose-fitting, lightweight, and light-colored clothing in hot weather and during exertion, with as much skin exposed as possible to allow evaporative dissipation of heat. Instruct children to rest often and seek shade in warm weather. Tell them to modify physical activity in the face of high ambient temperature and humidity and to drink frequently. Assure that athletes are well hydrated before initiating physical activity and that they continue to consume cold water throughout the exercise period and after exercise has been completed to avoid dehydration. In warm weather, ensure at least a 2-hour break between same-day events. Athletes should participate in a preseason conditioning program and allow a period of acclimation when exercising in the hot summer months. Athletes should be restricted from playing while experiencing a febrile illness.

60. **How can clinicians help prevent pediatric deaths in hot cars?**
    Clinicians can educate caregivers that it does not have to be a very hot, sunny day for the passenger compartment of a car to develop deadly temperatures. Advise caregivers of children to lock their car doors when not in use. About 27% of deaths are due to children finding their way into a hot car and becoming entrapped. Remind caregivers to never leave a child in a hot car intentionally. About 10% of deaths are related to caregivers not wishing to disturb a sleeping child, and then forgetting the child is in the car. Encourage caregivers to "Look Before You Lock." Most deaths occur when a well-meaning caregiver just forgets the infant is in the back seat (usually not visible in a rear-facing car seat). It is recommended that the driver leave a handbag, briefcase, or cell phone near the infant so they are more likely to check the back seat before exiting the car. Continue to advocate for the development and installation of technology that will alarm and alert drivers to check the back seat for an infant passenger. The technology exists and legislation can achieve such advances in automobiles.

61. **How much should a child drink during physical activity to stay well hydrated?**
    A child aged 9 to 12 years should drink 100 to 250 mL (3-8 ounces) every 20 minutes. The adolescent needs to drink 1 to 1.5 L (34-50 ounces) each hour.

62. **Besides environmental, what are other causes of hyperthermia?**
    Even though environmental is the number one cause of hyperthermia, neuroleptic malignant syndrome, serotonin syndrome, and malignant hyperthermia should be in your differential diagnosis.

KEY POINTS: PREVENTION OF HEAT-RELATED ILLNESS

1. Wear loose-fitting, lightweight clothing.
2. Rest often.
3. Seek shade.
4. Avoid exercise or strenuous activity, especially during the hottest part of the day.
5. Drink frequently.

KEY POINTS: SYMPTOMS OF HEAT EXHAUSTION

1. Severe thirst
2. Excessive sweating
3. Dilated pupils
4. Lightheadedness
5. Nausea/vomiting

KEY POINTS: SYMPTOMS OF HEAT CRAMPS

1. Sweating
2. Muscle spasms or cramps
3. Weakness
4. Lightheadedness
5. Can mimic an acute abdomen

KEY POINTS: PHYSICAL EXAMINATION FINDINGS OF HEAT STROKE

1. Anhidrosis
2. Fever
3. Red skin
4. Constricted pupils
5. Rapid shallow breathing
6. CNS dysfunction

KEY POINTS: TREATMENT OF HEAT-RELATED ILLNESS

1. Remove clothing.
2. Move the patient to a cooler location.
3. Increase salt intake.
4. Provide fluid replacement and maintenance.
5. Make active cooling available—use evaporation with fans after spraying the patient with cold water.
6. Give cardiovascular support.

Acknowledgment

The author wishes to thank Dr. Howard M. Corneli for his contributions to the section on hypothermia in the previous edition.

BIBLIOGRAPHY

1. Bergeron MF, Devore C, Rice SG. Climatic heat stress and exercising children and adolescents. Council on Sports Medicine and Fitness and Council on School Health. *Pediatrics.* 2011;128:e741–e747.
2. Brown DJ, Brugger H, Boyd J, Paal P. Accidental hypothermia. *N Engl J Med.* 2012;367:1930.
3. Connes P, Reid H, Hardy-Dessources MD, et al. Physiological responses of sickle cell trait carriers during exercise. *Sports Med.* 2008;38(11):931–946.
4. Corneli HM. Accidental hypothermia. *Pediatr Emerg Care.* 2012;28(5):475–480.
5. Danzl DF, Huecker MR. Auerbach's wilderness medicine. In: Auerbach PS, Cushing TA, Harris NS, eds. *Accidental Hypothermia.* 7th ed. Elsevier Publishers; 2017;1:135.

6. Dunn RJ, Kim TY. Pediatric heat-related illness: recommendations for prevention and management. *Pediatr Emerg Med Pract.* 2017;14(8):1–20.
7. Fatteh N, Naranjo CD. Association of hypothermia with increased mortality rate in SARS-CoV-2 infection. *Int J Infect Dis.* 2021;108:167–170.
8. Hammett DL, Kennedy TM, Selbst SM, Rollins A, et al. Pediatric heatstroke fatalities caused by being left in motor vehicles. *Pediatr Emerg Care.* 2021;37(12):e1560–e1565.
9. Heller JL. *Heat Emergencies.* Medline Plus Medical Encyclopedia. Available at http://www.nlm.nih.gov/medlineplus/ency/article/000056.htm.
10. Hughes A, Riou P, Day C. Full neurological recovery from profound (18.0 degrees C) acute accidental hypothermia: successful resuscitation using active invasive rewarming techniques. *Emerg Med J.* 2007;24:511.
11. Koutroulis I, Agrawal D. Environmental emergencies, radiological emergencies, bites and stings. In: Shaw KN, Bachur RG, eds. *Fleisher & Ludwig's Textbook of Pediatric Emergency Medicine.* 8th ed. Wolters Kluwer; 2021:680–723.
12. Mangus CW, Canares TL. Heat-related illness in children in an era of extreme temperatures. *Pediatr Rev.* 2019;40(3):97–107.
13. Maron BJ, Doerer JJ, Haas TS, et al. Sudden deaths in young competitive athletes: analysis of 1866 deaths in the United States, 1980-2006. *Circulation.* 2009;119:1085.
14. Paul P, Pasquier M, Darocha T, Lechner R, et al. Accidental hypothermia-2021 update. *Int J Environ Res Public Health.* 2022;19(1):501.
15. Westwood CS, Fallowfield JL, Delves SK, et al. Individual risk factors associated with exertional heat illness: a systemic review. *Exp Physiol.* 2021;106:191.

CHAPTER 66

HIGH-ALTITUDE ILLNESS

Lalit Bajaj

1. **What are the mechanisms that cause high-altitude illness (HAI)?**
   At sea level, a large pressure gradient exists so inspired oxygen can flow from inspired air into the tissues. As altitude increases, this pressure gradient is reduced, and this leads to a form of tissue hypoxia known as hypobaric hypoxia. This drives physiological changes and can initiate HAI.

2. **Is there a particular altitude threshold that is considered high altitude from a clinical concern standpoint?**
   The effects of altitude are usually first seen at 1500 m (5000 ft), with hyperventilation resulting in respiratory alkalosis, being one of the first responses. Longer-term mechanisms such as increased red blood mass; and increasing bicarbonate excretion from the kidneys take several days to weeks to develop. More serious clinical concerns, such as acute mountain sickness (AMS) and high-altitude pulmonary edema (HAPE), usually do not occur until above 2500 m (8000 ft). However, there are reports of AMS and HAPE down to 1400 m (4600 ft).

3. **What is the most common HAI?**
   By far, AMS is the most common HAI. Symptoms tend to develop within 6 to 48 hours of arrival to altitudes of 2500 m (8000 ft) or greater. Headache is the defining symptom of AMS and is usually bilateral and worsened with Valsalva. In addition, one or more of the following is needed to support the diagnosis: insomnia, dizziness, fatigue, nausea, vomiting, or loss of appetite. Overall estimates of incidence of AMS are 25% of those traveling higher than 2500 m (8000 ft).

4. **Is it true that children are more susceptible to AMS versus adults?**
   There is considerable debate about whether children have a higher incidence of AMS versus adults. At this time, the data would point to a similar incidence, although preverbal children are likely undercounted as their symptoms are vague (irritable, fussy, vomiting, poor sleep, poor oral intake) and the symptoms have significant overlay with other common illnesses.

5. **What is the management of AMS?**
   Children who develop AMS can often remain at their current altitude and be managed with acetaminophen or ibuprofen. If the child is vomiting, antiemetics can be helpful. The use of acetazolamide may be helpful but seems to be more helpful in prevention; and side effects (paresthesia, more frequent urination, and metallic taste) may not be well tolerated. The preferred treatment for children with more moderate-to-severe AMS is descent.

6. **Is there an AMS severity scale available?**
   Yes, the Lake Louise Scoring System is available to make the diagnosis and severity via scoring in eight clinical domains (Table 66.1). It has been modified to include a "Pediatric Symptom Score" and a "Fussiness Score" for younger and preverbal children. Utility of the scoring system may be limited clinically.

7. **Is AMS related to high-altitude cerebral edema (HACE)?**
   HACE is distinguished from AMS by the presence of neurological findings such as ataxia, confusion, or altered mental status during ascent to high altitude. It can follow AMS, but the mechanisms are not well understood. While increased intracranial pressure is thought to be related to tissue hypoxia, other aspects such as decreased cerebral venous flow may also contribute. HACE is very rare and almost unheard of at altitudes below 4000 m (13,000 ft).

8. **How is HACE managed?**
   The management of HACE where medical care can be provided is oxygen, dexamethasone, and immediate descent. If no access to medical care is available, immediate descent is indicated.

9. **What is High-Altitude Pulmonary Edema (HAPE)?**
   HAPE is formally defined as noncardiogenic pulmonary edema caused by hypobaric hypoxia. HAPE presents with dyspnea, reduced exercise tolerance, cough, hemoptysis, tachycardia, cyanosis, and rales on examination. It is estimated to occur in 0.5% of individuals and can occur even after just 2 hours at altitudes over 2500 m, which may be more common in children. It can be fatal. While much more common over 2500 m, HAPE has been reported to occur as low as 1400 m, so it is important to consider the diagnosis even at lower altitudes. There

Table 66.1 Lake Louise Scoring System for the Diagnosis of Acute Mountain Sickness (AMS), 2018 Revision

Headache

0–None at all
1–A mild headache
2–Moderate headache
3–Severe headache, incapacitating

Gastrointestinal Symptoms

0–Good appetite
1–Poor appetite or nausea
2–Moderate nausea or vomiting
3–Severe nausea and vomiting, incapacitating

Fatigue and/or Weakness

0–Not tired or weak
1–Mild fatigue/weakness
2–Moderate fatigue/weakness
3–Severe fatigue/weakness, incapacitating

Dizziness/Light-Headedness

0–No dizziness/light-headedness
1–Mild dizziness/light-headedness
2–Moderate dizziness/light-headedness
3–Severe dizziness/light-headedness, incapacitating

Adapted from Roach RC, Hackett PH, Oelz O, et al. The 2018 Lake Louise acute mountain sickness score. *High Alt Med Biol.* 2018;19(1):4–6. doi:10.1089/ham.2017.0164.
A score of 3 or greater, including at least one point from the headache parameter, is indicative of AMS. The sleep disturbance metric has been removed from this latest revision because of inconsistencies of sleep being correlated with other important indices of AMS (particularly headache). While sleep disturbance, including Cheynes-Stokes respiration, is a common finding at acute ascent in those who have AMS, it is also common in subjects who otherwise do not meet AMS criteria and is likely an effect of hypoxia alone.

are data suggesting that HAPE is more common in children versus adults as they may have increased pulmonary vasoreactivity and altered control of breathing especially at high altitudes. Data also suggest that males are at increased risk; and that there is likely a genetic-based susceptibility in some patients.

10. **Are there different types of available for HAPE?**
    Yes, there are three types of HAPE. Classic HAPE occurs in persons who reside in low-altitude locations and then travel to high altitudes. Children with respiratory illnesses have been shown to be at higher risk for classic HAPE, likely because of increased pulmonary vascular permeability. Reentry HAPE occurs in persons who reside at a high altitude, travel to a lower altitude (even if just for 1-2 days), and then develop HAPE upon returning to high altitude. There is some evidence suggesting that reentry HAPE is more common in children than adults. High-altitude resident pulmonary edema is a relatively new recognized entity where a child who resides at high altitude develops pulmonary edema without any change in elevation. It is poorly understood and difficult to diagnose.

11. **Are there diagnostic tools available for HAPE?**
    The Lake Louise criteria for HAPE requires a recent gain in altitude associated with two of the four symptoms of dyspnea at rest, cough, lowered exercise performance, and chest tightness/congestion. In addition, there must be two of the four signs of crackles/wheezes, central cyanosis, tachypnea, and tachycardia. There is a pediatric adaptation of the Lake Louise score but it has not been evaluated rigorously.

12. **Is chest radiography helpful for HAPE?**
    Chest radiographs are recommended to confirm the presence of pulmonary edema and "fluffy infiltrates" (Figs. 66.1 and 66.2). There are reports of lung ultrasound being used with the now-classic finding of "lung comets" (intraparenchymal edema) being diagnostic. Chest radiographs can also be helpful in evaluating predisposing conditions such as congenital heart disease. Concurrent pneumonia is also often diagnosed but likely s an overdiagnosis with radiograph findings being nonspecific at times.

13. **How is HAPE managed?**
    The mainstay of treatment for HAPE is descent in order to increase the partial pressure of inspired oxygen that will relieve pulmonary vasoconstriction and hypoxemia. Supplemental oxygen should also be delivered especially

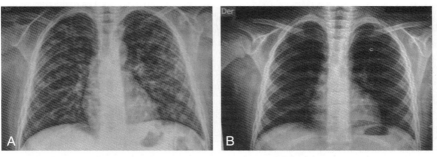

Fig. 66.1 Chest radiograph findings during a high-altitude pulmonary edema episode (A) and after recovery (B). (From Villca N, Asturizaga A, Heath-Freudenthal A. High-altitude Illnesses and Air Travel: Pediatric Considerations. *Pediatr Clin North Am.* 02 2021;68(1):305–319. (Courtesy of Adriana Asturizaga, MD, La Paz, Bolivia.)

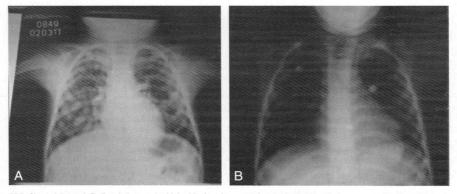

Fig. 66.2 Chest radiograph finding during reentry high-altitude pulmonary edema episode (A) and after recovery (B). (From Merino-Luna A, Vizcarra-Anaya J. Acute lung edema as a presentation of severe acute reentry high-altitude illness in a pediatric patient. *Case Rep Pediatr.* 2020;2020:8871098. https://doi.org/10.1155/2020/8871098.)

as the patient is awaiting transport and while in transport to a lower altitude. HAPE can be fatal, so the decision to have children remain at altitude should be made with extreme caution.

14. **Are there particular pediatric populations at higher risk for HAPE?**
    Certain pediatric populations are at greater risk of HAPE, especially at lower altitudes (Box 66.1). Patients with sickle cell anemia, cystic fibrosis, bronchopulmonary dysplasia, and cardiac disease that includes increased pulmonary blood flow such as atrial septal defect (ASD), ventricular septal defect (VSD), and patent ductus arteriosus (even without pulmonary hypertension) are all at higher risk. Pulmonary hypertension is a strong risk factor for the development of HAPE in general. Children with obstructive sleep apnea (OSA) who have hypoventilation are at increased risk as well. Children with Trisomy 21 (even in the absence of congenital heart disease) are at higher risk likely due to increased pulmonary vascular reactivity and often OSA. Infants less than 6 weeks old are also considered to be at higher risk as pulmonary pressures may still be elevated as prenatal to postnatal circulation transitions. Patients with sickle cell trait have also been found to be at higher risk of HAI, with the additional risk of solid organ infarct, particularly the spleen. Recommendations for children with preexisting illnesses are listed in Box 66.2. Interestingly, patients with asthma often see their symptoms improve at higher altitudes and are at no higher risk for HAI.

15. **Should children who develop HAPE be evaluated for underlying heart disease and/or pulmonary hypertension?**
    Evaluation for structural heart findings and pulmonary hypertension is recommended following a HAPE episode (all types). Many conditions can be clinically silent at sea level and the development of HAPE may be the way these children clinically present. Diagnoses such as unilateral absence of one pulmonary artery, ASD, coarctation of the

---

BOX 66.1 ASCENT RISK ASSOCIATED WITH UNDERLYING MEDICAL CONDITIONS

- Full-term infants less than 6 weeks old and premature infants less than 46 weeks post-conceptual age
- Premature infants greater than 36 weeks post-conceptual age with a history of oxygen requirement, BPD, or pulmonary hypertension
- Morbid obesity
- Cystic fibrosis (FEV, 30%-50% of predicted)
- Poorly controlled chronic conditions (asthma, diabetes, seizure disorder, hypertension, arrhythmia)
- CHDs, such as ASD, VSD, and pulmonary hypertension
- Down syndrome, especially with obstructive sleep apnea
- Sickle cell trait
- Systemic diseases with respiratory compromise (e.g., severe scoliosis, neuromuscular disease, obstructive sleep apnea)
- Premature and full-term infants who have experienced respiratory distress in the immediate postnatal period; infants up to 1 year of age with a history of oxygen requirement or pulmonary hypertension

ASD, Atrial septal defect; BPD, bronchopulmonary dysplasia; CHD, congenital heart disease; FEV_1, forced expiratory volume in 1 s; VSD, ventricular septal defect.
Adapted from Hackett PH, Shlim DR. *Chapter 3, CDC Yellow Book.* Oxford University Press; 2020, with permission.

BOX 66.2 RECOMMENDATIONS FOR CHILDREN WITH PREEXISTING ILLNESSES

Infants and children with certain underlying diseases are at particular risk for serious complications, including exacerbation of their preexistent condition or life-threatening illnesses:
- Sickle cell disease—these patients should ascend cautiously if at all, because sickle cell crisis may occur at altitudes as low as 1500 m (4920 ft).
- Asthma—these patients may find that their symptoms improve because of a relative lack of allergens at high altitudes. They seem to have no higher risk of HAI than patients without asthma. These patients do not need to avoid high altitudes.
- Other chronic lung disease—children with cystic fibrosis or BPD are at increased risk of significant hypoxemia and should undergo oxygen saturation monitoring during altitude travel.
- Cardiac diseases with increased pulmonary artery blood flow—patients with cardiac lesions involving an increase in pulmonary blood flow, such as ASD, VSD, and PDA, with or without pulmonary hypertension, are at risk of developing HAPE. Patent foramen ovale is not considered a contraindication to HA exposure.
- Children with trisomy 21 have increased pulmonary vascular reactivity and a higher risk of pulmonary hypertension than healthy children, in addition to their increased risk of congenital cardiac defects. They are also more likely to have obstructive sleep apnea and hypoventilation. These factors place them at a higher risk for HAPE, even at low altitudes. Thus traveling to high altitude with these patients should be handled cautiously or avoided, if possible.
- Infants with a history of oxygen therapy or pulmonary hypertension—infants younger than 6 weeks of age and those younger than 1 year of age with a history of oxygen requirement or pulmonary hypertension have several physiological limitations that place them at risk for hypoxemia, pulmonary hypertension, and, even right heart failure when rapidly exposed to high altitude. They should get the consent of the specialist before traveling to HA.

ASD, Atrial septal defect; HA, high altitude; HAI, high-altitude illness; PDA, patent ductus arteriosus; HAPE, high-altitude pulmonary edema; VSD, ventricular septal defect.
Data from Hackett P, Gallaher SA. High altitude disease: unique pediatric considerations. *UpToDate*; June 2020.

---

aorta, and VSD may be found. Patent foramen ovale is a risk factor for HAPE and is present in 10% to 35% of the population. While elevated pulmonary pressure is to be expected during an episode of HAPE, persistent elevation after recovery or with hypoxic challenge should be further investigated.

16. **What is the recurrence risk of HAPE?**
    The exact recurrence risk is unknown as many patients do not return to high altitude after an episode of HAPE. Children with underlying diagnoses such as those mentioned above should carefully consult with their medical provider team before returning to high altitude.

17. **Are there effective preventive measures for HAI?**
    The most effective preventive strategy is a gradual ascent. In Colorado, we often recommend that a family stay one to two nights in Denver (1600 m) before ascending to greater than 2500 m. Children with concurrent respiratory illnesses and young infants may benefit from the time acclimating at a somewhat lower altitude. Pharmacological prevention is not recommended in children with no history of HAPE.

KEY POINTS: HIGH-ALTITUDE ILLNESS

1. AMS is very common and can usually be safely managed with analgesics and antiemetics.
2. Classic HAPE should be managed with descent and supplemental oxygen.
3. Reentry HAPE should be considered and is more common in children than adults.
4. Patients with certain conditions, such as those with increased pulmonary blood flow with or without pulmonary hypertension have a greater risk of HAPE.
5. Children with an episode of HAPE should be evaluated for underlying structural heart disease and pulmonary hypertension.

BIBLIOGRAPHY

1. Bebic Z, Brooks Peterson M, Polaner DM. Respiratory physiology at high altitude and considerations for pediatric patients. *Paediatr Anaesth.* 2022;32(2):118–125. https://doi.org/10.1111/pan.14380.
2. Garlick V, O'Connor A, Shubkin CD. High-altitude illness in the pediatric population: a review of the literature on prevention and treatment. *Curr Opin Pediatr.* 2017;29(4):503–509. https://doi.org/10.1097/MOP.0000000000000519.
3. Giesenhagen AM, Ivy DD, Brinton JT, Meier MR, Weinman JP, Liptzin DR. High altitude pulmonary edema in children: a single referral center evaluation. *J Pediatr.* 2019;210:106–111. https://doi.org/10.1016/j.jpeds.2019.02.028.
4. Kelly TD, Meier M, Weinman JP, Ivy D, Brinton JT, Liptzin DR. High-altitude pulmonary edema in Colorado children: a cross-sectional survey and retrospective review. *High Alt Med Biol.* 2022;23(2):119–124. https://doi.org/10.1089/ham.2021.0121.
5. Liptzin DR, Abman SH, Giesenhagen A, Ivy DD. An approach to children with pulmonary edema at high altitude. *High Alt Med Biol.* 2018;19(1):91–98. https://doi.org/10.1089/ham.2017.0096.
6. Scott LS. Sickle cell trait at high altitudes as a response to summit on exercise collapse associated with sickle cell trait: finding the "way ahead". *Curr Sports Med Rep.* 2022;21(5):163. https://doi.org/10.1249/JSR.0000000000000957.

CHEMICAL AND BIOLOGICAL TERRORISM

Sarita Chung and Carl R. Baum

1. **Why is terrorism (particularly chemical and biological terrorism) relevant to those treating children in the emergency department (ED)?**

   As demonstrated by past events, children can become victims of acts of terrorism as direct targets or as the result of a community attack. In 1984 members of the Rajneeshee cult used *Salmonella* Typhi (*Salmonella enterica* serotype Typhi) in a series of intentional poisonings that affected 751 persons in The Dalles, Oregon, including 142 teenage patrons of a popular pizza parlor. In 1995 the Aum Shinrikyo cult killed 12 and caused thousands to become ill by intentionally releasing sarin nerve agent in the Tokyo subway system. In October 2001 anthrax spores were disseminated via the US mail, killing 5 and injuring 17 (including a 7-month-old boy) in an attack upon a nation deeply troubled by the 9/11 attacks of the previous month. As recently as 2018 there have been reports of chemical attacks in Syria affecting children.

   These incidents illustrate the potential for biological or chemical terrorist attacks and thus drive the imperative that health care workers, particularly first responders and ED personnel, be familiar with the expedient diagnosis and management of chemical and biological terrorist events. Although biological agents have incubation periods of days to weeks, making it possible that some victims will seek care through primary care providers, chemical agents are likely to produce effects immediately upon exposure, and ED personnel are almost certain to be called upon to respond to attacks with these agents. Anatomical and physiological vulnerabilities place children at greater risk for exposure and harm. Management and treatment of children including decontamination may need to be tailored to incorporate the developmental level of the child.

2. **Why might terrorists choose chemical and biological weapons?**

   The term *weapons of mass destruction* (WMD) has been used to denote weapons using chemical, biological, or nuclear agents in devices intended to injure or kill large numbers of victims. US military and counterterrorism experts believe that chemical and biological weapons constitute a likely mode of WMD attack on civilian populations by terrorist groups. These agents are relatively inexpensive and technically less difficult to produce and deploy than nuclear weapons; furthermore, the raw materials for their production are less regulated, and there is wide access to chemical and biological agent information via the Internet.

   Chemical and biological weapons can be deployed easily, using relatively simple devices, such as garden sprayers, aerial crop-dusting equipment, and insect control vehicles. In addition, a conventional attack on factories, chemical production facilities, or tank cars may lead to the release of toxic industrial chemicals, with effects similar to those of an attack by military chemical warfare agents. Biological agents may involve aerosol dispersal or possible contamination of food or water supplies.

3. **What did we learn from the anthrax outbreak of 2001?**

   This outbreak was characterized by 22 confirmed or suspected cases (11 inhalational, 11 cutaneous), with five deaths resulting from known or presumed exposure to anthrax-contaminated mail. At least five letters containing anthrax spores were sent from Trenton, New Jersey to government and business offices in Florida, Washington, DC, and New York City. This means of dispersal represents one mode of attack, but many bioterrorism defense experts express greater fear over the possibility of a widespread aerosol release (e.g., from a small crop duster-type airplane) that could potentially sicken hundreds of thousands. As it was, even the 2001 attack resulted in enormous public anxiety and major demands for medical care and public health resources. Antibiotic prophylaxis was prescribed for over 30,000 persons, and decontamination of the Hart Senate Office Building alone took months and cost more than $20 million.

   The one pediatric case from the outbreak was a 7-month-old boy who developed hemolytic anemia, coagulopathy, and hyponatremia from cutaneous anthrax despite early antibiotic treatment. Systemic manifestations resolved after a month of corticosteroids.

4. **What are the potential medical consequences of a chemical attack?**

   Chemical attacks combine elements of traditional mass disasters, in which large numbers of casualties occur almost immediately (e.g., earthquakes), and traditional hazardous materials (HAZMAT) incidents. However, they have the potential to be more catastrophic because chemical attacks:

   - Inflict mass casualties without warning or identification of hazardous materials
   - Involve hazardous materials of extreme lethality that can be toxic to rescue workers

- Include overwhelming numbers of patients requiring emergency medical services (EMS) and even larger numbers of mildly affected or "worried-well" patients self-transporting to EDs, placing additional demands on the health care system
- Promote mass hysteria and panic

5. What is an example of a chemical attack?

In 1995 the Aum Shinrikyo cult released canisters of sarin gas in the Tokyo subway. One ED close to the scene received more than 500 patients, including 3 in cardiopulmonary arrest. Citywide, over 5000 persons sought emergency medical treatment at more than 200 facilities within a few hours, and about 25% required hospitalization. Of note, 90% of the victims went to hospitals by taxi, private vehicles, or on foot rather than by formal EMS transport, further compounding the initial chaos. There were no significant efforts at patient decontamination initially, until the agent was identified, and numerous hospital staff developed mostly mild but noticeable symptoms.

6. How would a biological attack differ from a chemical attack?

Biological agents require incubation periods to cause illness, and therefore biological attacks must be viewed differently than conventional and chemical terrorist attacks. The scenario is more like that of a public health crisis than an EMS or HAZMAT emergency. Exposed persons may be unaware of the attack and disperse from the site of initial exposure. Many diseases caused by high-threat agents begin with nonspecific febrile syndromes. The first indication of a biological attack is likely to be an epidemic of an unusually large number of persons presenting to diverse locations, possibly several days after exposure, with either early nonspecific clinical findings or later findings of severe disease. Thus, patients may present to various medical offices and EDs in piecemeal fashion, reporting, for example, flu-like symptoms. This situation was clearly illustrated by the mail-borne anthrax outbreak in the fall of 2001. When such features are noted, pediatric emergency medicine providers should immediately report suspicion of such an attack to appropriate public health authorities. Electronic syndromic surveillance systems were developed to analyze health data (e.g., from EDs) in real-time and to provide early warning of outbreaks but have shown limited capabilities in small-scale events. However, these systems can enhance traditional public health surveillance and direct physician reporting.

7. What clues suggest a biological attack?

Pediatricians and emergency physicians must maintain an index of suspicion if a biological attack is to be diagnosed in time for useful measures to be undertaken. Several epidemiological features may suggest a bioagent attack. Immediately report suspicion of such an attack to appropriate public health authorities when these are noted:

- Epidemic presentation in a relatively compressed time frame (because most persons are exposed at the same time) and high infection rate among exposed persons
- Diseases that are rare or are not endemic in the area of exposure (e.g., anthrax in a nonrural area or plague in the northeastern United States)
- More respiratory forms of disease than usual
- Particularly high morbidity and mortality rates
- Several epidemics occurring simultaneously
- Infection rates lower in persons sheltered from the suspected route of exposure
- Infected or dying animals
- Discovery of suspicious actions or potential delivery systems
- Large numbers of cases of unexplained disease or death
- Diseases in an atypical age group or population, such as anthrax in children

8. Why may children be disproportionately affected by both chemical and biological agents?

There are a number of physiological, developmental, and logistical reasons that render children at greater risk from exposure to chemical and biological agents.

- Children's larger surface-area-to-body-weight ratio allows for greater exposure to toxicants that can be absorbed transdermally.
- Children have higher minute ventilation rates and breathe closer to the ground, which enhance respiratory exposure to aerosolized agents.
- Children have relatively smaller blood volumes, rendering them more susceptible to volume losses associated with enteric infections such as cholera.
- Children have immature blood-brain barriers, which may heighten the risk of central nervous system toxicity from nerve agents.
- Children have age-related developmental vulnerabilities that may hamper their ability to escape exposure from a contaminated site.
- Children may suffer unique psychological trauma in the context of separation from parents or witnessing the death of family members.

- Pediatric experience with several of the relevant antibiotics, antidotes, and vaccines is limited.
- Procedures are more difficult, especially with small children, if providers are garbed in protective gear.
- EMS systems may be unable to handle pediatric patients.
- Massive numbers of pediatric casualties would overwhelm hospital transport teams.
- Pediatric centers probably would be overwhelmed with local patients and those transferred.

9. **What are the principal biological agent threats, and what is the general approach to their management?**
   The major biological agents of concern are categorized by the Centers for Disease Control and Prevention as the most serious Category A agents:
   Variola virus
   Bacillus anthracis
   Yersinia pestis
   Francisella tularensis
   Botulinum toxin
   Filoviruses and arenaviruses (viral hemorrhagic fevers)
   The diseases caused by these agents are summarized in Table 67.1, which outlines the principal clinical findings, appropriate diagnostic measures, and specific antimicrobial or antitoxin therapies. Regarding initial ED management, in most circumstances, patients will present after a significant time interval from their exposure, and thus specific decontamination procedures are unnecessary. In the event of an announced attack, patients may present to the ED immediately after exposure and decontamination should be considered. In most cases, simple removal of outer garments and washing with soap and water provide for the safe removal of biological agents.

10. **What are the signs and symptoms of inhalational anthrax exposure?**
    After inhalation of anthrax spores, infection begins with pulmonary macrophage uptake and subsequent carriage to mediastinal lymph nodes, where necrotizing lymphadenitis and sepsis ensue. *Inhalational anthrax* has an incubation period of 1 to 6 days and then begins with a flu-like illness characterized by fever, myalgia, headache, cough, and chest "tightness." A brief period of improvement is sometimes seen 1 to 2 days later, but rapid deterioration follows with high fever, dyspnea, cyanosis, and shock. Hemorrhagic meningitis is present in up to 50% of cases. Chest radiographs obtained late in the course of illness may demonstrate a widened mediastinum or prominent mediastinal lymphadenopathy; infiltrates or pleural effusions may also be present. With this clinical picture, a widened mediastinum on chest radiograph and positive blood cultures confirm the diagnosis. The prognosis for patients with inhalational anthrax is grave; classically, death was universal in untreated cases and still may occur in as many as 95% of treated cases if therapy is begun more than 48 hours after symptom onset. Even in the 2001 outbreak, with modern intensive care and the availability of the latest generation antibiotics, only 6 of 11 patients with inhalational anthrax survived.

11. **What are the signs and symptoms of cutaneous anthrax exposure?**
    Cutaneous anthrax occurs when organisms gain entry to the skin, particularly through abrasions or cuts. The development of a papule at the inoculum site is characteristic; the lesion then progresses over days to a vesicle, then an ulcer, and finally to a depressed, black eschar. The surrounding tissue becomes markedly edematous, but not particularly tender, distinguishing this infection from more typical staphylococcal or streptococcal cellulitis. It is quite amenable to therapy with a variety of antibiotics; with timely institution of treatment, it is rarely fatal. In the fall 2001 outbreak, all 11 patients with cutaneous anthrax survived. The only pediatric victim of that attack was a 7-month-old boy with cutaneous anthrax on his arm, presumably contracted after a brief visit to a New York City television news studio that had received contaminated mail. He was initially suspected of having a brown recluse spider bite, and the correct diagnosis was confirmed only after the discovery of anthrax contamination at another television studio. Of note, he also developed hemolysis, thrombocytopenia, and renal insufficiency, features not usually observed in otherwise uncomplicated cases of cutaneous disease. This case raised the possibility of vulnerability in infancy.

12. **Why is smallpox of special concern?**
    As smallpox is highly contagious, the protection of health care workers and the prevention of secondary transmission are important considerations. Smallpox was globally eradicated in 1980, and children are no longer vaccinated; most American adults and all children are therefore susceptible. Smallpox produces a prodrome of fever; a characteristic centrifugal rash that follows and progresses synchronously from macules to papules to vesicles to pustules; fatality rates approach 30% in unimmunized patients. Smallpox mandates the use of the airborne isolation technique. Treatment consists of vaccination if it can be given within 2 to 3 days of initial exposure. There are three antiviral therapies that have shown effectiveness in animal and in vitro studies: tecovirimat (ST-246), brincidofovir, and cidofovir.

Table 67.1 Critical Biological Agents

DISEASE	CLINICAL FINDINGS	INCUBATION PERIOD (DAYS)	ISOLATION PRECAUTIONS	INITIAL TREATMENT	PROPHYLAXIS
Anthrax (inhalational)*	Febrile prodrome, then rapid progression to mediastinal lymphadenitis and mediastinitis, sepsis, shock, and meningitis	1-5	Standard	Consider vaccination under EUA. Ciprofloxacin 10-15 mg/kg IV q12 hr (max 500 mg/dose) or levofloxacin 8 mg/kg IV/PO q12 hr (max 250 mg/dose) or doxycycline 2.2 mg/kg IV q12 hr (max 100 mg/dose) and clindamycin§ 10 mg/kg IV q8 hr (max 900 mg/dose) and penicillin G‖ 400-600 kU/kg/day IV in divided doses q4 hr.	Ciprofloxacin 10-15 mg/kg PO q12 hr (max 1.5 g/day) or doxycycline 2.2 mg/kg PO q12 hr (max 100 mg/dose)
Plague (pneumonic)	Febrile prodrome, then rapid progression to fulminant pneumonia, hemoptysis, sepsis, disseminated intravascular coagulation	2-3	Droplet (for first 3 days of therapy)	Gentamicin 2.5 mg/kg IV q8 hr or doxycycline 2.2 mg/kg IV q12 hr (max 100 mg/dose) or ciprofloxacin 15 mg/kg IV q12 hr (max 500 mg/dose) or levofloxacin 8 mg/kg IV/PO q12 hr (max 250 mg/dose).	Doxycycline 2.2 mg/kg PO q12 hr (max 100 mg/dose) or ciprofloxacin 10-15 mg/kg PO q12 hr (max 1.5 g/day) or levofloxacin 8 mg/kg PO q12 hr (max 250 mg/dose)
Tularemia	Pneumonic: abrupt onset of febrile, fulminant pneumonia Typhoidal: fever, malaise, abdominal pain	2-10	Standard	Gentamicin 2.5 mg/kg IV q8 hr or doxycycline 2.2 mg/kg IV q12 hr (max 100 mg/dose) or ciprofloxacin 15 mg/kg IV q12 hr (max 500 mg/dose). Patients who are clinically stable after 14 days may be switched to a single oral agent (ciprofloxacin or doxycycline) to complete a 60-day course.†	Doxycycline 2.2 mg/kg PO q12 hr (max 100 mg/dose) or ciprofloxacin 20 mg/kg PO q12 hr (max 500 mg/dose)

	Clinical features	Incubation (days)	Isolation	Treatment	Postexposure prophylaxis
Smallpox	Febrile prodrome, then synchronous, centrifugal, vesiculopustular exanthema	7-17	Airborne (+ contact)	Supportive care. Antivirals include tecovirimat (ST-246), brincidofovir, and cidofovir.	Vaccination may be effective if given within 2-3 days after exposure
Botulism	Afebrile, then descending symmetrical flaccid paralysis and with cranial nerve palsies	1-5	Standard	Supportive care; antitoxin may halt the progression of symptoms but is unlikely to reverse them.	None
Viral hemorrhagic fevers	Febrile prodrome, then rapid progression to shock, purpura, and bleeding diatheses	4-21	Contact (consider airborne in cases of massive hemorrhage)	Supportive care; ribavirin may be beneficial in select cases.	None

*In a mass-casualty setting, in which resources are severely constrained, consider the substitution of oral therapy for the preferred parenteral option.

†Assuming organism sensitivity, children may be switched to oral amoxicillin (80 mg/kg/day in divided doses q8h) to complete a 60-day course. We recommend that the first 14 days of therapy or postexposure prophylaxis, however, include ciprofloxacin, levofloxacin, or doxycycline, regardless of age.

§Rifampin or clarithromycin may be an acceptable alternative to clindamycin as a drug that targets bacterial protein synthesis. If ciprofloxacin, levofloxacin, or another quinolone is used, doxycycline may be used as a second agent, because it also targets protein synthesis.

‖Ampicillin, imipenem, meropenem, and chloramphenicol may be acceptable alternatives to penicillin as drugs with good central nervous system penetration.

EUA, emergency use authorization.

Adapted from Henretig FH, Cieslak TJ, Eitzen EM. Biological and chemical terrorism. *J Pediatr.* 2002;141:311–326.

13. **What are the concerning features of plague?**
Plague is highly contagious. Inhalational exposure causes a severe, hemorrhagic pneumonia (pneumonic plague) with respiratory distress and hemoptysis. Plague is highly lethal in untreated patients. Antibiotics, including aminoglycosides and fluoroquinolones, are effective if begun within 24 hours of the onset of illness. Droplet precautions are necessary for managing patients with plague.

14. **How dangerous is ricin?**
Ricin is a biological protein toxin (toxalbumin) derived from the castor bean plant (*Ricinus communis*) that inhibits ribosomal protein synthesis. It is very toxic in animal studies when inhaled and may lead to delayed onset of respiratory distress, pulmonary edema, and acute respiratory failure. A case series of eight persons from the 1940s described a febrile respiratory illness after inhalational exposure. Ingestion can lead to severe gastroenteritis. If injected, ricin may cause a sepsis-like syndrome that may progress to a multiorgan system failure; ricin was suspected in the "umbrella" assassination of dissident Georgi Markov in 1978. Ricin-containing letters were mailed to a US Senate office building in 2004, and again to President Obama and New York City Mayor Bloomberg in 2013. Fortunately, no one became ill in these attacks via the postal service.

15. **What are the primary chemical threats?**
The primary chemical threats are summarized in Table 67.2.

16. **Describe the general approach to the management of chemical threats.**
The general approach to these exposures begins with the stabilization of life-threatening effects, with appropriate decontamination following as soon as possible. Decontamination capability should be deployed rapidly, typically using an outdoor facility with multiple patient stations, arranged so that parallel lines of ambulatory and nonambulatory patients may be processed simultaneously. One problem with outdoor decontamination units is the protection of victims from inclement weather in temperate climate zones, an issue especially important in the management of young children. An outdoor facility must optimally provide adequate water, some temperature control during environmental extremes, and measures to maintain personal modesty, such as curtains or other privacy barriers between shower lines. An alternative is the use of an enclosed facility, optimally adjacent to, but separate structurally from, the main ED, with a separate, high-volume ventilation system vented directly outdoors.
　　Medical personnel in appropriate personal protective equipment (PPE) should staff an initial triage station at the entrance to the decontamination area. Such PPE that is generally recommended for hospital personnel is Occupational Safety and Health Administration "Level C" (see Question 20), which consists of a nonencapsulated, chemically resistant body suit, gloves, and boots, with a full-face air purifier mask containing a cartridge with both an organic-vapor filter for chemical gases and vapors and a high-efficiency particulate air (HEPA) filter to trap aerosols of chemical and biological agents. These triage personnel facilitate the rapid identification of patients requiring immediate antidotal or other lifesaving intervention, as well as the diversion of nonambulatory patients to the appropriate area with medical assistance. Ambulatory patients who are old enough should be instructed in self-decontamination. Children should not be separated from parents or other caregivers whenever possible, but unaccompanied children should receive assistance.

17. **How is decontamination for chemical threats best accomplished?**
Decontamination starts with the removal of clothing; victims should disrobe themselves when possible. Preserve all clothing in labeled plastic bags for law enforcement. Consider dry (scraping, vacuuming, use of absorbent/adsorbent materials, or pressurized air in addition to clothing removal) or wet (shower) decontamination. Victims should have skin and hair washed thoroughly with water and soap, and should then be given replacement clothing, as some agents left on skin or clothing pose a serious threat to the patient as well as to first-responder and ED personnel. As noted above, make efforts to prevent hypothermia during and after showers, particularly among younger children, using warm water (around 100°F or 38°C at a pressure of 60 PSI), heat lamps, and blankets. Ocular exposure requires copious eye irrigation with saline or water.

18. **How is cyanide exposure evaluated and managed?**
Cyanide is a cellular poison with multiple clinical manifestations. Cyanide inhibits cytochrome a_3 interfering with normal mitochondrial oxidative metabolism, leading to cellular anoxia and lactic acidosis. Cyanide's volatility and relatively low lethality in open air limit its efficacy as a chemical terrorism agent in comparison with nerve agents. Generated in a fire or released intentionally in a closed space, however, cyanide can have devastating effects, as evidenced by its use in the Nazi gas chambers during World War II. Initially, cyanide toxicity would likely manifest as tachypnea and hyperpnea, as well as tachycardia, flushing, dizziness, headache, diaphoresis, nausea, and vomiting. As exposure increases, seizures, coma, apnea, and cardiac arrest may follow within minutes. An elevated anion gap metabolic acidosis, with increased serum lactate, is typically present, and decreased peripheral oxygen utilization leads to an elevated mixed venous oxygen saturation value.
　　Therapy for cyanide exposure includes removal of the patient to fresh air and intensive supportive care. In significant cases, specific antidotes are administered. The classic cyanide antidote relied on a two-step

Table 67.2 Critical Chemical Agents

AGENT	TOXICITY	CLINICAL FINDINGS	ONSET	DECONTAMINATION*	MANAGEMENT
Nerve Agents					
For example, tabun (GA), sarin (GB), soman (GD), VX	Anticholinesterase: muscarinic, nicotinic, central nervous system effects	Vapor: miosis, rhinorrhea, dyspnea Liquid: diaphoresis, vomiting Both: coma, paralysis, seizures, apnea	Vapor: seconds Liquid: minutes-hours	Vapor: fresh air, remove clothes, wash hair Liquid: remove clothes, wash skin and hair with copious soap and water, ocular irrigation	ABCs Atropine: 0.05 mg/kg IV,[†] IM[‡] (min 0.1 mg, max 5 mg), repeat q2-5 min PRN for marked secretions, bronchospasm Pralidoxime: 25 mg/kg IV, IM[§] (max 1 g IV; 2 g IM), may repeat within 30-60 min PRN, then again q1 hr for one or two doses PRN for persistent weakness, high atropine requirement Diazepam: 0.3 mg/kg (max 10 mg) IV; lorazepam: 0.1 mg/kg IV, IM (max 4 mg); midazolam: 0.2 mg/kg (max 10 mg) IM PRN for seizures or severe exposure
Blistering Agents (Vesicants)					
For example, Mustard gas (HD)	Alkylation	Skin: erythema, vesicles Eye: inflammation Respiratory tract: inflammation	Hours	Skin: soap and water Eyes: water (effective only if done within minutes of exposure)	Symptomatic care
Lewisite (L)	Arsenical		Immediate pain		Consider British antilewisite (BAL) 3 mg/kg IM q4-6 hr for systemic effects of lewisite in severe cases
Irritants/Corrosives					
Ammonia, bromine, chlorine	Liberate hydrochloric acid, alkylation	Eye, nose, and throat irritation (especially chlorine) Respiratory: bronchospasm, pulmonary edema	Minutes: eye, nose, and throat irritation, bronchospasm Hours: pulmonary edema	Fresh air Skin: water	Primarily symptomatic care

	CO$_2$) and acylation	irritation; cough and wheeze; noncardiogenic pulmonary edema	airway irritation); 12–24 hr (pulmonary edema)	Liquid: remove clothing; soap and water irrigation	
Asphyxiants					
Cyanide	Cytochrome oxidase inhibition	Tachypnea, coma, seizures, apnea, anoxia, lactic acidosis	Seconds	Fresh air Skin: soap and water	ABCs, 100% oxygen; Hydroxocobalamin 70 mg/kg IV (max 5 g) Sodium bicarbonate PRN for metabolic acidosis
Disabling Agents (Incapacitators)					
3-Quinuclidinyl benzilate (BZ)	Peripheral and central antimuscarinic	Anticholinergic toxidrome	Up to 24 hr	Fresh air	Supportive care; physostigmine
Fentanyl derivatives	Opioid	Opioid toxidrome	Seconds	Fresh air	Naloxone, ABCs
Lacrimators (chloroacetophenone, CN; chlorobenzylidene/capsaicin, CS)	Alkylation of tissue enzymes	Eye, mucous membrane, skin irritation, pulmonary edema	Seconds	Fresh air Eye: copious irrigation Skin: soap and water	Cycloplegics, oral analgesics; ABCs for pulmonary edema

*Decontamination, particularly for patients with significant nerve agent or vesicant exposure, should be performed by health care providers garbed in adequate personal protective equipment. For emergency department staff, recommended equipment consists of a nonencapsulated, chemically resistant body suit, boots, and gloves with a full-face air purifier mask/hood.

†Intraosseous route is likely equivalent to IV route.

‡Atropine might have some benefit via endotracheal tube or inhalation, as might aerosolized ipratropium. See also Table 67.3.

§Pralidoxime is reconstituted to 50 mg/mL (1 g in 20 mL of water) for IV administration, with the total dose infused over 30 min, or it may be given by continuous infusion (loading dose 25 mg/kg over 30 min, and then 10 mg/kg/hr). For IM use, see also Table 67.3.

ABCs, airway, breathing, and circulatory support; IM, intramuscular; IV, intravenous; max, maximum; min, minimum; PRN, as needed.

Table 67.3 Pralidoxime Autoinjector Therapy

APPROXIMATE AGE RANGE (YEAR)	APPROXIMATE WEIGHT (KG)	NUMBER OF AUTOINJECTORS	PRALIDOXIME DOSE (MG/KG)
3-7	13-25	1	24-46
8-14	26-50	2	24-46
>14	>50	3	<35

Consider autoinjector use for mass casualties when IV (intravenous) access or more precise mg/kg IM (intramuscular) dosing is logistically impractical. The initial dose using atropine autoinjectors is one autoinjector of the recommended size. The initial dose using pralidoxime autoinjectors is the recommended number of (adult-intended, 600 mg) autoinjectors. These pralidoxime autoinjectors may also be injected into an empty sterile vial; the contents redrawn through a filter needle into a small syringe may then provide a ready source of concentrated (300 mg/mL) pralidoxime solution for IM injection in infants. Although not US Food and Drug Administration–approved for patients <41 kg as of 2018, the atropine-pralidoxime combo autoinjector can be used in children older than 1 year.

process, first using nitrite to generate methemoglobin to bind with the cyanide anion, then sodium thiosulfate to convert cyanide to thiocyanate, a far-less toxic compound excreted in the urine. The antidote hydroxocobalamin, approved for use in the United States in 2006, avoids the toxicity of the intermediate methemoglobin, and instead exchanges its hydroxyl group for a cyano group, forming harmless cyanocobalamin (vitamin B_{12}) that subsequently undergoes renal excretion. Its efficacy and safety profile make hydroxocobalamin the cyanide antidote of choice, especially for children. See Table 67.2 for details.

KEY POINTS: SPECIFIC BIOLOGICAL AND CHEMICAL TERRORIST AGENTS

1. The prognosis for victims of inhalational anthrax is grave.
2. Cutaneous anthrax may present as a papule → vesicle → ulcer →finally a black eschar.
3. Few American adults and no children have been vaccinated for smallpox and are susceptible.
4. Plague is highly contagious and leads to hemorrhagic pneumonia and respiratory distress.
5. Cyanide toxicity involves tachypnea, tachycardia, vomiting, seizures, coma, and cardiac arrest.

19. **What are the clinical presentations of Ebola in children?**
    The 2014 to 2015 Ebola outbreak in West Africa has provided more insight into the clinical manifestations in children; however, due to outbreak conditions including an overwhelmed health care system, capture of clinical data remained limited. Travel history or known exposures should be elicited immediately. Symptoms and signs of Ebola virus disease in children may be difficult to differentiate from other infectious illnesses and include fever (63%-100%), anorexia (55%-99%), weakness (74%-98%), diarrhea (42%-80%), and vomiting (36%-70%). Less commonly, patients present with unexplained bleeding. Laboratory findings include abnormalities in electrolytes, as well as hypoglycemia and renal dysfunction. Supportive care includes attention to hydration and treatment for coinfections such as malaria.

20. **What do EDs need to consider when evaluating patients during an outbreak such as Ebola or COVID-19?**
    EDs will continue to be on the frontlines in the evaluation of patients with concerns about symptoms due to an outbreak. In fact, during the early COVID-19 period, many primary care offices referred sick patients to EDs. EDs will need to work with hospital leadership and public health departments to evaluate local surveillance and to develop triage screening protocols to identify those at risk. Once identified, protocols regarding proper isolation of the patient(s), such as negative pressure rooms, and staff protection (PPE) must remain up to date. If decontamination is needed, incorporate pediatric principles into plans (see Question 16). Offer staff training regarding potential chemical and biological agents as well as decontamination procedures on an ongoing basis.

21. **What level of PPE is needed for emergency responders in various situations?**
    The selection of PPE is one of several steps that employers take to ensure safety and health among emergency responders. First, there should be an assessment to determine which hazards the workers may encounter. If the hazards cannot be eliminated, then appropriate training and PPE should be provided to workers. There are four levels of PPE, from the most-protective Level A (self-contained breathing apparatus; chemical-protective suit, gloves, and boots) to Level D (standard work clothes without a respirator, but with surgical mask, gown, and gloves).

KEY POINTS: OVERVIEW OF CHEMICAL AND BIOLOGICAL TERRORISM

1. Children can be victims of chemical or biological terrorist attacks as direct targets or as part of a community attack.
2. Chemical and biological weapons are easily deployed using the letter/mail system, garden sprayers, aerial crop-dusting equipment, and insect control vehicles.
3. Chemical attacks can inflict mass casualties without warning and hazardous materials can endanger rescue workers.
4. Large numbers of casualties and even more mildly affected or "worried-well" patients can overwhelm EDs.
5. The first indication of a biological attack is likely an epidemic, or a large number of patients, with nonspecific symptoms (e.g., flu-like illness) presenting to various locations.
6. Rare diseases or those not endemic to the area, with high morbidity, suggest a biological attack.
7. Children are vulnerable due to anatomic differences, inability to escape contaminated sites, and psychological trauma when separated from their parents.

Acknowledgment

The authors thank Frederick M. Henretig and Theodore J. Cieslak for their contributions to previous editions.

BIBLIOGRAPHY

1. Berger T, Eisenkraft A, Bar-Haim E, et al. Toxins as biological weapons for terror–characteristics, challenges and medical countermeasures: a mini-review. *Disaster Mil Med.* 2016;2:7.
2. *CDC.* Bioterrorism agents/diseases. <https://emergency.cdc.gov/agent/agentlist-category.asp> Accessed 19.04.22.
3. *CDC.* Smallpox. <https://www.cdc.gov/smallpox/index.html>. Accessed 19.04.22.
4. Chung S, Baum CR, Nyquist A-C, Disaster Preparedness Advisory Council Council on Environmental Health Committee on Infectious Diseases American Academy of Pediatrics Technical report: chemical-biological terrorism and its impact on children. *Pediatrics.* 2020;145(2):e20193750.
5. Dixit D, Masumbuko Claude K, Kjaldgaard L, Hawkes MT. Review of Ebola virus disease in children – how far have we come? *Paediatr Int Child Health.* 2021;41(1):12–27. https://doi.org/10.1080/20469047.2020.1805260.
6. Freedman A, Afonja O, Chang MW, et al. Cutaneous anthrax associated with microangiopathic hemolytic anemia and coagulopathy in a 7-month-old infant. *JAMA.* 2002;287(7):869–874. https://doi.org/10.1001/jama.287.7.869. PMID: 11851579.
7. Kaufman Z, Shohat T. Syndromic surveillance in public health practice–an updated view. *Harefuah.* 2014;153(3–4):188–191.
8. Nelson CA, Meaney-Delman D, Fleck-Derderian S, et al. Antimicrobial treatment and prophylaxis of plague: recommendations for naturally acquired infections and bioterrorism response. *MMWR Morb Mortal Wkly Rep.* 2021;70(3):1–27.
9. Occupational Safety and Health Administration, US Department of Labor. PPE for emergency response and recovery workers. Emergency preparedness and response: getting started. <https://www.osha.gov/emergency-preparedness/getting-started#ppeemer>. Accessed 30.03.22.
10. Okumura T, Suzuki K, Fukuda A, et al. The Tokyo subway sarin attack: disaster management, part 2: hospital response. *Acad Emerg Med.* 1998;5:618–624.
11. Sanders KN, Aggarwal J, Stephens JM, et al. Cost impact of hydroxocobalamin in the treatment of patients with known or suspected cyanide poisoning due to smoke inhalation from closed-space fires. *Burns.* 2022;48(6):1325–1330. 00304-1.
12. Scarfone RJ, Madsen J, Cieslak TJ, Eitzen EM. Biological and chemical terrorism. In: Shaw KN, Bachur RG, eds. *Fleisher & Ludwig's Textbook of Pediatric Emergency Medicine.* 8th ed. Wolters Kluwer/Lippincott Williams & Wilkins; 2021.chapter 132, e-book.
13. Sivakumar A, Kalimuthu A, Munisamy M. Cutaneous anthrax. *JAMA Dermatol.* 2022;158(9):1065.
14. *Arms Control Association.* Timeline of Syrian chemical weapons activity, 2012-2022. <https://www.armscontrol.org/factsheets/Timeline-of-Syrian-Chemical-Weapons-Activity>. Accessed 07.04.22.
15. Tin D, Pepper M, Hart A, Hertelendy A, Ciottone G. Chemical warfare agents in terrorist attacks: an interregional comparison, tactical response implications, and the emergence of counterterrorism medicine. *J Spec Oper Med.* 2021;21(3):51–54.

DISASTER PREPAREDNESS

Katie Giordano

1. **What are some unique features of children that must be considered when caring for pediatric patients in a disaster?**
   - Increased respiratory rate
   - Unique drug metabolism
     - Need for weight-based doses
   - Smaller equipment size
   - Increased skin absorption due to body surface area
   - Increased risk of dehydration
   - Different organ proportions
   - Due to developmental differences, children fail to escape a dangerous scene

2. **Explain why children are vulnerable in a disaster.**
   Due to higher respiratory rates, children have a higher minute ventilation and will breathe in more of a chemical or biological toxin when exposed. With a higher heart rate, a young child will quickly circulate an absorbed toxin. The child's short stature means they will be closer to the ground and may be more likely to inhale some chemical agents like sarin and chlorine, which settle closer to the ground. Because of a child's larger skin-to-body mass ratio, they are at a higher rate of transdermal toxin absorption and injury. They are also at high risk of hypothermia during decontamination. With lower fluid reserves, children are more likely to suffer from dehydration in a food-borne terrorist attack. Due to the size of the child, the larger head size when compared to the body, and the larger organ size when compared to body surface area, a child is at higher risk of blunt trauma from debris or blast injury blunt trauma, especially traumatic brain injuries.

3. **How does developmental behavior affect a child in a disaster?**
   Children depend on their parent, guardian, or teacher for guidance. If they are separated from the adult, or the adult they are with is injured, they cannot escape from the threat. Infants cannot physically escape, toddlers and young children although may be able to walk away from the incident, they do not have the cognitive ability to understand the risks and needs to get away. This leads to higher exposures and risks. A young child may even go toward the hazard out of curiosity.

4. **True or false: most pediatric emergency department (ED) visits are at specialized pediatric hospitals.**
   FALSE. Most children in the United States who present for emergency care present to a general ED versus a pediatric ED. Per the National Hospital Ambulatory Medical Care Survey of 2019, there were 141 million ED visits. Approximately 20% of these visits are of children less than 15 years old. The majority of children who seek care in an emergency are seen by an ED that sees less than 15 pediatric patients a day.

5. **Are hospitals prepared for a disaster involving pediatric patients?**
   In 2013 the Pediatric Readiness Assessment noted that less than half of the hospitals in the United States have written policies that address the needs of children in a disaster. In response, the Checklist of Essential Pediatric Domains and Considerations for Every Hospital's Preparedness Policies was created by a national multidisciplinary workgroup. All hospitals and emergency medical service (EMS) agencies must have age and size-appropriate equipment, staff, training for staff, and policies to provide high-quality care for children. Hospitals also need to have written policies for interfacility transfers when necessary. Communities must also have pediatric equipment and medications in their stockpile. The Centers for Disease Control and Prevention Strategic National Stockpile contains pediatric-specific equipment and medications but there is a large disparity between the children's and adult's needs. The American Academy of Pediatrics (AAP) continually addresses these concerns.

6. **What is pediatric readiness?**
   The APP provided a policy statement in 2018 to address the unique needs of pediatric patients and take into account the notion that many children when faced with an emergency may not be cared for by a pediatric specialist. This statement provides the resources necessary to prepare any EDs to care for pediatric patients. The National Pediatric Readiness Project, which launched in 2013 is an ongoing quality improvement (QI) project and involves stakeholders in the federal EMSC program, such as AAP, American College of Emergency Physicians, and Emergency Nursing Association.

This project highlighted some key areas of improvement. The policy statement provides recommendations for clinical and administrative leadership to improve the hospital readiness for children of all ages. The identification of a pediatric emergency care coordinator (PECC) physician and nurse roles is key to the hospital's readiness abilities. These leaders will promote skills and knowledge, facilitate pediatric emergency medical and nursing education, develop and facilitate QI activities, develop and review ED policies, serve as a liaison in the community and regional EMS and emergency preparedness coordinators, and collaborate with hospital leadership to ensure equipment and supply needs are met. The statement goes into detail for each of these topics for which the PECC is responsible. Included in these recommendations are pediatric disaster planning, surge planning, and drills for these activities.

7. **What is EMSC?**
EMSC refers to the Emergency Medical Services for Children. The Mission statement of EMSC is as follows: "Ensuring all children and adolescents, no matter where they live, attend school or travel, receive appropriate emergency medical care."

8. **What are some organizations and resources involved in pediatric readiness and pediatric disaster management?**
- Pediatric Readiness Project
- EMSC: Emergency Medical Services for Children
- EIIC: EMSC Innovation and Improvement Center: Mission to optimize outcomes for children across the emergency care continuum by leveraging QI science and multidisciplinary, multisystem collaboration
- NEDARC: The National Emergency Medical Services for Children Data Analysis Resource Center. A national resource center helping state and territory EMSC managers and EMS offices develop capabilities to collect, analyze and utilize EMS data
- AAP Children and Disaster website (www.aap.org/disaster/educationandtraining)

9. **What is a mass casualty incident (MCI)?**
An MCI is any event where the need for medical resources exceeds the resources that are available. This can range from a multivehicle car accident with several victims to a terrorist attack or a large-scale natural disaster like a tornado or hurricane. We have learned about the impacts on children from several historical events such as 1995 sarin attack in Tokyo, Japan, and the 2017 sarin attack and the 2018 chlorine attack in Syria. Since the September 11, 2001 terrorist attacks and subsequent anthrax releases in the United States, the AAP recognized the need to address the impact of terrorism on children and appointed the AAP Disaster Preparedness Advisory Council, which collaborates with federal partners. The AAP website has comprehensive information on terrorism and its impact on children: www.aap.org/disasters/terrorism.

10. **What is disaster triage?**
During a mass casualty event, triage systems must adjust from providing the best care for an individual patient to the best possible care for the community at large. Disaster triage will prioritize those with the highest likelihood of survival after immediate care, from those that are most critically ill. The goal of mass casualty triage is to preserve medical resources so that the total mortality and morbidity caused by the incident are minimal.

There are numerous triage systems available but limited data to show one is superior to another. Two systems have been widely used in pediatric disaster triage: SALT (Sort, Assess, Lifesaving Treatment) and JumpSTART. Heffernan et al. found SALT slightly superior in accurately applying a triage level while Nadeau et al. found JumpSTART to be more accurate. JumpStart adapts the START triage system (widely used by EMS systems for adult mass casualty triage) to account for the physiological differences in pediatric patients and that respiratory arrest accounts for most pediatric cardiac arrests. This allows five rescue breaths to be given if the patient is apneic with a pulse to assess a change.

Disaster triage sorts patients into acuity by color; this terminology is nationally recognized. Green patients are the walking wounded. Yellow patients have sustained serious injuries that require urgent but not immediate care for survival. Red patients have sustained serious life-threatening injuries that are treatable with immediate medical attention. Black patients are dead or are likely to die despite immediate interventions (expectant).

11. **What federal agencies are responsible for addressing children's needs in a disaster?**
- US Department of Health and Human Services Office of the Assistant Secretary for Preparedness and Response
- Center for Disease Control
- Department of Homeland Security/Federal Emergency Management Agency (FEMA)
- Administration for Children and Families/Office of Human Services Emergency Preparedness and Response.

12. **Who advocates for children in disaster preparedness?**
Pediatricians, child experts in and out of government agencies, and the AAP Disaster Preparedness Advisory Council advocate to ensure that children's needs are specifically addressed in national planning documents. The government at the federal level is responsible for policy-making and coordination, but the implementation is the

responsibility of the state, local government, tribal programs, and community organizations. Local emergency operations centers (EOC) will bring together key players for the care of those affected in a disaster, but it is very important that pediatricians get involved to advocate for children to be taken into consideration in these disaster plans. The National Pediatric Readiness Project recommends that disaster drills include a pediatric MCI every 2 years.

13. **How can a community prepare for a disaster involving pediatric patients?**

Community, state, and federal disaster exercises should be routinely performed. The goal of a drill is to become more prepared for a real event. To increase comfort in caring for children involved in a mass casualty event, pediatric patients must be involved in the mass casualty disaster drill. These events allow for the discovery of potential problems and the education of the care of a child in a disaster. Families of children with special needs should also be involved in disaster drills. Adolescents can be involved in the disaster drill as mock patients and responders to the incident. There are groups that involve teens in disaster response, and these include the Teen Community Emergency Response teams (Teen CERT) and the FEMA Youth Preparedness Council. Public participation in a disaster drill will help the community during the disaster and also educate the individual on how to be prepared for a disaster before it occurs.

Pediatricians play an important role in advocating for their patients before, during, and after a disaster. They can educate families on being prepared for a disaster and work with local agencies to ensure children are included in disaster plans. They can also care for patients during the disaster through telephone triage and increased acute visits, to see minor injuries and relieve the local ED of these encounters.

14. **How can the pediatrician get involved in disaster preparedness?**

- Register your credentials with your state Emergency System for Advanced Registration of Volunteer Health Professionals (ESAR_VHP)
- Enroll in the local medical reserve corp (MRC)
- Participate on a federal disaster medical assistance team (DMAT)
- Participate on a state medical assistance team (SMAT)
- Familiarize yourself with the Incident Command System—free online courses are available through FEMA

15. **What are the standard disaster principles to guide the planning and management of an incident?**

The mnemonic D.I.S.A.S.T.E.R. developed by the National Disaster Life Support Education Consortium provides a framework for EDs to prepare for a disaster involving pediatric patients. D = detection, I = Incident Command, S = Safety, and Security, A = Assess Hazards, S = Support, T = Triage and Treatment, E = Evacuation, and R = Recovery.

16. **How will an ED know they are about to care for patients in a disaster?**

The first step of a disaster plan needs to include a mechanism to detect or declare an event. This may occur through biosurveillance systems or triage algorithms when an infectious or bioterrorism attack is occurring. EMS notification or the media may be the first indication of a mass casualty event either man-made or natural. The institution must predetermine its threshold for declaring an MCI event by planning its trauma care capacity, decontamination abilities and knowing its regional resources. The declaration of an event will start the formal process of activating the Hospital Incident Command System (HICS).

17. **What is an incident command system?**

The incident command system model is a well-established incident management leadership structure. This terminology is accepted nationally. It includes an incident commander and four section chiefs, which are operations, planning, logistics, and finance/administration.

The HICS was created specifically for hospitals and has requirements laid out by the Joint Commission. In the HICS model, the incident commander works with a Safety Officer, Liaison Officer, Public Information Officer, and Medical/Technical specialist. These roles are filled by positions and not specific personnel so that they can be timeless. The Safety Officer role is filled by either the hospital's Safety Manager, Director of Facilities, Director of Security, Radiation Safety Officer, or designee. The Liaison Officer is covered by Government Relations, Legal/Counsel, Community Relations Director, or designee. The Public Information Officer role is held by the Public Relations Director, Media & Public Relations Manager, or designee.

The Operations Section manages all incident tactical activities and implements the Emergency Operation Plan. This section is typically the largest due to the role of management and coordination of immediate resources needed to respond to the incident. Branches and units are implemented as needed to maintain a manageable span of control and streamline organizational management.

The Planning Section collects, evaluates, and disseminates situational information and intelligence regarding incident operations and assigned resources, conducts planning meetings, and prepares the Incident Action Plan for each operational period. The effectiveness of the Planning Section has a direct impact on the availability of information needed for the critical strategic decision-making done by the Incident Commander and the other general staff positions.

The Logistics Section provides for all the support needs of the incident. These responsibilities include acquiring resources from internal and external sources, using standard and emergency acquisition procedures as well as requests to other hospitals, corporate partners, and the local EOC or the Hospital Preparedness Coalition.

The Finance/Administration Section coordinates personnel time, orders items and initiates contracts, arranges personnel-related payments and Workers' Compensation, and tracks response and recovery costs and payment of invoices.

18. **What is hazardous vulnerability analysis?**
    Many hospitals perform a yearly hazardous vulnerability analysis. There are guidelines for the hospital to follow and to plan for natural events like hurricanes, tornados, floods or blizzards, chemical, biological, radiological, and nuclear events, internal power failure, cyberattacks, infectious surges like the COVID-19 pandemic and H1N1 surge in 2009, and the countermeasures for all of these events. Hospitals, and particularly EDs, should identify any gaps in caring for pediatric patients during these events.

19. **What supplies must always be considered at a hospital to be prepared?**
    It is estimated that for every critical care patient seeking care during a disaster, there will be five unaffected patients presenting for treatment. Hospitals must have surge capacity plans in place to care for large numbers of patients. This includes personal protective equipment for their staff, decontamination facilities, and alternative care sites. Medication stockpiles must be planned. This may involve utilizing state and federal resources. Staff, and the family of staff, must be considered in this need as you must have staff who can care for the influx of patients. In the cases of terrorist attacks, remember that all patients must be considered a victim of crime, and evidence collection will be needed.

20. **Should disaster planning include a plan for evacuation?**
    YES. A disaster will come in many forms. A natural disaster or terrorist event can directly involve a hospital structure leading to the need to fully or partially evacuate the patients. This was highlighted in 2005 with Hurricane Katrina and in 2011 after a tornado damaged the St. John's Regional Medical Center in Joplin, Missouri. The ED can facilitate interfacility transportation for patients. The hospital must have a relationship with the local health care coalition to support evacuation efforts in an emergency.

21. **How do you know when disaster care is complete?**
    The incident does not end when the last victim arrives at the hospital by EMS. There may still be victims arriving by private vehicle, although these victims are often the first to arrive. The patient's needs and hospital needs continue after the patient has left the emergency department. Further efforts and support may be needed by the operating room staff, critical care units, and inpatient floors to care for the influx of patients. Recovery is needed to restore the ED and hospital's ability to care for routine patients.

22. **What is reunification?**
    A key component of recovery after a disaster is the reunification of family members. Greater than 60 million children, including about 12 million infants and toddlers are in school or daycare every weekday. These children will be very vulnerable if a disaster occurs as they will be without a guardian who knows them well. Hurricane Katrina brought to light the need for reunification efforts. During this disaster, it took 6 months to reunite the last child. All efforts to keep families together for medical care should be initiated at the scene. Proper planning can help reunification occur in a timely fashion, minimizing the negative impact that separation can have on a child. The AAP has a reunification toolkit available with helpful strategies to identify verbal and nonverbal children. Local and state agencies such as the division of family services or child protection agencies can be called upon to aid with reunification. Proper discharge with a legal guardian must be ensured. Improper discharge could put children in the hands of former abusers or traffickers.

23. **What will increase the resilience of a hospital team during a disaster?**
    One study interviewed the staff of the hospital that cared for the victims of the Manchester Arena Bombing in 2017. It found five themes of adaptations to practice that enhanced the resilient performance of the hospital: teamwork; psychologically supporting patients, families, and staff; reconfiguring infrastructure; working around the electronic medical record; and maintaining hospital safety.

    Consider evaluating the walking wounded in an alternate care site within or near the hospital. Utilizing psychologists, social workers, pastoral care personnel, and child life staff will minimize trauma to pediatric patients and their families. Utilize these same resources to help the hospital staff in processing and recovering from the trauma of the event. Consider a buddy system for staff who will check in on each other during and after the disaster event.

24. **What will help a hospital most during a disaster?**
Preparation and *Training*. Have plans in place, include pediatric patients within your plan, then practice those plans. Consider plans to help your staff with childcare for their own children so that they can come to work. Consider plans to shelter the families of your staff during a disaster so the staff can work. Understand the comfort levels of your staff to care for critically ill pediatric patients. The Joint Commission requires that hospitals perform disaster drills twice a year. They do not mandate the performance metrics of these drills. The drills can range from tabletop to simulation or full-scale disaster scenarios. The goals of the drill should be to test the system, identify weaknesses, train staff, and review the hospital's response to the disaster.

KEY POINTS: DISASTER PREPAREDNESS

1. Pediatric patients are often not included in disaster preparedness plans.
2. Children are especially vulnerable to natural and man-made disasters.
3. Pediatricians must advocate for their patients to be included in local disaster plans.
4. Prepare yourself and your patients before a disaster occurs.
5. Incident command and hospital incident command are the leadership framework for a disaster.
6. Reunification is difficult but remains important. Plans utilizing support staff will better the outcome.
7. Preparation will help with community and staff resilience.

BIBLIOGRAPHY

1. Burke RV, Iverson E, Goodhue CJ, Neches R, Upperman JS. Disaster and mass casualty events in the pediatric population. *Semin Pediatr Surg.* 2010;19(4):265–270. https://doi.org/10.1053/j.sempedsurg.2010.06.003.
2. Chung S, Baum CR, Nyquist AC. Disaster Preparedness Advisory Council, Council on Environmental Health, Committee on Infectious Diseases. Chemical-biological terrorism and its impact on children. *Pediatrics.* 2020;145(2):e20193750. https://doi.org/10.1542/peds.2019-3750.
3. Chung S, Shannon M. Hospital planning for acts of terrorism and other public health emergencies involving children. *Arch Dis Child.* 2005;90(12):1300–1307. https://doi.org/10.1136/adc.2004.069617.
4. Disaster Preparedness Advisory Council Committee on Pediatric Emergency Medicine Ensuring the health of children in disasters. *Pediatrics.* 2015;136(5):e1407–e1417. https://doi.org/10.1542/peds.2015-3112.
5. Gilchrist N, Simpson JN. Pediatric disaster preparedness: identifying challenges and opportunities for emergency department planning. *Curr Opin Pediatr.* 2019;31(3):306–311. https://doi.org/10.1097/MOP.0000000000000750.
6. Gubbins N, Kaziny BD. The importance of family reunification in pediatric disaster planning. *Clin Pediatr Emerg Med.* 2018;19(3):252–259. https://doi.org/10.1016/j.cpem.2018.08.007.
7. Heffernan RW, Lerner EB, McKee CH, Browne LR, Colella MR, Liu JM, Schwartz RB. Comparing the accuracy of mass casualty triage systems in a pediatric population. *Prehosp Emerg Care.* 2019;23(3):304–308. https://doi.org/10.1080/10903127.2018.1520946.
8. MacKinnon RJ, Slater D, Pukk-Härenstam K, von Thiele Schwarz U, Stenfors T. Adaptations to practice and resilience in a paediatric major trauma centre during a mass casualty incident. *Br J Anaesth.* 2022;128(2):e120–e126. https://doi.org/10.1016/j.bja.2021.07.024.
9. Remick K, Gausche-Hill M, Joseph MM, Brown K, Snow SK, Wright JL. American Academy of Pediatrics Committee on Pediatric Emergency Medicine and Section on Surgery; American College of Emergency Physicians Pediatric Emergency Medicine Committee; Emergency Nurses Association Pediatric Committee. Pediatric readiness in the emergency department. *Pediatrics.* 2018;142(5):e20182459. https://doi.org/10.1542/peds.2018-2459.

CHAPTER 69

EMERGENCY MEDICAL SERVICES AND TRANSPORT MEDICINE

Emine M. Tunc and George A. (Tony) Woodward

1. **What are the links in the American Heart Association's pediatric chain of survival?**
   Prevention/early recognition → activation of emergency response system → high-quality cardiopulmonary resuscitation (CPR) → advanced resuscitation → postcardiac arrest care → recovery.

2. **What is enhanced 911?**
   Enhanced 911 automatically provides computerized identification of the telephone number and location of the caller, regardless of the quality of information provided.

3. **What is an emergency medical dispatcher (EMD)?**
   An EMD is a specialized communication specialist who gathers essential information regarding the location, nature, and severity of the emergency and relays this information to the emergency medical services (EMS) system for dispatch of a first responder or ambulance. When critical conditions are identified, the EMD may assist the caller in providing advice and guiding interventions prior to EMS arrival, such as opening the airway, providing CPR, controlling hemorrhage, and assisting with childbirth based on the dispatched protocols.

4. **Describe the four classifications of prehospital EMS personnel.**
   1. Emergency Medical Responder (EMR): EMRs administer life-saving techniques including CPR and mouth-to-mouth resuscitation, usually while awaiting the arrival of more qualified EMS professionals. EMRs provide assistance to other EMS professionals at the scene and/or during transport. EMRs can perform basic interventions with minimal equipment.
   2. Emergency Medical Technician (EMT): EMTs have received the training and skills needed to stabilize and safely transport patients who are stable or have life-threatening emergencies. These skills include such as basic airway interventions, controlling bleeding, stabilizing fractures, and addressing shock. EMTs perform interventions with the basic equipment typically found in an ambulance.
   3. Advanced Emergency Medical Technician (AEMT): AEMTs provide the same services as an EMT, plus have the additional training to administer fluids, limited medications and can use the advanced medical equipment carried in the ambulance.
   4. Paramedic: Paramedics provide advanced medical care for critical and emergent patients in the EMS system. This includes triage with sophisticated medical equipment and the administration of multiple types of medications.
      The classifications vary in levels of training and degrees of capabilities. At the federal level, the National Highway Traffic Safety Association (NHTSA) has developed the National Standard Curricula for certification for each category, but state or local requirements may supersede these standards. Intermediate levels of providers with varied capabilities have evolved, as many jurisdictions offer supplemental training modules.

5. **What are ALS providers?**
   ALS providers are usually referred to as paramedics. They can administer a high level of care in the field. They undergo 1000 to more than 3000 hours of training, internship, and clinical hospital time. They are trained to perform advanced resuscitation techniques, such as ventilatory support, vascular access, and drug administration. They are capable of general diagnostic skills, rhythm disturbance recognition and treatment, and advanced airway management, including endotracheal intubation. In some areas, they can perform medication-assisted intubations using sedatives and paralytics and can place emergent surgical airways. Some ALS provider educational programs have advanced to a 2-year associate or a 4-year baccalaureate degree.

6. **Are there recommendations for standard pediatric equipment for basic life support (BLS) and ALS units and protocols for the management of children?**
   A list of equipment in ambulances to safely manage pediatric emergencies was collaboratively developed and endorsed by the American College of Surgeons Committee on Trauma, the American Academy of Pediatrics (AAP), the American College of Emergency Physicians, the National Association of EMS Physicians (NAEMSP), and the Pediatric Equipment Guidelines Committee—Emergency Medical Services for Children (EMSC) Partnership for Children Stakeholder Group. The EMSC National Resource Center and AAP Field Guide for Air and Ground Transport of Neonatal and Pediatric Critical Care Transport Medicine provide model pediatric protocols.

7. **What is medical command?**
   Medical command is the entity responsible for the supervision of EMS services in the community. In general, prehospital personnel are assigned to a specific operational base or base station, and these base stations are responsible for medical command. Medical control provides medical direction to prehospital personnel. Medical control can be offline/indirect or online/direct.

8. **Differentiate offline/indirect and online/direct medical control.**
   Offline/indirect medical control consists of patient care protocol development, personnel education and training, prospective and retrospective patient care review, and other process improvement activities. **Online/direct medical control** involves real-time interaction between a physician or designee and an on-site field provider. Online medical control can be centralized or decentralized. In a *centralized* system, a designated hospital is responsible for all direct medical control orders and notifications, regardless of the receiving facility. In a *decentralized* system, each receiving hospital provides direction to prehospital personnel transporting patients to their facility.

9. **What are standing orders?**
   Standing orders are policies or protocols issued by a medical director of an EMS system that authorizes EMTs to perform particular skills in certain situations.

10. **Describe the difference between single-tiered and multitiered EMS systems.**
    In a **single-tiered** system, every response, regardless of the call type, involves the same level of personnel expertise and equipment (all BLS or ALS). The advantage of this design is the provision of an advanced level of care to all calls, and it potentially circumvents under- or over-triaging by EMS dispatchers. **Multitiered** systems respond with an ALS- or BLS-level unit depending on the nature of the call. This design reserves ALS units for higher-priority calls and aims to ensure that an ALS unit is always available for potentially critical responses.
    The ideal EMS system design provides appropriate patient care to each situation in the briefest possible period of time. Therefore the efficiency of adopting a single-tiered versus multitiered response is affected by the availability of BLS and ALS providers in the community and the distance from the scene to the nearest receiving hospital. Regardless of the response design, EMS systems often include EMR services, often provided by the police or fire department, as part of the response.

11. **What is EMSC?**
    EMSC (Emergency Medical Services for Children) is a federally funded program administered by the Health Resources and Services Administration's Maternal and Child Health Bureau and NHTSA that provides grant funding to states or medical schools in all 50 states, the District of Columbia, and five territories, to support pediatric emergency care initiatives at the state and local levels. Funding supports all the components of the program, namely, education and training, systems development, data analysis and research, and public policy and future planning. EMSC partners with numerous national organizations involved in the care of acutely ill or injured children.

12. **What is family-centered prehospital care?**
    Family-centered prehospital care is a systematic approach to building collaborative relationships between prehospital personnel and the patients' families during on-site treatment, transport, and transition of care. The goal is to provide the best outcome for the patient through collaboration with his or her family members.

13. **What should a 911 dispatcher or EMS provider do when caring for a patient (and/or family) who primarily or exclusively speaks a language other than English?**
    Based on the US Department of Justice Civil Rights Act of 1964 and Executive Order (13166), everyone is entitled to receive equitable care despite the race, religion, color, and language. To ensure equitable care for all patients, 911 dispatcher services and EMS agencies should utilize audio and/or video language interpreter services. Patients with limited English proficiency (LEP) are less likely to receive bystander CPR and less likely to survive. Providers should not rely on the caller's LEP and always offer to use an interpreter as the medical condition of the patient allows.

14. **How should a prehospital care provider respond to an advance directive?**
    Advance directives, such as do not resuscitate orders, are utilized for many pediatric patients. Most states require that prehospital care providers honor legitimate advance directives unless the legal guardian allows resuscitation. The legal guardian may revoke the advance directive at any time. If there is an advance directive (e.g., a certified do not resuscitate order or the patient is wearing a "do not resuscitate" medical bracelet), the prehospital provider with support from online medical control should try to communicate with the legal guardian (and perhaps providers of record) to determine their current wishes. If an advance directive cannot be verified, transportation with all appropriate emergency treatment measures is advised.

15. **Is it safe to use an automated external defibrillator (AED) for pediatric patients without a pediatric attenuator?**

    Yes. AEDs recognize rhythms amenable to shock and direct the user to deliver the shock to a pediatric patient. Some are equipped with a pediatric attenuator, which decreases the energy delivered and is preferred for use in infants and children younger than 8 years. If this is not available, an AED without a dose attenuator may still be used. AEDs without a dose attenuator may deliver higher energy doses, but they have been successfully used in infants with minimal myocardial damage and good neurologic outcomes.

16. **What is the doctrine of implied consent?**

    This doctrine permits the treatment of minors without parental consent when an emergency exists. A minor with a condition that threatens either life or limb is viewed as having an emergency and must be treated and transported.

17. **How should prehospital care providers respond if the legal guardian refuses transport?**

    Prehospital care providers and online medical control should try to persuade caregivers to allow transport to a hospital. Most children whose caretaker refuses transport receive medical care within a week of the refusal and typically have good outcomes. However, about 10% are admitted to the hospital. Hospital transport cannot be refused if the legal guardian is intoxicated or otherwise incompetent, if child abuse is suspected, or if the child appears to be in imminent danger.

    If the guardian refuses transport, prehospital care providers should complete a medical screening evaluation, contact medical command, follow all local regulations, document carefully, and have the legal guardian sign an "against medical advice" form.

18. **What action should be taken if a prehospital care provider suspects child abuse?**

    When a prehospital care provider suspects child abuse, the medical control physician must ensure that appropriate treatment and transport occur. Notify the receiving facility of the concern for child abuse. Prepare a mandatory report to child protection agencies in accordance with prevailing laws of the jurisdiction. Do not allow the caregiver to refuse transport when child abuse is suspected. Police protection may be required to ensure the safety of the prehospital provider and the patient and to ensure that medical transport occurs.

19. **Are EMS providers at great risk of acquiring COVID-19 infections when transporting patients?**

    Although there is reason for concern, paramedics are very unlikely to acquire COVID-19 infection from patients if they anticipate the need and adhere to standard infection prevention protocols. One study from Seattle/King County, WA, where EMS protocols called for a mask (surgical mask in most cases, N-95 masks if aerosol-generating procedures [AGP] involved), eye protection, gloves and gown, found only a single COVID-19 infection related to a patient. (One provider of 3710 provider-patient encounters, 0.28 cases/10,000 person-days at risk.) In that study, COVID-19 accounted for 1% of all 911 EMS responses and 16% of those involved AGP. Almost all of the COVID-19 infections in paramedics during the study period were not related to patients, but rather to encounters in the community or occupational settings. This suggests that even AGP can be safely delivered by EMS providers if proper personal protective equipment (PPE) is deployed.

20. **List the goals of interfacility transport.**

    Goals of interfacility transport are as follows:
    - To meet the unique needs of ill and injured infants and children
    - To meet the needs of the medical community
    - To allow for regionalization
    - To provide high-quality care
    - To deliver the patient to the receiving center in stable or improved condition

21. **List the advantages and disadvantages of different levels of ground transport.**

    The advantages and disadvantages of different levels of ground transport are listed below.

METHOD	ADVANTAGES	DISADVANTAGES
Private vehicle	Immediate transport	Potential for nondirect transport, likely no medical care en route (even if provider accompanies patient)
Taxi	Direct transport to hospital	No medical care
Volunteer ambulance	Direct transport to hospital	Minimal to no medical care

METHOD	ADVANTAGES	DISADVANTAGES
Basic life support (BLS) ambulance	Direct transport to hospital	Basic medical care, limited pediatric experience and expertise
Advanced life support (ALS) ambulance	Direct transport to hospital, emergency resuscitative care, some interventions available	Variable pediatric experience, limited diagnostic and interventional capabilities
Critical care ambulance	Direct transport to hospital, sophisticated medical care	Possibly limited or minimal pediatric expertise
Pediatric specialty critical care transport	Direct transport to hospital, pediatric expertise	Limited resources, may not be immediately available

22. **True or false: When choosing an ambulance service or interfacility transport provider, the receiving hospital is legally responsible for ensuring the adequacy of transport service.**
False. Under Emergency Medical Treatment and Active Labor Act (EMTALA) regulations, the *referring hospital* and clinicians are responsible for ensuring that the quality of care during transport does not diminish and that an unstable patient is not placed in a less sophisticated environment. The transporting system is responsible for ensuring that the medical care it delivers meets the defined standard of care.

23. **What are the advantages and disadvantages of ambulance transport?**
Advantages include the ambulance leaving from a referring facility and traveling directly to the receiving facility. Ambulances can stop or redirect if problems arise during transport. Team composition changes and personnel additions are easy and safe. Ambulance transport is relatively inexpensive in comparison to air transport, family member(s) can accompany the patient, backup vehicles are often available, and there are few weather restrictions. Disadvantages include noise, vibration, motion sickness, road conditions, traffic, detours, delays, and accident risk.

24. **Describe the advantages and disadvantages of transport by helicopter.**
Helicopters offer the advantage of rapid transport (often one-third to one-half of ground transport time to the same location). Helicopters can access difficult locations and avoid traffic. A major disadvantage is the need for a local landing zone or helipad, without which the speed advantage may be diminished. Size and space limitations may limit patient assessment or intervention. Altitude physiology, including pressure changes and hypoxia, is important but may not be an issue for low-altitude helicopter transport. Other flight issues include stress on equipment, humidity, fatigue, gravitational forces, weight restriction, and emergency survival, as well as increased noise and vibration. Helicopter travel may be limited by weather; many systems are regulated by visual flight rules rather than instrument flight rules (the capability for instrument flight rules enables safe flight in weather with diminished visibility). Helicopter transport is expensive.

25. **What are the advantages and disadvantages of transport with fixed-wing aircraft?**
Fixed-wing (jet, airplane) transport offers the advantage of speed and is appropriate for transports over 100 to 150 miles. An airplane often can fly over or around bad weather. The cabin can be pressurized to diminish problems with altitude physiology and often offers more room than a helicopter for patient assessment and intervention. A disadvantage is that the airport location may not be convenient to the hospital. Required additional patient transitions via ground or helicopter transport can increase transport time, complexity, and cost, as well as the risk to the patient.

26. **Can a minor be transported without parental consent?**
If a parent or legal guardian is not available for consent, the treating physician may decide and document that the benefits of transport exceed the risks of waiting for parents and may provide emergency consent. This emergency consent applies to the treatment and transport of that emergent issue only. Seek and obtain consent from the legal guardians as soon as possible.

27. **What are key elements of a pediatric transport system?**
Adequate preparation for transport involves designing and developing a transport process before it is needed. It is imperative to educate all levels of providers, provide appropriate patient care during transport, and review and address systems and quality issues during and after transport. Other key elements include medical supervision and involvement during transport, experienced on-site personnel, cooperation between referring and receiving hospitals and personnel, and adequate quality assurance and improvement.

28. **In what areas of interfacility transport is medical oversight important?**
Qualified and experienced medical oversight may be the most important element of the transport system. Knowledgeable physicians must be involved at all levels:
- **Organizational physicians** help design the transport system and evaluate operations.
- **Referring physicians** should be experts in recognition of illness/injury, provision of initial care, and stabilization. They should recognize limitations in local care opportunities (personnel, logistic, current or projected) and request assistance when needed. They should know how and when to refer patients to an appropriate transport service.
- **Medical control ("command" or "supervising") physicians** should be immediately available to the transport system for questions or issues that arise during transport.
- **Receiving physicians** must be aware of the patient's arrival and capable of streamlining the transition to care at the receiving hospital.

29. **What degree or level of education should pediatric transport personnel possess?**
No singular optimal degree or level has been established. The most important qualifications are experience in pediatric critical care or neonatal care and an appropriate skill level, as determined by routine competency assessments. Personnel must have specific training and experience in the care of critically ill children. These may include physicians, registered nurses, nurse practitioners, paramedics, and respiratory therapists. All who are involved must be familiar with the transport environment and capable of recognizing and stabilizing any problems that arise in that transport population.

30. **What logistical activity significantly increases the risk for transported patients?**
Whenever the patient is moved from one location to another (e.g., between vehicles [plane/helicopter to ambulance], bed to stretcher) the risk for line or tube displacement increases. Movement can cause appropriately immobilized patients to become malpositioned, perhaps decreasing desired protection, impeding respiratory efforts, or even worsening an existing injury. Multiple modes of transport increase movement and potential risk to the patient. If a patient deteriorates during or shortly after movement, immediately consider sequelae of the move as a potential cause.

31. **What equipment is important in a critical care ambulance environment?**
The answer depends on the patient population. Minimal required equipment includes appropriate pediatric interventional supplies, medication, monitors, and communication equipment (radios, phones, and other modalities). Monitoring capability should include pulse oximetry, respiratory rate, blood pressure, temperature, end-tidal carbon dioxide, and electrocardiography. Point-of-care laboratory testing, which allows rapid analysis of blood gases, chemistries, hemoglobin, and glucose, is imperative.

32. **How can referral for transport be streamlined?**
Development of a designated and advertised access number or specialized communication center with a centralized number is important. The ability to triage incoming calls efficiently in a standard fashion to appropriate command physicians and transport personnel is vital. Simultaneous logistic planning is more easily accomplished with the use of a dedicated communication center than with direct referral to a receiving physician when operational communications and arrangements will happen in sequence rather than in parallel. Transfer agreements and up-to-date knowledge of bed availability can markedly decrease time necessary for patient acceptance.

33. **What are the responsibilities of the referring physician during the transport process?**
The referring physician must assess and stabilize the patient to the best of his or her ability. He or she must ensure that the chosen transport service has the appropriate skills and equipment to avoid a decrease in the provided level of care. Discuss plans for stabilization and intervention with the receiving hospital or transport service, and, if possible, follow these recommendations. Discuss disagreements about patient stability or inability to perform a task for other reasons with the command physician. If the patient's condition changes, notify the transport service. The family must consent to the transport, a particular type of transport (air, ground) and to the receiving hospital. Document the consent in writing. Place a written order for transport services if relevant. The referring physician and care team should be available for discussion in person or by telephone when the transport service arrives.
   In addition, the referring physician and team must ensure the following:
- Vascular access is provided and secured as indicated.
- All tubes and lines are secured to help avoid dislodgement during transport.
- A copy of medical records, radiographs (hard copy, disk, or electronic transmission), and laboratory results accompanies the patient or is sent as soon as possible after acute transfer.
- A medical summary is completed and included with transfer materials.
- Blood products/medications ordered and available if use is considered during transport.

34. **When does the accepting facility become medicolegally responsible for the transport?**
Once the referring facility contacts the accepting facility and the accepting facility provides recommendations and accepts the patient, medical liability becomes a shared process. Most of the liability is still on the referring provider until the transport team leaves the facility. Most transport providers do not have privileges at the referring facility and therefore act under the supervision of the referring physician.

KEY POINTS: FACTORS THAT INCREASE EFFICIENCY OF TRANSPORT

1. Centralized phone number
2. Central communication center
3. Transport-literate personnel capable of triaging incoming calls
4. Predetermined transport agreements
5. Current awareness of bed availability

---

35. **Can a general rather than a pediatric transport service adequately transport children?**
The optimal decisions on mode and staffing for pediatric transport depend on patient acuity and resource availability. If a pediatric critical transport service is available, it potentially offers the highest level of pediatric-specific experienced care. If a pediatric transport service is not available, a general transport service may adequately transport the child. Many general critical care services are quite experienced with pediatric critical care transport, while others may not be. If the general critical care transport service is not trained or experienced with pediatric/neonatal issues, gains in availability and efficiency of response may be affected by limited abilities to assess and appreciate disease progression or clinical deterioration and to intervene for the pediatric patient. Referring and receiving physicians should take the opportunity to increase the pediatric expertise of general transport services to ensure adequate care.

36. **How can a transport service develop pediatric expertise?**
Many options are available. One is to visit and identify the best practices of other services. The AAP section on Transport Medicine is a great resource for collegial pediatric transport assistance and expertise, publishes the *Guidelines for Air and Ground Transport of Neonatal and Pediatric Patients*, and *Field Guide for Air and Ground Transport of Neonatal and Pediatric Critical Care Transport Medicine* and also provides a course in pediatric education for prehospital professionals. Introduction to pediatric advanced life support (ALS) is provided by the American Heart Association. The Committee on Accreditation of Medical Transport Systems offers standards and an accreditation process for transport systems.

37. **List the core critical quality metrics of neonatal and pediatric transport.**
    1. Unplanned dislodgement of therapeutic devices
    2. Verification of tracheal tube placement
    3. Average mobilization time of the transport team
    4. First-attempt tracheal tube placement success
    5. Rate of transport-related patient injuries
    6. Rate of medication administration errors
    7. Rate of patient medical equipment failure during transport
    8. Rate of CPR performed during transport
    9. Rate of serious reportable events
    10. Unintended neonatal hypothermia on arrival at destination
    11. Rate of transport-related crew injury
    12. Use of standardized patient care handover

38. **What major goal should be considered in determining the specifics of a critical care transport?**
Determine whether the immediate goal is to transport the patient to an intensive care setting or to bring intensive care capabilities to the patient. The answer may help to determine the type of transport and level of sophistication necessary for the transport personnel and service.

39. **How does EMTALA affect the transport of pediatric patients?**
EMTALA places clear duties on both referring and receiving hospitals. The referring clinicians must stabilize the patient's medical condition to the best of their abilities prior to transport unless the facility cannot provide an adequate level of care. Patient or parent consent for transport must be obtained. EMTALA requires receiving hospitals to accept a patient for transport if space and an appropriate level of care are, or can be, available. The patient's ability to pay should not be considered by the referring or receiving hospital for an unstable patient. When

considering critical care transport for an acute medical or surgical need, do not discuss the financial ramifications of the decision to transport with the patient or family.

40. **What are two major concerns about altitude physiology?**
    - According to **Boyle's law**, an increase in altitude brings a decrease in barometric pressure. Decreased barometric pressure (P) results in an increase in volume (V) of gas (Boyle's law: $P_1V_1 = P_2V_2$). Boyle's law has ramifications for air in enclosed spaces, such as ear canals, endotracheal tube and blood pressure cuffs, intestinal gas, pneumothorax, and pneumocranium. There is approximately a 20% increase in gas volume between sea level and 5000 feet and a 100% increase between sea level and 18,000 feet.
    - **Dalton's law**, or the law of partial pressure ($P_{total} = P_1 + P_2 + P_3 \ldots$), states that the total pressure of a gas is a sum of its components. Although the concentration of oxygen in air is always 21%, the air is less dense at higher altitudes; therefore an increase in altitude results in a decrease in ambient oxygen available to the patient.

41. **How concerning are issues related to altitude?**
    Most patients do not have problems related to air physiology at the relatively low altitudes at which helicopters usually fly, or with pressurized fixed-wing transport. However, if the patient has an unrecognized air collection, decompression sickness, diving illness, or if the air transport involves significant altitude changes, associated problems may develop. The decrease in ambient oxygen is usually not a factor because of the availability of supplemental oxygen and positive-pressure support. For patients already receiving maximal oxygen and pressure support at sea level, however, an increase in altitude may be of significant concern.

42. **Is there value to exposing residents and fellows to interfacility transport?**
    The transport environment provides an opportunity for senior pediatric and emergency medicine residents as well as critical care/emergency medicine fellows to apply skills developed during the first part of their training program. Although the patient population and disease processes are similar to those in the hospital, the environment in which care is given is markedly different. Significant preparation is required for optimal participation in the transport process, including the development of skills for communicating with transport team personnel and receiving and referring physicians and families. Trainees will also learn about transport vehicles (ambulance and aircraft) and equipment (medications, monitors, interventional equipment). Trainees on transport will learn to anticipate and respond to issues that do not occur within the hospital, including delays in transport, traffic, mechanical factors, and differences in skill levels and personalities at referring and receiving hospitals. These are often enlightening and rewarding growth experiences.

43. **Should a parent accompany their child on transport?**
    Whenever possible, allow parents to be part of the transport process. Their presence can be invaluable for information and for patient comfort. It is also important to maintain the family support unit as much as possible during these transfers. If, however, parental involvement puts the patient at risk (weight or space limitations of the vehicle; a parent who is abusive, inebriated, or belligerent; or a parent who may distract medical attention from the patient during the transport), reconsider their accompaniment.

44. **Identify potential care personnel participants for pediatric transport.**
    Transport personnel can include physicians, nurses, nurse practitioners, respiratory therapists, and emergency medical services personnel who hold variable titles, including volunteer, EMR, emergency medical technician (EMT), advanced medical technician (AEMT), paramedic and critical care emergency medical transport paramedic.

45. **Should seat belts and restraint devices be used by transport personnel during transport?**
    Yes. Safety of the transport patient and personnel is paramount. *Unless an acute patient change dictates that personnel are temporarily mobile*, personnel must be restrained at all times when in a moving transport vehicle. In addition, secure any objects that might move during a rapid acceleration or deceleration to help ensure a safe environment. Move any objects that are in an area where one's head might strike them during a motor vehicle accident.

46. **What are some strategies for restraining an infant and pediatric patient during the transport?**
    For infants and children up to about 18 kg, if their medical condition allows for semiupright position, they can be secured in their own car seat in a forward-facing seat in the ambulance. This also helps ensure an appropriate car seat is available to help promote safe discharge from the hospital. Alternatively, they can be restrained on the stretcher with various approved commercial child safety seats or devices.

47. **What are some strategies for follow-up to a stressful transport or patient care experience?**
    Critical incident stress management helps personnel to understand and cope with stressful events. These preparations and interventions include understanding stressful issues in the transport environment and education

regarding coping skills prior to involvement, as well as defusing (discussing) and debriefing (formal incident review) processes after an incident has occurred.

48. **Does ambulance use of lights and sirens improve patient outcomes and decrease risk to occupants?**
No. Accidents, unfortunately, are not uncommon when using ambulances for transport. Most accidents occur in intersections and involve the use of lights and sirens. While the ambulance staff/patients/occupants may have the impression that lights and sirens are providing ample warning to others, that may not always be appreciated by other drivers. For most patients, the time saved when using lights and sirens for increased speed is not significant or impactful for the patient's care.

49. **Should an ambulance circumvent traffic laws while transporting emergency ill patients?**
In general, ambulances should adhere to standard traffic laws. Do not assume that the use of lights and sirens allows for disregard of speed limits or need to stop at lights and intersections. Many of the injuries and fatalities with ground transport are related to disregard for standard safety traffic expectations and are preventable with appropriate adherence to normal traffic rules/patterns.

50. **Do pediatric specialty transport teams impact outcome?**
Compelling evidence suggests that the use of rapid initiation of goal-directed therapy, and use of specialty transport teams that can continue therapy en route, provide safer care with less unplanned care events and better outcomes for critically ill children. Calhoun et al. suggest that outcomes were similar for trauma patients, after noting that younger and sicker children were transported by pediatric specialty teams. Although specialty teams are not always an option owing to their availability, always consider the use of these teams for a critically ill pediatric patient.

51. **What are some specific considerations for neonatal transport?**
Goals of patient care for neonatal transport are similar to that for pediatric patients, including securing an airway, adequate oxygenation and ventilation, and maintaining normal blood pressure. Some considerations emphasized more in neonatal transport include normoglycemia (50-200 mg/dL), thermoregulation (36°C-37°C, except for indicated otherwise for hypoxic-ischemic encephalopathy), initiating and maintaining umbilical vascular access as well as administration of surfactant, prostaglandin E_1 and inhaled nitrous oxide for specific circumstances.

52. **How can one evaluate the effectiveness of their transport system?**
Surveying constituents and stakeholders is a good place to start and can occur after every transport or in a more general approach. Evaluate responsiveness, efficiency, medical care delivery, and outcomes. Having an outside reviewer evaluate the system and providers is also invaluable. Obtaining certification through an accreditation agency such as the Commission on Accreditation of Medical Transport Systems can help ensure that the team is aware of and functions to expected transport safety standards. A current list of accredited transport programs is available at https://www.camts.org/services/.

KEY POINTS EMS AND TRANSPORT MEDICINE

- Awareness of capability of teams is imperative in delivery of appropriate EMS and interfacility transport care.
- Knowledge of EMTALA is important in stabilization and transport of pediatric patients.
- Awareness of consent laws guides appropriate EMS and transport decisions.
- Knowledge of benefits and limitations between modes of transport (e.g., ground vs. air ambulance) informs appropriate transport responses.
- A working knowledge of BLS versus ALS and the specifics of prehospital provider capabilities are important when determining EMS options and the level of care to be provided during the transport process.

BIBLIOGRAPHY

1. AAP Section on Transport Medicine Meyer K, Schwartz HP, Fernandes CJ, eds. *Field Guide for Air and Ground Transport of Neonatal and Pediatric Critical Care Transport Medicine.* American Academy of Pediatrics; 2018.
2. AAP Section on Transport Medicine *Guidelines for Air and Ground Transport of Neonatal and Pediatric Patients.* 4th ed. AAP Section on Transport Medicine; 2016.
3. Topjian AA, Raymond TT, Atkins D, et al. Part 4: Pediatric basic and advanced life support: 2020 American Heart Association guidelines for cardiopulmonary resuscitation and emergency cardiovascular care. *Circulation.* 2020;142(16_suppl 2):S469–S523.
4. Ali A, Miller M, Cameron S, Gunz A. Paediatric Transport Safety Collaborative (PTSIC): critical events with family presence during paediatric critical care transport. *J Paediatr Child Health.* 2020;25(suppl 2):e1.
5. Billimoria Z, Woodward GA. Chapter 19: Neonatal transport. In: Gleason CA, Juul S, eds. *Avery's Diseases of the Newborn.* 11th ed. Elsevier, Inc.; 2023:217–230.

6. Bradley SM, Fahrenbruch CE, Meischke H, Allen J, Bloomingdale M, Rea TD. Bystander CPR in out-of-hospital cardiac arrest: the role of limited English proficiency. *Resuscitation*. 2011;82(6):680–684.
7. Brown A, Schwarcz L, Counts CR, Barnard LM, et al. Risk of acquiring coronavirus disease illness among emergency medical services personnel exposed to aerosol generating procedures. *Emerg Infect Dis*. 2021;27(9):2340–2348.
8. Calhoun A, Keller M, Shi J, et al. Do pediatric teams affect outcomes of injured children requiring inter-hospital transport? *Prehosp Emerg Care*. 2017;21(2):192–200.
9. Carroll LN, Calhoun RE, Subido CC, Painter IS, Meischke HW. Serving limited English proficient callers: a survey of 9-1-1 police telecommunicators. *Prehosp Disaster Med*. 2013;28(3):286–291.
10. Giardino AP, Tran XG, King J, Giardino ER, Woodward GA, Durbin DR. A longitudinal view of resident education in pediatric emergency interhospital transport. *Pediatr Emerg Care*. 2010;26(9):653–658.
11. Gross TK, Walls TA, Woodward GA. Prehospital care. In: Shaw KN, Bachur RG, eds. *Fleisher & Ludwig's Textbook of Pediatric Emergency Medicine*. 8th ed. Lippincott, Williams and Wilkins; 2021:e134.
12. Murray B, Kue R. The use of emergency lights and sirens by ambulance and their effect on patient outcomes and public safety: a comprehensive review of the literature. *Prehosp Disaster Med*. 2017;32(2):209–216.
13. National Highway Traffic Safety Administration. *Working Group Best Practice Recommendations for the Safe Transportation of Children in Emergency Ground Ambulances. NHTSA*. U.S. Department of Transportation; 2012. Available at: www.nhtsa.gov.
14. O'Mahony L, Woodward GA. Chapter 28: Neonatal transport. In: Gleason CA, Juul S, eds. *Avery's Diseases of the Newborn*. 10th ed. Elsevier, Inc.; 2018:347–360.
15. Orr RA, Felmet KA, Han Y, et al. Pediatric specialized transport teams are associated with improved outcomes. *Pediatrics*. 2009;124:40–48.
16. Ayub EM, Sampayo EM, Shah MI, Doughty CB. Prehospital providers' perceptions on providing patient and family centered care. *Prehosp Emerg Care*. 2017;21(2):233–241.
17. Lyng J, Adelgais K, Alter R, et al. Recommended essential equipment for basic life support and advanced life support ground ambulances 2020: a joint position statement. *Pediatrics*. 2021;147(6): e2021051508.
18. Schwartz HP, Bigham MT, Schoettker PJ, et al. Quality metrics in neonatal and pediatric critical care transport: a national Delphi project. *Pediatr Crit Care Med*. 2015;16(8):711–717.
19. Committee on Pediatric Emergency Medicine and Committee on Bioethics Consent for emergency medical services for children and adolescents. *Pediatrics*. 2011;128(2):427–433. (reaffirmed 2021).
20. Tate RC. The need for more prehospital research on language barriers: a narrative review. *West J Emerg Med*. 2015;16(7):104–105.
21. Wall J, Woodward GA, Tsarouhas N. Stabilization and transport. In: Shaw KN, Bachur RG, eds.*Fleisher & Ludwig's Textbook of Pediatric Emergency Medicine*. 8th ed. Lippincott, Williams and Wilkins; 2021:e11.
22. Watanabe BL, Patterson GS, Kempema JM, et al. Is use of warning lights and sirens associated with increased risk of ambulance crashes? A contemporary analysis using national EMS information systems (NEMSIS) data. *Ann Emerg Med*. 2019;74(1):101–109.
23. Woodward GA, Fleegler EW. Should parents accompany pediatric interfacility ground ambulance transports? The parents' perspective. *Pediatr Emerg Care*. 2000;16:383–390.
24. Woodward GA, Fleegler EW. Should parents accompany pediatric interfacility ground ambulance transports? Results of a national survey of pediatric transport team managers. *Pediatr Emerg Care*. 2001;17:22–27.

WEBSITES

https://cpr.heart.org/-/media/CPR-Files/Training-Programs/AED-Implementation/AED-Programs-QA-ucm501519.pdf
https://emscimprovement.center/
https://www.ems.gov/pdf/EMS_Education_Standards_2021_v22.pdf
https://www.ems.gov/projects/safe-transportation-of-children-in-ground-ambulances.html
https://www.faa.gov/sites/faa.gov/files/2021-11/Air_Ambulance_Operations_Data_2019_PL_115-254_Sec314d.pdf
https://www.justice.gov/crt/executive-order-13166

PATIENT SAFETY AND QUALITY IMPROVEMENT

Arezoo Zomorrodi

1. **What is health care quality and quality improvement?**

   The Institute of Medicine defines quality of care as the "degree to which health services for individuals and populations increase the likelihood of desired health outcomes and are consistent with current professional knowledge." Quality is considered to be high when expectations of patients, physicians, organizations, regulators, payers, and communities are met. Medical outcome expectations are set through professional organizations and adopted as standards of care. Quality improvement is the framework used to systematically improve care through the standardization of processes to reduce variation, achieve predictable results, and improve outcomes for patients and health care organizations.

2. **What is the model for improvement?**

   The model for improvement asks teams to answer three fundamental questions and use the Plan-Do-Study-Act (PDSA) cycle to test change.

   Question 1: What are we trying to accomplish?

   At the outset of an improvement project, teams should set SMART aims that are specific, measurable, achievable, relevant, and time-specific to define and guide their work.

   Question 2: How will we know that a change is an improvement?

   Identify quantitative measures to determine if a change actually leads to an improvement. These measures should be realistic and easily tracked, using small samples collected sequentially within time intervals as close to when the work was done as possible. They should be graphed visually over time to show that improvements are temporally correlated to interventions.

   Question 3: What change can we make that will result in improvement?

   Ideas for change can come from local experts who work in the system/emergency department (ED) or from the experience of others who have successfully improved in other settings. Change concepts should attempt to automate work, reduce variation, and eliminate unnecessary steps when possible.

   The Plan-Do-Study-Act (PDSA Cycle) is a scientific method to learn from tests of change. It involves planning the intervention, performing the change concept, studying the results, and acting on the learnings. After testing a change on a small scale and making refinements through several PDSA cycles, the change may be scaled up and implemented more broadly.

3. **How does standardization improve quality?**

   Taiichi Ohno, the father of the Toyota Production System management methodology said, "Without standards, there can be no improvement." It is difficult to improve a process that is not documented and consistently used. Variation allows more errors to occur and makes those errors more difficult to notice, track, and improve. Standardization to best practice allows for predictable and measurable results, thereby setting the foundation for quality improvement.

4. **What is the triple aim?**

   In 2008 the Institute for Healthcare Improvement developed a framework for optimizing health system performance. The intent of the Triple Aim initiative is to transition to population health while lowering health care costs. The three aims are to
   1. improve the patient experience and satisfaction
   2. improve the health of populations
   3. reduce the cost of health care

   Pursuing these objectives together allows health care organizations to work on problems such as poor coordination of care and overuse of medical services while paying attention to resources that have the greatest impact on health. The goal is to shift from a focus on acute care to preventative and population-based care.

   In 2014 it was recommended to add a fourth aim, improved clinician experience, to highlight that achievement of the Triple Aim requires an engaged and productive workforce who sees joy in their work. In 2022, other thought leaders proposed adding an additional aim of advancing health equity because quality improvement efforts without a focus on disparity may unintentionally worsen them.

5. **What is patient safety?**

According to the World Health Organization, patient safety includes prevention of diagnostic errors, medical errors, injury, or other preventable harm to a patient during health care encounters. Patient safety is foundational to delivering quality health care. In 2001 the Institute of Medicine announced that the American health care delivery system needed fundamental change. Effective health care must be brought to all Americans while avoiding harmful interventions and preventable complications. They proposed six domains for health care improvement:

- Safe—without preventable errors and harm
- Effective—evidence-based care that ensures the right care for the right patient such that only those who would benefit from care will receive it
- Patient-centered—respectful of and responsive to individual patient preferences, needs, and values
- Timely—occurs when it is necessary for optimal quality care delivery thus preventing harm from delays
- Efficient—without waste of equipment, supplies, ideas, and energy
- Equitable—giving all patients the care they need with the same level of quality, without variation based on gender, ethnicity, geographic location, and socioeconomic status

6. **How extensive is the problem of medical errors?**

The Institute of Medicine estimated in 1998 that 44,000 to 98,000 deaths per year are due to medical errors. A landmark publication by Makary in 2016 suggested that medical errors account for 250,000 deaths a year, making it the third leading cause of death in the United States. Shojania et al. disputed these numbers because the report did not distinguish between deaths where error was the primary cause from deaths where errors occurred but did not directly cause a fatal outcome. They believed more accurate articles reported 25,000 deaths a year from errors. Overestimation of such high magnitudes runs the risk of disengaging clinicians and damaging their confidence in interventions intended to improve patient safety. There is less literature on the frequency of pediatric mortality from medical errors. One study showed that 4500 deaths annually occurred in pediatrics as a result of medical errors.

7. **What is the difference between a medical error and an adverse event?**

According to the Institute of Medicine, a *medical error* is defined as the "failure of a planned action to be completed as intended or the use of a wrong plan to achieve an aim." While medical errors can be harmful, they often do not result in patient injury. As an example, giving a scheduled medication 2 hours after it is due is a medical error that may not necessarily lead to patient harm. Errors that do not lead to harm are called *near misses*, close calls, or simply mistakes. Medical errors can lead to *adverse events* when they are associated with unintended harm to the patient through either omission or commission and are not related to the natural course of an illness.

8. **What is a sentinel event?**

The Joint Commission has labeled a *sentinel event* as a patient safety event that reaches a patient and results in death, permanent harm, or severe temporary harm, which requires intervention to sustain life. An event can also be considered sentinel if it highlights the need for immediate investigation and countermeasure implementation to prevent recurrence.

9. **What is Reason's Swiss Cheese Model?**

The Swiss cheese model of accident causation shows that actual hazards occur as a result of multiple smaller failures. It likens human systems to multiple slices of Swiss cheese stacked side by side. The different layers of defenses against errors are stacked against each other so that weaknesses in one part of the system (a single point of failure) do not lead to a safety event because they are prevented by the next layer of defenses. Each hole in the cheese represents weaknesses in individual parts of the system. However, when the holes all line up, a "trajectory of accident opportunity" ensues and a hazard passes through all the holes in all the slices and leads to a failure.

10. **What are latent and active errors?**

Latent errors are design flaws or failures inherent in the tools or systems and work environment that produce circumstances in which a worker (nurse, physician) is likely to err. Latent errors may persist for long periods of time before they are discovered and corrected. *Active errors* are the actual events that result in harm. Latent errors contribute to the occurrence of active errors.

11. **What can we learn about errors in the pediatric ED from incident reports?**

Incident reports are necessary for the prevention of harm. Incident reporting allows underlying root causes to be explored and systems enhancements to be implemented. ED staff must be encouraged to report incidents in a nonpunitive environment.

Safety incidents are grossly underreported through voluntary incident reporting systems. One study collected more than 3000 incident reports from 18 different pediatric EDs in 1 year. The most common incidents reported are laboratory errors (25%), medication errors (20%), and process variances (14%), (e.g., delay in care). Only 15% of reported events resulted in harm to the patient. Almost 70% of incidents were related to human factors, and most of them were due to the lack of adherence to established protocols. Very few reports involve sentinel events. It is possible these events are rare and reported through other mechanisms. A subanalysis of the near misses and unsafe conditions from these incident reports revealed that the most common near misses were medication-related, followed by laboratory-related, radiology-related, and lastly process-related. Human factor issues from noncompliance with procedures accounted for 66%.

12. What is root cause analysis (RCA)?

RCA is a method used to analyze serious adverse events. The goal of RCA is to determine underlying problems that increase the likelihood of errors. A multidisciplinary team uses a systems approach to identify both active and latent errors. The analysis usually begins with data collection and reconstruction of the event through chart reviews and interviews of health care providers involved with the adverse event. Interviews should be structured and performed free of bias and accusation. The team then uses this information to understand the sequence of events that led to the error and to determine how and why the event happened. Countermeasures are identified and implemented to strengthen the system, eliminate latent errors, and prevent future harm. Effective analysis requires involvement of organizational leadership and specialized experts in safety science. Success requires implementation of strong systems-level solutions and measurement of the impact on outcomes.

13. What factors inherent to the ED contribute to medical errors?

- Time pressures
  - Failure to understand and assess severity of patient's status during rapid triage
- Incomplete/unavailable medical and drug histories
- Unscheduled care
- Inconsistency of patient arrival
- High-risk patients (high acuity)
- Environment in flux, patients have varied locations (rooms, x-ray department, hallway)
- 24-hour activity in the ED
  - No time to restore order and "reset" the environment
  - Circadian rhythm of staff is challenged
- Transition of patient care among staff (consultants, change of shift)
- Inadequate and poor communication
- Overcrowding
  - Presence of an excess number of patients waiting for care
- Lack of organization and supervision of work processes

14. Why are children in the ED at particular risk for error?

- Variety of patient sizes and ages
- Need to calculate most medication doses by weight
  - Errors in calculation
  - Errors in obtaining or recording correct weights
  - Errors in diluting certain stock solutions
- Limited time for pharmacist review of medication orders
- Pediatric patients are often seen in community emergency departments where staff are less familiar with specific pediatric needs

15. What are potential causes of patient misidentification?

- Similar or same patient names
- Language barriers
- Patient answers with wrong name
- Identification (ID) bands removed
- ID bands illegible or incorrect
- Lack of patient ID processes or failure to comply

16. How common are medication errors in the ED?

A systematic review of ED adverse events revealed a paucity of literature in this area, particularly in pediatrics. Medication errors are among the most common reported errors. Medication-related problems have been reported in up to 11% of ED visits. The volume of medications given in the ED makes it ripe for errors. The weight-based dosing and calculations required for prescribing medications to children make medication errors in a pediatric ED a real issue. In a study by Kozer and colleagues, 10% of all patients seen in a pediatric ED had a prescribing error. In a study by Nelson and coworkers, 16% of electronic prescriptions in a pediatric ED contained an error.

17. **What are transitions and handoffs?**

Transition is the transfer of care between care providers and includes communication of important data. Examples of transitions in the ED are arrival of patients via emergency medical services, "change of shift," a visit by a speciality consultant, admission of the patient to an inpatient unit, and a resident or student presenting the patient to an attending physician. Transitions interrupt continuity of care and are a source of potential error. Staff should be educated on the risks created by the transfer of a patient's care, and best practices for safe transitions should be promoted.

Handoff is an effective communication surrounding the transfer of patient care responsibilities and acts to pass important patient information from one team of caregivers to another. Handoffs have been reported to contribute to up to 80% of serious medical errors from miscommunication. Due to their importance, the Association of American Medical Colleges has included handoffs as one of the 13 core entrustable professional activities for entering residency. Patient safety can likely be improved with standardized handoffs and face-to-face communication, especially at the bedside.

18. **What information is essential for an I-PASS handoff?**

I-PASS is a commonly used standardized handoff tool. A large multicenter study showed incorporation of standardized education, the I-PASS mnemonic, and electronic adoption reduced medical errors by 26% in the inpatient setting. I-PASS incorporates the following elements:

- **I**llness severity
- **P**atient summary
- **A**ction list
- **S**ituation awareness and contingency plans
- **S**ynthesis by receiver

A mixed-method needs assessment reported that emergency medicine providers generally endorsed the order and content of the I-PASS tool in their practice setting. They recommended the patient summary should include anticipated disposition and wording changes for brevity and clarity.

19. **Why is emergency department discharge important for patient safety?**

The discharge process is a high-risk handoff transition where patients are expected to understand their diagnosis and treatment plan. Patients and families are quickly given new and complex information during a stressful period. Variable literacy levels and language barriers also contribute to understanding and compliance with expectations. The four domains of discharge instructions include (1) diagnosis and cause, (2) care given in the ED, (3) care after the ED visit, and (4) instructions on when to return to the ED. Many studies have shown that patients have poor understanding of their discharge instructions in the various domains, with the greatest deficits in home care and return to the ED. This lack of understanding and poor teaching by the health care professional leads to preventable return ED visits.

20. **How can emergency department discharge be improved?**

Verbal discharge instructions can be enhanced with the addition of written discharge instructions. Written instructions should use health literate language and contain simplified text that is free of unnecessary information. Illustrations can assist in patient understanding. Use interpretive services when there are language barriers. In a pooled meta-analysis, while video instructions showed improved understanding, it was not statistically significant. Teach-back has been shown to improve understanding of discharge instructions even after adjusting for age and education level. Teach-back methodology involves asking patients to repeat information that has been given to them. It allows the educator to check for deficits in understanding and to reteach until the patient/parent exhibits comprehension.

21. **How common are interruptions in the ED?**

There is an association between interruptions in workflow and medical errors. Studies show interruption rates of 10 to 12 an hour for ED nurses and providers. The ED staff members perform between 1 and 8 other activities before returning to the original task. High rates of interruptions are correlated with lower rates of situational awareness. Interruptions by telephone/pager, technical malfunctions, and interruptive communication are further correlated with lower situational awareness. Some interruptions are unavoidable, as in the case of deteriorating patients or critical findings.

22. **How does computer provider order entry (CPOE) affect patient safety?**

CPOE, the process by which orders for patient care are directly entered into the computer by the treating provider, can make medication ordering safer. The software can provide decision support, check allergies and weights and eliminate transcription errors. CPOE avoids omitted information on generated prescriptions, and the prescriptions can be sent electronically to a given pharmacy, enhancing efficiency. Implementation of CPOE in one intensive care unit setting decreased medication errors by 99% and adverse drug events by 40%. Unfortunately, there can be new types of errors inherent in the system due to human-computer interaction. Alerts have been reported to fire 0.06-0.76 times per encounter in a study of six pediatric hospitals, which can lead to "alert fatigue" and overriding of important warnings. There can also be adverse events if allergy information is not updated. Incorrect human data entry can result in mistaken weight, order, or dose entry or other typographical errors. Wrong order-wrong patient errors are created by selecting a chart or laboratory result that is not for the intended patient prior to placing an order. Physicians spend as much time on the computer as they do interacting with patients, contributing to burnout, which can threaten patient safety. The US Emergency Medicine Information Technology Consensus Conference concluded that if there is a weakness in a CPOE system, it will first fail in the ED because of the complex, high-risk, fast-paced setting.

23. **Why are children with special health care needs vulnerable to errors in emergency care?**
Children with medical complexity account for <1% of the pediatric population but more than one-third of pediatric health care costs. Hospitalized CMC are at increased risk for medical errors for several reasons:
- Some of their problems are difficult to recognize, thus delaying care.
- Some conditions are recognizable but refractory to standard therapy.
- Their baseline condition (e.g., vital signs, mental status) may not be known to the ED provider. Thus severity of illness can be underestimated or overestimated.
- They often have rare conditions that are unfamiliar to the emergency care provider.
- Many require technological devices that are not available to ED providers.

24. **What can be done to make children with medical complexity more safe when receiving emergency care?**
An emergency information form can help ED physicians provide more efficient and appropriate care to patients with medical complexity. The form may contain contact information, past medical history and procedures, common presenting problems, and suggestions for management strategies.
   Hospitals should provide clear mechanisms for families to share safety concerns. Families of children with medical complexity have reported adverse events not otherwise detected in the medical record.

25. **When caring for a patient with limited English proficiency in the ED, would a family member interpreter be sufficient?**
No, it would not be ideal. In one pediatric study, one clinical encounter generated 31 errors in medical interpretation. Most errors were of omission and had potential for clinical consequences. Errors committed by ad hoc interpreters (hospital staff, family members, and other patients in the ED) as opposed to hospital interpreters were more likely to have clinical consequences. A systematic review reported that quality of care is compromised when patients with limited English proficiency need, but do not get, interpreters. Trained professional interpreters and bilingual health care providers positively impact patient satisfaction, quality of care, and outcomes. In-person, telephone, video, and interpretation provided by a bilingual physician confer the same patient satisfaction. However, in-person interpreters lead to shorter ED throughput compared to telephone interpreters. Video interpretation improves understanding of diagnoses when compared to phone interpretation.

KEY POINTS: MEDICAL ERRORS IN THE PEDIATRIC EMERGENCY DEPARTMENT

1. The largest threat to children in the ED is medication errors, most of which are dosing errors.
2. The ED environment is a challenge, largely because of its unstructured and hurried environment, and patients of varied sizes that present with unpredictable issues, and different levels of urgency, at unscheduled times.
3. Better ED systems, communication, and teamwork can reduce errors.

---

26. **Why would physicians conceal a medical error?**
According to Kaldijian et al., factors that impede physician disclosure include:
   Attitudinal barriers
      Perpetuating perfectionism
      Belief that others do not need to know about one's errors
      Arrogance and pride
      Placing self-interests before patient interests
      Competition with peers
      Doubt about the benefits of disclosure

Uncertainties
  How to disclose
  Which errors to disclose
  Disagreement about whether an error occurred
Helplessness
  Lack of control over what happens to information once disclosed
  Lack of confidentiality
  Lack of collegial support
  Belief error reporting is punitive
  Lack of time to disclose
Fears and anxieties
  Legal, financial liability
  Professional discipline
  Patient/family anger
  Admitting negligence
  Possibility of looking foolish
  Negative publicity
  Possibility of falling out with colleagues
  Sense of personal failure

27. **Are physicians ethically obligated to disclose medical errors to patients?**
The American Medical Association Code of Medical Ethics states, "It is a fundamental ethical requirement that a physician should at all times deal honestly and openly with patients. Patients have a right to know their past and present medical status and to be free of any mistaken beliefs concerning their conditions. Situations occasionally occur in which a patient suffers significant medical complications that may have resulted from the physician's mistake or judgment. In these situations, the physician is ethically required to inform the patient of all the facts necessary to ensure understanding of what has occurred. Only through full disclosure is a patient able to make informed decisions regarding future medical care." Even minor errors should be discussed with patients to maintain an honest and open relationship. "This obligation holds even though the patient's medical treatment or therapeutic options may not be altered by the new information."

28. **Are physicians legally obligated to disclose medical errors, and do these disclosures lead to malpractice lawsuits?**
Most patients, when asked, would be more likely to distrust a doctor, take their care elsewhere, or bring a lawsuit against a physician who conceals an error, as opposed to one who is truthful and forthcoming with information. They prefer acknowledgment of even minor errors. Some states have laws mandating full disclosure of all unanticipated outcomes. Hospitals are implementing policies that support disclosure, called compensation and resolution programs. Unanticipated outcomes and medical errors are disclosed, and patients are offered compensation upfront. The University of Michigan's Health System decreased their average monthly rate of new claims from 7.03 to 4.52 per 100,000 and lawsuits from 2.13 to 0.75 per 100,000 patient encounters after they adopted a compensation and resolution program. Communication and resolution programs in four Massachusetts hospitals did not cause an increase in liability trends.

29. **What is the second victim syndrome?**
The second victim syndrome is the suffering of health care professionals who are involved in a medical error. This is manifested by psychological, cognitive, and/or physical reactions that have a personal negative impact. Health care providers often respond to their own mistakes with anger and projections of blame, similar to acute stress disorder. Scott et al. described six predictable stages of the second victim syndrome:
1. Chaos and accident response
2. Intrusive reflections
3. Restoring personal integrity
4. Enduring the inquisition
5. Obtaining emotional first aid
6. Moving on

30. **What are the National Patient Safety Foundation's recommendations to improve patient safety?**
1. Ensure that leaders establish and sustain a safety culture
2. Create centralized and coordinated oversight of patient safety
3. Create a common set of safety metrics that reflect meaningful outcomes
4. Increase funding for research in patient safety and implementation science

5. Address safety across the entire care continuum
6. Support the health care workforce
7. Partner with patients and families for the safest care
8. Ensure that technology is safe and optimized to improve patient safety

31. How can patient safety be improved in the ED?

Safety culture can be improved by considering human, managerial, and organizational factors. Individual performance metrics and incentives to improve care should be combined with education on core patient safety concepts. Leadership support and prioritization of patient safety are important to nurturing safety culture. Formal processes geared toward promoting patient safety and error prevention such as standardized handoffs and team communication training are also important for strengthening a patient safety culture.

Many *processes can be implemented* to directly improve patient safety. Implementation and utilization of a voluntary safety event reporting system can enable tracking, trend recognition, and countermeasure development. Morbidity and Mortality (M&M) conferences allow for a nonpunitive environment to review and learn from medical errors. M&M conferences also serve as an important didactic tool for trainees and are an Accreditation Council for Graduate Medical Education requirement. Lastly, patient safety walk rounds performed by ED leadership allow open communication about safety concerns and help escalate opportunities for improvement.

Structural mechanisms can support *systems-based improvement* in patient safety. For instance, use of clinical guidelines can reduce variability in patient management and ensure evidence-based care is delivered. In addition, CPOE can decrease errors by standardizing orders such as lab panels for certain conditions. CPOE can also decrease the need for performing manual mathematical calculations when ordering medication for pediatric patients. Additionally, CPOE can integrate clinical decision support, which promotes the use of evidence-based practice. Another structural mechanism to improve patient safety is the integration of patient- and family-centered care through the use of standardized introductions, joint decision-making, acknowledgment of patients' emotions, reflective listening, expectation setting, clear communication, and interpretive services when needed.

32. What is a high-reliability organization (HRO)?

High-reliability organizations (HROs) promote a culture of safety by being constantly aware of potential safety gaps. Errors are inevitable and result from system breakdowns, not individual flaws. Everyone in the organization needs to maintain safety as their highest priority and work relentlessly to reduce failures and errors. HROs are based on five principles:
1. Sensitivity to operations—vigilant to possibilities of risk and unreliability of processes
2. Preoccupation with failure—mindful that small failures can add up to big ones
3. Deference to expertise—hierarchies may lead to mistakes
4. Resilience—recover from setbacks
5. Reluctance to simplify—simple answers are not provided for complex problems

33. What resources are available to learn about patient safety?

- Agency for Healthcare Research and Quality (AHRQ) (https://www.ahrq.gov/patient-safety/resources/index.html): a division of the US Department of Health and Human Services with a mission to improve the quality, safety, efficiency, and effectiveness of health care for all Americans

KEY POINTS: PATIENT SAFETY AND QUALITY IMPROVEMENT IN THE ED

1. Patient safety includes prevention of diagnostic errors, medical errors, injury, or other preventable harm to a patient.
2. Quality improvement is the framework used to systematically improve care through the standardization of processes to reduce variation, achieve predictable results, and improve outcomes for patients and health care organizations.
3. Handoffs, language barriers, computer order entry, medical complexity, and patient identification can all contribute to patient safety threats.
4. Incident reporting and root cause analyses are important ways to improve transparency and to learn from and prevent future safety events.
5. A culture of safety requires a total systems approach that attributes errors to inevitable system breakdowns rather than failures caused by individuals. Everyone in the organization needs to maintain safety as their highest priority and work relentlessly toward it.

- National Guideline Clearinghouse (www.guideline.gov): a public resource for evidence-based clinical practice guidelines and an initiative of the AHRQ
- National Patient Safety Foundation (www.npsf.org): nonprofit organization devoted to understanding patient safety issues and how to improve them, as well promoting public awareness and fostering communication
- Institute for Safe Medication Practices (www.ismp.org): nonprofit organization devoted entirely to medication error prevention
- The Leapfrog Group (www.leapfroggroup.org)
- The American Hospital Association (www.aha.org)
- Institute for Healthcare Improvement (www.ihi.org)
- Joint Commission on Accreditation of Healthcare Organizations (www.jointcommission.org)

BIBLIOGRAPHY

1. Al-Harthy N, Sudersanadas KM, Al-Mutairi M, et al. Efficacy of patient discharge instructions: a pointer toward caregiver friendly communication methods from pediatric emergency personnel. *J Family Community Med.* 2016;23(3):155–160.
2. Alimenti D, Buydos S, Cunliffe L, Hunt A. Improving perceptions of patient safety through standardizing handoffs from the emergency department to the inpatient setting: a systematic review. *J Am Assoc Nurse Pract.* 2019;31(6):354–363.
3. Alshyyab MA, FitzGerald G, Dingle K, et al. Developing a conceptual framework for patient safety culture in emergency department: a review of the literature. *Int J Health Plan Manage.* 2019;34(1):42–55.
4. Amaniyan S, Faldaas BO, Logan PA, Vaismoradi M. Learning from patient safety incidents in the emergency department: a systematic review. *J Emerg Med.* 2020;58(2):234–244. https://doi.org/10.1016/j.jemermed.2019.11.015.
5. Berwick DM, Nolan TW, Whittington J. The triple aim: care, health and cost. *Health Aff.* 2008;27:759–769.
6. Boylen S, Cherian S, Gill FJ, Leslie GD, et al. Impact of professional interpreters on outcomes for hospitalized children from migrant and refugee families with limited English proficiency: a systematic review. *JBI Evid Synth.* 2020;18(7):1360–1388.
7. Brixey JJ, Tang Z, Robinson DJ, Johnson CW, et al. Interruptions in a level one trauma center: a case study. *Int J Med Inform.* 2008;77(4):235–241.
8. Chamberlain JM, Shaw KN, Lillis KA, Mahajan PV, et al. Pediatric Emergency Care Applied Research Network. Creating an infrastructure for safety event reporting and analysis in a multicenter pediatric emergency department network. *Pediatr Emerg Care.* 2013;29(2):125–130.
9. Cohen E, Berry JG, Camacho X, Anderson G, et al. Patterns and costs of health care use of children with medical complexity. *Pediatrics.* 2012;130(6):e1463–e1470.
10. Dlugacz YD. *Chapter 5: Improving patient safety. Introduction to Health Care Quality: Theory, Methods, and Tools.* Jossey-Bass; 2017:133–172.
11. Heilman JA, Flanigan M, Nelson A, Johnson T, et al. Adapting the I-PASS handoff program for emergency department inter-shift handoffs. *West J Emerg Med.* 2016;17(6):756–761.
12. Hoek AE, Anker SCP, van Beeck EF, Burdorf A, et al. Patient discharge instructions in the emergency department and their effects on comprehension and recall of discharge instructions: a systematic review and meta-analysis. *Ann Emerg Med.* 2020;75(3):435–444.
13. Im D, Aaronson E. Best practices in patient safety and communication. *Emerg Med Clin North Am.* 2020;38(3):693–703.
14. Institute of Medicine (US) Committee on Quality of Health Care in America. In: Kohn LT, Corrigan JM, Donaldson MS, eds. *To Err Is Human: Building a Safer Health System.* Washington (DC): National Academies Press (US); 2000.
15. Institute of Medicine (US) Committee on Quality of Health Care in America. *Crossing the Quality Chasm: A New Health System for the 21st Century.* Washington (DC): National Academies Press (US); 2001.
16. Joseph C, Garruba M, Melder A. Patient satisfaction of telephone or video interpreter services compared with in-person services: a systematic review. *Aust Health Rev.* 2018;42(2):168–177.
17. Kachalia A, Sands K, Niel MV, et al. Effects of a communication-and-resolution program on hospitals' malpractice claims and costs. *Health Aff (Millwood).* 2018;37(11):1836–1844.
18. Kaldjian LC, Jones EW, Rosenthal GE, Tripp-Reimer T, Hillis SL. An empirically derived taxonomy of factors affecting physicians' willingness to disclose medical errors. *J Gen Intern Med.* 2006;21(9):942–948.
19. Khan A, Coffey M, Litterer KP, et al. The Patient and Family Centered I-PASS Study Group. Families as partners in hospital error and adverse event surveillance. *JAMA Pediatr.* 2017;171(4):372–381.
20. Khan A, Furtak SL, Melvin P, et al. Parent-reported errors and adverse events in hospitalized children. *JAMA Pediatr.* 2016;170:4.
21. Kozer E, Scolnik D, Macpherson A, Keays T, et al. Variables associated with medication errors in pediatric emergency medicine. *Pediatrics.* 2002;110(4):737–742.
22. Makary MA, Daniel M. Medical error-the third leading cause of death in the US. *BMJ.* 2016;353:i2139.
23. Mercer AN, Mauskar S, Baird J, et al. Family safety reporting in hospitalized children with medical complexity. *Pediatrics.* 2022;150:2.
24. Navanandan N, Schmidt SK, Cabrera N, DiStefano MC, et al. The caregiver perspective on unscheduled 72-hour return visits to pediatric acute care sites: a focus on discharge processes. *Acad Pediatr.* 2017;17(7):755–761.
25. Nelson CE, Selbst SM. Electronic prescription writing errors in the pediatric emergency department. *Pediatr Emerg Care.* 2015;31(5):368–372.
26. Nundy S, Cooper LA, Mate KS. The quintuple aim for health care improvement: a new imperative to advance health equity. *JAMA.* 2022;327(6):521–522.
27. O'Neill KA, Shinn D, Starr KT, Kelley J. Patient misidentification in a pediatric emergency department: patient safety and legal perspectives. *Pediatr Emerg Care.* 2004;20(7):487–492.
28. Orenstein EW, Kandaswamy S, Muthu N, et al. Alert burden in pediatric hospitals: a cross-sectional analysis of six academic pediatric health systems using novel metrics. *J Am Med Inform Assoc.* 2021;28(12):2654–2660.
29. Palojoki S, Mäkelä M, Lehtonen L, Saranto K. An analysis of electronic health record-related patient safety incidents. *Health Inform J.* 2017;23(2):134–145.
30. Ruddy RM, Chamberlain JM, Mahajan PV, Funai T, et al. Pediatric Emergency Care Applied Research Network. Near misses and unsafe conditions reported in a Pediatric Emergency Research Network. *BMJ Open.* 2015;5(9):e007541.

31. Sacchetti A, Sacchetti C, Carraccio C, Gerardi M. The potential for errors in children with special health care needs. *Acad Emerg Med.* 2000;7(11):1330–1333.
32. Scott SD, Hirschinger LE, Cox KR, McCoig M, et al. The natural history of recovery for the healthcare provider "second victim" after adverse patient events. *Qual Saf Health Care.* 2009;18(5):325–330.
33. Selbst SM, Levine S, Mull C, Bradford K, Friedman M. Preventing medical errors in pediatric emergency medicine. *Pediatr Emerg Care.* 2004;20(10):702–709.
34. Shojania KG, Dixon-Woods M. Estimating deaths due to medical error: the ongoing controversy and why it matters. *BMJ Qual Saf.* 2017;26(5):423–428.
35. Slater BA, Huang Y, Dalawari P. The impact of teach-back method on retention of key domains of emergency department discharge instructions. *J Emerg Med.* 2017;53(5):e59–e65.
36. Starmer AJ, Spector ND, Srivastava R, et al. Changes in medical errors after implementation of a Handoff program. *N Engl J Med.* 2014;371(19):1803–1812.
37. Weigl M, Catchpole K, Wehler M, Schneider A. Workflow disruptions and provider situation awareness in acute care: an observational study with emergency department physicians and nurses. *Appl Ergon.* 2020;88:103155.
38. Wu AW. Medical error: the second victim. The doctor who makes the mistake needs help too. *BMJ (Clinical Res Ed).* 2000;320(7237):726–727.

CHAPTER 71

RISK MANAGEMENT AND LEGAL ISSUES

Steven M. Selbst

1. **Which diagnoses involving pediatric patients in an emergency department (ED) are most likely to result in malpractice suits?**
   Specific diagnoses associated with malpractice claims against physicians in pediatric emergency medicine have evolved overtime. Most malpractice lawsuits involving children in an ED are related to the significant morbidity and mortality of cardiac conditions and cardiorespiratory arrest. Many others result from failure to diagnose appendicitis and testicular torsion. In the past, failure to diagnose meningitis was a leading etiology for malpractice lawsuits, but this condition is now less common and thus malpractice lawsuits related to meningitis are infrequent. In addition, failure to diagnose sepsis (especially meningococcemia), medication errors, and errors in wound management often result in lawsuits. Furthermore, failure to diagnose and manage fractures, slipped capital femoral epiphysis, myocarditis, dehydration, pneumonia, and child abuse are among the common conditions leading to lawsuits in pediatric emergency medicine.

2. **Why are emergency physicians at high risk for involvement in a malpractice suit?**
   Whenever the outcome is poor, an emergency physician is likely to be the subject of a malpractice suit, especially if the family is angry during their visit to the ED. Anger is a major force in initiating a lawsuit. Families in the ED may be dissatisfied before they even interact with the physician. They may be angry because of a long waiting time to see the physician. Sometimes they are angry with a discourteous staff member. The impersonal setting in the ED may be another contributing factor. It is often difficult to establish rapport with a family during a brief visit to the ED, which also puts the physician at a disadvantage if the outcome is poor.

3. **Why are cases of testicular torsion so often involved in malpractice lawsuits?**
   Testicular torsion can sometimes be difficult to diagnose. Histories and physical examinations are not always protective against a missed diagnosis. About 5% to 12.5% of patients with testicular torsion (found upon surgical exploration) did not present with testicular pain as the chief complaint. In one study of malpractice cases related to testicular torsion, 31% of patients listed abdominal pain as the chief complaint rather than scrotal pain. Furthermore, examination findings may be inconsistent in patients with testicular torsion. For instance, the cremasteric reflex is usually absent but has been present even in confirmed cases of testicular torsion.

   History of minor trauma to the scrotum can confuse the picture. Additionally, other conditions such as torsion of the appendix testes or epididymitis may mimic testicular torsion.

   Unfortunately, no single test is always diagnostic for torsion. Doppler ultrasound is about 89% to 96% sensitive and 98% specific for torsion, but false-negative ultrasound reports have been cited in malpractice cases involving torsion.

   In many cases, the emergency physician fails to examine the genitalia (perhaps when a boy complains of abdominal pain rather than scrotal pain). It is imperative to get every male completely undressed and examine the genital region when they have testicular or abdominal complaints.

   Also, emergency physicians may not realize that testicular torsion is found in young infants as well as older boys. Testicular torsion should be considered in the differential diagnosis of the irritable infant and should be suspected if the infant has scrotal swelling or inflammation.

   Finally, delay in consultation or delay in action by the urologist can lead to a bad outcome. Time is of the essence. When clinical suspicion is high, a urologist should be consulted immediately. Do not delay consultation while waiting for the ultrasound result.

4. **Why are cases of appendicitis frequently involved in malpractice lawsuits?**
   - Numerous conditions can cause abdominal pain and mimic appendicitis.
   - Young children may have nonspecific signs of pain such as irritability, lethargy, and poor feeding.
   - Appendicitis may not be considered in a young child.
   - Physical examination of a child can be challenging because of the lack of cooperation.
   - Features of "classic" appendicitis may be absent; atypical cases are common.
   - Diarrhea may confuse the picture with gastroenteritis.
   - The examination can be misleading; tenderness in the right lower quadrant may be absent. (An appendix in the lateral gutter can cause flank pain and lateral abdominal tenderness. An appendix that lies toward the left can cause hypogastric tenderness. Pain may be elicited only on deep palpation if the appendix is retrocecal.)
   - Diagnostic studies may be unhelpful. (Leukocytosis and pyuria are nonspecific; the appendix may not be visualized with ultrasound.)
   - Failure to observe the child, consult a surgeon, or arrange follow-up are common flaws.

- Failure to document findings makes it difficult to defend actions.

A malpractice claim is likely to result from failure to diagnosis appendicitis when there are negative consequences like perforation, abscess formation, bowel obstruction, sepsis, or death.

5. **How can a case of child abuse result in a medical malpractice lawsuit?**

A malpractice lawsuit can result if child abuse is missed and the patient returns with a more serious injury or death. If an emergency physician fails to view an injury as suspicious for child abuse and fails to report the case to child protective services, the infant/child may remain in the care of the abuser and suffer further injury. The family could then file a lawsuit and claim the physician should have recognized the red flags of abuse at the initial visit and taken precautions to prevent subsequent injuries. Physicians must be aware of injuries that should arouse suspicion for child abuse (see Chapter 51). Failure to report these cases could result in a misdemeanor offense as well as a costly lawsuit.

It is very rare that a physician will be sued for reporting suspected abuse when the report is later found to be unsubstantiated. All states provide some immunity to physicians who report abuse in good faith.

6. **How is the "standard of care" defined?**

The standard of care is defined as care that a reasonable physician in a particular specialty would give to a similar patient under similar circumstances. Physicians generally are held to the same standard of care across the country—a national level of competence. It is assumed that all physicians have the same knowledge of current procedures, treatments, and practices. Although not every doctor has the same access to specialists and technology, it is usually expected that an emergency physician will recognize a medical condition and attempt to get the proper care for the child as soon as reasonably possible.

7. **In addition to civil charges, can criminal charges be brought against an emergency physician in a malpractice setting?**

Very rarely. In some cases, such as failure to report a case of drug abuse, child abuse, or injury by a weapon, an emergency physician may be charged with a misdemeanor. Such charges usually are not made unless it is believed that the doctor was deliberately uncooperative. If a patient has died, the doctor can be charged with manslaughter if it is believed that an extreme or unusual breach of the physician's duty took place. The court may determine that the physician's actions were reckless or disregarded the rights and safety of others. Again, this event is very rare.

8. **What is the statute of limitations?**

The statute of limitations sets the length of time in which a person may bring a lawsuit for an alleged injury. Each state sets its own statute of limitations, but most states set a limit for adult patients of 2 to 3 years from the time that an injury due to alleged negligence is discovered or should have been discovered. After that time has passed, a malpractice suit cannot be initiated, regardless of the merits of the case. In a malpractice case involving a child, the time period does not begin until the child has reached the age of majority (18-21 years of age) in many states, because the child is unable to initiate legal action on his or her own behalf. Thus it is possible for a lawsuit to be filed 18 to 20 years after the alleged injury occurred.

9. **What percentage of malpractice lawsuits are brought to a jury for a verdict?**

Only about 8% to 10% of malpractice cases involving children in the emergency department reach a jury verdict. Most are settled out of court, and some are dropped altogether. Nonetheless, a malpractice lawsuit, once initiated, is a long and stressful event for the physicians involved.

10. **How are plaintiffs rewarded in malpractice lawsuits involving children in the ED?**

Although millions of dollars are paid out in malpractice lawsuits each year, money is actually paid to plaintiffs who initiate the lawsuit in less than one-third of closed claims. The overwhelming majority of payments occur in pretrial settlements. If a case proceeds to trial, the plaintiff is rarely rewarded. One recent study showed only 3% of cases result in judgment for the plaintiff. Claims involving major permanent injury more often result in payment.

11. **What is the impact of a malpractice lawsuit on the doctor who is sued?**

The outcome of most malpractice claims favors the physicians. However, malpractice litigation stress can be devastating for some doctors. Emergency medicine physicians involved in malpractice litigation find themselves in a contentious, adversarial situation, very different from their usual work environment. The duration of claims against physicians can last for 11 to 43 months. Physicians undergoing litigation stress often feel isolation, sadness, anger, disbelief, and a sense of betrayal. About 95% have some "emotional disequilibrium" and will report frustration, anger, and anxiety. Many sued physicians will suffer headaches, abdominal pain, and other gastrointestinal symptoms. About 30% of physicians who have been sued report symptoms of depression, such as insomnia, loss of energy, and feelings of hopelessness. It is understandable that physicians worry about their honor and professional reputation when they are named in a malpractice lawsuit. They are often embarrassed and feel shame. Many tend to doubt their skills. They are frequently concerned about their finances and perhaps their medical license. Social isolation or self-medication can be serious "side effects" of a lawsuit. Some physicians will even retire from medical practice after they are named in a lawsuit. Fortunately, thoughts of suicide are rare.

12. **What role does good communication play in reducing malpractice suits?**
Good communication with patients and families is crucial. A lawsuit is more likely when there is poor communication between family members and the medical staff. It is important for a patient or family to perceive that the physician has a caring attitude, professional integrity, openness, and high standards of excellence. It is essential to explain your thought process to families and acknowledge uncertainty about a diagnosis when appropriate. Tell families that symptoms of serious illness (e.g., appendicitis or meningitis) can develop later and encourage them to seek care if the child's condition worsens. Unfortunately, communication at the time of discharge from the ED is not always adequate.

13. **What factors lead to medical errors and missed diagnoses, ending in malpractice lawsuits? How can they be reduced?**
Most missed diagnoses in the ED are related to cognitive errors. These can result from:
- Challenging patients (atypical presentations, poor historians, changing clinical conditions, nonadherence to instructions, cultural or language barriers)
- The need for rapid clinical decisions
- Constant multitasking and frequent interruptions
- Busy, noisy, chaotic environment
- Fatigue (physicians, nurses, other staff)
- Frequent transfer of care (inadequate handoffs)
- Lack of technical competence
- Poor communication with other clinicians

To prevent some of these errors, emergency physicians should have a high index of suspicion when a child "just doesn't look right" to the parent or the clinician. If there is a worrisome history or a suspicious physical examination, it is wise to observe the child in the ED for a period of time. Observation in the ED is advised for children with persistent vomiting, irritability, lethargy, or inability to drink fluids, as these can be early signs of serious illness.

14. **How important is it to arrange for a follow-up examination of a child seen in the ED?**
Physicians have been found liable when they failed to instruct parents, instructed them inadequately, or could not prove that they gave instructions to return to the ED or to seek care elsewhere. In one case, a patient successfully sued because a doctor did not document that an incidental finding of hypertension had been addressed and follow-up arranged. The child eventually developed end-stage renal disease. Discharge instructions for patients or parents should include specific information about when to seek follow-up care with the child's primary care physician or specialist or when to return to the ED.

One study showed that even when instructions are given, only 60% of guardians for pediatric patients complied with discharge instructions to follow up with a physician after leaving the ED.

15. **What is the physician's obligation to inform parents about a procedure or treatment?**
Physicians are obligated to obtain informed consent from parents. Most states follow a "patient-focused" concept of informed consent. That is, the doctor must give the consenting person (guardian) a description of the procedure along with the risks and alternatives so that a reasonably prudent person would be able to make an informed decision about the procedure. A physician must speak in "lay language" so that the guardian understands the information. A guardian or patient is entitled to know the diagnosis, nature of the proposed treatment or procedure, risks and side effects of the procedure, available alternatives, and risks involved with alternatives. Guardians or patients also are entitled to know the prognosis with and without treatment. A physician should disclose all but the most remote risks if the outcome may be serious, but only common risks if they are likely to result in only minor harm to the child.

16. **How important is it to get parents to sign a consent form for a procedure?**
A signed consent form has some value. It provides documentation that an attempt was made to educate the guardian about a procedure. However, signing a form does not always equate with informed consent. A parent may still claim that risks and benefits were not adequately explained. If used, the consent form must be clearly written in language that most parents would understand. If a signed consent form is not used, the medical record should contain documentation that specific risks and benefits were explained to the guardian before the procedure was performed.

17. **When is it permitted to treat a minor in the ED without consent from a parent or guardian?**
    Any minor can and should receive medical care in the event of a true emergency. Most states define an emergency in vague terms such as one that "threatens life and limb" or "life and health" of a child. Such vague definitions are meant to protect a well-meaning physician. In reality, because an emergency is often difficult to define, every patient who presents to the ED should receive a medical screening examination, even if parents or guardians are not available to give consent. Furthermore, parental consent for treatment is generally not needed if a child presents to the ED with a chief complaint related to venereal disease, pregnancy, testing for HIV, or drug and alcohol abuse. However, many states require that the child be over the age of 14 before treatment can be rendered for these conditions.

KEY POINTS: COMMUNICATING WITH PARENTS/FAMILIES IN THE ED

1. Demonstrate compassion and professionalism (try to appear unhurried).
2. Apologize for the wait time.
3. Be a good listener.
4. Sit in the examination room, at eye level with the family.
5. Speak clearly in a language the family will understand.
6. Hide your own frustrations.
7. Keep the family informed, and tell them what to expect.
8. Use an interpreter if needed.

18. **What is an emancipated minor?**
    An emancipated minor is one who can seek and receive medical care without the consent of parents. In almost all 50 states, an emancipated minor is defined as one who is:
    - Over the age of 18 years
    - Has been married or self-employed
    - Has graduated from high school
    - Has served in the armed forces
    - Is otherwise independent of parental care or control
        Many states consider a pregnant minor to be emancipated and allow her to give consent for care for herself and her unborn baby.

19. **What is the "mature minor doctrine?"**
    This law, recognized by less than half of all states, allows a minor over the age of 14 years (not necessarily emancipated) to consent to medical or surgical treatment even if it is not a true emergency. In the judgment of the treating physician, the minor must be "sufficiently mature to understand the nature of the procedure and its consequences." The treatment must be intended to benefit the minor rather than someone else and must not involve serious risks. For example, the mature minor doctrine was applied to the case of a 17-year-old girl who consented to receive treatment for a minor finger laceration without parental consent.

20. **In which situations do parents *not* have the right to refuse treatment for their child?**
    If a life-threatening situation exists and the emergency physician believes that it is unsafe for a patient to leave the ED to seek care elsewhere, a family cannot sign out against medical advice or refuse care for their child. Likewise, if the patient or parent is under the influence of drugs or alcohol and cannot understand the risks and benefits of receiving or refusing care, the patient cannot be permitted to leave the ED. Finally, if child abuse is suspected, a guardian may not refuse care for the child.

21. **Can parents refuse emergency care for their child based on their religious beliefs?**
    Usually not. Most courts in the United States will not allow a parent to impose his or her religious beliefs on a minor, especially in a life-threatening situation. In such situations, it is generally unclear whether the child has the same religious beliefs and is "autonomous" or free from coercion or manipulation by the family. A young child may also be unable to comprehend the risks of refusing recommended treatment. Therefore if a blood transfusion is essential for treatment, give the blood. If parents object, report the situation as medical neglect to the appropriate agency and obtain a court order for permission to treat, while simultaneously delivering the emergency care. When it is unclear if an emergency situation exists, err on the side of treatment.

22. **List guidelines for documentation in the medical record of a child who presents to the ED.**
    - Always document the child's chief complaint, even if it seems trivial.
    - Be sure to record the child's medical history, allergies, immunization status, and current medications.
    - Carefully describe the child's general appearance (active, playful) and state of hydration.

- Include important positive and negative findings, rather than just noting that the examination was "normal."
- Document only parts of the examination that were actually performed. (Be careful when clicking on templates or dropdown lists.)
- When appropriate, record a "progress note" to indicate a child has improved prior to discharge.
- Avoid derogatory or self-serving statements in the record.
- *Never enhance or alter the record* after the child leaves the ED. Additions should be made cautiously. With electronic medical records, it is immediately known when the record was entered and what information was added or deleted. Altered, missing, or "misplaced" records create the appearance of a "cover-up" and can result in sanctions.

23. **How should an ED physician proceed if the referring primary care doctor disagrees with the ED physician's assessment and plan for the child?**
It is not uncommon for a referring physician to have a specific plan in mind for a pediatric patient. However, once the child arrives in the ED, the emergency physician probably will have some liability if the outcome is poor. The ED physician may be considered in a better position to determine the child's need for treatment and hospital admission, especially if the referring doctor has not actually examined the patient. Thus do not automatically defer to the referring doctor on the telephone. Try to reach an agreement about the child's care without compromising what you believe is the best plan for the child. If the referring doctor does not agree with the decision to admit a child, it is best for that doctor to come to the ED (if he or she has staff privileges) to examine the child and assume responsibility for the disposition. Do not delay emergency care while waiting for a primary care physician or specialist requested by the primary care physician to arrive in the ED. Hospital policies should be in place to guide the staff in such situations.

24. **What role do consultants play in malpractice lawsuits in the ED?**
Malpractice suits that originate in the ED frequently involve consultants, especially radiologists. The ED and hospital radiologists must have a system in place where the ED is contacted whenever there is a discordant reading or a change in the official reading of the x-ray. Likewise, ED physicians and other specialists/consultants must communicate clearly during a telephone consultation. There is a legal risk whenever information is given or requested by telephone. Finally, sometimes an ED physician disagrees with the recommendations of a specialist. The ED physician can be sued with the specialist if the patient has a bad outcome. When an ED physician has concerns about telephone advice of the consultant, he/she should insist that the specialist come to the ED to evaluate the patient directly. For all phone consultations, record the essence of the phone conversation with the specialist in the patient's chart.
 The ED physician is not obligated to accept the advice of a consultant, but the recommendations of the specialist should not be rejected without careful consideration and discussion. The recommendations of the specialist will have great weight in court. When applicable, document why the consultant's recommendations are not followed.

25. **What is Emergency Medical Treatment and Active Labor Act (EMTALA)?**
The EMTALA states that all hospitals that receive Medicare funds and have an ED must provide an "appropriate medical screening examination" to all patients who present to the ED to determine whether a medical emergency exists. EMTALA was developed to protect patients without medical insurance from being "dumped" by some hospitals, but the law applies to patients with insurance as well as to those who belong to a managed care plan. Many experts recommend that an emergency physician perform the medical screening examination rather than a nurse. However, hospitals may allow nonphysicians to perform the screenings as long as hospital policies define in writing that such individuals are authorized to perform the screenings. The acuity of the patient's illness may indicate whether a physician should perform the screening. A medical screening examination may range from a brief history and physical examination to a complex process involving ancillary studies and procedures. Triage assessment is not considered a medical screening examination. The screening examination must include all appropriate ancillary tests and services normally available to any patient. The tests must be ordered regardless of the patient's insurance if they are needed to determine whether an emergency exists.

KEY POINTS: TIPS TO PREVENT MALPRACTICE LAWSUITS IN PEDIATRIC EMERGENCY MEDICINE

1. Use caution in treating children with fever and abdominal pain.
2. Use caution if the patient is unable to ambulate upon discharge without a good explanation.
3. Use caution in performing a lumbar puncture (LP) in a small infant, especially if the baby is in respiratory distress (risk of apnea when the baby is curled up for a LP.
4. Remember that care given by others in the hospital (and prehospital) will affect the liability of the ED staff.
5. Communicate carefully with colleagues, especially around change of shift.

6. Consider pathology beyond the gastrointestinal tract if a child has vomiting.
7. Do not allow consultants to avoid cases when their help is needed.
8. Ask for help when managing complex wounds.
9. Read the notes of others involved in the child's care.
10. Document patient improvement in a progress note or discharge note.

26. **When is transfer of a child from the ED in compliance with EMTALA?**
A patient may be transferred from the ED if the transfer is medically indicated and the patient needs a level of care that is not available at the transferring hospital. A patient is considered stable when "no material deterioration of the emergency medical condition is likely, within reasonable medical probability, to result from or occur during the transfer of the individual from the facility." An unstable child may be transferred if the patient or parents make the request. Informed consent should be obtained if the patient or parent requests the transfer. If the transfer is medically indicated, the emergency physician must document that the benefits of transfer outweigh the risks and must arrange for an "appropriate" or safe transfer.
    Before transfer of the patient, obtain an agreement to accept the patient from a physician or responsible individual at the receiving hospital. When a patient requires a higher level of care that cannot be provided at the transferring facility, a hospital with the capability and capacity to provide the higher level of care may not refuse any request for transfer. Send an appropriate medical summary and other pertinent records with the patient to the receiving facility or have these records electronically transferred as soon as is practical.

27. **Is a pediatric ED responsible for an adult with an emergency according to EMTALA?**
If a patient is within 250 yards of the hospital, EMTALA rules apply. Thus if a person (child or adult) collapses on the parking lot or sidewalk outside the ED, or in the hospital gift shop, the hospital is obligated to screen and appropriately stabilize the individual, regardless of the person's age or ability to pay. Pediatric ED staff should screen and attempt to stabilize the adult patient within their capabilities. Staff should not just call emergency medical services without first starting to treat the adult. The hospital should generate a medical record for the adult patient, and the physician may wish to certify that benefits of transfer to a hospital for adults outweigh the risks of continuing treatment in the pediatric hospital, which has limited capabilities.

28. **What are the most important factors in patient satisfaction in the ED?**
Patient satisfaction depends primarily on prompt treatment, the caring nature of the emergency nurses and physicians, and the degree of organization of the medical staff. If the patient and family perceive the staff had a caring attitude, openness, professionalism, integrity, and standards of excellence, a lawsuit may be preventable despite a bad outcome.

29. **What are the most common sources of complaints resulting from pediatric visits to the ED?**
Most patients' or parents' complaints concern waiting time, quality of medical care (including an incomplete medical examination or failure to order enough tests), attitude of the ED staff, and misdiagnosis. In a general ED, complaints about billing are frequent, but billing accounts for only about 20% of complaints from a pediatric ED. Other complaints from families involve an unclean appearance and lack of privacy in the ED. Complaints from parents in the ED are inevitable, but many are preventable. It generally requires less work to prevent a complaint than to manage a family after they have formally complained about their ED visit. Developing rapport with families is essential.

30. **What are some tips to prevent complaints in the pediatric ED?**
See Table 71.1.

Table 71.1 Tips to Prevent Complaints in the Pediatric Emergency Department
1. Meet or exceed the expectations of the patient and family.
2. Introduce yourself to the family.
3. Pay attention to the patient and family.
4. Tell them why they are waiting.
5. Make the patient and family comfortable while they wait.
6. Defuse potential complaints during the visit.

31. **What are "Good Samaritan statutes"?**

    Good Samaritan statutes exist in almost every state and provide immunity to physicians and others who err while administering emergency medical care to ill or injured people. The Good Samaritan laws were passed to encourage physicians and others to stop at the scene of an emergency and offer assistance without fear of a malpractice suit. These statutes require that aid be given without compensation. They generally apply to care at the scene of an accident rather than in the ED or elsewhere in the hospital. Physicians are obligated to act in good faith but are not expected to put their own lives or their families in danger. Many statutes exclude "gross negligence" or "willful misconduct," but a physician who makes an "honest mistake" while providing emergency care at the scene is likely to be protected. A lawsuit still may be initiated if the patient suffers a poor outcome after treatment at the scene of an accident, but the suit is very unlikely to be successful if the physician acted in good faith.

32. **How should you manage a medical error?**

    - Follow hospital policies
    - Contact the hospital Risk Management office
    - Do not attempt to cover up
    - Investigate errors thoroughly
    - Disclose errors to families
    - Apologize when appropriate

33. **Should a medical error be disclosed to the family?**

    If an error has occurred, it is best to disclose this to the family. Physicians often assume that error disclosure will increase the risk of a malpractice suit, but there is no evidence for this. In fact, error disclosure may reduce the likelihood of a malpractice lawsuit. If the patient and family perceive the staff had a caring attitude, openness, professionalism, integrity, and standards of excellence, a lawsuit may be preventable despite a bad outcome. Error disclosure is endorsed by the American College of Emergency Physicians (ACEP), the American Medical Association, and the Joint Commission. Seven states mandate disclosure of medical errors and 36 states have "apology" laws that preclude some or all information used in a practitioner's apology from being used in a malpractice suit.

34. **What should you do if named in a malpractice lawsuit?**

    Do not panic. However, if you receive a letter of "Complaint" from a plaintiff's attorney, take this matter seriously. Even if you disagree with everything in the complaint (charges are often exaggerated), *do not ignore this*. The complaint may list statements that are demoralizing or insulting, but they are only unproven accusations. Contact your insurance carrier as soon as possible about any potential lawsuit, even a threatening letter from an attorney. Early notification allows the insurance carrier to investigate the claim, assign an attorney to assist you, and prepare a defense. Your attorney, once assigned to the case, will send an **"Answer"** to the Complaint (generally denying the allegations) within a certain time frame. It is possible that a "default judgment" against the physician may result if the doctor fails to notify his or her carrier and the defense team is not given adequate time to answer a claim.

    Tell your attorney everything about the case and help him/her develop the defense. Make some recommendations for a possible expert witness for your case. Do not discuss the case with colleagues. Do not call the patient or his/her family.

35. **Does the presence of family members at the resuscitation of a relative increase the risk of litigation for emergency physicians?**

    No data exist on family member presence and litigation. However, most families who witness a resuscitation report favorable opinions of the medical personnel involved. Family satisfaction after witnessing cardiopulmonary resuscitation may actually lower the risk of a malpractice lawsuit, even in the event of a poor outcome. Family members build trust in health care professionals when they are present for resuscitation in the ED. Also, health care providers are more likely to consider the privacy of a patient and pain management when family members are present. Attention to these details may also reduce the risk of malpractice lawsuits.

36. **What steps can be taken to avoid adverse outcomes and potential malpractice lawsuits when sedating a child in the ED?**

Follow hospital policies and procedures
Provider must be qualified and credentialed
Provider must have skills to rescue the patient
Provider must have knowledge of medications used and potential complications
Provider must be prepared for a deeper level of sedation than anticipated
Perform a presedation evaluation
Consult anesthesia for high-risk cases
Check medications and dosages prior to administration
Observe patients until they are back to baseline

37. **What guidelines exist for emergency physicians who serve as expert witnesses? Why is this important?**

The outcome of many, if not all, medical malpractice cases is related to testimony and opinions of expert witnesses. Expert witnesses have the potential to establish the standards of medical care with their testimony. Thus the outcome of a malpractice lawsuit often comes down to a "battle of the experts." Guidelines from the ACEP note that experts testifying in a case involving an emergency physician should be certified by a recognized certifying body in the field. The expert should be currently licensed and active in clinical practice for at least 3 years preceding the date of the incident that gives rise to the case. ACEP further states that the expert's opinion should reflect the state of medical knowledge at the time the event leading to the suit took place. Furthermore, the expert should not provide testimony that is false, misleading, or without foundation. The expert should be willing to submit transcripts of the testimony or depositions for peer review and may face disciplinary action if the testimony is found to be false or misleading. Finally, an expert witness should never accept a compensation arrangement that is contingent on the outcome of the litigation.

BIBLIOGRAPHY

1. Katz AL, Macauley RC, Mercurio MR, et al. American Academy of Pediatrics Committee on Pediatric Emergency Medicine and Committee on Bioethics. Informed consent in decision-making in pediatric practice. *Pediatrics.* 2016;138:e20161484.
2. American College of Emergency Physicians. *Expert witness guidelines for the specialty of emergency medicine*; revised June 2021, <www.acep.org>
3. Cronan K. Pediatric complaints in a pediatric emergency department: Averting lawsuits. *Clin Pediatr Emerg Med.* 2005;4:235–242.
4. Dresinger N, Zapolsky N. Ethics in the pediatric emergency department: when mistakes happen. *Ped Emerg Care.* 2017;33:128–131.
5. Edwards BL, Dorfman D. High-risk pediatric emergencies. *Emerg Med Clin NA.* 2020;38:383–400.
6. Glerum KM, Selbst SM, Parikh PD, et al. Pediatric malpractice claims in the emergency department and urgent care settings from 2001-2015. *Pediatr Emerg Care.* 2021 Jul 1;37(7):e376–e379.
7. Leske JS, McAndrew NS, Brasel KJ. Experiences of families when present during resuscitation in the emergency department after trauma. *J Trauma Nurs.* 2013;20(2):77–85.
8. Rappaport DI, Selbst SM. Medical errors and malpractice lawsuits: impact on practitioners. *Pediatr Emerg Care.* 2019;35:440–442.
9. Samuels-Kalow ME, Stack AM, Porter SC. Effective discharge communication in the ED. *Ann Emerg Med.* 2012;60:152–159.
10. Scarfone RJ, Nagler J. Cognitive errors in pediatric emergency medicine. *Ped Emerg Care.* 2021;37:96–103.
11. Selbst SM, Friedman MJ, Singh SB. Epidemiology and etiology of malpractice lawsuits involving children in US emergency departments and urgent care centers. *Ped Emerg Care.* 2005;21:165–169.
12. Studdert DM, Bismark MM, Mello MM. Prevalence and characteristics of physicians prone to malpractice claims. *NEJM.* 2016;374:354–362.
13. Weinstock MB, Joliff H. High-risk medicolegal conditions in pediatric emergency medicine. *Emerg Clin NA.* 2021;39:479–491.
14. Yu KT, Green RA. Critical aspects of emergency department documentation and communication. *Emerg Med Clin NA.* 2009;77:641–654.

CHAPTER 72

SEDATION AND ANALGESIA

Richard J. Scarfone

1. Why is it important to set patient management goals for sedation and analgesia?
Establishing clear patient management goals must be the primary consideration when determining the need for sedation and/or analgesia for children in the Emergency Department (ED). For some patients, providing local pain relief with the use of a topical anesthetic agent will be the main goal. For others, providing anxiolysis or moderate sedation will be the primary objective. For example, you may be caring for a young child needing to remain still and cooperative for a diagnostic imaging procedure and you may choose to use a pure sedative-hypnotic agent such as a benzodiazepine to accomplish this. Another child may have significant pain from a scald injury requiring an analgesic agent such as an opioid. For your patient needing reduction of her significantly displaced radius fracture, you will choose from several medications that will allow her to achieve deep sedation and analgesia. Deep sedation is a drug-induced depression of consciousness. She won't be easily aroused but will respond to painful stimuli. Most children who are deeply sedated in the ED maintain a patent airway and can ventilate normally.

2. Why has pain been inadequately addressed in children?
- Lack of available data in children. The Food and Drug Administration studies and approves medications for use in adults. Physicians must extrapolate this information for pediatric patients. Thus there are fewer clinical trials assessing the safety and efficacy of sedatives and analgesics in children compared to adults.
- Fear of addiction from opioids. In both adult and pediatric patients, physicians have been overly concerned about inducing addiction with the use of opioid analgesics. In fact, addiction is a rare consequence of the short-term ED use of opioids for medical purposes in children.
- Belief that neonates and young children do not experience pain to the same degree as adults because of their immature nervous systems. Any physician who has attempted to intubate the trachea of an awake neonate or to perform a lumbar puncture (LP) in a struggling toddler can testify to the contrary.

In fact, young children cannot understand the purpose of a painful procedure or comprehend its time-limited nature. Therefore, they are likely to experience a greater degree of pain and anxiety compared to older children or adults and are more likely to benefit from the liberal use of procedural sedation and analgesia (PSA).

3. Under what circumstances should I consider a topical anesthetic?
Intact skin (e.g., venipuncture, LP, or joint aspiration).
Lidocaine is a commonly used topical anesthetic for minor painful procedures, but this requires insertion of a needle through intact skin. Techniques that may reduce the pain of injection include using a needle of small caliber, buffering the lidocaine with bicarbonate, warming the drug, injecting slowly, and providing counterstimulation to the adjacent skin. You can avoid the pain of a lidocaine injection by applying either liposomal 4% lidocaine (LMX) cream or a mixture of lidocaine-prilocaine cream (EMLA) to intact skin. 4% lidocaine takes effect in about 30 minutes while maximal effects from lidocaine-procaine are achieved in about an hour.
Nonintact skin.
For most lacerations, lidocaine, epinephrine, and tetracaine (LET) liquid or gel should be applied directly to the wound, 20 to 30 minutes prior to a suture repair. A blanching of the circumference of the wound is expected due to the vasoconstriction caused by epinephrine. In many cases, additional administration of injected lidocaine is not needed. Traditionally, fingertips, toes, nose, and penis have been described as areas to avoid administration of LET due to concern of tissue injury from intense vasoconstriction; however, there is little data to support this concern.

4. What are the key elements of the medical history of a child about to receive PSA?
Before drug administration, obtain a complete review of systems including timing and content of the child's most recent meal, current medications, allergies, pregnancy status, comorbid conditions, and history of complications with sedation or general anesthesia. If the child was transported from another institution, verify whether he/she received sedation or analgesia at the referring hospital and, if so, what was given and when. In addition, ask questions related to specific contraindications to the medication that is about to be given. For example, a patient with a history of psychosis should not receive ketamine.

5. What are the key elements of the physical examination for a child about to receive PSA?
You must carefully monitor the patient's vital signs (especially blood pressure), mental status, and cardiac and pulmonary status before, during, and after the procedure. If your patient is receiving PSA due to traumatic injuries, these need to be addressed. It is imperative to first rule out potentially life-threatening injuries such as

an intracranial or intraabdominal bleed before proceeding with the PSA. Other features of the exam may influence medication choice. Patients who are borderline hypotensive will need fluid resuscitation prior to PSA. Ketamine, which causes a catecholamine release, would be a good choice for those with borderline hypotension needing an emergent procedure; propofol would be a poor choice. Similarly, agents that may cause hypoventilation and hypoxemia are poor choices for any child with respiratory distress.

6. **What is the American Society of Anesthesiologists' (ASA) physical status system?**
   This system was developed to assess preanesthesia medical comorbidities to help predict perioperative risks. It is useful to consider this classification prior to administering PSA medications:
   - **Class I:** Normally healthy patient
   - **Class II:** Mild systemic disease (e.g., asthma without exacerbation)
   - **Class III:** Severe systemic disease (e.g., poorly controlled epilepsy)
   - **Class IV:** Severe systemic disease that is a constant threat to life (e.g., symptomatic congenital heart disease)
   - **Class V:** Moribund patient who is unlikely to survive without the operation (e.g., victim of massive trauma)
        Strongly consider consulting an anesthesiologist for all Class III patients. All Class IV and V patients should be managed by an anesthesiologist.

7. **How much time should elapse between the last oral intake of food or liquid and PSA for my patient?**
   - This has been an area of controversy in the administration of PSA to children in the ED. Traditionally, ASA fasting guidelines have been fairly conservative with a 6-hour fasting recommendation following ingestion of milk, formula, or a light meal. These guidelines have been criticized for not being evidence-based, being more appropriate for fasting prior to general anesthesia, and not acknowledging that aspiration following moderate or deep sedation in the ED is extremely rare. The American Academy of Pediatrics has said: "The risks of sedation and the possibility of aspiration must be balanced against the benefits of performing the procedure promptly." The Pediatric Sedation Research Consortium found an aspiration rate of just 1/10,000 PSAs outside of the operating room and that fasting status was not a predictor of aspiration. In making such decisions, balance various factors including patient comorbidities, procedure urgency, targeted depth of sedation, and nature and timing of recent oral intake.

8. **During PSA, which equipment do I need to monitor the patient and to be immediately available at the bedside?**
   The risks of sedating children are significant and include hypoventilation, apnea, airway obstruction, hypotension, and less commonly aspiration. Ensure that the following equipment is immediately available at the bedside:
   - Cardiorespiratory monitor
   - Pulse oximeter
   - Capnograph to measure exhaled carbon dioxide
   - Blood pressure cuff
   - Suction catheters
   - Oxygen source
   - Airway equipment, such as self-inflating breathing bags with masks, oropharyngeal and nasopharyngeal airways
        In addition, make sure that advanced airway equipment, such as laryngoscopes and endotracheal tubes, are readily available in the ED.

9. **Explain the importance of capnography during PSA.**
   Capnography allows you to monitor the concentration of carbon dioxide (CO_2) during the inspiratory and expiratory phases of respiration of a sedated patient, plotted over time. In particular, measurement of exhaled CO_2 allows for an indirect assessment of the partial pressure of arterial CO_2; these values closely approximate one another. Although pulse oximetry indicates oxygen saturation, it does not assess ventilation. In contrast, capnography provides a graphic display of the effectiveness of ventilation. A common practice is to administer supplemental oxygen to a deeply sedated patient. This practice can delay the detection of hypoventilation or even apnea in a patient who is not being monitored by capnography since oxygen administration will prolong the delay between hypoventilation and desaturation.

10. **What is the optimal staffing for PSA?**
    Ideally, a physician experienced in pediatric advanced life support should administer the medications and closely observe the child's response. The risk of respiratory depression is minimized by administering agents slowly, over about 60 seconds. The physician should remain at the bedside at least until the period of peak sedation and cardiorespiratory side effects has passed (typically about 20 minutes, depending on the agent administered). A second physician should perform the procedure. In this way, a single physician is not dividing attention between two important tasks. A nurse should be available to assist in suctioning or administering oxygen or reversal agents and to document the patient's response to medications. Medications given, times administered, doses, routes, and

name of the person who gave the drugs must all be recorded. A flow chart should depict the patient's vital signs, oxygen saturation, exhaled CO_2, and mental status, with recordings documented every 5 minutes for the first 30 minutes after drug administration. Provide one-on-one nursing staff for clinical monitoring until the child is well into the recovery phase.

11. **Describe the characteristics of the ideal medication for PSA.**
    - Painless administration
    - Onset of action within minutes
    - Adequate and predictable sedation, analgesia, anxiolysis, and amnesia
    - Excellent safety profile
    - Duration of action exceeds the procedure time
    - Rapid recovery
    - Ready reversibility

    In fact, no single medication possesses all of these desirable attributes. You must determine what agent or combination of agents can safely and efficiently achieve the goals for a particular clinical situation.

12. **Are there any disadvantages to the transmucosal route of drug administration?**
    The main advantage of transmucosal (oral, intranasal, rectal), as compared to parenteral (intravenous [IV], intramuscular [IM]), drug administration is its painless nature. It seems counterintuitive to cause pain with a needle puncture in an attempt to ultimately relieve pain. However, important disadvantages of transmucosal administration include delayed onset of action, less predictable results, and difficulties in titrating the dose to the desired effect. It can be frustrating to the child, parents, and clinicians if the child is fully alert 40 minutes after an oral sedative has been administered. Atomizers convert liquid medications to aerosols. When employed to administer drugs intranasally, they result in enhanced tissue delivery and more rapid onset of action of drugs such as midazolam or fentanyl. However, when more potent sedation and/or analgesia is required, the parenteral route is preferred because it allows administration of additional doses of the medication or reversal agents if needed, as well as the ability to support blood pressure by giving fluids concurrently.

13. **What are some of the more serious adverse effects of medications commonly used for PSA?**
    Most clinicians prefer to develop a strong working knowledge of a subset of PSA drugs including recommended starting doses (Table 72.1). Midazolam, pentobarbital, propofol, fentanyl, and ketamine are often included within that subset of frequently used agents. Midazolam, pentobarbital, and propofol are classified as pure sedative-hypnotics. Midazolam is versatile in that it may be administered via multiple routes. Its principal adverse effect

Table 72.1 Recommended Doses for Procedural and Sedation Medications

DRUG	ROUTE	DOSE (MAX)
Midazolam	IV	0.05-0.1 mg/kg (2.5 mg)
Midazolam	IN	0.4 mg/kg (10 mg)
Midazolam	PO, PR	0.5 mg/kg (15 mg)
Pentobarbital	IV	2 mg/kg (100 mg) Additional doses: 2 mg/kg/dose every 3-5 min to a max total dose 6 mg/kg (including initial dose)
Propofol	IV	2 mg/kg bolus (100 mg) Continuous infusion: 200 mcg/kg/min
Etomidate	IV	0.2 mg/kg (10 mg) Additional doses: 0.05 mg/kg every 3-5 min to a max total dose 0.6 mg/kg
Ketamine	IV	1.5-2 mg/kg (100 mg) Additional doses: 0.5 mg/kg every 10-15 min prn
Ketamine	IM	4 mg/kg (200 mg)
Morphine	IV	0.1 mg/kg (4 mg; lower in young infants)
Fentanyl	IV	1-2 mcg/kg (100 mcg)
Fentanyl	IN	2 mcg/kg (100 mcg)

IM, intramuscular; IN, intranasal; IV, intravenous; PO, oral; PR, rectal.

is hypoventilation, especially if combined with fentanyl. Patients given pentobarbital must be monitored closely for hypotension. Propofol is a nonbarbiturate ultra-short-acting hypnotic agent. It has an extremely short onset (within 1 minute) of effect and duration of action, necessitating delivery by continuous IV infusion or frequent readministration for most procedures. Respiratory depression with hypoxemia, hypotension, and injection pain are common side effects. Its use requires vigilance on the part of clinicians because of the potential for adverse effects. Given the depth of sedation achieved with propofol, in many cases, it is not necessary to add an analgesic even for painful procedures such as joint relocations or fracture reductions. However, given its safety profile, propofol may not be a good choice for sedating a child who will be leaving the ED unaccompanied by a physician, such as for a radiologic study.

Fentanyl is a synthetic opioid. Compared to morphine, it is 100 times more potent and has a more rapid onset of action but a shorter duration of analgesia. Its principal adverse effect is hypoventilation, especially if combined with midazolam. Chest wall rigidity is an adverse effect seen with doses that are considerably higher than those used in the ED. Ketamine causes dissociation between the cortical and limbic systems, resulting in potent sedation, analgesia, and amnesia. Unlike most other agents, it does not cause cardiovascular depression. In fact, patients typically experience increased heart rate and blood pressure with its use. Two uncommon but potentially serious side effects are laryngospasm and hallucinatory emergence reactions. Incidence of laryngospasm is approximately 3 to 4 per 1000 sedations and the incidence is not decreased with coadministration of atropine or glycopyrrolate.

14. Can I safely use opioids in neonates?

The greatest experience with the use of opioids in neonates is with the use of morphine. Morphine may be indicated to reduce the pain associated with a strangulated inguinal hernia or from an inflicted injury, such as a fracture. Because a smaller proportion of an administered dose of morphine is protein-bound in young infants compared to older children, the proportion of drug reaching the brain is increased and the elimination half-life is prolonged. Thus, very young infants are particularly susceptible to apnea and respiratory depression with morphine. For those younger than 6 months, you should use a starting dose that is one-quarter to one-third the dose recommended for older infants and children. Age from birth, rather than duration of gestation, determines how premature and full-term infants metabolize narcotics. Thus a 4-month-old infant who was born at term metabolizes narcotics at the same rate as a 4-month-old infant who was born prematurely. You may judge the infant's facial expressions, heart rate, and blood pressure to determine whether to administer additional morphine for the desired effect.

15. How can sucrose be helpful for neonates during a painful procedure?

Sucrose is a safe and effective agent to help manage pain in infants younger than 6 months. It has the greatest effect on newborns and decreases gradually over the first 6 months of life. It is most effective for short painful procedures such as a heel stick or venipuncture. It has also been noted that infants can be calmed during an LP while sucking on a pacifier dipped in sucrose. It is recommended to use 25% sucrose solution and give 2 mL orally, by allowing the infant to suck on a pacifier. Alternatively, give 1 mL orally on each cheek with a syringe. The dose can be repeated; there are almost no side effects. Give the sucrose no more than 2 minutes before the painful procedure begins.

16. A bead is located in the ear canal of a 4-year-old boy. Initial attempts to remove it cause considerable anxiety and discomfort, preventing successful removal. What are your sedation options for this patient?

Because the boy does not have an inherently painful condition, and because he does not require an IV line for any other reason, a pure sedative-hypnotic such as midazolam given orally may be a reasonable option. It will take about 30 minutes for the full effects to be realized and the depth of sedation after oral administration is not predictable. Intranasal midazolam administered with an atomizer may be preferred since it will result in more rapid sedation compared to a dose given orally.

Another option would be nitrous oxide, an odorless gas that patients inhale. Nitrous oxide causes mild analgesia, anxiolysis, sedation, and amnesia. Its ease of delivery and rapid onset of action make it ideal for sedation before foreign body removal. However, at a ratio of 50% nitrous oxide to 50% oxygen, it is not likely to be effective for more painful procedures, such as incision and drainage of an abscess.

For young children, you can couple anxiolysis with distraction techniques. For example, engaging the child in viewing a video or blowing bubbles will greatly increase the likelihood of cooperation and successful foreign body removal.

17. A 3-year-old girl fell down five cement steps and struck her head on the pavement. She has vomited repeatedly since the injury but is fully alert and awake in the ED. You want to

perform a CT of the head to rule out an intracranial injury. What are some sedation options for this patient?

Because the desired goal is to prevent the child from struggling and moving during the study, you wish to achieve sedation rather than analgesia. Commonly used pure sedative-hypnotics include propofol, benzodiazepines, barbiturates, and etomidate. In addition to providing sedation before imaging studies, these drugs may also be useful as adjuncts to narcotics prior to painful procedures. For this patient, midazolam or pentobarbital may be the best choices. Their safety profiles and longer durations of action offer advantages over propofol and etomidate.

Midazolam may be administered by the IV, IM, oral, nasal, or rectal routes. Its onset is within minutes after IV administration, and clinical effectiveness usually lasts about 30 minutes. One may expect mild reductions in blood pressure and dose-related respiratory depression. Significant hypoventilation is rare unless the drug is given concurrently with a narcotic or pushed too rapidly. Its effects may be reversed with the competitive antagonist flumazenil.

Pentobarbital is a short-acting barbiturate that produces sedation within 5 minutes, lasting 30 to 60 minutes. As with midazolam, hypoventilation may occur but responds readily to gentle stimulation. Hypotension is a common side effect; do not use the drug in children with possible cardiovascular compromise.

18. **An adolescent girl needs an LP to assess for meningitis. What are some of your PSA options for this patient?**

IV sedation alone does not provide adequate analgesia for the painful LP. She will need a local anesthetic in the lumbar region, and administration of this will be painful. Topical anesthetics alone do not provide a great enough depth of analgesia for the LP. In response to the injection of the local anesthetic, an anxious patient may arch her back and move enough that it will be nearly impossible to perform the LP.

You should apply a topical anesthetic such as 4% lidocaine or lidocaine-prilocaine to the lower back. Regarding sedation and analgesia for this patient, you have several options to choose including ketamine or propofol but you may decide to use midazolam with fentanyl. Fentanyl's onset and duration of action closely parallel those of midazolam, making this combination particularly potent. Fentanyl provides analgesia and potentiates the sedative effect of midazolam. Respiratory depression is common with this combination but may be minimized by administering each agent over 60 seconds with a 60-second interval in between, and by titrating doses carefully. Gentle stimulation of the patient and supplemental oxygen almost always prevents hypoxemia.

Fentanyl has a more rapid onset and shorter duration of action than morphine, making it a better choice for most procedural analgesia. When more prolonged analgesia is desired (e.g., for vaso-occlusive crisis), morphine is the better choice. The combination of midazolam and fentanyl is also useful for laceration repair, burn care, and reduction of minimally displaced fractures.

19. **A 10-year-old boy has significantly displaced and angulated fractures to his ulna and radius that require closed reduction. What are some of your PSA options for this patient?**

Clearly, the primary goal, in this case, is to achieve potent analgesia for what is anticipated to be a very painful procedure. With the midazolam/fentanyl combination, it will be difficult to achieve the depth of analgesia required without producing significant hypoventilation. Therefore, in this case, ketamine is a good choice. Onset of action after IV administration is 3 to 5 minutes, with return of coherence in 30 to 45 minutes. It may also be administered IM. In a study assessing the ED use of IM ketamine among more than 1000 children, over 90% achieved acceptable sedation within 10 minutes, and 4 young children experienced transient laryngospasm.

You should anticipate that the child's eyes may remain open while sedated and he may develop nystagmus. In addition, catecholamine release will produce tachycardia and a clinically insignificant blood pressure elevation. He may grimace and/or verbalize during the actual reduction but will likely not remember any part of the procedure upon emerging from the PSA. A small proportion of patients will develop a rash or will vomit. This typically occurs during the emergence phase and children maintain their gag reflex when sedated with ketamine making aspiration highly unlikely.

20. **A 17-year-old boy dislocates his right shoulder while playing football. What are some of your PSA options for this patient?**

As noted above, there are several medication options to consider for this patient. Although ketamine is a reasonable option, it will increase the patient's muscle tone, potentially making a successful reduction more difficult. The combination of midazolam and fentanyl could be considered but the overall potency of the analgesia achieved may be insufficient for this patient.

Propofol may be the optimal choice for this patient. It is contraindicated for those with anaphylaxis to eggs or soy and it should be avoided for any patients with a history of a difficult airway, cardiac disease, or hypotension. Apnea, hypoventilation, and hypotension are potential adverse effects; a common practice is to give the patient a 20 cc/kg bolus of IV normal saline before giving propofol. Although it may be infused continuously, for a brief procedure such as a shoulder reduction, a series of IV propofol boluses may be preferred. For example, you can give a 2 mg/kg bolus followed by smaller 0.5 mg/kg boluses of propofol as needed after that.

21. **For what period of time should you observe your patient in the ED after PSA, before being discharged home?**

A recent report of over 1300 sedation events in children found that 92% of adverse events occurred during the procedure and serious adverse events rarely occurred after 25 minutes from the final medication administration. In another study of over 1000 children who had received IM ketamine, four experienced laryngospasm. Onset of this complication ranged from 15 to 25 minutes after ketamine administration.

Ideally, a child should return to his or her baseline verbal and motor skills and mental status before ED discharge. However, if the drugs are administered to a young child in the late evening or beyond, this state may not be achieved until the following morning. More practical endpoints are the ability to maintain normal spontaneous respirations and oxygen saturation for a period beyond the peak effect of the drugs, coupled with easy arousability. For most of the agents discussed previously, the child will be ready for discharge 45 to 90 minutes after drug administration.

22. **What are the top 10 pitfalls you need to avoid in administering sedation and analgesia to children in the ED?**
    1. Undersedation
    2. Oversedation
    3. Using reversal agents to speed recovery
    4. Choosing a short-acting narcotic when prolonged pain relief is required
    5. Combining two opioids or two sedative agents
    6. Choosing a sedative when analgesia is required or vice versa
    7. Choosing an improper route of administration
    8. Failure to document appropriately
    9. Failure to have proper equipment immediately available
    10. Not including parents in the discussion about the need for sedation and analgesia

KEY POINTS: SAFE SEDATION AND ANALGESIA

1. Determine your management goals and choose one or more medications that will safely achieve those goals.
2. Prior to medication administration, know the timing and content of the child's most recent meal, current medications, allergies, pregnancy status, comorbid conditions, and history of complications with sedation or general anesthesia.
3. Review the American Society of Anesthesiologists' (ASA) physical status classification of your patient and follow the recommendations regarding when it is appropriate for the sedation to be managed by an anesthesiologist.
4. When making sedation decisions, consider the child's last oral intake and balance factors including patient comorbidities, procedure urgency, targeted depth of sedation, and nature and timing of recent oral intake. (The appropriate elapsed time from the patient's most recent oral intake prior to sedation has been an area of disagreement.)
5. Have knowledge of several different sedative and analgesic medications, including recommended doses and side effect profiles.

BIBLIOGRAPHY

1. Bhatt M, Johnson DW, Taljaard M, et al. Association of preprocedural fasting with outcomes of emergency department sedation in children. *JAMA Pediatr.* 2018;172(7):678–685.
2. Cote CJ, Wilson S. Guidelines for monitoring and management of pediatric patients before, during, and after sedation for diagnostic and therapeutic procedures: update 2016. *Pediatrics.* 2016;138(1): e20161212.
3. Green SM, Leroy PL, Irwin MG, et al. An international multidisciplinary consensus statement on fasting before procedural sedation in adults and children. *Anesthesia.* 2020;75(3):374–385.
4. Green SM, Roback MG, Kennedy RM. Clinical practice guideline for emergency department ketamine dissociative sedation: 2011 update. *Ann Emerg Med.* 2011;57(5):449–461.
5. American Society of Anesthesiologists Task Force on Moderate Procedural Sedation and Analgesia, American Association of Oral and Maxillofacial Surgeons, American College of Radiology, American Dental Association, American Society of Dentist Anesthesiologists, Society of Interventional Radiology. Practice guidelines for moderate procedural sedation and analgesia 2018. Anesthesiology. 2018;128:437–479.
6. Stevens B, Yamada J, Lee GY, et al. Sucrose for analgesia in newborn infants undergoing painful procedures. *Cochrane Database Syst Rev.* 2013;1 CD001069.

CHAPTER 73

POINT-OF-CARE ULTRASOUND

Matthew P. Kusulas

1. What exactly is point-of-care ultrasound (PoCUS)?

PoCUS, sometimes referred to as "bedside ultrasound" or "focused ultrasound" is a diagnostic imaging modality. Unlike comprehensive radiology-performed ultrasound (US) studies, PoCUS studies are not designed to fully evaluate any given organ or body area. Instead, PoCUS aims to answer specific questions that inform immediate care at the bedside. To emphasize that focus, PoCUS practitioners are often encouraged to frame their PoCUS questions in a "yes/no" format.

In general, PoCUS is designed to be a "rule-in" test, rather than a "rule-out" test. As such, it is not uncommon to obtain comprehensive imaging after a "negative" PoCUS examination. In some settings, though, PoCUS can be used to eliminate certain diagnostic possibilities. A strong understanding of the strengths and limitations of PoCUS is needed to safely rely on PoCUS in medical decision-making.

2. What is the scope of PoCUS?

In pediatric emergency medicine (PEM), there are extensive PoCUS applications. Although variation exists between consensus statements and recommendations for the scope of PoCUS training for newly trained PEM physicians, most would agree that the following are among the basic applications:

- Bladder volume evaluation
- Lung US to identify pneumothorax or consolidation
- Focused Cardiac Ultrasound (FoCUS) to identify gross cardiac dysfunction or pericardial effusion
- Focused Assessment with Sonography in Trauma (FAST) to identify free fluid

3. How is a US image created?

PoCUS uses sound waves that are sent into the body by the US probe. The US probe then listens for echoes as some of that sound energy is reflected back. Some body structures reflect sound strongly, appear white, and are termed "echogenic." Some do not reflect sound at all, appear black, and are termed "anechoic." Examples of strongly echogenic structures include bones, gallstones, and the pericardium. Fluid-filled structures are anechoic, as fluid allows most sound waves to pass unobstructed. The most commonly used US imaging mode is "brightness mode" (also called "B-mode" or "2D"). In this mode, the strength of the reflected sound energy received by the probe is mapped onto the screen.

4. Why are there multiple probes?

Sound waves differ in their frequency. Sounds with higher frequencies have shorter wavelengths. Short wavelength allows for more interaction of that sound wave with body structures, resulting in images that show finer detail. However, as energy interacts with matter, energy is dissipated. As such, higher frequency sound waves are not able to reach as deeply into the body. High-frequency probes, therefore, are designed to evaluate superficial structures by providing good spatial resolution, at the expense of penetration. The typical high-frequency probe on a PoCUS system is the linear probe.

Low-frequency probes, on the other hand, are designed to penetrate deeply into the body, at the expense of spatial resolution. The phased array and curvilinear probes are the typically low-frequency probes used on PoCUS systems.

If penetration is needed, a low-frequency probe would be the right choice. If resolution is needed for a superficial structure, a high-frequency probe would be the appropriate choice.

5. How does the probe orientation correlate with the orientation of the PoCUS image?

On any US image, you will see an indicator. In PoCUS images, this is typically on the upper left side of the screen. The indicator tells you what part of the image correlates with the probe marker, which physically exists on each probe. By convention, in diagnositic imaging, the probe marker points to either the patient's head or the patient's right side.

When a probe sends energy into the body, it does so in a way that slices the body in half along the long axis of the probe. This creates two mirror images that can be displayed. The decision as to which of those two images to display is determined by the probe marker. By rotating the probe 180 degrees or by switching the position of the marker on the screen (i.e., to the right), the images displayed will be the mirror image of the original. If you switch both, the image will be identical.

In both mirror images, the footprint of the probe (typically at the top of the screen where the probe marker is located) represents where the probe is touching the body. Structures that are close to the probe are closer to the footprint and are typically more superficial. As you get further from the footprint (typically toward the bottom of the screen), the structures being represented are deeper structures.

6. **How do I know if an image has been optimized?**
   When starting to perform PoCUS, you will need to take the following steps to optimize a B-mode image:
   - Select a probe
   - Choose an application
   - Set the depth
   - Set the gain

   The probe you select will depend on whether your focused PoCUS question requires good resolution or penetration. If penetration is needed, a low-frequency probe would be the right choice. If resolution is needed for a superficial structure, a high-frequency probe would be the appropriate choice.

   Applications (on some units termed "exams") are presets that optimize many advanced settings that can be tweaked (and are beyond the scope of most PEM clinicians to worry about) and give the best image for the type of PoCUS you are performing.

7. **How do I optimize depth?**
   Typically, you want your structure of interest to be in the middle third of the screen. On most US machines, this is where structures will be most crisp and detailed. In addition, this allows the image to evaluate surrounding tissue and structures which, in many PoCUS questions, provides additional information.

8. **How do I optimize gain?**
   Gain can be compared to the exposure of a photograph. Like an overexposed photo, overgained images are washed out and too bright, while undergained images are too dark. As a rule of thumb, fluid-filled structures should be black, strongly echogenic structures should be white, and everything else should have a gradation of grays.

9. **How can PoCUS of the bladder be used clinically?**
   Two common reasons that a clinician may want to perform a PoCUS of the bladder would be to compare pre- and postvoid volumes or to determine if there is an adequate volume to obtain a sample prior to performing bladder catheterization.

10. **How can we determine the bladder volume using PoCUS?**
    Most PoCUS machines have a "calculation" feature for volume. The clinician must obtain views of the bladder and measure the required dimensions in order for the machine to perform the calculation. Typically, the two views obtained are the transverse view (which provides both anterior-posterior and left-right measurements of the bladder) and the sagittal view (which provides both anterior-posterior and head-foot measurements). A common mistake is to count the anterior-posterior measurement in both views. To avoid this, a common teaching is to think "+" and "−" when choosing dimensions (Fig. 73.1).

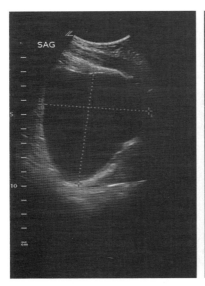
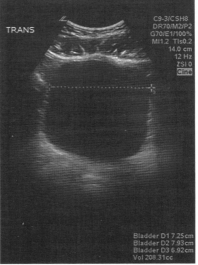

Fig. 73.1 Images demonstrating dimensions required to calculate bladder volume. In this example, the anterior-posterior dimension and cephalad-caudad dimensions are measured in the sagittal view, the left-right dimension is measured in the transverse view. This example demonstrates the "+" and "−" rule.

11. **How is lung PoCUS used clinically?**

PoCUS of the lung is utilized for the evaluation of pneumothoraces, pleural effusions, and pneumonias. The literature shows that PoCUS outperforms x-ray in the evaluation of pneumothorax. The evidence of pneumonia has been harder to establish.

12. **I tried to image the lung and it did not look like any structures I saw in my anatomy atlas. What is the deal?**

Air is the enemy of the US, and thus, the lung itself is difficult to evaluate. The pleura provides an air interface, which reflects sound waves strongly back to the probe. Pleura is so reflective that when the sound is directed perpendicularly to it, the wave may bounce multiple times between the probe and the pleura. An US machine does not know that a sound wave has bounced more than once and so interprets that sound energy as having come from a structure twice the distance or triple the distance. When creating an image, the US machine will represent that as multiple, equidistance lines that are parallel to the pleura. These are called A-lines. An A-line pattern is the US artifact that is characteristic of a normal, air-filled lung.

13. **How do we identify the pleural line and the A-line?**

In the sagittal plane, the probe will slice multiple ribs in cross section. Like air, solid bone does not allow sound waves to pass but reflects most of its energy back to the probe. Unlike sound, this does not create a reverberation. Therefore, on a US image, the periosteum appears bright, and behind is a dark shadow. Just under the two ribs is the pleural line. In normal lungs, you will see a shimmering along that line as the parietal and visceral pleural slide on each other during the respiratory cycle. This is known as lung slide.

Together, the periosteum of two adjacent ribs and the pleural line make up what is known as the "bat sign," where each periosteum represents the wings of a bat, the pleural line represents the stomach of the bat, and the intercostal muscle represents the body of the bat (Fig. 73.2).

14. **What features of lung US would help identify a pneumothorax?**

On a US image of a pneumothorax, you will not see the normal shimmering motion of the lung slide as the pleura is separated by air. Additionally, if you image at the point of separation, you will see the lung slide on half of your image, but no slide on the other half. This is known as a lung point and is highly suggestive of a pneumothorax.

To avoid a false-negative result, a sonographer needs to ensure that they are imaging the chest at the point where free air is most likely to be present. As air rises, this will be the most nondependent area of the chest. So, in a supine patient during a trauma evaluation, this would be the anterior chest. In a seated patient, this would be at the lung apex.

15. **You told me about A-lines, but what are B-lines?**

B-lines are bright lines that originate from the pleural line and extend down toward the bottom of the screen, cutting across A-lines. They are created by irregularities at the pleural line and can represent an accumulation of interstitial fluid in the underlying airspaces. One or two in any given lung, fields can be normal. But, as the number increases, it is more likely to represent pathology.

The pattern of B-lines can help give clues as to what lung pathology may be present. For example, evidence of B-lines in all lung fields suggests that a diffuse process is present such as a lower respiratory tract inflammatory process, fluid overload, and acute respiratory distress syndrome. A more localized B-line pattern suggests a local process such as mucous plugging, atelectasis, or focal bacterial pneumonia.

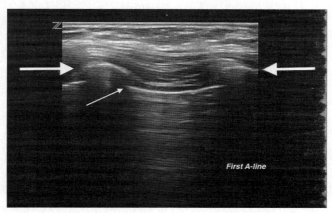

Fig. 73.2 The "bat sign," which is found in point-of-care ultrasound images of normal lungs. Thick arrows show the rib periosteum (making up the wings of the bat), and the thin arrow shows the pleural line (making up the belly of the bat).

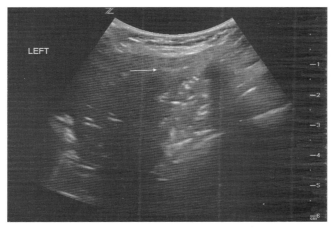

Fig. 73.3 A point-of-care ultrasound image which demonstrates pneumonia. This consolidation has multiple air bronchograms, one of which is indicated by the arrow.

16. **What does pneumonia look like on the US?**

    In pneumonia, the alveolar tree begins to fill with fluid, bacteria, and white blood cells. Because that region is no longer air-filled, A-lines no longer are created. Instead, US images begin to have the appearance of solid organs such as the liver and are described as "hepatization" of the lung. Additionally, within the alveolar tree, small air bubbles may get trapped within the inflammatory fluid. This is represented as bright, white lines and dots that take the pattern of the bronchial tree and are described as "air bronchograms" (Fig. 73.3).

17. **What is FoCUS?**

    FoCUS is focused cardiac ultrasound. In the emergency setting, details such as valve competency and pressure gradients are not clinically relevant, and taking the time to obtain it would likely be counterproductive to initiating emergent care. Instead, in the most basic forms of FoCUS, sonologists aim to answer two main questions: is there a pericardial effusion, and is there diminished left ventricular function?

18. **What is special about imaging the heart?**

    Unlike most body structures, the heart is dynamically in motion while being imaged. If imaged using typical US probes, motion creates a graininess that would make it hard to visualize fine detail. To overcome this challenge, the "phased array" probe was created. Unlike most other probes, the phased array has the ability to send out sounds in sequence, rather than simultaneously. As such, it is able to listen for echoes created by sounds sent at different times. This feature (which is enabled when one selects a "cardiac" application) provides "temporal resolution," which improves visualization of structures in motion.

19. **What does the heart look like on FoCUS?**

    There are four commonly obtained views of the heart in a FoCUS examination—the parasternal long axis (PSL) view, parasternal short axis (PSS) view, subxyphoid (Sx) view, and apical four-chambered (A4) view. The last of these views, A4, is the most challenging to obtain and is not needed to answer the two basic questions of FoCUS listed above. Thus, we will focus on the other three views: PSL, PSS, and Sx.

    The parasternal views are obtained by placing the probe in the "parasternal position" or just to the patient— left of the sternum. Because the ribs at that location are cartilaginous, especially in young infants, rib shadows do not provide as much of an obstacle as we encountered in the lung US. To start, we place the probe nipple line but may have to adjust up or down a few rib spaces. Once the appropriate parasternal position is identified, a practitioner has the choice of cutting the heart along the long axis of the heart from base to apex (creating the "parasternal long axis" view or PSL) or cutting the heart along the short axis, slicing the left and right ventricles in cross section (creating the "parasternal short axis" view or PSS).

    In the PSL view (Fig. 73.4), the practitioner aims for the right ventricle (which is the chamber closest to the probe), left ventricle, and left ventricular outflow tract (which leads to the aorta). The depth should be set so that the pericardium and the descending aorta (viewed in cross section outside of the pericardium) are visualized.

    In the PSS view (Fig. 73.5), the practitioner should aim to fully view the level of the left ventricular chamber, such that the papillary muscles are seen on either side. If the probe is properly positioned, the left ventricle should appear circular, while the right ventricle creates a moon shape, wrapping around the left ventricle.

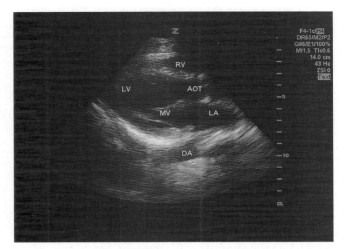

Fig. 73.4 Parasternal long view of the heart. Right ventricle (RV) is separated from the left ventricle (LV) by the intraventricular septum. The aortic outflow tract (AOT) leaves the LV. Blood flows from the left atrium (LA) to the LV via the mitral valve (MV). An important structure to differentiate pericardial effusions from pleural effusions in the descending aorta (DA), which is seen in cross section underneath the pericardium in the parasternal long view of the heart.

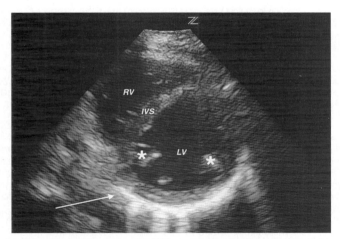

Fig. 73.5 Parasternal short view of the heart. The right ventricle (RV) is separated from the left ventricle (LV) by the interventricular septum (IVS). Within the LV, papillary muscles are visible (*). The pericardium is an echogenic structure surrounding the heart (indicated by an arrow).

To obtain the subxyphoid view (Sx), the probe is placed in the subxyphoid region and aimed up toward the left shoulder (Fig. 73.6). In this view of the heart, all four chambers of the heart can be viewed but attention remains on the pericardium.

20. **How do I identify a pericardial effusion?**
    Effusions are typically fluid filled and thus appear anechoic or black. The two views most useful to evaluate this are the PSL view and the Sx view. Further, the PSL view can help to differentiate a pericardial effusion from a pleural effusion. If the anechoic collection is above the descending aorta, and thus within the pericardium, we can conclude that the fluid is a pericardial effusion. If, on the other, the fluid surrounds the aorta, we know this is outside of the pericardial sac and therefore is more consistent with a pleural effusion.

21. **I am not a cardiologist. How do I evaluate cardiac function?**
    Studies have shown that a simple, gross evaluation of left ventricular contractility can identify significant degrees of diminished cardiac function. In an emergent setting, this is typically the degree of information needed to make

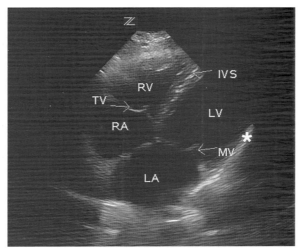

Fig. 73.6 Subxyphoid view of the heart. Right atrium (RA), right ventricle (RV), tricuspid valve (TV), intraventricular septum (IVS), left atrium (LA), left ventricle (LV), mitral valve (MV), and pericardium (*).

clinical decisions. For example, for a patient in shock, normal contraction can reassure a clinician that there is not a cardiogenic origin of the shock and thus inform a decision to perform aggressive fluid resuscitation. On the other hand, poor contractility may lead one to more quickly initiate vasoactive support. In the extreme, FoCUS can also be used to confirm asystole in a patient in cardiac arrest.

Contractility is best evaluated in the PSL and PSS views. In both, the left ventricular chamber size typically decreases by about 50% in normal systole. If one quadrant fails to contract as well as the others, this is concerning for ischemic changes in that area of the heart. By looking grossly at the contractions of the left ventricle, a clinician can determine with reliability whether the contractility is adequate, diminished, or absent.

22. **What is the FAST examination?**
The Focused Assessment with Sonography in Trauma, or FAST, was designed to detect free fluid in the setting of trauma care, specifically hemoperitoneum, hemothorax, or hemopericardium. More recently, the extended FAST, or eFAST, has included views to evaluate for traumatic pneumothorax. In the pediatric literature, the test characteristics of the eFAST for pneumothorax and hemothorax are both strong. However, the use of both a positive or negative FAST when evaluating for free peritoneal and pleural fluid is less clearly delineated by the literature. Despite these limitations, many argue that the FAST plays a role in the evaluation of critically injured children, but a clear understanding of the limitations of the FAST is needed.

23. **What does blood look like on a FAST examination?**
Like all fluids, fresh blood is anechoic and appears black on the FAST examination. However, if a patient arrives at the emergency department (ED) sometime after the initial bleed, the blood may have some fibrinous changes due to clotting. These collections are less uniformly anechoic and thus may have some shades of gray.

24. **What are the four views required for a full FAST examination, and what do they evaluate?**
   - Right upper quadrant (RUQ): right hemothorax or hemoperitoneum
   - Left upper quadrant (LUQ): left hemothorax or hemoperitoneum
   - Subxyphoid view of the heart (Sx): hemopericardium
   - Suprapubic region (SP): hemoperitoneum

25. **Within each of the upper quadrant FAST views, where do we see fluid collect?**
On the right side, there are four areas to investigate:
   - Above the diaphragm
   - Between the diaphragm and liver
   - Between the liver and kidney (an area called "Morison pouch")
   - The inferior pole of the kidney and caudal tip of the liver
      The first of these areas—above the diaphragm—evaluates for a right-sided hemothorax. The remaining three areas evaluate for hemoperitoneum. Any one of these areas can be positive in isolation, so omitting any of them may lead to a false-negative study and thus decrease your sensitivity. Experienced sonologists will also fan

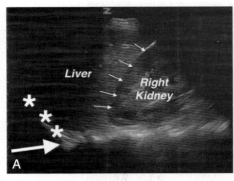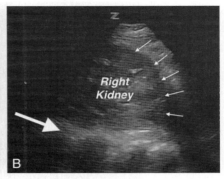

Fig. 73.7 Normal right upper quadrant Focused Assessment with Sonography in Trauma view. Visible are the spine (large arrows), diaphragm (*), Morrison pouch (small arrows in image A), and the inferior pole of the kidney (small arrows in image B).

through the kidney to ensure minor amounts of collecting fluid are not missed (Fig. 73.7). The left upper quadrant is similar to the right upper quadrant but replaces the liver with the spleen.

In children, the pelvis is the most sensitive area of the abdomen to detect free fluid. Due to the lordosis of the lumbar spine, fluid settles in the pelvis even from injuries higher in the abdomen. As such, a full evaluation of the pelvis includes a full fan through the bladder in both the sagittal and transverse planes.

26. **How might posterior acoustic enhancement affect the evaluation of free fluid in the pelvis?**
Sound waves pass through fluid with minimal absorption or other interference. These sound waves, therefore, reach structures behind fluid more unencumbered compared to sound waves that have to pass through more solid structures. Therefore, the tissue immediately behind a fluid-filled structure will appear brighter. This is typically a good thing, providing a good window to view structures, but when looking for free fluid behind the bladder, this enhancement can actually "white out" fluid that is present. In order to prevent a false-negative result, experienced sonologists must pay careful attention to adjust gain as needed.

27. **What is the spine sign?**
When interrogating the upper quadrants, we do so in the caudal plane in the posterior axillary line, usually using a curvilinear probe. The curvilinear probe "splays" out its sound waves. Some are aimed upwards toward the diaphragm, some go directly into the abdomen toward the spine, and others are aimed downwards toward the feet.

The sound waves that go directly perpendicular to the abdomen hit the spine and are imaged as a bright white structure.

The sounds that are directed toward the diaphragm travel through the liver before reaching the diaphragm. Once those sound waves go through the diaphragm, they encounter air-filled lungs. Sound waves are never able to reach the spine above the diaphragm because of this reflection. As a result, in a normal patient, the spine appears to stop at the diaphragm. As the patient breaths, it appears to be a curtain over the spine, making it appear or disappear at different portions of the respiratory cycle.

In the setting of a hemothorax, sound waves cross the diaphragm, and no longer encounter air, but rather fluid. The sound waves are no longer reflected, but rather continue through the thorax, eventually reaching the spine, and are visualized similarly to what is seen in the abdomen. The spine, therefore, no longer stops at the diaphragm. This is known as the spine sign (Fig. 73.8) and is indicative of fluid in the chest cavity.

28. **What is an intussusception?**
An intussusception is a "telescoping" of one piece of bowel into an adjacent piece of bowel. The portion of the bowel that is inside is termed the intussusceptum, and the outer portion of the bowel is termed the intussuscipiens. The most clinically significant form of intussusception is ileocolic intussusception, in which the terminal ileum (intussusceptum) telescopes into the adjacent cecum and ascending colon (intussuscipiens). When this happens, patients classically present with intense abdominal pain, often putting themselves in the fetal position. Sometimes, they present with altered mental status.

29. **How does an intussusception appear in the US?**
When the intussuscipiens and intussusceptum are viewed in cross section, their alternative layers are organized in concentric rings, creating the "target sign" (Fig. 73.9), which is perhaps the most classic US image for learners. When viewing the intussusception in the long view, you can sometimes view the actual telescoping of the bowel into itself, but more often, a "pseudo-kidney" sign is obtained.

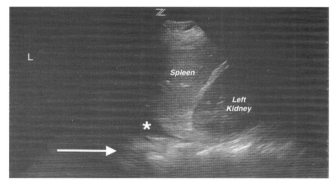

Fig. 73.8 The "spine sign," which is indicative of free fluid in the thorax (*). Notice that the spine (arrow) continues above the diaphragm.

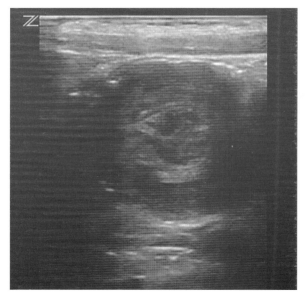

Fig. 73.9 The "target sign," which can be seen in intussusception.

30. **What else can I do with the US?**
    If you are looking for your next PoCUS study to learn, consider skin/soft tissue evaluation for cellulitis, abscess, or foreign body; confirming first-trimester pregnancy; and US-guided vascular access. More advanced PoCUS practitioners may consider evaluation of the inferior vena cava, musculoskeletal US, ocular US, evaluation of the right-upper quadrant, US for appendicitis, US for pyloric stenosis, renal US, US-guided nerve blocks, ovarian US, and scrotal US. Novel uses of PoCUS are constantly being evaluated and shared in the literature.

KEY POINTS: POINT-OF-CARE ULTRASOUND IN THE ED

1. When performing a PoCUS study in B-mode, follow four simple steps: Select a probe, select an appropriate application, optimize depth, and optimize gain.
2. Choice of probes depends on the frequency: high-frequency probes provide good resolution of superficial structures. Low-frequency probes can penetrate more deeply.

3. When measuring dimensions to calculate bladder volume, think "+" and "−" in both measurements of sagittal and transverse views.
4. Normal lung is characterized by an A-line pattern with lung slide at the pleural line.
5. When performing a FAST, make sure to interrogate all areas where fluid can collect to avoid a false negative.
6. FoCUS is not a replacement for an echocardiogram performed by cardiology. FoCUS is used to assess gross cardiac function and identify asystole or pericardial effusion.

Acknowledgment
Special thanks to Gina Pizzitola, William Sokoloff, and Lindsay Tishberg for their assistance in obtaining illustrative images.

BIBLIOGRAPHY

1. 5 Minute sono – basic ultrasound physics. <https://www.coreultrasound.com/basic_physics/>; Accessed 02.06.22.
2. 5 Minute sono – knobology. <https://www.coreultrasound.com/knobology/>; 2020 Accessed 02.06.22.
3. Alerhand S, Gulalp B. Lung. ACEP sonoguide. <https://www.acep.org/sonoguide/basic/lung/>; Accessed 02.06.22.
4. Au A, Zwank M. Ultrasound physical and technical facts for the beginner. ACEP sonoguide. <https://www.acep.org/sonoguide/basic/ultrasound-physics-and-technical-facts-for-the-beginner/>. Accessed 02.06.22.
5. Blavias M, Lyon M, Duggal S. A prospective comparison of supine chest radiography and bedside ultrasound for the diagnosis of traumatic pneumothorax. *Ann Emerg Med.* 2005;12(9):844–849.
6. Chen L, Hsiao AL, Moore C, Dziura JD, et al. Utility of bedside bladder ultrasound before urethral catheterization in young children. *Pediatrics.* 2005;115(1):108–111.
7. Constantine E, Levine M, Arroyo A, Ng L, et al. Core content for Pediatric Emergency Medicine Ultrasound Fellowship Training: a modified Delphi consensus study. *AEM Educ Train.* 2019;4(2):130–138.
8. Deschamps J, et al. Lung ultrasound made easy: step-by-step guide. POCUS 101. <https://www.pocus101.com/lung-ultrasound-made-easy-step-by-step-guide/>; Accessed 02.06.22.
9. Doniger S. Bedside emergency cardiac ultrasound in children. *J Emerg Trauma Shock.* 2010;3:282–291.
10. Frazen D. "FAST exam." Clerkship directors in emergency medicine – MS3 curriculum. <https://www.saem.org/about-saem/academies-interest-groups-affiliates2/cdem/for-students/online-education/m3-curriculum/bedside-ultrasonography/fast-exam>; Accessed 02.06.22.
11. Holmes JF, Kelley KM, Wooton-Gorges SL, Utter GH, et al. Effect of abdominal ultrasound on critical care, outcomes, and resource use among children with blunt torso trauma: a randomized clinical trial. *JAMA.* 2017;317(22):2290–2296.
12. Jones BP, Tay ET, Elikashvili I, Sanders JE, et al. Feasibility and safety of substituting lung ultrasonography for chest radiography when diagnosing pneumonia in children: a randomized control trial. *Chest.* 2016;150(1):131–138.
13. Kessler DO. Abdominal ultrasound for pediatric blunt trauma: FAST is not always better. *JAMA.* 2017;317(22):2283–2285.
14. Lichetenstein DA, Meziere GA. Relevance of lung ultrasound in the diagnosis of acute respiratory failure: the BLUE Protocol. *Chest.* 2008;134:117–125.
15. Lichtenstein D, Meziere G, Biderman P, Gepner A. The "lung point": an ultrasound sign specific to pneumothorax. *Intensive Care Med.* 1998;24(12):1331–1334.
16. Marin JR, Abo AM, Arroyo AC, Doniger SJ, et al. Pediatric emergency medicine point-of-care ultrasound: summary of the evidence. *Crit Ultrasound J.* 2016;8(1):16.
17. Moore C, Liu R. Not so FAST-let's not abandon the pediatric focused assessment with sonography yet. *J Thorac Dis.* 2018;10(1):1–3.
18. Moore CL, Rose GA, Tayal VS, Sullivan DM, et al. Determination of left ventricular function by emergency physician echocardiography of hypotensive patients. *Acad Emerg Med.* 2002;9(3):186–193.
19. Shah VP, Tunik MG, Tsung JW. Prospective evaluation of point-of-care ultrasonography for the diagnosis of pneumonia in young adults. *JAMA Pediatr.* 2013;167(2):119–125.
20. Sharon MJ, End B, Findley S, Kraft C, et al. Definitive diagnosis before leaving the room: PoCUS for pediatric intussusception. *J Emerg Med.* 2019;57:247–248.
21. Shefrin AE, Warkentine F, Constantine E, Toney A, et al. Consensus point-of-care ultrasound applications for pediatric emergency medicine training. *AEM Educ Train.* 2019;3(3):251–258.
22. Richards JR, McGahan JP. Focused Assessment with Sonography in Trauma (FAST) in 2017: what radiologist can learn. *Radiology.* 2017;283(1):30–48.
23. Tayal VS, Rose Ga, Kline JA. Emergency echocardiography to detect pericardial effusion in patients in PEA and near-PEA states. *Resuscitation.* 2003;59(3):315–318.
24. Vargas CA, Quintero J, Figueroa R, Castro A, et al. Extension of the thoracic spine sign as a diagnostic marker for thoracic trauma. *Eur J Trauma Emerg Surg.* 2021;47(3):749–755.
25. Bregmann KR, et al. Diagnostic accuracy of point-of-care ultrasound for intussusception: a multicenter, noninferiority study of paired diagnostic tests. *Ann Emerg Med.* 2021;78(5):606–615.

INDEX

Note: Page numbers followed by *b* indicate boxes, *f* indicate figures and *t* indicate tables.